CURRENT
RESPIRATORY CARE

Other Titles in the Current Therapy Series

CURRENT
RESPIRATORY CARE

ROBERT M. KACMAREK, PH.D., RRT

Director, Respiratory Care
Massachusetts General Hospital
Boston, Massachusetts

JAMES K. STOLLER, M.D.

Attending Staff Physician
Department of Pulmonary Disease
The Cleveland Clinic Foundation
Cleveland, Ohio

1988

B.C. Decker Inc • Toronto • Philadelphia

Publisher   B.C. Decker Inc   B.C. Decker Inc
                     3228 South Service Road   320 Walnut Street
                     Burlington, Ontario   L7N 3H8   Suite 400
                                                                        Philadelphia, Pennsylvania   19106
Sales and Distribution

United States   The C.V. Mosby Company   Asia   Info-Med Ltd.
and Possessions   11830 Westline Industrial Drive   802–3 Ruttonjee House
                     Saint Louis, Missouri   63146   11 Duddell Street
                                                                       Central Hong Kong

Canada   The C.V. Mosby Company, Ltd.
                     5240 Finch Avenue East, Unit No. 1   South Africa   Libriger Book Distributors
                     Scarborough, Ontario   M1S 5P2   Warehouse Number 8
                                                                       ''Die Ou Looiery''
United Kingdom, Europe Blackwell Scientific Publications, Ltd.   Tannery Road
and the Middle East   Osney Mead, Oxford OX2 OEL, England   Hamilton, Bloemfontein 9300

Australia and   Harcourt Brace Jovanovich Group   South America Inter-Book Marketing Services
New Zealand   (Australia) Pty Limited   Rua das Palmeriras, 32
                     30–52 Smidmore Street   Apto. 701
                     Marrickville, N.S.W. 2204   222–70 Rio de Janeiro
                     Australia   RJ, Brazil

Japan   Igaku-Shoin Ltd.
                     Tokyo International P.O. Box 5063
                     1–28–36 Hongo, Bunkyo-ku, Tokyo 113, Japan

---

NOTICE

The authors and publisher have made every effort to ensure that the patient care recommended herein, including choice of drugs and drug dosages, are in accord with the accepted standards and practice at the time of publication. However, since research and regulation constantly change clinical standards, the reader is urged to check the product information sheet included in the package of each drug, which includes recommended doses, warnings, and contra-indications. This is particularly important with new or infrequently used drugs.

Current Respiratory Care   ISBN 1-55664-049-8

Library of Congress catalog card number: 87-72968   10 9 8 7 6 5 4 3 2 1

For
My daughter Darla,
My parents, Irene and George,
and Gram

RMK

For
My wife Terry, and
My parents, Nickie and Al

JKS

CONTRIBUTORS

MUZAFFAR AHMAD, M.D.

Chairman, Department of Pulmonary Disease, Cleveland Clinic Foundation, Cleveland, Ohio
Therapeutic Bronchoscopy

JEFFREY ASKANAZI, M.D.

Assistant Professor, Department of Anesthesia, Columbia University College of Physicians and Surgeons, New York, New York
Nutritional Considerations in Respiratory Failure

MICHAEL J. BANNER, M.Ed., RRT

Assistant in Anesthesiology, Department of Anesthesiology, University of Florida College of Medicine, Gainesville, Florida
Clinical Use of Inspiratory and Expiratory Waveforms

ROBERT H. BARTLETT, M.D.

Professor of General and Thoracic Surgery, University of Michigan Medical School; Director, Surgical Intensive Care Unit, University of Michigan Medical Center, Ann Arbor, Michigan
Incentive Spirometry

MICHAEL J. BELMAN, M.D.

Associate Professor, University of California School of Medicine; Associate Director, Division of Pulmonary Medicine and Director, Pulmonary Physiology Section, Cedars-Sinai Medical Center, Los Angeles, California
Ventilatory Muscle Training

PHILIP G. BOYSEN, M.D.

Professor of Anesthesiology and Medicine, University of Florida College of Medicine, Gainesville, Florida
Postoperative Ventilatory Management

RICHARD D. BRANSON, RRT

Clinical Instructor of Surgery, University of Cincinnati College of Medicine; Attending Staff, University Hospital Medical Center, Cincinnati, Ohio
Bland Aerosol Therapy

NORMA M. T. BRAUN, M.D.

Associate Professor of Clinical Medicine, Columbia University College of Physicians and Surgeons; Associate Attending Physician, St. Luke's-Roosevelt Hospital Center, New York, New York
Positive Pressure Mechanical Ventilation: Alternative Approaches

ROBERT BROWN, M.D., C.M.

Assistant Professor of Medicine, Harvard Medical School, Boston; Chief, Department of Pulmonary Medicine, Brockton/West Roxbury VA Medical Center, West Roxbury, Massachusetts
Spinal Cord Injury

MERI BUKOWSKYJ, B.Sc., M.Sc., M.D., F.R.C.P.(C), F.C.C.P.

Private Practice, Kingston, Ontario, Canada
Methylxanthines

GEORGE G. BURTON, M.D.

Clinical Professor of Medicine and Anesthesiology, Wright State University School of Medicine; Medical Director, Respiratory Care Services, Kettering Medical Center, Dayton, Ohio
Exacerbations of Chronic Obstructive Pulmonary Disease: Pharmacologic Management

GRAZIANO C. CARLON, M.D.

Associate Professor of Anesthesiology, Cornell University Medical College; Chief, Critical Care Medicine Service, Department of Anesthesiology and Critical Care Medicine, Memorial Sloan-Kettering Cancer Center, New York, New York
High Frequency Jet Ventilation

BART CHERNOW, M.D., F.A.C.P.

Associate Professor of Anesthesia (Critical Care), Harvard Medical School; Associate Director, Respiratory-Surgical Intensive Care Unit and Co-Director, Henry K. Beecher Memorial Anesthesia Research Laboratories, Massachusetts General Hospital, Boston, Massachusetts
Mechanical Ventilation: Fluid and Pharmacologic Management of Hypotension

KENT L. CHRISTOPHER, M.D., RRT

Assistant Clinical Professor of Medicine, University of Colorado Health Sciences Center School of Medicine; Director, Institute for Transtracheal Oxygen Therapy, AMI Presbyterian-Denver Hospital, Denver, Colorado
At-Home Administration of Oxygen

BOB DEMERS, B.S., RRT

Consultant, Demers Consulting Services, Stanford, California
Humidification Systems

HAROLD J. DeMONACO, M.S.

Assistant Professor, Massachusetts General Hospital
Institute of Health Professions; Director of Pharmacy,
Massachusetts General Hospital, Boston, Massachusetts
Other Drugs Administered Via the Respiratory Tract

SANDRA DINGUS, M.A.

Consultant, Denver, Colorado
Smoking Cessation Techniques

JOHN B. DOWNS, M.D.

Professor and Vice Chairman, Department of
Anesthesiology, Ohio State University College of
Medicine, Columbus, Ohio
F_IO_2 *and PEEP*

STEVEN R. DUNCAN, M.D.

Clinical Instructor and Physician Specialist, Division of
Respiratory Medicine, Stanford University Medical Center,
Stanford, California
Status Asthmaticus: Ventilatory Management

CHRISTOPHER H. FANTA, M.D.

Assistant Professor of Medicine, Harvard Medical School;
Associate Physician, Brigham and Women's Hospital,
Boston, Massachusetts
*Acute Exacerbations of Asthma and Status Asthmaticus:
Pharmacologic Management*

MICHAEL J. GUREVITCH, M.D.

Assistant Clinical Professor of Medicine, Department of
Pulmonary Medicine, University of Southern California
School of Medicine, Los Angeles; Staff Physician,
Huntington Memorial Hospital, Pasadena, California
Selection of the Inspiratory:Expiratory Ratio

CHARLES A. HALES, M.D.

Associate Professor of Medicine, Harvard Medical School;
Associate Physician, Massachusetts General Hospital,
Boston, Massachusetts
Corticosteroids

KATHRYN W. HARRIS, B.A., RRT

Associate in Anesthesia (Respiratory Care), Harvard
Medical School; Associate Director, Respiratory Care,
Massachusetts General Hospital, Boston, Massachusetts
Respiratory Care Quality Assurance Program

RONALD A. HARRISON, M.D.

Associate Professor of Clinical Anesthesia, Department of
Anesthesia, Northwestern University Medical School;
Attending Staff Physician, Northwestern Memorial
Hospital, Chicago, Illinois
Chest Trauma

PAUL HASSOUN, M.D.

Research Fellow, Harvard Medical School; Clinical and
Research Fellow, Department of Medicine, Massachusetts
General Hospital, Boston, Massachusetts
Corticosteroids

DEAN HESS, M.Ed., RRT

Program Director, School of Respiratory Therapy,
York Hospital and York College of Pennsylvania,
York, Pennsylvania
Aerosolized Drug Delivery: Technical Aspects

THOMAS L. HIGGINS, M.D., F.A.C.P.

Staff Anesthesiologist, Cardiothoracic Intensive Care Unit,
Cleveland Clinic Foundation, Cleveland, Ohio
*Anesthetic and Paralytic Techniques in the
Intensive Care Unit*

JOHN E. HODGKIN, M.D.

Clinical Professor of Medicine, University of California,
Davis; Medical Director, Center for Health Promotion and
Rehabilitation, St. Helena Hospital, St. Helena, California
Pulmonary Rehabilitation

LEONARD D. HUDSON, M.D.

Professor of Medicine and Head, Division of Pulmonary
and Critical Care Medicine, University of Washington
School of Medicine; Attending Physician, Division of
Pulmonary and Critical Care Medicine, Harborview
Medical Center and University Hospital,
Seattle, Washington
Weaning Techniques

T. SCOTT JOHNSON, M.D.

Assistant Professor, Department of Medicine, Harvard
Medical School; Associate Physician, Brigham and
Women's Hospital, Boston, Massachusetts
Sleep Apnea and Hypoventilation Syndromes

ROBERT M. KACMAREK, Ph.D., RRT

Assistant Professor, Department of Anesthesia
(Respiratory Care), Harvard Medical School; Director,
Respiratory Care, Massachusetts General Hospital,
Boston, Massachusetts
In-Hospital Administration of Oxygen
Noninvasive Monitoring Techniques in the Ventilated Patient

MARCIA S. KEMPER, B.A., CRTT

Senior Staff Associate of Research, Department of
Anesthesiology, Columbia University College of Physicians
and Surgeons, New York, New York
Nutritional Considerations in Respiratory Failure

COLLEEN M. KIGIN, M.S., RPT

Assistant Professor, Massachusetts General Hospital Institute of Health Professions and Associate in Anesthesia, Harvard Medical School; Director, Cardiopulmonary Physical Therapy, Massachusetts General Hospital, Boston, Massachusetts
Chest Physical Therapy

ROBERT R. KIRBY, M.D.

Professor of Anesthesiology, University of Florida College of Medicine; Staff Anesthesiologist, Shands Hospital at the University of Florida, Gainesville, Florida
Modes of Mechanical Ventilation

PETER A. KIRKPATRICK, M.D.

Medical Director, Program for Ventilator-Assisted Patients, Shaughnessy-Kaplan Rehabilitation Hospital and Associate Director of Pulmonary Medicine, Salem Hospital, Salem, Massachusetts
Home Discharge of the Ventilator-Assisted Patient

ISABELLE C. KOPEC, M.D.

Fellow, Critical Care Medicine, Department of Anesthesiology and Critical Care, Memorial Sloan-Kettering Cancer Center, New York, New York
High Frequency Jet Ventilation

SAMSUN LAMPOTANG, M.E.

Graduate Research Assistant, Department of Anesthesiology, University of Florida College of Medicine, and Department of Mechanical Engineering, University of Florida College of Engineering, Gainesville, Florida
Clinical Use of Inspiratory and Expiratory Waveforms

JACOB LOKE, M.D.

Associate Professor of Medicine, Director of Pulmonary Function Laboratory, Yale University School of Medicine; Attending Physician, Yale–New Haven Hospital, New Haven, Connecticut
Diaphragm Pacing

NEIL R. MacINTYRE, M.D.

Assistant Professor of Medicine, Duke University School of Medicine; Medical Director, Respiratory Care Services, Duke University Medical Center, Durham, North Carolina
Pressure Support: Inspiratory Assist

THEODORE W. MARCY, M.D.

Assistant Professor of Medicine, University of Minnesota Medical School; Attending Pulmonary Physician, Section of Pulmonary and Critical Care Medicine, Saint Paul-Ramsey Medical Center and Ramsey Clinic, Minneapolis, Minnesota
Stable Asthma

JOHN J. MARINI, M.D.

Associate Professor of Medicine, Vanderbilt University School of Medicine; Medical Director of Respiratory Care, Vanderbilt University Hospital, Nashville, Tennessee
Work of Breathing

RICHARD A. MATTHAY, M.D.

Professor of Medicine and Associate Director, Department of Pulmonary Medicine, Yale University School of Medicine, New Haven, Connecticut
Stable Asthma

ATUL C. MEHTA, M.D., F.C.C.P., F.A.C.P.

Staff Physician, Department of Pulmonary Disease, Cleveland Clinic Foundation, Cleveland, Ohio
Laser Applications in Respiratory Care

STEPHEN C. MELIA, RRT

Chief, Respiratory Therapy Department, Brockton/West Roxbury VA Medical Center, West Roxbury, Massachusetts
Spinal Cord Injury

ANIL S. MENON, Ph.D.

Research Fellow, University of Toronto Faculty of Medicine, Toronto, Ontario, Canada
High Frequency Ventilation: Current Use and Future Perspectives

WILLIAM F. MILLER, M.D., F.A.C.C.P., F.A.C.P.

Professor, Internal Medicine, Pulmonary Research Division, University of Texas Southwestern Medical Center; Consultant in Pulmonary Diseases, University Affiliated Hospitals, Dallas, Texas
Intermittent Positive Pressure Breathing (IPPB)

LOUISE M. NETT, R.N., RRT

Instructor in Medicine and Clinical Associate Professor of Nursing, Webb-Waring Lung Institute, University of Colorado Medical School, Denver, Colorado
Smoking Cessation Techniques

MICHAEL S. NIEDERMAN, M.D.

Assistant Professor of Medicine, Department of Medicine, State University of New York, Stony Brook; Director, Medical and Respiratory Intensive Care Unit, Winthrop-University Hospital, Mineola, New York
Pneumonia

P. PEARL O'ROURKE, M.D.

Assistant Professor of Anesthesia (Pediatrics), Harvard Medical School; Associate Director, Multidisciplinary Intensive Care Unit, Children's Hospital, Boston, Massachusetts
Choosing a Home Care Mechanical Ventilator

THOMAS L. PETTY, M.D.

Professor of Medicine, University of Colorado School of Medicine; Director, Webb-Waring Lung Institute, University of Colorado Health Sciences Center, Denver, Colorado
Stable Chronic Bronchitis and Emphysema (COPD)

DAVID J. PIERSON, M.D.

Associate Professor of Medicine, University of Washington School of Medicine; Medical Director, Respiratory Care Department, Harborview Medical Center, Seattle, Washington
Exacerbation of Chronic Bronchitis and Emphysema: Ventilatory Management

THOMAS A. RAFFIN, M.D.

Associate Professor and Assistant Chief, Department of Medicine and Medical Director of Respiratory Therapy, Stanford University Medical Center, Stanford, California
Status Asthmaticus: Ventilatory Management

COLE RAY Jr., A.A.S., RRT

Adjunct Clinical Lecturer, Respiratory Therapy Programs, Department of Allied Health, Borough of Manhattan Community College, City University of New York; Technical Director, Respiratory Care Services, Memorial Sloan-Kettering Cancer Center, New York, New York
Independent Lung Ventilation

ANTHONY S. REBUCK, M.B., B.S., M.D.

Professor of Medicine, University of Toronto Faculty of Medicine; Chief of Respiratory Medicine, Toronto Western Hospital, Toronto, Ontario, Canada
High Frequency Ventilation: Current Use and Future Perspectives

S. DAVID REGISTER III, Major, U.S.A.F.(M.C.)

Staff Anesthesiologist, Department of Anesthesiology, Wilford Hall USAF Medical Center, Lackland AFB, San Antonio, Texas
FIO_2 and PEEP

THOMAS W. RICE, B.A.Sc., M.D.

Staff Surgeon, Department of Thoracic and Cardiovascular Surgery, Cleveland Clinic Foundation, Cleveland, Ohio
Extracorporeal Membrane Oxygenation

STEVEN M. SCHARF, M.D., Ph.D.

Assistant Professor of Medicine, Harvard Medical School; Attending Physician, Department of Pulmonary Medicine, Brockton/West Roxbury VA Medical Center, West Roxbury, Massachusetts
Spinal Cord Injury

RICHARD M. SCHWARTZSTEIN, M.D.

Instructor in Medicine, Harvard Medical School; Associate Physician, Beth Israel Hospital, Boston, Massachusetts
Sympathomimetic Bronchodilators, Anticholinergics, and Cromolyn Sodium

SANDRA M. SEGER, CRRT

Clinical Therapist, Department of Respiratory Care, Children's Hospital Medical Center, Cincinnati, Ohio
Bland Aerosol Therapy

MARISSA SELIGMAN, Pharm.D.

New Product Training Specialist, Pharmaceutical Division, Miles, Inc., West Haven, Connecticut
Mucolytics

BARRY A. SHAPIRO, M.D.

Professor of Clinical Anesthesia and Director, Division of Respiratory/Critical Care, Department of Anesthesia, Northwestern University Medical School; Medical Director, Respiratory Care Services, Northwestern Memorial Hospital, Chicago, Illinois
Management of Adult Respiratory Distress Syndrome (ARDS)

EDWARD D. SIVAK, M.D.

Director, Medical Intensive Care Unit, Section of Pulmonary Disease, Cleveland Clinic Foundation, Cleveland, Ohio
Home Care Patient: Ventilatory Management

ARTHUR S. SLUTSKY, M.D.

Associate Professor of Medicine and Surgery, University of Toronto Faculty of Medicine; Senior Scientist, Mount Sinai Hospital Research Institute and Staff Physician, Mount Sinai Hospital, Toronto, Ontario, Canada
High Frequency Ventilation: Current Use and Future Perspectives

ROBERT A. SMITH, M.S., RRT

Director of Critical Care Medicine, Experimental Research and Training Laboratory, Memorial Medical Center of Jacksonville, Jacksonville, Florida
Mask and Nasal Continuous Positive Airway Pressure

CHARLES B. SPEARMAN, B.S., RRT

Assistant Professor, Department of Respiratory Therapy, School of Allied Health Professions, Loma Linda University, Loma Linda, California
Appropriate Ventilator Selection

DANIEL M. STEIGMAN, M.D.

Clinical and Research Fellow in Medicine, Harvard Medical School and Massachusetts General Hospital, Boston, Massachusetts
Mechanical Ventilation: Fluid and Pharmacologic Management of Hypotension

JAN A. STEINEL, R.N., RRT

Home Care and Rehabilitation Respiratory Therapist,
Section of Pulmonary Disease, Cleveland Clinic
Foundation, Cleveland, Ohio
Home Care Patient: Ventilatory Management

JAMES K. STOLLER, M.D.

Attending Staff Physician, Department of Pulmonary
Disease, Cleveland Clinic Foundation, Cleveland, Ohio
Preoperative Preparation of the Patient

JOHN E. THOMPSON, RRT

Associate in Anesthesia, Harvard Medical School;
Director, Department of Respiratory Care, Children's
Hospital, Boston, Massachusetts
Choosing a Home Care Mechanical Ventilator

ALAN L. VanDERVORT, M.D.

Fellow, Critical Care Medicine, Department of
Anesthesiology and Critical Care, Memorial Sloan-
Kettering Cancer Center, New York, New York
High Frequency Jet Ventilation

JANETTE JONES WALSH, R.N., RRT

Respiratory Care Specialist, New England Health
Resources, Home Care Providers, Boston, Massachusetts
Home Discharge of the Ventilator-Assisted Patient

SCOTT T. WEISS, M.D., M.S.

Associate Professor of Medicine, Harvard Medical School;
Associate Physician, Beth Israel Hospital,
Boston, Massachusetts
*Sympathomimetic Bronchodilators, Anticholinergics, and
Cromolyn Sodium*

HERBERT P. WIEDEMANN, M.D.

Staff Physician, Department of Pulmonary Disease and
Head, Section of Respiratory Therapy, Cleveland Clinic
Foundation, Cleveland, Ohio
Invasive Monitoring Techniques in the Ventilated Patient

ROBERT L. WILKINS, M.A., RRT

Assistant Professor and Coordinator of Clinical Education,
Department of Respiratory Therapy, School of Allied
Health Professions, Loma Linda University,
Loma Linda, California
Suctioning and Airway Care

DONNA J. WILSON, R.N., RRT

Respiratory Care Consultant, Respiratory Care
Department, Massachusetts General Hospital,
Boston, Massachusetts
Airway Appliances and Management

CYNTHIA COFFIN ZADAI, P.T., M.S.

Assistant Professor, Massachusetts General Hospital
Institute of Health Professions; Director, Chest Physical
Therapy, Beth Israel Hospital, Boston, Massachusetts
Exercise Techniques During Pulmonary Rehabilitation

PREFACE

Faced with an increasing frequency of serious lung disease in the United States, respiratory care practitioners are constantly challenged to update the skills needed to care for patients with pulmonary disease. To meet this ongoing challenge, this volume in the Current Therapy series has been organized as a collection of "consultations" from recognized experts in respiratory care. Above all, the text is designed to be practical and to help in the everyday management of respiratory patients. In keeping with this practical spirit, we have asked the contributors to avoid detailed discussions of physiology and pathophysiology in preference to useful bedside clinical information. We have also asked the contributors to provide their personal approaches to problems, even when—and especially when—the respiratory care literature provides no straightforward answers. We have also asked contributors to shun exhaustive lists of references in favor of shorter lists of key readings for the specific chapters. As the editors, we think the product is an especially useful and practical text for the respiratory care practitioner.

The text is organized into two major parts: (1) technical and therapeutic applications and (2) patient management approaches. In the first part, emphasis is placed on individual, technical, pharmacologic, and clinical approaches to patient care—each chapter addressing one specific issue, such as aerosol delivery, oxygen delivery, and negative pressure ventilation. The second part of the text addresses management of specific clinical conditions and calls upon contributors to provide personal perspectives on the management of specific clinical problems.

We hope you will find this text a useful and especially practical approach to the management of patients requiring respiratory care.

This book would not have been possible without the help of several key people, to whom we offer our heartfelt thanks: Gertrude Shaw, Mary Kalil, and Sherry Rubins, whose secretarial help was invaluable.

Robert M. Kacmarek, Ph.D., RRT
James K. Stoller, M.D.

CONTENTS

HOME CARE AND PULMONARY REHABILITATION

PATIENT MANAGEMENT APPROACHES

OXYGEN THERAPY TECHNIQUES

IN-HOSPITAL ADMINISTRATION OF OXYGEN

ROBERT M. KACMAREK, Ph.D., RRT

Oxygen is one of the most common pharmacologic agents administered to patients with cardiopulmonary disease. However, controversy still exists over capabilities of commonly used oxygen delivery systems as well as indications and end points of therapy. In this chapter I discuss the indications, delivery systems, and clinical application of oxygen therapy.

INDICATIONS

Oxygen therapy, as with most aspects of respiratory care, is only supportive. It can help prevent or reverse tissue hypoxia. Thus, indications for oxygen therapy evolve about clinical manifestations of actual or potential tissue hypoxia. As a result, hypoxemia is the primary clinical indication for oxygen therapy. As the PaO_2 falls below the lower limit of normal (80 mm Hg), the need for supplemental oxygen becomes great. The effect of oxygen on hypoxemia and the quantity of oxygen required to reverse it are dependent on its cause. Excluding exposure to environments with less than 20.95 percent O_2, ventilation/perfusion ($\dot{V}/\dot{Q}$) mismatching and true intrapulmonary shunting are the primary causes of hypoxemia.

$\dot{V}/\dot{Q}$ mismatching is probably the most common cause of hypoxemia. Most patients admitted to general medical units requiring oxygen therapy manifest $\dot{V}/\dot{Q}$ mismatches. The origin of the mismatch may be pulmonary (COPD, retained secretions, bronchoconstriction) or cardiovascular (recent myocardial infarction, congestive heart failure). It is not uncommon for these patients to present with ventilatory patterns that accentuate the mismatch; that is, rapid shallow breathing.

Hypoxemia caused by $\dot{V}/\dot{Q}$ mismatch is normally responsive to increases in FIO_2. Even small changes in FIO_2 may have dramatic effects on oxygenation. In addition to improving the PaO_2 in poorly ventilated areas, improved oxygenation often normalizes ventilatory patterns, further decreasing the extent of the mismatch.

True intrapulmonary shunting ($\dot{Q}s/\dot{Q}t$) presents a significant challenge to oxygen therapy. The hypoxemia caused by intrapulmonary shunting is little affected by increases in FIO_2 (i.e., refractory to oxygen). In general, the greater the shunt, the less effective oxygen therapy is in reversing hypoxemia. With severe Qs/Qt (greater than 30 percent) even 100 percent oxygen may have little effect on the hypoxemia, because at atmospheric conditions it is impossible to dissolve enough O_2 in normally ventilated blood to provide O_2 sufficient to saturate the hemoglobin in the shunted blood.

In addition to hypoxemia, increased myocardial work and increased work of breathing are indications for oxygen therapy. If tachycardia and hypertension are required to maintain a specific PO_2, the administration of oxygen therapy should relieve the tachycardia and hypertension as it improves the PO_2. In many cases PO_2 may not be markedly changed but vital signs are significantly improved.

Oxygen therapy should also decrease the work of breathing. The normal response to hypoxemia is hyperventilation, because given a specific $P(A-a)O_2$, a higher PaO_2 can be achieved if hyperventilation occurs. Rapid deep breathing with use of accessory muscles indicates increased ventilatory work. As oxygen therapy relieves hypoxemia, normalization of ventilatory pattern and a decrease in work of breathing are expected.

OXYGEN DELIVERY SYSTEMS

Two general categories can be used to define oxygen delivery systems: high-flow and low-flow systems. The major distinction between these systems is the gas flow sufficient to meet the patient's peak inspiratory demands.

High-Flow Systems

Theoretically, high-flow gas delivery systems provide the total environment a patient inspires. In order to do this, the system must normally provide flows in excess of 40 L per minute. In some severely hypoxemic patients with strong ventilatory drives, flows up to 90 L per minute are required to ensure a precise and constant FIO$_2$. If designed properly, high-flow systems have the advantage of maintaining a constant environment (humidity and FIO$_2$). However, they are usually bulky and poorly tolerated by patients.

Air Entrainment Masks (Ventimasks)

Air entrainment masks can deliver a specific FIO$_2$ by entraining room air before gas flow reaches the patient. The jet drag effect, varying flow rates, and variation in the size of either the air entrainment port or the jet orifice (Fig. 1) allows commercially available masks to deliver different FIO$_2$ from about 0.24 to 0.50 (Table 1).

As with all high-flow systems, a particular mask qualifies as a high-flow system only if the total system flow meets patient demands. Systems delivering low FIO$_2$ normally qualify; however, the likelihood that the patient's needs will exceed the flow capabilities of the system increases as system FIO$_2$ increases. At higher oxygen settings (greater than or equal to 40 percent), consistent and accurate delivery of FIO$_2$ should be questioned. These systems can be applied via a mask or Briggs "T" piece and also allow for the entrainment of an aerosol.

Mechanical Aerosol Systems

The jet drag effect is used in mechanical aerosol systems (Fig. 2) to create an aerosol as well as vary the delivered FIO$_2$ (see Table 1). These systems have the added advantage of delivering particulate water to the airway. Nondisposable aerosol generators allow little variability in possible FIO$_2$ delivered (commonly

TABLE 1 Entrainment Ratios and Outputs of Specific Air Entrainment Systems*

Entrainment ratio	FIO$_2$	Minimal flow at which operated†	Total flow (L/min)
1–25	0.24	4	104
1–10	0.28	4	44
1–7	0.31	6	48
1–5	0.35	8	48
1–3	0.40	8	32
1–1.7	0.50	12	32
1–1	0.60	12	24
1–0.6	0.70	12	19

* Minor variations in delivery of FIO$_2$ may exist with disposable systems.

† Maximal operated flow depends on size of jet orifice.

0.40, 0.70, and 1.0), but disposable systems theoretically allow variation from 0.21 to 1.0. Regardless of the FIO$_2$ setting, these systems are commonly powered by more than 10 L per minute of 100 percent O$_2$; thus, at low FIO$_2$ they are capable of very high flows because of entrainment ratios (see Table 1). At higher FIO$_2$, desired flow may be achieved by using two aerosol generators in tandem (see Fig. 2). These systems can be applied via an aerosol mask, facehood, trach collar, or Briggs "T" piece (Fig. 3). For most consistent FIO$_2$s, a Briggs "T" piece with a 15- to 20-inch reservoir tube to prevent further entrainment of room air should be employed.

High-Flow Humidifier Systems

Humidifier systems (Fig. 4) are capable of delivering a consistent and accurate FIO$_2$ at any level

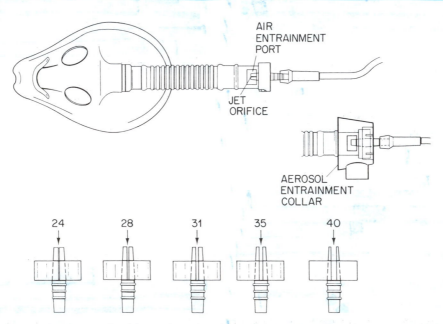

Figure 1 Air entrainment mask with various jet orifices. Each orifice provides a specific delivered FIO$_2$.

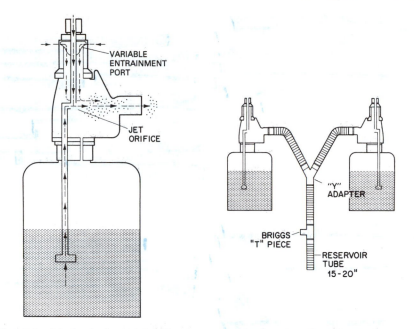

Figure 2   Mechanical aerosol delivery systems: single unit and tandem arrangement.

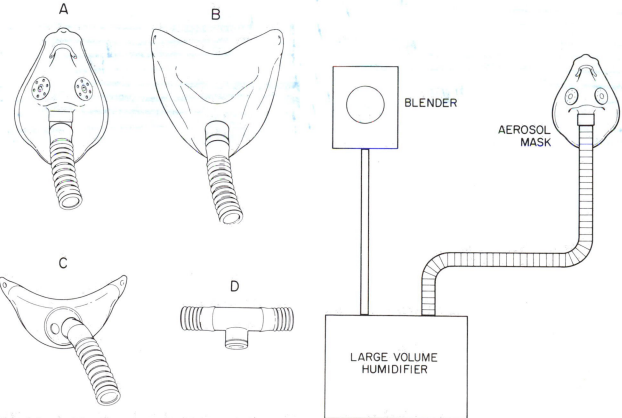

Figure 3   *A*, Aerosol mask; *B*, facehood; *C*, trach collar; *D*, Briggs "T" piece.

Figure 4   High-flow humidifier system.

desired and can deliver more than 100 L per minute if needed. Their primary drawback is the noise created as higher flows move through large-bore tubing. As with all high-flow systems, they can be easily applied to patients with or without artificial airways. When they are applied to patients with artificial airways, a 15- to 20-inch reservoir tube (see Fig. 4) should be used to decrease the likelihood of entraining room air into the system.

Continuous Positive Airway Pressure (CPAP) Systems

Figure 5 depicts a continuous-flow CPAP system, which is a modification of the high-flow humidifier system. Because work of breathing is a primary concern, a 5 to 10 L anesthesia bag is included, acting as a reservoir to ensure minimal airway pressure change during inspiration (less than or equal to 2 cm H_2O). In addition, an O_2 analyzer, a high and low pressure alarm, and a pressure manometer are included. The positive end-expiratory pressure (PEEP) device chosen should be of low flow resistance to prevent excessive pressure increase during exhalation. However, all PEEP devices have varying degrees of flow resistance. As a result, CPAP on the device should be adjusted only after attachment to the patient and appropriate adjustment of system flow. System flows should be maintained at or above 60 L per minute. At this level, 3 to 5 cm H_2O CPAP is generated as a result of flow resistance of the PEEP valve used. It is important to remember that with any continuous-flow system the CPAP level is a result of both system flow and PEEP device setting. Ideally, total system pressure should not fluctuate by more than 2 cm H_2O in either direction if imposed work of breathing is to be kept at a minimum.

Low-Flow Systems

With low-flow systems the delivered FIO_2 is based on the following variables: flow rate, size of anatomic and mechanical reservoir, and most important, patient ventilatory pattern. In general, delivered FIO_2 is increased as patient tidal volume, peak inspiratory flow rate, and minute ventilation decrease and is decreased as these variables increase. That is, at any one point in time a cannula at 2 L per minute may be providing an FIO_2 of 0.24 or 0.32 or 0.40, totally dependent on patient ventilatory pattern. Table 2 lists *calculated* FIO_2s provided by various low-flow systems. These values are determined at a respiratory rate of 20 per minute, tidal volume of 500 ml, and inspiratory time of 1 second. They provide only gross guidelines of FIO_2 delivered. Clinically, actual FIO_2 is difficult, if not impossible, to assess at the bedside. It is essential to realize that when these systems are used, consistent and precise FIO_2 is impossible to achieve.

Nasal Cannula

The most commonly used oxygen delivery device is the nasal cannula (Fig. 6A). This is true not because of range or accuracy of FIO_2, but because of patient tolerance. Regardless of the accuracy of the delivery system, it must be used properly to be of benefit. Few patients have difficulty tolerating a nasal cannula, and compliance in patients without artificial airways is highest with this device. Flow rate settings vary from 0.25 to 6 L per minute. The FIO_2 delivered at any setting depends primarily on the patient's ventilatory pattern. Flows higher than 6 L per minute do not appear to increase delivered FIO_2. In addition, flows of 4 L per minute or more for prolonged periods of time may dry the nasal mucosa, resulting in irritation

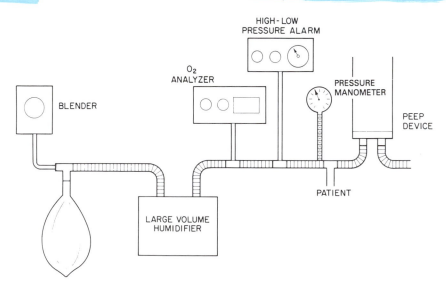

Figure 5　Continuous-flow CPAP system.

TABLE 2 **Approximate Delivered FIO_2 with Low-Flow Systems**

System	Flow range (L/min)	Approximate FIO_2
Cannula	0.25–6.0	0.24 to 0.44
Simple mask	5–8	0.40 to 0.60
Partial rebreathing mask	≥8	≥0.60
Nonrebreathing mask	>10	≥0.80

FIO_2s are based on calculations at respiratory rate of 20/min. V_T 500, inspiratory time 1 sec. Actual FIO_2 is dependent on patient's ventilatory pattern.

and bleeding and should always be administered with a humidifier. The nasal passages must be patent whenever a cannula is used. Ideally, the patient should be a nose breather; however, data indicate that FIO_2 is maintained in mouth breathers as long as nasal patency is assured.

Simple Masks

A simple mask (Fig. 6B) provides FIO_2s higher than those provided by nasal cannulas because of the mechanical reservoir of the mask itself. Thus, in addition to the delivered flow, the O_2 accumulated in the mask at end exhalation is inhaled by the patient.

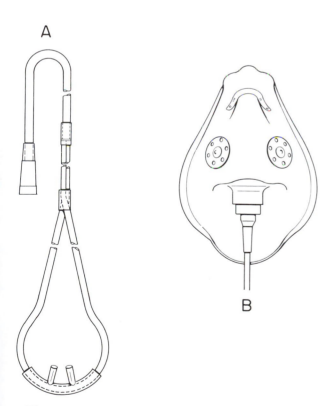

Figure 6 *A,* Nasal cannula; *B,* Simple oxygen mask.

To ensure O_2 accumulation and prevent CO_2 buildup in the mask, a *minimum* of 5 L per minute flow should be employed. Flows of greater than 8 L per minute do not appear to increase delivered FIO_2. At settings of 5 to 8 L per minute an FIO_2 of 0.40 to 0.60 can be expected, depending on the patient's ventilatory pattern.

Partial Rebreathing Masks

A partial rebreathing mask system adds a 750 to 1,000 ml reservoir bag to the simple O_2 mask, and as a result it may deliver over 60 percent oxygen, depending on the patient's ventilatory pattern (Fig. 7). For proper function, during inspiration the reservoir bag should not collapse completely. If it collapses completely, gas exhaled from the lung parenchyma may enter the bag. This system is designed to allow the first part of exhalation (anatomic deadspace gas) to enter the reservoir. If the bag collapses completely on inspiration, CO_2 rebreathing is likely. This system should run at 8 L per minute or more to prevent total collapse. Regardless of flow rate, it is unlikely that this mask will approach the patient's peak inspiratory demands. It is thus doubtful that FIO_2s greater than 0.80 can be provided with this system.

Nonrebreathing Masks

At first glance a nonrebreathing mask and a partial rebreathing mask appear identical. However, a nonrebreathing mask incorporates valves, allowing one-way gas flow into and out of the mask and between the mask and the reservoir bag (see Fig. 7). These valves are included in an attempt to deliver 100 percent O_2. Theoretically, the combination of the gas volume in the reservoir bag and the delivered liter flow (10 to 15 L per minute) provide the patient's entire inspired volume. However, spontaneously breathing, nonintubated patients requiring 100 percent oxygen normally have strong inspiratory drives with very high peak inspiratory flow rates. As a result, these patients exceed the nonrebreathing mask's capability of gas delivery. Because today's nonrebreathing masks are disposable and do not provide a tight facial seal, room air is inspired. This mask should always be set above 10 L per minute and may provide more than 80 percent O_2, depending on the patient's ventilatory pattern. Use of the older, tight-fitting, nondisposable nonrebreathing masks may result in higher FIO_2 delivered but may also increase inspiratory work of breathing. All nondisposable nonrebreathing masks include a spring-loaded safety valve that opens if the patient evacuates the system. Because of the design, the effort required to open these valves and establish a high flow of gas into the system can be excessive, resulting in marked increases in work of breathing.

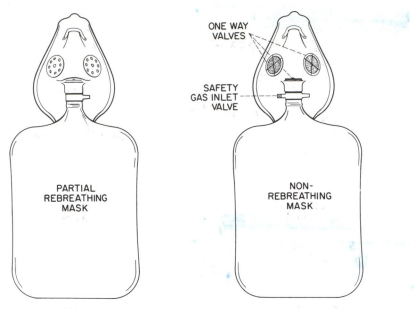

ONE WAY VALVES

SAFETY GAS INLET VALVE

PARTIAL REBREATHING MASK

NON-REBREATHING MASK

Figure 7 Partial rebreathing and nonrebreathing masks.

SELECTION OF SYSTEM

A number of factors enter into the decision of which oxygen delivery system to employ. The placement of an artificial airway normally narrows the selection to a high-flow system, but the primary factor is whether a need exists for accurate and constant FIO_2. In addition, the actual FIO_2 required as well as patient tolerance and compliance must be considered.

Patients with Artificial Airways

Only high-flow systems are adaptable to artificial airways. Compliance is normally not a concern with these patients, but comfort is important. If an endotracheal tube is in place, attachment to the system is always via a Briggs "T" piece; however, with tracheostomy tubes a Briggs "T" piece or trach mask can be used. If accurate and consistent FIO_2 is required, I always use a Briggs "T" piece with reservoir. However, if heated humidified gas is the primary concern, with constant and accurate FIO_2 unnecessary, I use a trach collar to increase patient comfort. When 40 percent or less oxygen is needed, either a mechanical aerosol system or a high-flow humidifier system may be employed. I prefer the mechanical aerosol system because of ease of setup and maintenance and because of its ability to humidify the airway. When FIO_2s above 0.40 are required, mechanical aerosol systems become impractical, even tandem set-ups. In this situation I always use a high-flow humidifier system because of its accuracy, versatility, and flow capacity. When CPAP is required, I prefer the use of a continuous-flow CPAP system.

Patients without Artificial Airways

All systems discussed may be employed when the patient does not have an artificial airway. Here, the important questions are whether accurate and consistent FIO_2 is required, how high an FIO_2 is needed, and most important, whether the patient will tolerate the system applied.

In spite of the fact that high-flow systems can be delivered to patients without artificial airways, I prefer using low-flow systems. Patient tolerance and compliance with high-flow systems are normally low unless constantly monitored. As a result, the nasal cannula is the system I most commonly employ with this group. Even in patients with chronic obstructive pulmonary disease in whom the use of a Ventimask would be ideal, I frequently use a nasal cannula. These patients are very claustrophobic, have a difficult time keeping the mask in place, and must take the mask off for eating, shaving, and oral hygiene. If patients can tolerate a Ventimask, if they have frequent changes in their ventilatory pattern, and if small changes in FIO_2 affect their $PaCO_2$, I use a Ventimask. However, most non-ICU, nonemergency patients are easily maintained on a nasal cannula.

In the emergency room I use a simple O_2 mask or a partial rebreathing mask for immediate application of FIO_2 unobtainable with a cannula. Most of these patients requiring high FIO_2 are sent to the ICU; some are intubated. In the ICU, if accurate and constant FIO_2s are required, I prefer to use a high-flow system. Ventimasks or unheated mechanical aerosol systems are normally used if low FIO_2s are needed. Here, I base my decision on the need for supplemental humidity. If high FiO_2 (greater than 0.40) is needed, a high-flow humidifier system is preferred.

In the recovery room an unheated mechanical aerosol system with either a face mask or a facehood is ideal, depending on the need for O_2 and patient tolerance.

MONITORING O_2 THERAPY

Arterial blood gas analysis and pulse oximetry are most commonly employed to monitor O_2 therapy, but because O_2 can be expected to decrease the work of the myocardium and of breathing, clinical signs of work must also be monitored.

Figure 8 depicts the oxyhemoglobin dissociation curve with key levels highlighted. Note that an increase in Po_2 from 40 to 60 mm Hg (steep aspect of the curve) results in a percent oxyhemoglobin increase from 75 to 90 percent, whereas a Po_2 increase from 60 to 100 mm Hg (flat aspect of the curve) results in a saturation change of 90 to 98 percent. Oxygen therapy results in the greatest increase in oxygen carriage when a patient's Po_2 is on the steep aspect of the HbO_2 saturation curve. Thus, regardless of patient, attaining a PaO_2 of at least 60 mm Hg is always the primary goal of therapy. I attempt to maintain a PaO_2 between 60 and 80 mm Hg. Some prefer to maintain the PaO_2 between 80 and 100 mm Hg. This is acceptable depending on the FiO_2 required. If a Po_2 of 100 mm Hg can be obtained at an FiO_2 of 0.40 or less, there is no compelling reason to decrease FiO_2. However, if greater than 40 percent oxygen is re-

quired, I maintain the Po_2 between 60 and 80 mm Hg rather than risk the toxic effects of a high FiO_2.

Maintaining a Po_2 over 100 mm Hg can be justified only when the oxygen carrying capacity is markedly decreased (e.g., carbon monoxide poisoning or severe anemia). The increase in O_2 content for a Po_2 increase from 100 to 200 mm Hg is, at maximum, about 0.7 volumes percent, normally a clinically insignificant increase.

In addition to arterial blood gases, careful assessment of the patient's cardiopulmonary status is necessary any time oxygen is applied. Frequently, an apparently small increase in Po_2 markedly reduces cardiopulmonary stress. A Po_2 increase from 55 to 62 mm Hg accompanied by decreases in pulse (110 to 84 per minute), blood pressure (140/100 to 118/84), respiratory rate (28 to 20 per minute), and use of accessory muscles of ventilation has a marked positive effect on a patient's clinical status, even though the Po_2 changes by only 7 mm Hg. If clinical signs of decreased work are absent, the 7 mm Hg increase in Po_2 may not be viewed as adequate.

USE OF 100 PERCENT OXYGEN

Use of 100 percent oxygen is avoided because of the threat of O_2 toxicity, absorption atelectasis, and oxygen-induced hypoventilation. However, 100 percent FiO_2 is indicated in certain situations, primarily during cardiac arrest, during transport, in acute cardiopulmonary instability, and whenever carboxyhemoglobin levels are greater than 10 percent. In these

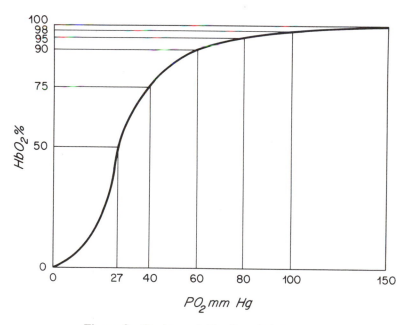

Figure 8 Oxyhemoglobin dissociation curve.

situations, 100 percent oxygen is applied until the condition is stabilized, at which time the F_{IO_2} should be reduced to an appropriate level.

Suggested Reading

Burton GG, Hodgkin JE. Respiratory care: a guide to clinical practice. 2nd ed. Philadelphia: JB Lippincott, 1984.

Concerns Conference. National conference on oxygen therapy report. Chest 1984; 86:234–247.

Eubanks DH, Bone RC. Comprehensive respiratory care: learning system. St Louis: CV Mosby, 1985.

Kacmarek RM, Mack C, Dimas S. Essentials of respiratory therapy. 2nd ed. Chicago: Year Book, 1985.

McPherson SP. Respiratory therapy equipment. 3rd ed. St. Louis: CV Mosby, 1986.

Shapiro BA, Harrison RA, Kacmarek RM, et al. Clinical application of respiratory care. 3rd ed. Chicago: Year Book, 1985.

Spearman CB, Sheldon RL, Egan OF. Egan's fundamentals of respiratory therapy. 4th ed. St Louis: CV Mosby, 1982.

AT-HOME ADMINISTRATION OF OXYGEN

KENT L. CHRISTOPHER, M.D., RRT

SCIENTIFIC FOUNDATIONS FOR HOME OXYGEN THERAPY

Priestly discovered oxygen in 1774, and shortly thereafter, Beddoes described medical applications of oxygen. Over 150 years later, Barach began using oxygen in the treatment of hospitalized patients. Finally, in 1970, Neff and Petty proposed that long-term continuous oxygen therapy might be efficacious in the treatment of outpatients with hypoxemia due to chronic obstructive pulmonary disease (COPD). Subsequent studies suggested that home oxygen therapy improved exercise tolerance, decreased pulmonary hypertension, reduced erythrocytosis, and improved neuropsychologic function in patients with COPD. More recently, the Medical Research Council Working Party demonstrated that mortality was reduced when nocturnal oxygen was used compared with no oxygen. This extensive investigation was paralleled by the Nocturnal Oxygen Therapy Trial (NOTT), which showed nearly a twofold reduction in mortality when continuous use of ambulatory oxygen was compared with nocturnal therapy only. Long-term continuous oxygen therapy improves survival and quality of life in patients with COPD; there is probably a similar beneficial effect in the treatment of other diseases causing chronic hypoxemia.

An increasing number of patients have been placed on this form of therapy since the efficacy of home oxygen has been clearly established. Exact figures are not known, but it is estimated that between 500,000 and 800,000 patients currently receive home oxygen. As a result, the cost of continuous oxygen delivery has increased dramatically. Guidelines for establishing the medical need for home oxygen therapy have evolved based on previous studies. The Health Care Financing Administration (HCFA) has also set guidelines for reimbursement for oxygen. Our task is to offer home oxygen therapy to qualified patients in the most efficacious and cost-effective manner.

GUIDELINES FOR LONG-TERM HOME OXYGEN THERAPY

Only patients who demonstrate chronic hypoxemia should receive long-term oxygen therapy. Because hypoxemia may be transitory in some individuals, a commitment to a lifetime of treatment should not be made unless inadequate oxygenation can be demonstrated on more than one occasion (preferably over a period of 2 or 3 weeks). Patients with an acute illness such as pneumonia, pulmonary embolism, the adult respiratory distress syndrome, asthma, bronchitis, left ventricular failure, or any other acute cardiopulmonary disorder may have transient hypoxemia that resolves with treatment of the underlying illness. Furthermore, patients with chronic lung disease may have a significant improvement in hypoxemia following aggressive medical therapy, even though a specific superimposed acute illness cannot be identified. For example, oxygenation in patients with COPD may improve with aggressive treatment of air flow obstruction with inhaled bronchodilators, anhydrous theophylline, or other oral beta agonists, antibiotics, or a trial of corticosteroids. If hypoxemia is caused by alveolar hypoventilation, medications that stimulate ventilatory drive may be of value (e.g., anhydrous theophylline, acetazolamide [Diamox], or medroxyprogesterone [Provera]). In this regard, 21 percent of the hypoxemic patients screened for entry into the NOTT study were later excluded because oxygenation significantly improved following aggressive medical therapy.

The clinical definition of hypoxemia is not always clear-cut. An arterial blood gas measurement obtained while breathing room air showing a PaO_2 of 55 torr or less was established as a definition of hypoxemia for entry into the NOTT study, and HCFA has adopted this value in the reimbursement guidelines for continuous oxygen therapy. However, the PaO_2 measurement does not totally reflect the adequacy of oxygenation. Three different room air arterial blood gas results theoretically obtained on one individual are shown in Table 1. The PaO_2 readings range from 48 to 60 torr. The degree of hypoxemia, as expressed by the alveolar-to-arterial oxygen tension gradient, is exactly the same in each situation. The difference in PaO_2 is due entirely to differences in alveolar ventilation, or the $PaCO_2$. According to current Medicare guidelines, home oxygen would be reimbursed based on the results in examples one and two but denied in example three, even though all three measurements were obtained on the same patient.

Arterial oxygen saturation can also be used to assess the adequacy of oxygenation. Noninvasive finger probe or ear oximetry has now been accepted by the HCFA as acceptable documentation of hypoxemia. However, the room air oximetry cutoff for oxygen

TABLE 1   Serial Room Air Arterial Blood Gases Obtained on One Patient

	Example 1	Example 2	Example 3
PaO_2 (torr)	48	53	60
SaO_2 (%)	83	88	93
$PaCO_2$ (torr)	52	48	42
pH	7.38	7.42	7.49
A-a DO_2 (torr)	12	12	12
HCO_3	30.3	30.8	31.9
BE (Base excess)	4.2	5.4	7.7

saturation was set at equal to or less than 85 percent. Assuming a normal pH, an 85 percent saturation is much less than expected for a PaO_2 of 55 torr. Therefore, it is possible that a patient might be excluded for Medicare reimbursement by oximetry but may have been eligible according to arterial blood gas measurement, as shown in example two of Table 1. Alkalemia may elevate the saturation through a leftward shift of the oxyhemoglobin dissociation curve (example three of Table 1). Other factors, such as the presence of carboxyhemoglobin, may increase the saturation reading by oximetry.

Patients with a PaO_2 of 56 to 59 torr may be candidates for continuous administration of supplemental oxygen if end-organ compromise due to hypoxemia can be demonstrated. Since the hematocrit may serve as a reflection of the overall adequacy of oxygenation, polycythemia (e.g., hematocrit greater than 56 ml per deciliter) qualifies a patient for continuous supplemental oxygen therapy if the room air arterial blood gas shows a PaO_2 of 56 to 59 torr. Peripheral edema or other signs of cor pulmonale (e.g., an electrocardiogram showing a P wave greater than 2 mm in leads II, III, or AVF) are evidence for the deleterious effects of chronic hypoxemia and would also justify continuous oxygen therapy for a patient with a PaO_2 of 56 to 59 torr. Patients with a resting room air PaO_2 of greater than 56 torr may also qualify for intermittent use of oxygen if hypoxemia can be documented either during exercise or sleep.

OXYGEN DELIVERY SYSTEMS

There are different sources of oxygen, different delivery devices, and a variety of modalities available for administering oxygen flow to the patient in the home.

Stationary Oxygen Sources

There are three different stationary sources of home oxygen. Large tanks of compressed gas have been used to deliver oxygen in the home for over 2 decades. The most frequently used have been the H or K tanks (Table 2). These huge compressed gas cylinders are very heavy, cumbersome, and visually unappealing. Duration of the oxygen supply is determined by the liter flow requirement, and the upper and lower limits of flow are determined by the characteristics of the flow meter used. Unlike the other oxygen sources described below, up to 15 L per minute can be administered in the home from these units, but this is obviously expensive and impractical.

The concentrator is another stationary source of home oxygen (Table 3). This electrically powered device uses molecular sieve beds to purify entrained ambient air. Concentrators are often more economical than oxygen reservoirs because they do not require periodic refilling. However, routine maintenance schedules are important to assure reliable perfor-

TABLE 2   Compressed Gas Cylinders

Manufacturer	Weight (lb)	Capacity (L)	Duration (hr) (at 2 L/min)
Standard Sizes			
E Cylinder	12	622	5.5
D Cylinder	10	415	3.5
H Cylinder	130	6600	55
Bunn			
Portalite 240	7	240	2
Portalite 406	9	406	3
Puritan-Bennett			
Companion 240	5.25	240	1.5
Companion 480	7.5	480	3.0

TABLE 3 Oxygen Concentrators

Manufacturer	Weight (lb)	Flow Range (L/min)	O_2 Concentration	
			(L/min)	(FiO$_2$ + 3%)
BUNN 3001	43	1–3	1	95
			2	94
			3	87
BUNN 5001	50	1–5	1–3	95
			4	93
			5	85
BUNN NATURAL	29	0.5–5	0.5–4	94
			5	90
INSPIRON 3500	54	1–4	1–2	94
			3	92
			4	90
DE VILBISS				
DEVO/44	44	1–5	1–3	95
			4	90
			5	82
DEVO/MC29	29	1–3	1	95
			2	93
			3	90
MOUNTAIN MEDICAL				
ECONO 2	114	1–5	1–4	95
			5	90
MINI O$_2$	56	1–3	1–2	95
			3	93
SUMMIT	59	1–5	1–3	95
			4	93
			5	85
SAGE	49	1–3	1–2	95
			3	93
ASPEN	35	1–2	1–2	93
INVACARE				
MOBILAIRE III	64	1–3	1–2	95
			3	93
PURITAN-BENNETT 492	49	1–4	1–4	92
HEALTHDYNE				
HEALTHAIRE 5000	54	0.5–5	0.5–4	90
			5	85
PENOX BX 5000	55	0.5–5	0.5–4	90
			5	85
LINDE MARK 4	62	1–3	1–2	93
			3	90

mance with adequate purity of the gas and accuracy of liter flow. The expense of routine maintenance schedules offsets the cost savings of the concentrator. Concentrators are much more attractive than compressed gas cylinders and can be camouflaged to appear like household furniture. The maximum liter flow may be up to 5 L per minute with some units, but efficiency is reduced at these higher flow rates. Consequently, the FiO$_2$ may drop into the mid 80s with concentrators when used at high flow rates. Under most circumstances this is of little clinical significance. Disadvantages are that they are often noisy, and insurance carriers generally do not reimburse for electricity used to power the concentrator, which may contribute $50.00 or more per month to the patient's electrical bill. Because of the possibility of electrical power failure or equipment malfunction, patients using a concentrator should have one of the small oxygen cylinders, described in the next section, as a back-up.

The third stationary oxygen source is the liquid reservoir (Table 4). This tends to be much more visually appealing than the compressed gas cylinder (Fig. 1). Pure oxygen is delivered at up to 8 L per minute with some systems. At high flow rates the units may occasionally freeze. Because oxygen is condensed into a liquid form, significantly more can be stored in the unit. Consequently, these systems require less frequent filling than the compressed gas cylinder. Unlike compressed gas cylinders, evaporative loss of oxygen occurs when a liquid source is used. If a patient is hospitalized for a prolonged period, one must make

TABLE 4 Liquid Oxygen Systems

	Stationary Units			Portable Units		
Manufacturer	Weight (lb)	Flow Range (L/min)	Duration (Days @ 2 L/min)	Weight (lb)	Flow Range (L/min)	Duration (hours @ 2 L/min)
BUNN	130	1–8	7–11	11	0.5–8	8–9
CRYO II						
Grandair	140	0.25–12	11			
Stationair	99	0.25–12	7			
Pulseair I				7.1	1–5	11.8
Pulseair II				10.4	1–5	25.5
Wanderair				6.5	1–5	3.3
Travelair I				9.5	1–5	7.3
Travelair II				13.5	1–8	13
CRYOGENICS						
Liberator 45	163	0.25–6	12			
Liberator 30	122	0.25–6	8			
Liberator 20	86	0.25–6	5			
Stroller				9.6	0.25–6	7.5
Sprint				6.9	0.25–6	4.3
INSPIRON	130	1–8	7–11	11	0.5–8	8–9
LINDE						
OR 212	70	0–15	4			
OR 303	116	1–5	8			
R-40	78	0–15	4			
R-70	115	0–15	8			
Large Walker				10	0.5–5	8
Small Walker				6.5	0.5–5	4
Mark 4 Walker				8.5	0.5–6	8
PENOX						
Large Base Unit	151	0–8	12			
Standard Base	116	0–8	8			
Mini Base	89	0–8	5			
Lightweight				5	0.25–5	2.75
1 Portable				6.5	0.25–5	3
2 Portable				8.5	1–5	6
3 Portable				12	1–5	11
PURITAN-BENNETT						
Companion 21	92	0.25–6	6			
Companion 31	125	0.25–6	8			
Companion 41	160	0.25–6	11			
Companion 1000				7.5	0.25–6	8.5

sure that significant evaporative loss of oxygen did not occur while the patient was in the hospital, so that the oxygen supply at the time of discharge is adequate.

One of the three stationary sources described above is placed in one room of the patient's residence and a 25 to 50 foot extension tubing is used to allow the patient to ambulate from room to room. A major disadvantage of the stationary source is that the patient is literally tethered to the unit. Patients must be careful that oxygen flow is not interrupted by the extension tubing's becoming kinked or crushed under furniture. The long tubing is awkward, and patients must be careful that they do not trip over the hose and injure themselves. It is difficult to adjust flow rates for rest and exertion when the oxygen source is a distance away. These inconveniences probably result in suboptimal patient compliance.

Portable Oxygen Sources

Smaller more portable units should accompany the large stationary oxygen delivery systems. The major indication for a portable system is the need for patient mobility. Even severely disabled patients must occasionally leave the home or nursing home for physician visits and should have one portable source. Portable oxygen units use either compressed gas or liquid oxygen. Small compressed gas cylinders can come in a variety of sizes (see Table 2). The most popular is the E cylinder, which requires a cart for portability because of its weight. As with the H cylinder, the duration of a portable compressed gas cylinder is determined by the oxygen flow rate. At a flow of 2 L per minute a full E cylinder can be expected to last about 5 hours. E cylinders are generally sup-

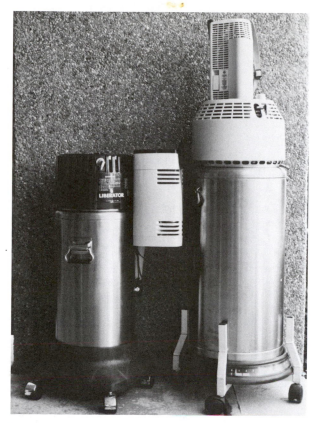

Figure 1 The two stationary liquid oxygen systems are shown with their transfillable portable units. The Liberator 20 (Cryogenic Associates, Indianapolis, IN) is shown on the left and the Companion 31 (Puritan-Bennett Corporation, Lenexa, KS) is presented on the right. Equipment courtesy of Glasrock Home Health Care, Atlanta, GA.

plied when either concentrators or large H cylinders are the stationary source.

The stationary liquid oxygen reservoirs can be safely used to transfill the smaller, more lightweight portable units (see Table 4). The temperature in the liquid phase is quite low, and patients must be careful not to burn their hands in the transfilling process. These liquid portable units are usually conveniently carried over the shoulder, which offers greater patient mobility (Fig. 2). However, patients with severe respiratory impairment may still choose to place the unit on a cart and either push or pull it like a compressed gas cylinder. Duration of the oxygen in the portable unit is related to both the liter flow requirement and the evaporative loss that occurs with liquid oxygen. Advantages and disadvantages of both stationary and portable oxygen sources are summarized in Table 5.

Oxygen Delivery Devices

Devices that have been used to administer oxygen in the home are the face mask, the trach collar, the T-piece, the nasal cannula, and the transtracheal catheter. The first patients to receive home oxygen often used a face mask. Today only rarely does a patient with extremely high oxygen requirements use a mask in the home. A trach collar and a T-piece can be used to administer oxygen to patients with tracheostomies in the hospital or the home, but adequate humidification must also be provided.

In the past, most patients received home oxygen by the standard nasal cannula or prongs. Short-term use of these devices during hospitalization has been described in the previous chapter. Although more comfortable than the face mask for long-term use, there are problems and complications of the standard nasal cannula, which are shown in Table 6.

In efforts to lengthen the duration of performance of a portable unit and reduce the cost of oxygen, devices designed to conserve oxygen have evolved over the past few years. One such device is the reservoir cannula, which contains small plastic reservoir bags that are located below the nasal prongs (Fig. 3). During exhalation, oxygen-enriched gas is stored in the bags and subsequently inhaled with the next inspiration. The storage of oxygen during exhalation, which would otherwise be wasted, allows equivalent oxygenation with a lower liter flow requirement. The major advantage of the reservoir cannula is that oxygen conservation of 50 to 75 percent can lengthen the duration of the oxygen source, which encourages ambulation. A disadvantage of this device is that it is much larger than the cannula and is cosmetically unappealing to many patients; it also requires frequent replacement. A variation on the concept of the reservoir nasal cannula has been developed in the form of a pendant (Fig. 4). The oxygen pendant has a reservoir that is positioned over the chest. The nasal prongs

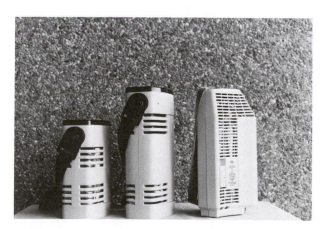

Figure 2 Portable liquid systems from left to right are the Stroller, Stroller Sprint (Cryogenic Associates, Indianapolis, IN) and the Companion 1000 (Puritan-Bennett Corporation, Lenexa, KS). Equipment courtesy of Glasrock Home Health Care, Atlanta, GA.

TABLE 5 Comparisons of Oxygen Delivery Systems

Stationary Oxygen Sources
  Compressed Gas Cylinder (e.g., H)
    Advantages
      High flow capabilities, no evaporative loss.
    Disadvantages
      Heavy, cumbersome, visually unappealing.
  Concentrator
    Advantages
      No refilling required, most attractive system.
    Disadvantages
      Routine maintenance required, noisy, electricity costs not reimbursed,
      lower flow capabilities, reduction in FIO_2 related to flow.
  Liquid Reservoir
    Advantages
      More visually appealing and fewer refills than the cylinder, higher
      flows than with a concentrator.
    Disadvantages
      Evaporative loss, unit can freeze.
Portable Oxygen Sources
  Compressed Gas Cylinder (e.g., E)
    Advantages
      No evaporative loss, higher flow capabilities.
    Disadvantages
      Heavier, more awkward, shorter duration, unattractive.
  Portable Liquid Unit
    Advantages
      Longer duration, more attractive.
    Disadvantages
      Evaporative loss.

and tubing of the device are larger than the standard cannula, but the pendant is much more cosmetically appealing. Like the reservoir cannula, the oxygen pendant needs to be replaced more frequently than the standard nasal cannula. Weekly replacement is currently recommended.

The third device for home oxygen delivery is the transtracheal oxygen catheter. The first device was a modification of a 16-gauge intravenous catheter that was placed percutaneously between the second and third tracheal rings using a 14-gauge breakaway needle. A 16-gauge catheter with a flange and Luer connector was later designed. Recently, a needle-wire guide-dilator technique was developed to create a tracheocutaneous fistula. One week after the procedure, supplemental oxygen is delivered through a 9 F polyurethane catheter that has one distal port, and the patient learns to clean it in place with a cleaning rod while the tract is maturing. After approximately 6 weeks the tract is mature, and the patient is taught to remove, reinsert, and clean a second catheter design that is No. 8 F. and has multiple side ports for the dispersion of oxygen flow (Fig. 5). As with the reservoir cannula and pendant, transtracheal oxygen delivery significantly reduces liter flow requirements. Results of investigators from Britain, France, and the United States show an overall reduction in flow rates of 50 percent. In addition to reduced flow requirements, the specific indications for transtracheal oxy-

TABLE 6 Complications of the Nasal Cannula

Skin irritation (ear and nose)
Cellulitis (bacterial and fungal)
Nasal crusting/postnasal drip
Recurrent nosebleeds
Septal perforation
Loss of sense of smell and taste
Acute sinusitis
Blockage of tear ducts
Serous otitis/acute otitis
Sore throat/hoarseness

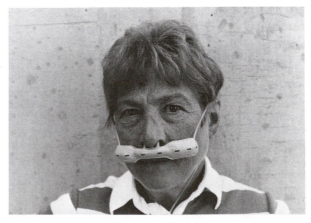

Figure 3 The Oxymizer Reservoir Cannula (Chad Therapeutics, Inc., Chatsworth, CA).

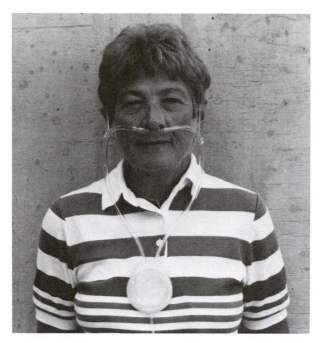

Figure 4 The Oxymizer Pendant (Chad Therapeutics, Inc., Chatsworth, CA).

gen delivery reduces oxygen flow requirements. Technology for "pulse" or demand oxygen delivery is growing rapidly (Fig. 6). One device is incorporated into a portable liquid oxygen unit (Pulsair II, $Cryo_2$, Ft. Pierce, FL) and can be adjusted to deliver a variable volume with each inspiratory effort. Another device (Oxymatic, Chad Therapeutics, Chatsworth, CA) can be interfaced with either liquid reservoirs or compressed gas cylinders and delivers a fixed volume. It can be adjusted to either cycle on each breath or on a variable breath basis. To date, demand oxygen has been delivered using a nasal cannula and has only been used with a portable source. Nasal pulse delivery has not been evaluated during sleep. Some

gen therapy are listed in Table 7. General indications are the same as for continuous supplemental oxygen therapy. The potential complications of transtracheal oxygen therapy are also listed in Table 7. Overall, transtracheal oxygen therapy has an acceptably low morbidity in properly selected patients.

Methods for Delivering Oxygen Flow

Until recently, supplemental oxygen could only be delivered as a continuous flow of gas. Studies have shown that oxygen can be "pulsed" in phase with inspiratory efforts using very sensitive thermistors or pressure transducers to sense respiratory effort. Oxygen is not wasted into the atmosphere during expiration. Results have shown that this method of oxy-

TABLE 7   Transtracheal Oxygen Therapy

Specific Indications
   Need for improved mobility
   Complications of nasal cannula
   Suboptimal compliance due to nasal oxygen
   Hypoxemia refractory to nasal oxygen
   Patient preference due to comfort or cosmesis
Potential Complications
   Bronchospasm
   Subcutaneous emphysema
   Keloids
   Pneumothorax
   Infection
   Bleeding

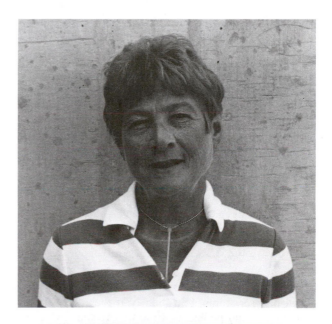

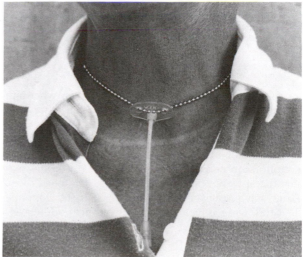

Figure 5 The SCOOP-2 Transtracheal Catheter (Transtracheal Systems, Denver, CO).

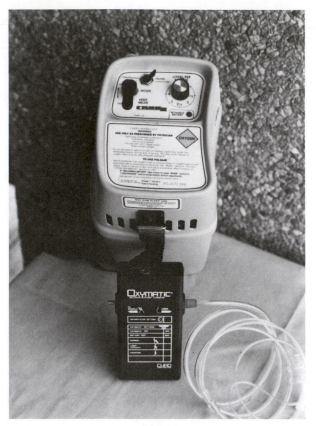

Figure 6 Examples of two portable pulse delivery systems. The Pulsair II (Cryo₂ Corporation, Ft. Pierce, FL) is shown on the top, and the Oxymatic (Chad Therapeutics, Inc., Chatsworth, CA) is shown on the bottom.

patients may have difficulty with reproducible cycling nasal pulse systems, particularly if there is nasal obstruction or the patient is a mouth breather. Mechanical failure of the pulse system may also be a concern. Studies are under way to evaluate pulse transtracheal oxygen delivery.

THE OXYGEN PRESCRIPTION

Careful consideration should be given when prescribing home oxygen therapy. It is often more complex than ordering supplemental continuous flow oxygen in the hospital. The commitment to oxygen therapy is usually for life, and cost implications of your prescription are considerable. Cost issues in home oxygen therapy are constantly changing. The most recent issues have been succinctly addressed by O'Donohue. The following issues should be routinely addressed.

Residence

The altitude at which the patient lives should also be taken into consideration when prescribing home oxygen. For example, a patient who is hospital evaluated in Denver (elevation of 5,280 feet above sea level) with a PaO_2 of 56 torr will be significantly more hypoxemic in his home in Evergreen, Colorado (elevation 7,278 feet above sea level). On the other hand, a patient seen in consultation in Denver with a PaO_2 of 54 torr may not require continuous supplemental oxygen therapy in his home town of Colby, Kansas (elevation 2,180 feet above sea level).

Patients from a rural area may be limited in the oxygen sources that are available to them. Though liquid or compressed gas may be preferable based on patient needs, those living in remote areas may only have access to concentrators. Home care providers in rural areas must generally service a broad territory, and frequent oxygen delivery is neither practical nor cost-effective.

Since patients receiving home oxygen are often disabled, the home situation must also be assessed, including the patient's ability to climb stairs. Patients on compressed gas cylinders or liquid may also pose a problem to the home care provider if they must routinely transport the heavy awkward stationary system refills to the bedroom on the second floor. Oxygen may be prescribed for patients in a nursing home. Unlike hospitals, nursing homes rarely have wall oxygen sources, and the same considerations for selection of a stationary home oxygen source apply.

Duration of Oxygen Use

As described earlier, patients with chronic hypoxemia at rest should be encouraged to use supplemental oxygen 24 hours per day. Patients randomized to 24-hour oxygen therapy only used oxygen an average of 19 hours per day in the highly supervised protocol of the NOTT study. The oxygen source, delivery device, and method of administration should be carefully tailored to the patient's needs in order to maximize compliance. Comfort and cosmesis should not be underestimated in terms of their impact on patient compliance.

Even though supplemental oxygen during sleep could be administered using a liquid, compressed gas, or concentrator source, liquid oxygen would be both wasteful and costly. Daytime evaporative loss while the system sits idle would be significant. Similarly, patients requiring supplemental oxygen only during brief and infrequent high levels of exercise would find the portability and convenience of a portable liquid reservoir appealing. However, the evaporative loss from the idle stationary source may be greater than the actual oxygen consumed by the patient. In this setting a stationary system is unnecessary, and the patient's needs may be best met by a supply of small compressed gas cylinders.

It is difficult to justify oxygen strictly on an as necessary basis, particularly when there is such a poor correlation between hypoxemia and dyspnea. It is common to see patients with profound hypoxemia who are unaware of their degree of compromise. Furthermore, patients may have an entirely normal PaO_2 during episodes of dyspnea.

Length of Time Needed

With careful selection of candidates for home oxygen therapy, the overwhelming majority of patients require supplemental oxygen for the remainder of their lives. Occasionally patients may require home oxygen for a few weeks to months while they are recovering from an acute illness. Unfortunately, health care financing regulations are encouraging earlier discharge of patients from the hospital and are requesting health care providers to manage ill patients in the home. As a result, the number of patients who will receive short-term home oxygen therapy may be on the increase.

Flow Requirements

Patients with high flow requirements can present a problem. Concentrators usually have lower flow capabilities than either liquid or compressed gas sources, and as noted earlier, oxygen concentration is flow-dependent. On the other hand, liquid and compressed gas can be expensive with high flow rates. Continuous flow nasal cannula delivery at high flows can be uncomfortable, and the short duration of portable systems markedly limits mobility. Transtracheal oxygen therapy has been shown to be practical and efficacious in patients with high liter flow requirements, particularly if oxygenation is refractory to nasal cannula use. Other oxygen conserving devices such as the reservoir and pendant cannula or a pulse delivery system may be considered.

The oxygen delivery system may need to deliver flow rates as low as one-quarter L per minute, particularly with treatment of infants, small children, and adults on transtracheal oxygen therapy.

Humidification

There is controversy in the literature as to whether or not the average patient on continuous flow nasal oxygen needs supplemental humidity provided by a bubble humidifier. Many contend that this humidifier is both inconvenient and an unnecessary expense. Since infection related to respiratory therapy equipment is thought to require the production of contaminated water aerosols, it is unlikely that these humidifiers (which produce only water vapor) are a potential source of infection. Many patients do not require a bubble humidifier. However, a humidifier should be used in the treatment of patients with high oxygen flow rates, those who reside in arid climates, and those who have a propensity to develop inspissated secretions.

Ambulation

Studies suggest that a regular program of medically supervised exercise is beneficial to those suffering from COPD and other chronic lung diseases. Even though pulmonary function will not show significant change, there may be improvement in cardiovascular fitness, exercise tolerance, and self-confidence. It can be argued that much of the improved survival in the NOTT study was due to use of continuous ambulatory oxygen (in contrast to providing only nocturnal therapy). Under ideal circumstances, all patients requiring continuous oxygen should have unlimited access to a portable source and a delivery device that encourages ambulation. However, this is both impractical and wasteful in patients who are too ill to leave the home. It is important to be aware of the fact that nearly all patients have a need for increased flow rates above their resting prescription when they engage in exercise. New portable oximetry equipment makes flow titration during ambulation both convenient and cost-effective.

Travel

Early on in the history of oxygen therapy the safety of automobile travel with oxygen was demonstrated. Networks of home care providers make it easier for patients to arrange for an oxygen supply at their destination as they travel throughout the United States by car, boat, train, or airplane. The physician must play an active role in facilitating airline authorization for in-flight oxygen. Currently, patients are not allowed to board the plane with their own oxygen supply, and an oxygen source before departure and after arrival must be arranged. Alterations in flow requirements due to altitude changes at destination point must be considered. International travel is possible but much more complicated.

HEALTH MAINTENANCE EVALUATION

As with any chronic medical therapy, supplemental oxygen delivery must be monitored. Routine evaluation by the physician and periodic laboratory assessment of the adequacy of the oxygenation are highly recommended. Flow requirements may increase over time as the underlying disease progresses. Changes in medication may translate into changes in oxygenation, and flow requirements may temporarily need to increase during an acute illness such as bronchitis or an upper respiratory infection.

THE HOME CARE PROVIDER

The home care provider must play an integral role in the management of your patient on home oxygen therapy. He or she must work closely with you in arranging the appropriate oxygen source, delivery device, and mode of delivery. Insurance reimbursement for oxygen therapy is intimately tied to the adequate documentation of oxygen need. Your assistance will be asked for in properly completing certificates of medical necessity. Based on current trends, it is likely that this documentation will become more complicated in the future and will vary from region to region.

An individual home care provider may not be able to offer the patient every available option in oxygen delivery. For example, most local home care companies can only provide a liquid system by one manufacturer. This is because capitalization costs of multiple liquid systems by different manufacturers are prohibitive, and the liquid oxygen sources in the delivery trucks are only compatible with transfilling units of the same manufacturer. Because of the rapid growth in home oxygen technology, the physician must continue to seek recommendations from experts in the home care field.

Home care providers commonly have the ability to make periodic clinical evaluations of the patient in the home and assess oxygenation and flow requirements by oximetry. The physician should specify whether or not he or she wishes these follow-up reports. Frequency of the visits depends both on clinical need and the home-care company's ability to provide the service.

THE FUTURE

The future of long-term home oxygen therapy is integrally related to a delicate balance between advances in technology and the necessity for appropriate cost containment.

Acknowledgments

The author wishes to thank John R. Goodman, B.S. RRT, Dawn C. McCarty, RRT, and Siobhan L. Zevin, Educational Coordinator, all of The Institute for Transtracheal Oxygen Therapy, for their expert technical and clinical assistance.

Suggested Reading

Christopher KL, Spofford BT, Brannin PK, Petty TL. Transtracheal oxygen therapy for refractory hypoxemia. JAMA 1986; 256:494–497.

Flenley DC. Long-term home oxygen therapy. Chest 1985; 87:99–103.

Medical Research Council Working Party. Long-term domiciliary oxygen therapy in chronic hypoxic cor pulmonale complicating chronic bronchitis and emphysema. Lancet 1981; 1:681–686.

Nocturnal Oxygen Therapy Trial Group. Continuous or nocturnal oxygen therapy in hypoxemic chronic obstructive lung disease: A clinical trial. Ann Intern Med 1980; 93:391–398.

O'Donohue WJ. Oxygen conserving devices. Respir Care 1987; 32:37–42.

HUMIDIFICATION

HUMIDIFICATION SYSTEMS

BOB DEMERS, B.S., RRT

Generically, two categories of humidification devices are in common use: nebulizers and true humidifiers. Nebulizers produce particulate water in the form of extremely small droplets, and the collective surface area of these droplets affords a vast air-liquid interface from which evaporation can take place. This results in a carrier gas that is usually fully saturated at whatever ambient temperature prevails. True humidifiers, on the other hand, evaporate water in the form of individual molecules or true water vapor. Particulate water is notably absent from the gases emanating from a humidifier. During continuous mechanical ventilation, humidifiers are commonly employed in lieu of nebulizers. Therefore, my comments will be confined to humidifiers as opposed to nebulizers.

HEAT AND MOISTURE EXCHANGE IN THE INTACT NORMAL AIRWAY

The upper airway is admirably well suited to its task of warming inspired gases to body temperature and humidifying those gases on their way to the lungs. Warming and humidification functions are facilitated by exposing the inspirate to a large surface area of mucous membrane, which is moist and highly vascular. Chatburn and Primiano have observed that, during normal, quiet breathing, tracheal inspired gas has a temperature within the range of 32 to 34° C and is saturated. This corresponds to an absolute water content of between 36 and 40 mg per liter. The quantitative moisture exchange characteristics of the airways appear to be widely misunderstood by clinicians. For example, insensible water loss via the respiratory tract is frequently invoked as a mechanism for weight loss in critically ill patients. As the subsequent calculations indicate, however, volumetric water losses over a 24-hour period are rather modest and are unlikely to account for appreciable variations in body weight. Insensible water losses from the respiratory tract will, of course, depend on the absolute

humidity of the inspired air. But we can calculate the maximum insensible water loss during normal, quiet breathing as follows.

Assuming a minute inspired volume of 6.00 L of completely dry air, warming of that gas to body temperature and complete saturation with water vapor will add 43.8 mg per liter, or

$$(6.00 \text{ L/min}) \times (43.8 \text{ mg/L}) = 263 \text{ mg/min}.$$

Over a 24-hour period, water vapor excretion is

$$(263 \text{ mg/min}) \times (60 \text{ min/hr}) \times (24 \text{ hr/day}) = 378,432 \text{ mg/day}.$$

This translates to a weight (mass) of 378 g per day, having a volume of 378 ml. An alternative method can be used to derive the same result, as outlined by Demers and Irwin.

Naturally, to the extent that inhaled gases are at least partially saturated with water vapor, this figure will necessarily decrease; it represents the upper limit of mass-volume when the subject breathes dry gas. At the other end of the spectrum, if inhaled gases were to be fully saturated and at body temperature before they were introduced into the upper airway, insensible water losses would be driven to zero. Conditions whereby a normal subject breathes saturated gases at body temperature through an intact upper airway are fortunately unusual. Most of us would shun an environment that provided an ambient temperature of 99° F and 100 percent humidity.

APPROPRIATE THERAPEUTIC AND PROPHYLACTIC END POINTS FOR HUMIDIFIERS

As noted earlier, inspired gases are not normally body temperature, pressure, and saturated (BTPS) during quiet breathing even well within the respiratory tract (at the site of the trachea). In view of these observations, it is somewhat puzzling that we clinicians often go to heroic lengths to provide inspired gases that are fully saturated and fully warmed to body temperature or even higher to intubated and tracheostomized patients. Gases introduced into the trachea at 32 to 34° C and saturated at that temperature (absolute humidity 36 to 40 mg per liter) mimic the conditions that prevail normally. The Emergency Care Research

Institute (ECRI) cites a minimum acceptable absolute humidity figure of 21 to 24 mg per liter for long-term ventilation of intubated or tracheostomized patients. Thus, it must be conceded that devices and methods that furnish an absolute humidity in excess of 24 mg per liter are preferable for most patients. Although devices that fully saturate inspired gases at body temperature are acceptable, such devices need not necessarily be employed for all patients, especially in view of their complexity and expense and the availability of cheaper effective alternative devices.

HEATED HUMIDIFIERS

Certain patients manifest signs and symptoms that suggest that one go the extra mile to provide BTPS inspirate. For example, a tracheostomized patient transferred from a nursing home who presents with crusty, inspissated secretions on admission would be a good candidate for a Cascade-type humidification device. Also, if a patient's prime indication for intubation is management of copious secretions, such a humidifier is well conceived. Such devices are available from multiple manufacturers (e.g., Puritan-Bennett, Respiratory Care, Inc., Bear Medical Systems, and Travenol), and tests of these units by independent laboratories such as ECRI reveal that they perform satisfactorily. Two features of this type of humidifier represent major drawbacks, however: their expense and their predilection for condensation (rainout). The expense of the heated humidifier resides not only in the initial expense of purchasing such a device but also in the sterile distilled water that must be purchased to feed the unit. Certain units require the purchase of a single-patient use heating element in addition to the water, which further escalates expense. For example, several years ago we performed an audit in a respiratory care department and found that we were paying $15.18 per patient for the water and Concha Column (Respiratory Care, Inc.) required to manage patients for 48 hours after surgery. The vast majority of these patients were good candidates for hygroscopic condenser humidifiers (HCHs), and the substitution of the HCH for the heated humidifier resulted in substantial cost savings for our department. The accumulation of rainout in the dependent loops of ventilator tubing is another shortcoming associated with the use of heated humidifiers. One might employ internal heated wire tubing circuits to prevent rainout, but this in itself is a rather costly solution. Alternatively, therapists can make it a practice to "milk" the tubes at frequent intervals. Of course, this approach is not free, although the hidden costs of more labor-intensive modes of practice are frequently discounted.

Despite the therapist's vigilance, condensate will pool in tubing loops periodically, and a bolus of the condensate will be inadvertently mobilized into the patient's endotracheal or tracheostomy tube. Such an event is, at the very least, uncomfortable for the patient. The possible presence of high concentrations of facultative organisms in such condensate renders such an event a potential infection control problem. Several years ago, we reported an outbreak of *Acinetobacter* that had occurred because the organism proliferated in the wet, warm environment of a bellows spirometer. This provided forceful evidence to us that condensate in ventilator circuit components can represent an infection hazard. In spite of these shortcomings, heated humidifiers are in widespread use and, as noted earlier, represent the humidification method of choice for certain patients.

These devices have fallen into such widespread use that most mechanical ventilators are fitted routinely with a heated humidifier during the normal setup procedure. This continues to be warranted, because a given patient might manifest a need for a heated humidifier at one time or another during his or her ventilator course. For example, if the physician were to write an order to convert a patient from assisted mechanical ventilation to intermittent mandatory ventilation (IMV), and if much or most of the patient's minute ventilation requirements were delivered during the spontaneous breathing component of the IMV mode, a heated humidifier would constitute the humidification device of choice. As will be discussed later, the dead space incorporated in alternative humidification apparatuses (hygroscopic condenser humidifiers and heat and moisture exchanging filters [HMEF]) would render them poor choices in such circumstances. This obliges most respiratory care departments to purchase a heated humidifier for each of their mechanical ventilators. Once this considerable initial expense has been incurred, subsequent cost-benefit decisions hinge on the differential costs of additional equipment (sterile water and disposable heating elements, for example) for use with the heated humidifier versus the cost of substitutable humidification devices.

HYGROSCOPIC CONDENSER HUMIDIFIERS

A hygroscopic condenser humidifier is a device that sequesters some or most of the water vapor that traverses it during a patient's exhalation and returns that moisture to the inspirate during the succeeding inspiration. Various brands of HCHs are available commercially (Siemens Servo 152, Engstrom Edith, Terumo Breath Aid, Portex Humidivent, Artec Humid). Of these, the Siemens, Engstrom, and Portex are the most efficient, providing an inspirate with an absolute humidity of 26, 26, and 24 mg per liter, respectively, according to the tests of Branson and Hurst. This level of performance qualifies the HCH for use with most patients for short- to moderate-term mechanical ventilation. The principal virtues of the HCH are its low expense (approximately $2.00 to $4.00 per unit) and its ability to rid the ventilator tubing of condensate. However, clinicians should remember that the HCH is contraindicated for use with certain categories of patients (Table 1). Patients who produce copious amounts of secretions should be ventilated with conventional heated humidifiers, because mobilization of secretions into the HCH will compromise its function in addition to impairing ventilation. The HCH's matrix has a finite capacity for water, such that its use should be limited to patients having a tidal volume below that cited by the manufacturer (for instance, the Siemens Servo 152 is recommended for use with patients having tidal volumes below 1,500 ml). It is imperative that the full volume of the previous expiration traverse the HCH so that it can capture a sufficient amount of water vapor to donate to the next inspiration. Thus, the HCH must not be used if the inspired volume appreciably exceeds the expired volume, such as might occur in the presence of a bronchopleural fistula or substantial amounts of leakage past an intratracheal inflatable cuff. Last, the volume of the HCH housing and its placement between the patient Y-piece and the endotracheal or tracheostomy tube contribute mechanical dead space (for example, both the Siemens Servo Humidifier 152 and the Engstrom Edith contribute a dead space volume of 90 ml to the circuit). Therefore, the HCH should not be used for patients breathing spontaneously and at low tidal volumes (all pediatric patients or certain adults) unless it is specifically configured for such patients. This caveat might apply, of course, to patients being ventilated in the IMV mode if the bulk of their minute ventilation is delivered during spontaneous breathing, as opposed to the positive-pressure component of that mode. In patients for whom the preceding contraindications do not apply, the HCH is a clinically useful and cost-effective alternative to heated humidifiers.

HEAT AND MOISTURE EXCHANGING FILTERS

A great many ventilator breathing circuit filters (so-called bacteria filters) are currently on the market. Most of these units consist of a single or double layer of porous filter material designed to filter organisms from the gases that traverse them.

As noted earlier, the presence of contaminated condensate in ventilator circuit tubing can potentially constitute an infection control hazard. In most cases, these organisms find their way into a given patient's tubing circuit precisely because the patient served as a source. In such a circumstance, it is the patient, not the tubing circuit, who might rightly be considered the reservoir for the organisms. Similarly, one need not be unduly concerned that such contaminated condensate represents a significant infection control hazard for the patient who served as the source. On the other hand, it would be naive to consider contaminated condensate as innocuous, because it does serve as a septic focus as far as staff members and other patients are concerned. The methods by which such condensate is discarded and the possible contamination of caregivers' hands by the condensate put other patients at risk of nosocomial infection. Patients' endotracheal tubes, expiratory tubing circuits, and inspiratory circuits, in that order, become contaminated during long-term use of a ventilator tubing circuit. On this basis, then, breathing circuit filters are considered standard components of the breathing circuit in some institutions. They prevent contiguous spread of organisms from the patient to the tubing circuit.

Pall Biomedical Products Corporation has marketed bacteria filters for many years. The configuration of the Pall filter is somewhat unique in that it consists of a large area of pleated filter material arranged in a multilayered matrix. The surface area provided by this matrix is very large, and this feature prompted Pall to adapt their design for use as a com-

TABLE 1   Contraindications for the Use of Hygroscopic Condenser Humidifiers and Heat and Moisture Exchanging Filters

Type of Contraindication	Rationale for Contraindication
Certain neonatal and pediatric patients	Mechanical dead space of the HCH or HMEF may be excessive relative to the patient's tidal volume
Patients who produce copious amounts of secretions	Secretions mobilized into HCH or HMEF compromise its humidification function and increase resistance
Patients who derive the majority of their minute ventilation via spontaneous breaths (IMV/SIMV*/CPAP† modes)	Mechanical dead space of the HCH or HMEF may be excessive relative to the patient's tidal volume
Patients whose tidal volume exceeds tidal volume specification listed by HCH or HMEF manufacturer	Finite capacity of HCH or HMEF for storage/delivery of water must not be exceeded
Patients who lose appreciable amounts of inhaled gas through a patent bronchopleural fistula	Volume of dry inspirate will exceed HCH's or HMEF's capacity to saturate it due to low recovery from expirate
Patients who lose appreciable amounts of inhaled gas due to leakage around their intratracheal inflatable cuff	Volume of dry inspirate will exceed HCH's or HMEF's capacity to saturate it due to low recovery from expirate

* Spontaneous intermittent mandatory ventilation
† Continuous positive airway pressure

bination bacteria filter and heat and moisture exchanger. This device, the HME 15-22 Heat and Moisture Exchanging Filter, is claimed to have a bacterial filtration efficiency in excess of 99.999 percent. By virtue of the large air-liquid interface provided by its filter element, it is capable of humidifying inspired gas to an absolute humidity of 25 mg per liter in the study of Branson and Hurst. This compares favorably with the specifications of the HCHs listed earlier. The internal volume of the unit (90 ml) is identical to that of the Siemens and the Edith HCH. The unit's ability to serve as a bacteria filter and its low price ($3.00) are obvious virtues. The reader should note, of course, that the contraindications for the use of this device are identical to those listed for the HCH (see Table 1). Specifically, it should not be used for (1) patients who produce copious secretions (Fig. 1); (2) patients whose tidal volumes are very large (Fig. 2); (3) patients whose inspired volumes appreciably exceed their expired volumes (bronchopleural fistula or leakage around inflatable cuff or both) (Fig. 3); and (4) spontaneously breathing (pediatric or adult) patients who exhibit low tidal volumes. The bacterial filtration feature makes the Heat and Moisture Exchanging Filter an attractive device for use with certain mechanically ventilated patients. This would include those harboring pathogens that can be transmitted via respiratory secretions (AIDS, herpes, virulent pneumonias, etc.).

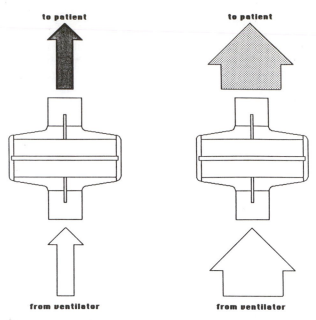

Figure 2 The HCH (or heat and moisture exchanging filter) matrix has a finite capacity for water. If tidal volume is excessively large, the unit is unable to humidify inhaled gases adequately.

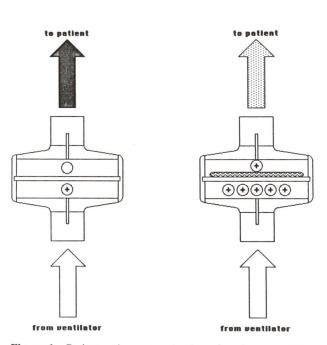

Figure 1 Patients who are productive of copious amounts of secretions can mobilize those secretions into HCHs (or heat and moisture exchanging filters). This would result in compromised humidification function and an increase in airflow resistance.

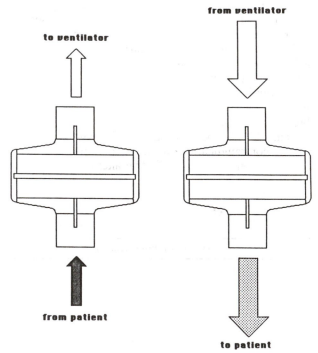

Figure 3 The volume exhaled through the HCH (or heat and moisture exchanging filter) must be equal to the subsequent inhaled volume so that it can capture a sufficient amount of water to donate to the inspirate. The presence of a substantial bronchopleural fistula or leakage around an inflatable cuff renders this impossible.

Suggested Reading

Argentieri M. Heat and moisture exchangers. Health Devices 1983; 12:155–167.

Branson RD, Hurst JM. Laboratory evaluation of moisture output of seven airway heat and moisture exchangers. Respiratory Care 1987; 32:741–747.

Chalon J, Markham JP, Ali MM, Ramanathan S, Turndorf H. The Pall Ultipor breathing circuit filter—an efficient heat and moisture exchanger. Anesth Analg 1984; 63:566–570.

Chatburn RL, Primiano FP Jr. A rational basis for humidity therapy (Editorial). Respir Care 1987; 32:249–254.

Craven DE, Goularte TA, Make BJ. Contaminated condensate in mechanical ventilator circuits. A risk factor for nosocomial pneumonia? Am Rev Respir Dis 1984; 129:625–628.

Demers RR, Irwin RS. Pulmonary hygiene and artificial airway management. In: Kirby RR, Smith RA, Desautels DA, eds. Mechanical ventilation. New York: Churchill Livingstone, 1985.

Irwin RS, Demers RR, Pratter MR, Garrity FL, Miner G, Pritchard A, Whitaker S. An outbreak of *Acinetobacter* infection associated with the use of a ventilator spirometer. Respir Care 1980; 25:232–237.

Gallagher J, Strangeways JEM, Allt-Graham J. Contamination control in long-term ventilation. Anaesthesia 1987; 42:476–481.

BRONCHIAL HYGIENE TECHNIQUES

BLAND AEROSOL THERAPY

RICHARD D. BRANSON, RRT
SANDRA M. SEGER, CRTT

Inhalation of aerosols, for pleasure or medicinal benefit, in the form of smoke (solid particles in gas) or steam (liquid in gas) is a technique humans have practiced for centuries. Similarly, relief of croup-like symptoms in children by placing them in a closed bathroom with the shower running can be verified by generations of anxious parents. Treatment of respiratory disease with "bland aerosol" or "mist therapy" is a common practice in respiratory care today; however, the basis for this therapy is often subjective opinion rather than scientific fact. Clinically, the addition of water or saline solutions to the respiratory tract has been reported to reduce upper airway edema, thin secretions, stimulate cough, and assist in obtaining sputum for cytologic examination. In this chapter, we will discuss the generation of aerosols, factors affecting their deposition, and potential clinical applications in respiratory care.

GENERATION OF AEROSOLS

Generically, a piece of equipment used to produce aerosols is known as a nebulizer. Selection of an appropriate nebulizer is based on the aerosol particle size required and the total volume to be delivered. Particle size is measured in microns (μm) and is a major determinant in the final deposition of the aerosol. Total volume is measured in cubic centimeters per minute (cm^3 per minute) or in milligrams of water per liter (mg H_2O per liter) and reflects not only particle size but also the total number of particles.

Nebulizers can be classified by reservoir size (large or small), power source (electrical or pneumatic), site of placement in the breathing system (mainstream, sidestream, slipstream), and method of aerosol production (spinning disk, mechanical, hydrodynamic, or ultrasonic). All nebulizers used for intermittent or continuous bland aerosol therapy have large reservoirs. All can be placed directly in the main flow of gas (mainstream), or added peripherally such that the aerosol travels into the main flow from a separate gas source (sidestream), or a combination of these (slipstream) according to clinician preference.

Types of Nebulizers

The simplest nebulizer is the spinning disk or centrifugal force nebulizer. It is electrically powered and operates on the principle of the archimedean screw. A disk rotates around a hollow shaft that is immersed in the reservoir. As the disk spins, water is drawn through the shaft and out an opening onto the disk. The centrifugal force of the spinning disk "hurls" the water against a series of baffles, breaking it up into smaller particles. Blades on the disk, similar to those on a fan, create an air current that carries the smaller particles out into the room. Larger particles coalesce and return to the reservoir. This type of nebulizer is often used for room humidification. A schematic of the centrifugal force nebulizer is shown in Figure 1.

The most common nebulizer used to deliver aerosol therapy is the mechanical or jet nebulizer. Operating on Bernouilli's theorem, a high-pressure gas source is directed through a jet orifice. Reduction in lateral pressure surrounding the jet draws water up a capillary tube, where the gas stream shatters it into small particles. The resultant aerosol is impacted on a ball baffle, where larger particles fall back into the reservoir. Further baffling occurs with the water's surface and sides of the reservoir container. The remaining aerosol exits the container and is delivered to the patient via standard corrugated tubing. Total volume output of the mechanical nebulizer can be increased by heating the reservoir, which allows the gas to carry a larger volume of water. Heating, however, increases the amount of rainout that occurs in the delivery tubing.

An important attribute of the mechanical nebulizer is its ability to blend room air with source gas, using Venturi's principle. This allows fairly accurate delivery of oxygen concentrations between 30 and 60 percent. Entrainment of room air also increases the total flow of gas in the system as well as the volume of aerosol. Set at 40 percent, the total flow of gas increases four-fold and aerosol output by approximately 50 percent. The density of the aerosol, however, decreases, since the increase in output is small

SPINNING DISK NEBULIZER

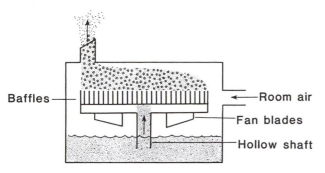

Figure 1 The spinning disk nebulizer. See text for principle of operation.

in comparison with the increase in gas flow. Particles produced by a mechanical nebulizer range in size from 2 to 20 μm, with 40 to 50 percent of particles between 2 and 4 μm. Total output is approximately 30 to 50 mg H_2O per liter, depending on gas flow and degree of air entrainment.

There are numerous models of disposable and nondisposable jet nebulizers. Differences in perfor-

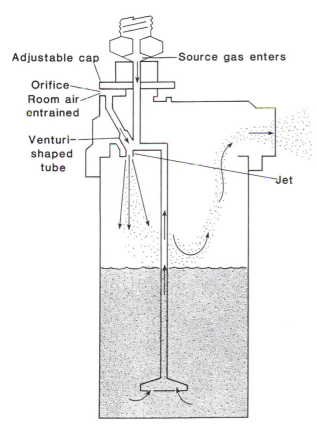

Figure 2 Diagram of a jet nebulizer, showing the path of gas flow from the source gas and the site of air entrainment. See text for a more detailed explanation of function.

HYDROSPHERE NEBULIZER

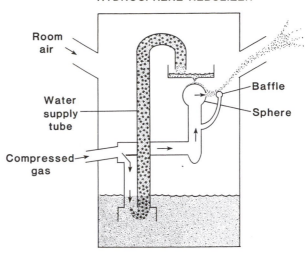

Figure 3 Schematic depicting gas flow and movement of solution in the Babbington or hydrosphere nebulizer. See text for further information.

mance among units are minimal. A typical jet nebulizer is shown in Figure 2.

The hydrodynamic, or Babbington, nebulizer is shown in Figure 3. Originally employed as a furnace jet for burning oil, the hydrodynamic nebulizer produces a dense aerosol, which has a mean particle size of 3 to 5 μm. Total output is between 60 and 70 mg H_2O per liter. A high-pressure gas source enters the nebulizer and travels in two directions. Part of the gas travels into the water reservoir and forces water up a capillary tube, where it flows into a container and drips down over the hollow glass sphere. The rest of the high-pressure gas is forced through a slit in the sphere, where it impacts the water and creates an aerosol. A ball baffle is placed directly in front of the slit and serves to remove the larger particles and return them to the reservoir. By placing a multiorificed cap on the room air inlet of the nebulizer, FiO_2 can be varied from 30 to 100 percent (no air entrainment).

The ultrasonic nebulizer is electrically powered and operates by changing an electric current into high frequency vibrations. It is composed of two separate parts, the electrical power unit and the nebulization unit. The electrical power unit converts standard alternating current into a high frequency current between 1.35 and 3.0 megacycles. The high frequency current is preset by the manufacturer and is not adjustable. From the electrical power unit a coaxial cable carries the signal to the nebulizing unit. The nebulizing unit consists of a piezoelectric transducer, couplant chamber, and nebulization chamber. The transducer receives the signal from the electrical power unit and converts it into high frequency vibrations. The vibrations are transmitted to water within the couplant chamber, which serves as a conductor between the transducer and the nebulization chamber. The bottom of the nebulization chamber is a very thin membrane that allows transfer of the vibrations into the solution to be nebulized. Water cannot pass through the membrane. The energy of the vibrations physically shatters the surface of the solution, creating a very fine aerosol. The particles are carried to the patient by a fan or blower.

The ultrasonic nebulizer creates particles between 1 to 10 μm with an average size of 3 μm. Its total volume output is between 60 to 100 mg H_2O per liter. Output is changed by increasing or decreasing the amplitude of the transducer vibrations through an adjustment on the electrical power unit. Particles also retain a slight electric charge, which helps to maintain stability. A schematic of an ultrasonic nebulizer is shown in Figure 4.

AEROSOL DEPOSITION AND STABILITY

Once an aerosol has been produced, final deposition in the respiratory tract is dependent on a variety of factors. Each of these will be considered below.

Particle Size

The upper airway is an efficient filter of environmental aerosols (e.g., dust and soot) and consequently will prevent penetration of any medical aerosol particle delivered to the bronchial tree that is larger than 40 μm. Particles in the range of 8 to 15 μm have a tendency to fall out in the bronchi and bronchioles. Alveolar deposition occurs with particles 2 to 5 μm. Smaller particles are so stable that they pass in and out of the respiratory tract. Clinically, smaller particles are used to deliver medications for topical effect and larger particles 8 to 15 μm are used to deliver larger volumes of bland aerosol at the bronchiolar level.

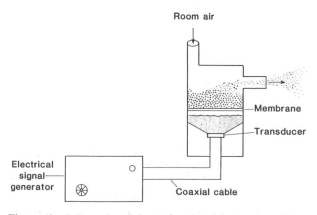

Figure 4 Schematic of the main components of an ultrasonic nebulizer. See text for more detailed information.

Gravity

Stokes' law states that the rate of sedimentation of a particle equals the density times the diameter squared. More simply, the larger the particle, the greater the effect of gravity, and the sooner the particle will be deposited. Viscosity of the carrier gas also plays a part in Stokes' law. When molecules of the carrier gas are small, the force of impaction with the aerosol particles will be decreased. Therefore, a gas such as helium is a less efficient carrier of an aerosol than is oxygen.

Inertia

As an aerosol particle travels through the delivery system and respiratory tract, inertia causes particles to be deposited. Since water molecules have a greater mass than gas molecules, changes in airflow, as a result of bifurcations, result in water molecules' tendency to continue traveling in a straight path. In the bronchi, the numerous branching areas cause inertial impaction at each bifurcation. The tendency toward inertial impaction is also affected by the position of the aerosol in the gas stream. Peripherally located particles are more likely to collide with the bronchial walls. The smaller the diameter of the conducting tube, the greater the incidence of inertial impaction.

Kinetic Activity

The fourth factor in aerosol deposition is the kinetic activity of gas molecules. Suspended in a liquid, particles can be seen continuously colliding with each other and the sides of the container. This movement, similar to brownian movement, applies mainly to particles smaller than 0.5 μm. The greater the kinetic energy, the more frequent the collisions and the greater the likelihood that the particles will coalesce.

Physical Nature of the Particles

Deposition of an aerosol can be influenced by three physical properties of the particles themselves: tonicity, electrical charge, and temperature.

With respect to tonicity, hypotonic solutions tend to lose water and, at least in theory, may evaporate. Hypertonic solutions tend to gain water, which would increase particle size and result in earlier deposition.

The electric charge of a particle is directly related to the energy used to produce it. Aerosols produced by an ultrasonic nebulizer carry a greater charge than those produced by a mechanical nebulizer. The positive charge helps prevent coalescence, since the particles tend to repel one another.

Changes in temperature and humidity can also affect particle size. If the particles are introduced into a warmer gas stream, they tend to increase in size and fall out earlier. This can be important in situations such as introducing a cool bronchodilator aerosol into a heated and humidified ventilator circuit.

Ventilatory Pattern

The final factor in determining aerosol deposition is ventilatory pattern. Generally, the amount of deposition is proportional to the tidal volume and inversely proportional to the inspiratory flow rate and respiratory frequency. Other factors enhancing aerosol deposition are mouth breathing (bypassing the filtration afforded by the nose) and use of an inspiratory hold (allows more efficient settling of particles).

CLINICAL USES OF BLAND AEROSOLS

The term "bland aerosol therapy" refers specifically to the addition of large volumes of water or saline solutions to the bronchial tree. The theoretical benefits of bland aerosol therapy are numerous, but hard clinical evidence is lacking. We will look at the proposed uses of aerosol therapy by anatomic region.

Environmental Modification

The uncomfortable effects of breathing dry gases can be appreciated by anyone who has lived in an old home with a gas forced-air furnace. These effects are even more noticeable to patients with respiratory disease. It is common practice in many areas of the country to use an ultrasonic or jet nebulizer to increase room humidity and make breathing more comfortable. Since the only benefits are subjective effects related to comfort, little scientific basis can be given to this type of therapy. In fact, since there is significant potential for bacterial contamination, this type of therapy is best avoided. Commercially available humidification systems for furnaces are preferred.

Upper Airway

As mentioned in the introduction, the use of steam and hence the medical application of aerosol therapy is a widely practiced modality of care for children with croup. Delivery of the aerosol is accomplished by mask or head hood. Early reports suggested that bland aerosol therapy reduced inflammation and resulted in easier and more quiet breathing. Recent evidence suggests that if the relative humidity of gases is maintained at 100 percent, the use of particulate water is unwarranted.

The use of bland aerosol delivered by mask, with or without an elevated FIO_2, is also common practice in adults after discontinuation of endotracheal intu-

bation. Again, the advantage is thought to occur by reducing inflammation in the upper airway. In our institution the use of aerosols following extubation is gradually being replaced by air-entrainment masks. The air-entrainment mask provides a high-flow system capable of meeting the patient's needs, and it delivers an accurate FIO_2 and reduces costs associated with water use and tubing changes. Additionally, rainout in the tubing does not occur and associated problems (bacterial colonization, fluctuating FIO_2, and therapist time spent emptying water) are avoided. When bland aerosol therapy is used for upper airway disease, a jet nebulizer is adequate, since it produces a range of particles likely to be deposited there.

Lower Airway

A majority of studies looking at aerosol therapy for lower airway disease were performed on children with cystic fibrosis. During the 1960s, all-night mist-tent therapy for children with cystic fibrosis was a popular modality. The beneficial effect was thought to be deposition of a large volume of water in the bronchial tree, resulting in liquefaction of retained airway secretions and improved expectoration. These observations were questioned both in vitro and in vivo. Dulfano and colleagues studied the effects of 100 percent relative humidity on expectorated secretions from patients with chronic bronchitis. After 3 hours, water content of the sputum increased only slightly, and there was no change in viscosity. Application of water aerosol for 3 hours increased water content by 29 percent and decreased viscosity by 35 percent. With most mist-tent therapy, aerosol was produced by a jet nebulizer, resulting in approximately 90 percent deposition in the upper airway. Matthews and co-workers and several other investigators failed to show any short- or long-term benefits in pulmonary function associated with mist-tent therapy.

A common but poorly documented use of bland aerosol therapy in lower airway disease is as an aid to bronchial hygiene. This form of therapy is intermittent and may be performed with heated mist from a jet nebulizer or room air mist from an ultrasonic nebulizer. When done three to four times a day, along with techniques designed to improve expectoration (coughing and deep breathing, postural drainage), some clinicians claim improved mobilization of dried, retained secretions. Whether aerosol therapy serves to liquefy secretions or simply to stimulate a cough in these situations is unknown. Controlled trials of postural drainage techniques with and without aerosol therapy are warranted to determine the causative factors. The best liquefying agent to use in these situations is also unknown. Water is a hypotonic irritant to the respiratory mucosa and has been associated with bronchospasm and swelling of retained secretions.

Hypertonic solutions stimulate cough but may cause water to exit the mucosal layer, resulting in further drying of secretions. The agents of choice are probably normal (0.9 percent) or half-normal saline (0.45 percent). At present we do not include intermittent aerosol therapy with standard treatments for mobilizing secretions.

Sputum Induction

Perhaps the most widely used form of bland aerosol therapy is ultrasonic nebulization to induce a sputum specimen. This therapy is usually performed with a hypertonic saline solution or water first thing in the morning. Both add moisture to the bronchial tree and act as irritants to induce cough in uncooperative subjects. Our experience suggests that when performed correctly, ultrasonic nebulizer therapy is effective in producing sputum specimens for bacteriologic or cytologic examination in the majority of patients. Whether the desired effect is accomplished through thinning of secretions, making them easier to expectorate, or through stimulation of the cough reflex by irritation is speculative.

Hazards and Complications

For a therapeutic modality with little scientific backing, bland aerosol therapy is fraught with potential complications. Addition of water to the respiratory tract may cause dried and retained secretions to swell and occlude major and minor airways. During aerosol therapy, the patient should never be left unattended, and means for clearing the airway and restoring ventilation should be close at hand.

Just as irritation of the bronchial tree may promote cough and mobilize secretions, it may also cause bronchospasm. This is particularly true with ultrasonic nebulization. Chronic exposure to ultrasonic nebulizers in animals has been shown to cause increased airway resistance and respiratory morbidity. Admin-istration of a bronchodilator prior to ultrasonic nebulizer therapy may help to alleviate this problem.

Fluid overload is often thought to be associated with continuous ultrasonic nebulizer therapy. However, this has only been reported in neonates receiving continuous therapy during mechanical ventilation. In adults this problem seems to be more theoretical than practical.

Perhaps the most serious and frequent complication of aerosol therapy is nosocomial infection. Since all nebulizers described in this chapter use room air to propel the aerosol, the risk of contamination is present. When heated systems are used and rainout settles in the delivery tubing, the risk becomes even greater. Proper sterilization, appropriate use of filters, and routine equipment changes are all a part of safe, effective aerosol therapy.

Suggested Reading

Chatburn RL, Lough MD, Klinger JD. An in-hospital evaluation of the sonic mist ultrasonic room humidifier. Respir Care 1984; 29:893–899.

Cheney FW, Butler J. The effects of ultrasonically produced aerosols on airway resistance in man. Anesthesiology 1968; 29:1099–1106.

Dulfano MJ, Adler K, Wooten O. Physical properties of sputum. IV. Effects of 100 per cent humidity and water mist. Am Rev Respir Dis 1973; 107:130–132.

Matthews LW, Doershuk CF, Spector S. Mist tent therapy of the obstructive pulmonary lesion of cystic fibrosis. Pediatrics 1967; 39:176–185.

Morrow PE. Aerosol characteristics and deposition: Proceedings of the conference on the scientific basis of respiratory therapy. Am Rev Respir Dis 1974; 110 (Part 2):88–99.

Pavia D, Thomson ML, Clarke SW. Enhanced clearance of secretions from the human lung after the administration of hypertonic saline aerosol. Am Rev Respir Dis 1978; 117:199–203.

Wolfsdorf J, Swift DL. An animal model simulating acute infective upper airway obstruction of childhood and its use in the investigation of croup therapy. Pediatr Res 1978; 12:1062–1065.

Wolfsdorf J, Swift DL, Avery ME. Mist therapy reconsidered: an evaluation of the respiratory deposition of labelled water aerosols produced by jet and ultrasonic nebulizers. Pediatrics 1969; 43:799–808.

INTERMITTENT POSITIVE PRESSURE BREATHING (IPPB)

WILLIAM F. MILLER, M.D., F.A.C.C.P., F.A.C.P.

HISTORICAL AND DEVELOPMENTAL CONSIDERATIONS

In spite of references to positive pressure breathing as early as 800 BC, it did not attain widespread use in anesthesia until the late 19th and early 20th centuries. The first basic physiologic evaluations of IPPB in humans were reported in 1947 and 1948 by Barach and co-workers and in 1952 by Cherniak and associates. In 1955 we reported comparisons of the administration of bronchodilator by compressor nebulizers versus IPPB in patients with severe chronic bronchitis. In most of these patients, no significant differences were noted; however, in a small group with severe hypoxemia, cor pulmonale, and copious secretions, IPPB resulted in greater improvement in spirometric and gas exchange function.

In 1959, we reported dramatic success using IPPB for pulmonary edema with severe hypoxemia that did not respond to conventional measures of treatment, including 100 percent inspired oxygen.

Until the 1960s, when the modern volume ventilators were widely available, we continued to treat all levels of ventilatory insufficiency with modified conventional pressure-limited IPPB devices, with or without tracheal intubation, as deemed appropriate.

During the late 1960s and 1970s, rapid technologic advances in respiratory diagnosis and care occurred; however, physician education and understanding of the rationale of mechanical physiologic therapy had not kept pace. As a result, many respiratory modalities were applied empirically so that overuse and improper use became common. This was especially true of IPPB used as a means of routinely administering bronchodilators or as a routine method of promoting deep breathing during the postoperative period. After the 1974 Sugar Loaf Conference on the Scientific Basis for Respiratory Therapy, it became fashionable to over-react against such therapy. In conference and in print, many were strongly opposed to all forms of respiratory therapy simply because in limited studies these techniques had not been firmly established on what were newly defined scientific grounds. Much of the over-reaction was just as irra-

tional as the promiscuous overuse and abuse that preceded it. Moreover, many of the most aggressive antagonists privately admitted they had their own criteria for application of IPPB, although they were advocating elimination of all use by others.

PHYSIOLOGIC BASIS FOR IPPB

Mechanical assistance in breathing is clearly indicated in those situations in which breathing is very difficult, causing the patient much discomfort, or the unassisted volume of ventilation is inadequate to maintain reasonably safe levels of gas exchange. The latter situation is generally accepted as requiring assistance, but the former is often not recognized as sufficient cause for ventilatory assistance, not only for patient comfort but also as a logical step to avoiding exhaustion and, ultimately, respiratory failure.

In the past 20 years, many studies have been done purporting to examine the merits of using IPPB as an adjunct to administration of bronchodilator aerosol. Unfortunately, most of these studies are flawed, since only stable, nonhypoxemic, nonhypercapnic patients without breathing difficulty were studied. Furthermore, therapy was applied in various and arbitrary ways without regard for the patient's need or for defined physiologic goals.

I know of no study that has demonstrated a special value for IPPB as a treatment or as an adjunct to treatment in patients for whom there is no physiologic basis for its use. Why, then, has so much importance been attached to the need for elaborately expensive long-term studies comparing bronchodilators administered three times daily by IPPB or by a compressor nebulizer to stable patients with chronic obstructive pulmonary disease without sound physiologic indications for the use of IPPB? The result of all the negative attention generated by these studies has been a failure to recognize those situations in which compromised ventilatory capacity, short of life-threatening ventilatory failure, may be a basis for ventilatory assistance by mask or mouthpiece.

Thus IPPB is simply a method for providing assisted or controlled mechanical ventilation for those patients who cannot, or for some reason will not, breathe deeply enough for optimal therapy or gas exchange. However, the special physiologic alterations of different disease states require that mechanical assistance be tailored to individual patients. Such therapy cannot be evaluated solely on the basis of whether the patient lives longer or shows lasting objective physiologic changes, even though these end points are important and desirable.

SPECIFIC CLINICAL APPLICATIONS

Volume-Limited Disorders

The pathogenesis of ventilatory impairments associated with neuromuscular disorders and thoracic cage defects is generally well known and will not be discussed here. Assuming there is no significant concomitant air flow limitation, the major physiologic concern is to provide sufficient volume at a frequency that does not cause hyperventilation.

Periodic assisted deep breathing may be indicated to accomplish one or more of the following goals:

1. Short-term alleviation of the work of breathing to reduce the onset of fatigue. During the 1950s, working with polio patients, we found that large mechanical tidal volumes at slow frequencies exercised the lung and thoracic cage, resulting in a decrease in the work of breathing that persisted for hours after each treatment. Moreover, when used on a regular basis, the progressive volume restriction and increased work of breathing were attenuated, allowing for smoother adaptation to the volume-limited state. Today, the same techniques are used to treat the respiratory consequences of spinal cord injury and during withdrawal from continuous mechanical ventilation.
2. Short-term improvement of alveolar ventilation to prevent respiratory failure that might require an artificial airway and continuous mechanical ventilation.
3. Deep breathing as an aid to improved bronchial hygiene. This is especially important in those patients who are prone to respiratory infections that result in an accumulation of secretions in the airways. The result is uneven distribution of ventilation and gas exchange impairment as well as bronchial plugging and further volume limitation. If this condition continues unabated, it could also lead to respiratory failure, necessitating an artificial airway and continuous mechanical ventilation.

Respiratory infections, atelectasis, and respiratory failure are very common in those patients who cannot maintain good regular bronchial hygiene without mechanical assistance. At the outset, it is important to assess the pressure-volume relationships of the respiratory apparatus by plotting inflation plateau pressure against volume. This can be repeated periodically thereafter as an index of change in total compliance. Problems are reflected by changes in compliance assessed at high frequencies (40 breaths per minute) and low frequencies (less than 15 breaths per minute). This allows for the detection of impairment

in distensibility of lung units and small airways flow limitation. The vital capacity is also a useful direct correlate of changes in compliance and muscle power. Maximum inspiratory and expiratory pressures are useful methods for monitoring muscle function in relation to restrictive or volume-limited defects. Volume-directed IPPB attempts to restore optimal total lung capacity with volume expansion and to rehabilitate inspiratory and expiratory muscle power through graded resistive exercises.

Adverse effects from using IPPB in these patients are rare. However, increasing intra-alveolar pressure can reduce pulmonary capillary blood flow and cardiac output as well as increase physiologic deadspace. These effects are most likely to be found in patients who are volume-depleted, obese, or have severe fixation of the thoracic cage.

In patients with nonuniform mechanical properties of the lung, IPPB may decrease perfusion to well ventilated lung units while diverting blood flow to poorly ventilated lung units, thus increasing intrapulmonary shunt. Careful physiologic monitoring is necessary with IPPB to ensure against hypoxemia. Nonuniform distribution of gas also creates the risk of focal overdistention, leading to alveolar rupture and pneumothorax. Monitoring total compliance (see above) identifies patients at high risk of barotrauma. Thus, control of frequency may enhance volume expansion in patients with variable volume limitation, such as acute lung injury, where the goal is volume expansion by recruitment of lung units that are well perfused but poorly ventilated. Moreover, these patients have both extreme volume and flow limitation that results not only in severe hypoxemia but also in a profound increase in the work of breathing and carbon dioxide retention. This situation is the classic indication for IPPB as well as for positive end-expiratory pressure.

The combination of continuous positive airway pressure (CPAP) with IPPB or intermittent mandatory ventilation (IMV) at low respiratory frequencies appears to be the ideal system for most instances of acute hypoxemic and hypercapnic respiratory failure. Certainly, the incidence of adverse effects such as barotrauma, inappropriate hyperventilation, and cardiovascular embarrassment is minimal with this system.

There is some difference of opinion as to how this is accomplished if the patient has carbon dioxide retention and may be less than optimally cooperative. A trial of effectively applied IPPB-CPAP-IMV by mask or mouthpiece is always appropriate before proceeding to intubation, especially if the problem has been of recent onset because the problem may be readily reversible, especially with the concomitant use of appropriate pharmacologic therapy. Although I know of no comparisons between conventional rate-controlled IPPB with a supplemental spontaneous breathing circuit (IMV) and pressure support ventilation (PSV), I suspect the latter system might be more convenient if not also more appropriate physiologically. During PSV, the ventilation is more precisely augmented in the inspiratory phase only. Both of these systems are more favorable to the circulation than simple assisted or controlled IPPB.

When treating the patient with acute dyspnea and respiratory difficulty, it is important to begin with inspiratory flows (80 to 100 L per minute) and pressures (40 to 80 cm H_2O) in order to sustain positive airway pressure and sufficient lung inflation until dyspnea is relieved. Once this is done, respiratory frequency decreases and inspiratory flow may be reduced.

FLOW-LIMITED (OBSTRUCTIVE) DISORDERS

For purposes of this discussion, patients are divided into several categories:

1. Patients with chronic stable disease who are without serious hypoxemia (PaO_2 greater than 55 mm Hg), are normocapnic ($PaCO_2$ less than 46 mm Hg), lack persistent productive cough or large volumes of tenacious secretions, and have dyspnea with minimal activity.

   Without exception, there is no indication for the use of IPPB under these circumstances.
2. Patients with frequently recurring or chronic serious hypoxemia, hypercapnia, severe productive cough, and dyspnea at rest or with minimal activity.

   IPPB may improve the quality of life for many of these patients and decrease the frequency of hospital and clinic visits. However, if IPPB is not used properly and regularly, little or no benefit is derived. For this group of patients, well controlled studies by current criteria have never been performed. However, experienced clinicians eventually find that intermittent mechanical breathing assistance with IPPB is necessary to sustain a good quality of life.
3. Patients with acute or subacute exacerbations of exhausting productive cough, severe dyspnea with hypoxemia and hypercapnia, and severely limited functional capacity who have reached a state of near exhaustion.

   As these patients come to the hospital, they may require immediate intubation and mechanical volume ventilation or they often reach that stage within 48 hours after admission. In such patients, if aggressive bronchial hygiene therapy is pursued with IPPB as an adjunct early enough in the course of their illness, intubation may be avoided. Many physicians have a very cavalier attitude toward this group of patients and intubate them immediately. Such an approach may well be justified if the physician and patient find themselves in a situation in which quality aggressive bronchial hygiene with

IPPB cannot be accomplished even in critical care areas.
4. Patients with combined flow-limited (obstructive) and volume-limited (restrictive) impairment who cannot or will not take deep breaths to facilitate bronchial clearance or adequate alveolar ventilation.

   Such patients are also candidates for IPPB. Early recognition of those patients who are heading toward exhaustion and respiratory failure is essential. In such patients, use of IPPB to provide intermittent rest with properly applied mechanical ventilatory assistance can avert the need for intubation and continuous mechanical ventilation.

Perhaps the single most significant physiologic consideration concerning flow limitation caused by airways obstructive disorders is that during inspiration airways expand and lengthen and during exhalation they shorten and decrease in diameter. When the major problem involves intrinsic obstruction of the smaller intrapulmonary airways or loss of elasticity of the supporting lung tissue, then forced expiration will exaggerate these dynamic changes in the airways, leading to closure of the smaller airways and air trapping. The net effect is to initiate the vicious cycle of impairment leading to dyspnea and exaggerated respiratory effort causing more air trapping and expiratory airways obstruction. Therefore, when IPPB is used, it must be employed with slow, relaxed breathing so the mechanical assistance serves to help the patient rather than merely to exaggerate air trapping and maldistribution of ventilation and perfusion. In my opinion, the use of CPAP or expiratory retard to implement slow exhalation is absolutely essential to achieve this goal. The use of a 2.5- to 3.0-mm expiratory retard, or about 5 cm of expiratory positive pressure, provides an appropriate amount of physiologic feedback to train the patient to use IPPB properly. If IPPB is not used properly its value will not be readily appreciated or its effects may be detrimental by worsening air trapping.

Even though reversal of airways obstruction is not expected, most patients with chronic obstructive pulmonary disease have hyper-reactive airways with bronchitis at times. Therefore, it is appropriate to make observations before and after the administration of aerosol bronchodilator to ascertain the value of bronchodilators as an adjunct to IPPB.

Since the inspiratory phase is the shortest time period of the breathing cycle and the expiratory phase is prolonged, it is desirable that nebulization occur only during inspiration so that medication is not wasted. With continuous nebulization, less than 10 percent of the medication is delivered to the patient; with nebulization on inspiration only, this amount increases to 30 percent or more, depending on the breathing pattern. Long, slow inspiration, with several seconds of inspiratory breath-holding, facilitates deposition and retention of aerosols.

In many publications authors mention the well known risk of contamination of reservoir nebulizers as a potential complication of IPPB. Quite simply, contamination has nothing to do with IPPB. Reservoir nebulizers may or may not be used with IPPB, but when they are used, the precautions appropriate to their safe use should be executed.

POSTOPERATIVE PERIOD

All the foregoing principles also apply to the postoperative period. When postoperative pain compromises deep breaths necessary to facilitate bronchial clearance, properly applied IPPB supplements impaired muscle power. The key to success is preoperative training in the use of IPPB. Relaxation techniques must also be taught so that patients do not resist inflation and allow expansion to desired inspiratory volumes. Few studies have ever controlled this very critical constraint to effective utilization of IPPB.

Suggested Reading

Anderson WH, Dossett BE Jr, Hamilton GL. Prevention of postoperative pulmonary complications. Use of isoproterenol and intermittent positive pressure breathing on inspiration. JAMA 1963; 186:763–766.

Ayres SM, Kozam RL, Lukas DS. The effects of intermittent positive pressure breathing on intrathoracic pressure, pulmonary mechanics, and the work of breathing. Am Rev Respir Dis 1963; 87:370–379.

Barach AL, Martin J, Eckman M. Positive pressure respiration and its application in the treatment of acute pulmonary edema. Ann Intern Med 1938; 12:754–795.

Cropp AJ, DiMarco AF, Altose MD. Effects of intermittent assisted ventilation in patients with severe chronic obstructive pulmonary disease (COPD). Am Rev Respir Dis 1984; 129:Part 2, A34.

Emmanuel GE, Smith WM, Briscoe WA. The effect of intermittent positive pressure breathing and voluntary hyperventilation upon the distribution of ventilation and pulmonary blood flow to the lung in chronic obstructive lung disease. J Clin Invest 1966; 45:1221–1233.

Miller WF, Johnston FF, Tarkoff MP. Use of ultrasonic aerosols with ventilatory assistors. J Asthma Res 1968; 5:335.

Miller WF, Sproule BJ. Studies on the role of intermittent inspiratory positive pressure oxygen breathing (IPPB/I-O$_2$) in the treatment of pulmonary edema. Dis Chest 1959; XXXV:5, 469–479.

Motley HL, Cournand A, Werko L, Dresdale DT, Himmelstein A, Richards DW. Intermittent positive breathing: A means of administering artificial respiration in man. JAMA 1948; 137:370–383.

Prakas O, Meij S. Cardiopulmonary response to inspiratory pressure support during spontaneous ventilation vs. conventional ventilation. Chest 1985; 88:403–408.

Wu N, Miller WF, Cade R, Richburg P. Intermittent positive pressure breathing in patients with chronic bronchopulmonary disease. Am Rev Tuberc 1955; 71:693–703.

MASK AND NASAL CONTINUOUS POSITIVE AIRWAY PRESSURE

ROBERT A. SMITH, M.S., RRT

Continuous positive airway pressure (CPAP) was originally introduced in 1878 as a treatment for pulmonary diseases that exhibited a reduction in the gas-exchanging surface area. Later, CPAP was specifically employed to treat intractable bronchial asthma, chronic obstructive pulmonary disease, constricting lesions of the larynx and trachea, pneumonia, and cardiogenic pulmonary edema. Although recently revived as a therapy to reduce airway resistance, inspiratory work, and paradoxical pulsus associated with severe refractory bronchospasm, contemporary threshold expiratory pressure therapy is primarily used for ventilatory insufficiency characterized by decreased functional residual capacity, ventilation-perfusion abnormalities, and pulmonary edema. Typically, this form of therapy is used in conjunction with mechanical ventilation and thus requires tracheal intubation. However, the use of nasal CPAP for infants with hyaline membrane disease and mask CPAP for children and adults with acute ventilatory insufficiency has, in many instances, obviated the need for tracheal intubation. Mask CPAP has also been advocated to improve gas exchange, to decrease venous return, and to reduce left ventricular afterload in patients suffering from congestive heart failure.

CPAP may also be applied to the nares via mask to reduce snoring and obstructive apnea in susceptible adults, thus normalizing sleep structure and preventing the development of severe hypoxemia and its consequences. The purpose of this chapter is to review the indications, the circuitry, the complications, and the therapeutic approach for administering mask and nasal CPAP in adults.

MASK CPAP THERAPY

Indications

Many patients with acute ventilatory insufficiency ($PaO_2/FIO_2 < 300$; $Q_{SP}/Q_T > 0.15$) and normal cardiac output are initially normo- or hypocapnic. Such patients may require little or no mechanical ventilation. Rather, hypoxemia, alveolar collapse, and interstitial pulmonary edema should be alleviated, none of which are materially benefited by intermittent positive pressure ventilation (IPPV). During the expiratory phase of IPPV, unstable alveoli recruited during insufflation collapse. Since the expiratory phase is generally longer in duration, desaturated blood traverses the collapsed region without being oxygenated (intrapulmonary shunting).

When mechanical ventilation is not indicated, ventilatory function may be improved with CPAP therapy, which is administered via an artificial airway. However, in awake and alert patients capable of protecting their airways, CPAP may be administered by a snugly fitting face mask. The indications for mask CPAP therapy are summarized in Table 1.

Circuitry

The CPAP system requires a continuous- or a demand-flow regulator. Since most demand valve systems exhibit a sluggish response and require significant inspiratory effort to initiate gas flow, I advocate a continuous flow system, which is detailed in Figure 1. Gas is mixed to desired FIO_2 by an air-oxygen blender and is then delivered from a flow meter to a 2- or 3-L capacity rubber reservoir bag attached to a humidifier via a unidirectional valve. A one-way valve is employed to prevent retrograde flow of expired gas and subsequent rebreathing. However, this valve is unnecessary if the humidifier allows only one-directional flow and/or when continuous gas flow provides sufficient circuit washout. A valve with 0.5 to 1.0 cm H_2O opening pressure is added to permit inspiration of ambient air should there be pneumatic source failure.

Since the normal conditioning mechanism of the upper airway is not circumvented, the humidifier need only be slightly above room temperature to facilitate humidification of inspired gas to approximately 70 percent relative humidity at continuous flow rates of 40 to 60 L per minute. The resistance to flow through the humidifier may be of considerable importance. If patient peak inspiratory flow rate exceeds that supplied by the CPAP circuit, the patient must work to draw sufficient gas from the reservoir through the system's humidifier. The work of breathing in such a circumstance increases proportionally to the flow resistance of the circuitry. The pressure gradient across the most commonly employed humidifiers is 3 to 6 cm H_2O at a flow of 60 L per minute. In and of itself this resistance may not pose significant work; however, in conjunction with the series resistance provided by the unidirectional valve, it could cause an intolerable inspiratory load for some patients.

One end of the inspiratory limb of the CPAP circuit is connected to the outflow port of the humidifier and the other to a T-adapter with a pressure measurement port. An anaeroid or mercury gauge is attached to the port via a small caliber plastic tube to monitor fluctuations in proximal airway pressure. The expiratory limb connects the distal end of the T-adapter to a threshold-type expiratory pressure valve. A soft, translucent face mask is connected to the patient side of the T-adapter. The face mask is held in place by a head strap. If a mask with extremely compliant contact surface is employed, little force is necessary to prevent leaks. In our hands, the Downs CPAP mask manufactured by Vital Signs, Inc. (East Rutherford, New Jersey) provides excellent results (Fig. 2). This mask incorporates a pliable pneumatic lip that is incrementally inflated to effect a custom fit. The mask also includes an inspiratory and an expiratory leaf valve, a pressure measurement port, and an adjustable head harness. Fresh gas is directed into the mask via the inlet port, and a nongravity dependent threshold-type expiratory pressure valve (Vital Signs, Inc.) is attached to the outlet port. Threshold pressure is developed via tension from two curved springs applied to a disc valve. Individual valves are available to provide threshold pressure from 2.5 to 20 cm H_2O.

Gas flow rate must be sufficient to prevent reservoir bag deflation during tidal ventilation. Precise regulation of the circuit flow can be achieved by ob-

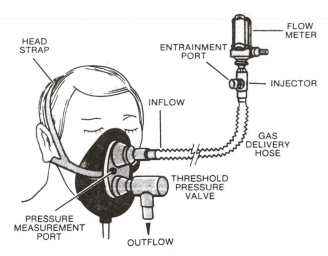

Figure 2 Downs mask CPAP system. Gas is metered to an injector that entrains ambient air, providing up to 45 to 50 L per minute to the mask inlet port. See text for further details.

serving the pressure manometer during the patient's inspiration and by adjusting the system flow to a level that produces the least pressure deflection toward ambient (Fig. 3).

When ability to titrate FiO_2 is not critical, a continuous gas flow can be provided by a high performance injector (see Fig. 2), (i.e., one with a high stall pressure). Source gas, usually oxygen, is metered to a constriction (jet). A subatmospheric pressure is created as gas is accelerated (Bernoulli principle), and thus gas is entrained into the tube (Venturi principle). The resultant delivered gas is a mixture of source (100% oxygen) and entrained (room air) gases, and its flow rate is equal to the sum of their individual flows. Entrainment is affected by fluctuation in pressure at the outlet of the injector. When pressure increases above atmospheric pressure in the delivery circuit (e.g., CPAP), the quantity of entrained air decreases while jet flow (100% oxygen) remains unaltered. Eventually, a pressure is achieved that prevents further entrainment (injector stall point), and delivered FiO_2 is then 1.0. Thus, as pressure rises a higher FiO_2 is delivered at a lower total flow. However, since gas exits

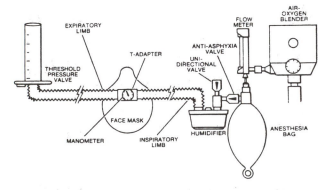

Figure 1 Continuous flow mask CPAP system.

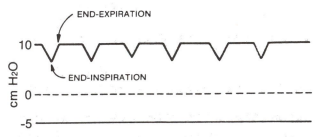

Figure 3 Airway pressure pattern during mask CPAP therapy.

the Downs injector at such high pressures, the effects of incremental CPAP titration on FIO_2 (about 0.45) and on flow rate (50 L per minute) are minimal. Another version of this injector includes needle valve control of metered jet flow and entrainment, and regulation of total flow delivery (up to 190 L per minute with a 50 psi compressed gas source) and of FIO_2 (about 0.45 to 0.88). Since ambient air somewhat increases the relative humidity of the compressed oxygen (or air), humidification may not be necessary. However, the relative humidity of inspired gas can be improved by interfacing a compressed-air powered nebulizer with the entrainment port of the injector.

Potential Complications

Several potential complications are associated with this form of therapy (Table 2). CPAP has been shown to decrease cadiac output. The degree of circulatory depression is more pronounced in hypovolemic patients and, with rational CPAP titration, may not occur at all in normovolemic patients.

All forms of positive pressure therapy may precipitate pulmonary barotrauma, and this remains a potential problem with mask CPAP therapy. However, the incidence of barotrauma appears to be increased when large volumes are insufflated with high peak pressure, neither of which is characteristic of CPAP therapy.

Probably the most important complication associated with mask CPAP is the aspiration of gastric contents. Aerophagia increases the potential for gastric reflux. However, since normal esophageal opening pressure is approximately 15 cm H_2O, aerophagia is minimized during CPAP therapy that is below that pressure in the absence of active swallowing. This hazard may be substantially diminished by inserting a nasogastric tube to maintain gastric decompression.

Another potential complication is hypoventilation. CPAP, if excessive, can increase the deadspace to tidal volume ratio, can predispose to sustained alveolar overdistention with subsequent compliance reduction, and can cause an increase in arterial PCO_2. Alveolar overdistention may manifest clinically as an increased respiratory rate with "active" exhalation. In addition, excessive CPAP levels may increase intrapulmonary shunting. This shunting can occur when

intra-alveolar pressure exceeds pulmonary venous pressure (estimated by pulmonary arterial occlusion pressure), thereby causing pulmonary capillary compression (Starling resistor effect). Blood may be shunted to a region of the lung with decreased ventilation, thus precipitating an increased venous admixture and a decreased PaO_2.

A potential complication associated with the mask is patient discomfort and erythema or skin erosion at surface contact points (particularly at the bridge of the nose and at the cheek bones), especially if the mask is too tight or not very pliable. These potential problems may be reduced by the use of a compliant, pneumatically adjustable lip, rather than a relatively fixed surface rubber mask.

CPAP can be applied via an endotracheal or a tracheostomy tube. Numerous additional complications are associated with tracheal intubation (e.g., occlusive mucous plugs, tracheal erosion, tracheoesophageal fistula, tracheal stenosis, and infection). The circulatory consequences of CPAP are identical whether a mask or an endotracheal tube is employed. When mechanical ventilation and positive end-expiratory pressure (PEEP) are utilized, mean airway pressure is higher than with a similar level of CPAP, and the potential risks of hemodynamic depression and of pulmonary barotrauma are theoretically greater.

Therapeutic Approach

Mask CPAP appears to be a reasonable mode of therapy for a selected group of awake, spontaneously breathing patients with mild to moderate ventilatory insufficiency. Since this mode of therapy is noninvasive, attendant complications with translaryngeal intubation are avoided, and the patient is able to talk. In some cases of mild ventilatory insufficiency (e.g., postoperative atelectasis and interstitial pulmonary edema) the mask can be removed periodically. We have also found mask CPAP to be extremely useful for patients who would otherwise receive frequent deep breathing maneuvers (i.e., either incentive spirometry or intermittent positive pressure breathing (IPPB) treatments) on a 24-hour basis. Most patients can sleep with the CPAP mask in place. The patient must be awakened periodically if deep breathing treatments are used, thus precipitating physical and mental consequences of altered sleep structure.

The CPAP level is customarily titrated in 3- to 5-cm H_2O increments until desired effect(s) are achieved (e.g., increased PaO_2 and/or normalized or reduced respiratory rate and/or radiologic improvement). Table 3 summarizes the results of mask CPAP therapy in 34 patients. All patients exhibited mild to moderate ventilatory insufficiency following postoperative extubation or traumatic injury. Two patients presented with multiple anterior rib fractures and bi-

TABLE 2 Potential Complications with Mask CPAP Therapy

Patient discomfort
Erythema, skin erosion
Aerophagia, gastric distention
Aspiration of gastric contents
Decreased cardiac output
Hypoventilation

TABLE 3   Results of Mask CPAP Therapy in 34 Patients with Acute Ventilatory Insufficiency

	Before	*After*	*p value*
PaO_2/FiO_2	186 ± 49	295 ± 61	$p < 0.001$
$PaCO_2$ (mm Hg)	35.5 ± 6.7	38.5 ± 5.5	$p < 0.05$
CPAP (cm H_2O)	0	9.8 ± 6.5	

lateral pulmonary contusions. One postoperative patient in the group did not respond to mask CPAP therapy and was subsequently intubated and ventilated. The range of CPAP employed was from 5- to 35-cm H_2O.

Mask CPAP therapy is a useful alternative to intubation and mechanical ventilation in some patients. The technique adds an effective mode of therapy to the expanding repertoire that enables respiratory care practitioners to individualize therapy for specific pathophysiologic settings.

NASAL CPAP THERAPY

Indications

Obstructive sleep apnea is characterized by periodic breathing and hypoxemia during sleep and by hypersomnolence while awake. In severe cases, cor pulmonale and polycythemia may be present. Functional airway occlusion at the level of the pharynx results from factors such as reduced airway caliber and increased resistance to air flow that necessitate the generation of extraordinary subatmospheric pressure in the upper airway and from reduced skeletal muscle tone during sleep (particularly REM). Obstructive sleep apnea can be eliminated by tracheostomy. However, since airway closure results chiefly from subatmospheric intrapharyngeal pressure, the application of positive airway pressure via the nasal cavity has been shown to obviate the obstruction in susceptible individuals. Nasal CPAP acts as a pneumatic splint, thus preventing airway collapse (Fig. 4).

The symptoms of obstructive sleep apnea syndrome are summarized in Table 4. Nearly 80 percent of patients presenting with sleep apnea exhibit at least five of these symptoms.

Circuitry

The circuitry used for administering both nasal and face mask CPAP is constructed similarly (Fig. 5). Continuous gas flow from 30 to 60 L per minute, usually air, is delivered to a nasal mask by a lightweight 22-mm diameter corrugated plastic hose. Source gas can be provided by a high output air blower or by an air compressor via a flow meter appropriately linked to a delivery hose. When compressor flow is inadequate to maintain CPAP, an injector (previously de-

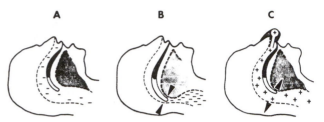

Figure 4   Mechanism of sleep-induced upper airway obstruction and its reversal with nasal CPAP. *A*, while the patient is awake pharyngeal muscle tone is sufficient to sustain airway patency in the face of subatmospheric ($-$) pressure developed during inspiration. However, *B*, during sleep the tongue and soft palate collapse against the posterior wall of the hypopharynx, thereby causing air flow obstruction. *C*, application of CPAP ($+$) to nares prevents occlusion via pneumatic splinting.

scribed) can be employed to augment flow to the mask. A threshold pressure valve is connected to the expiratory outlet of the nasal apparatus by large bore tubing. A nongravity dependent threshold pressure valve is recommended. The device utilized to generate gas flow may often be located outside the patient's room to minimize noise. When required, supplemental oxygen can be titrated into the delivery hose.

Problems related to applying nasal CPAP have centered around the development of a nasal mask that is comfortable and provides an adequate seal. Numerous apparatus have been described to interface the nares and the CPAP circuit. Each of these apparatus incorporate a custom-fitted mask with soft plastic tubes shaped to fit snugly in each nare (see Fig. 5).

Each nasal mask is held in place with a head strap, chiefly for positioning, rather than for enhancing the airtight seal. Whatever the approach, priority should

TABLE 4   Symptoms of Obstructive Sleep Apnea Syndrome Decreasing in Order of Prevalence

Altered sleep structure: snoring, agitation
Daytime hypersomnolence
Intellectual impairment
Alterations in personality
Morning headache
Hallucinations, automatic behavior
Dyspnea, particularly during exertion
Insomnia

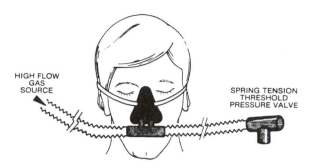

Figure 5 Schematic illustration of a nasal CPAP circuit.

be placed on ease of application, on durability, and on reliability.

Complications

Potential complications of nasal CPAP include patient discomfort and anxiety, nasal abrasions, and nasal drying or rhinitis. These latter side effects can sometimes be alleviated by the humidification of inspired gas or by the use of nasal decongestants. Ear pain and conjunctivitis may represent barotrauma to the inner ear and to the conjunctiva, respectively. The latter may be caused by a leak in the mask or by a gas leak through the lacrimal duct.

Nasal CPAP can occasionally cause hypoventilation accompanied by hypoxemia during REM sleep. As a result, supplemental oxygen administration is sometimes necessary. However, with prolonged use, this problem resolves without further need of supplemental oxygen.

Therapeutic Approach

Candidates for nasal CPAP therapy are observed and monitored over several consecutive nights in order to establish a baseline sleep pattern, the degree of oxyhemoglobin desaturation, and any changes in heart rhythm. Periods of snoring and/or apnea are best monitored via respiratory air flow changes that are detected with a thermistor placed at the airway. Events are recorded against time. Arterial desaturation can be measured and recorded by means of pulse or ear ox-

imetry. CPAP is then titrated to a level that prevents or that significantly reduces episodes of snoring and apnea, thereby improving the quality of sleep and reducing hypoxemic events. Generally, snoring is abated at a lower CPAP level than obstruction, which may require 10 to 15 cm H_2O.

Many unresolved questions remain since there are no large controlled trials of nasal CPAP. The major unresolved issue is how long and how frequently to use nasal CPAP to abate the effects of sleep apnea. Some patients find they do not need therapy every night after receiving nasal CPAP for a period of time. However, these symptoms seem to recur if CPAP is not reinstituted within several days. Thus, because nasal CPAP is reported to be effective with intermittent use, controlled studies that evaluate various treatment protocols are needed.

Suggested Reading

Barach AL, Martin J, Eckman M. Positive pressure respiration and its application to the treatment of acute pulmonary edema. Ann Intern Med 1938; 12:754–795.

Berry RB, Block AJ. Positive nasal airway pressure eliminates snoring as well as obstructive sleep apnea. Chest 1984; 85:15–20.

Covelli HD, Weled BJ, Beekman JF. Efficacy of continuous positive airway pressure administered by face mask. Chest 1982; 81:147–150.

Greenbaum DM, Millen JE, Eross B, Snyder JV, Grenvik A, Safar P. Continuous positive airway pressure without tracheal intubation in spontaneously breathing patients. Chest 1976; 69:615–620.

Ortel MJ. Respiratory therapeutics. In: Von Ziemssen's handbook of therapeutics. Volume 3. New York: William Wood, 1985:448.

Poulton EP, Oxon DP. Left-sided heart failure with pulmonary edema: treatment with the "pulmonary plus pressure machine." Lancet 1936; 2:981–983.

Remmers JE, Sterling JA, Thorasinsson B, Kuna ST. Nasal airway positive pressure in patients with occlusive sleep apnea: methods and feasibility. Am Rev Respir Dis 1984; 130:1152–1155.

Smith RA, Kirby RR, Gooding JM, et al. Continuous positive airway pressure (CPAP) by face mask. Crit Care Med 1980; 8:483–484.

Strohl KP, Cherniack NS, Gothe B. Physiologic basis of therapy for sleep apnea. Am Rev Respir Dis 1986; 134:791–802.

Sullivan CE, Issa FG, Berthon-Jones M, et al. Reversal of obstructive sleep apnea by continuous positive airway pressure applied through the nares. Lancet 1981; 1:862–865.

INCENTIVE SPIROMETRY

ROBERT H. BARTLETT, M.D.

The normal pattern of breathing includes inhalation to total lung capacity several times each hour. This periodic inflation occurs during waking and sleep states and prevents alveolar collapse in normal lungs. When the pattern of breathing is changed to one of tidal ventilation without periodic maximal inflation, atelectasis ensues within a few hours. This occurs with administration of narcotics, anesthetics, and other sedative drugs and following head injury and operation on the chest and abdomen. Therefore, any respiratory maneuver that is intended to prevent atelectasis and related pulmonary complications must achieve regular maximal inflation, that is, assure a normal pattern of breathing. Various respiratory maneuvers are compared in Figure 1. The optimal maneuver (sustained maximal inspiration) achieves maximal volume during periods of inflating pressure.

With this understanding of the pathophysiology of breathing, it is obvious that any prophylactic respiratory maneuver must emphasize breathing in rather than breathing out. Alveolar inflation cannot occur during coughing, tracheal suctioning, or blowing into gloves, bottles, or other devices. Expiratory maneuvers may serve to quantitate the gas volume inhaled before the maneuver, but this is a backwards way to approach maximal lung inflation.

It is also apparent that rapid breathing (as in CO_2-induced hyperventilation or rebreathing) and breathing against expiratory resistance (as in mask continuous positive airway pressure) correctly emphasize inhalation but do not achieve regular maximal lung inflation. Mechanical ventilation (intermittent positive pressure breathing or IPPB) can be used to achieve regular maximal inflation, but IPPB is rarely used with this specific goal in mind. Moreover, when IPPB is used to mechanically support tidal breathing without emphasis on volume, no benefit accrues.

The incentive spirometer was designed to study the pattern of breathing in postoperative patients by requiring them to inhale to total lung capacity frequently. Those studies led to a family of devices that emphasize inhalation to total lung capacity. The term "incentive spirometer" was coined to describe the active involvement of the patient and the emphasis on maximal volume inhalation. However, "voluntary inspiratory exerciser" would be a more accurate name.

The original studies on regular maximal inflation in postoperative patients using an incentive spirometer device showed a significant decrease in the incidence of pulmonary complications (Fig. 2). Subsequent studies using incentive spirometers and other techniques of assuring maximal lung inflation have produced similar results. The emphasis in pulmonary prophylaxis must be on frequent maximal inflation; the method used to achieve this pattern of breathing is less important than the frequency and volume of inhalation. When breathing exercisers have been used infrequently without volume measurement, any potential benefits are lost.

To be effective, an incentive spirometer maneuver should be based on inhaled volume, not flow rate. The original incentive spirometer is of a piston-canister design with a small leak incorporated in the piston. The patient must inhale to a given volume, at which time a light signifies successful inspiration. The patient is instructed to keep the light on by inhaling, thus achieving maximal volume inhalation. The current descendant of that device is the Volurex incentive spirometer (Fig. 3). This is an actual bellows that can be observed by the patient, and the specific inhaled volume can be quantitated.

There are several breathing exercisers on the market that respond to inspiratory flow, not volume. In these devices, a floating piston or ping pong ball is activated by the Venturi effect of inspiratory flow. The ball moves faster during rapid forced inspiration, but this maneuver is often painful in postoperative patients and may limit maximal inspiratory effort. On the other hand, a long, slow inspiratory maneuver (which is ideal in the postoperative patient) may not move the ball at all. It is not unusual to see patients with these devices taking a series of short, shallow, unmeasured breaths, thinking that they are doing some good, when actually no benefit will occur. If nonvolumetric flow-dependent devices are used as inspiratory exercisers, the patient should be instructed to breathe in at a rate that gets the ball or piston moving and then to sustain that effort for as long as possible (rather than trying to get the ball or piston progressively higher and higher).

Regular inflation to total lung capacity can certainly be achieved without the aid of incentive spirometers or other devices. Any maneuver that achieves total and regular inflation would be effective prophylaxis. Most postoperative patients find it difficult to make this effort spontaneously. Even with coached deep breathing, it is difficult to know when the basal alveoli have been fully inflated, unless the observer

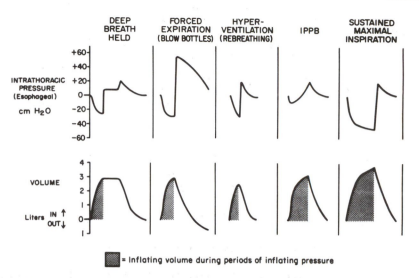

Figure 1   Pulmonary mechanics during respiratory maneuvers in normal subjects. The shaded areas indicated inspiratory volume during periods of inflating pressure. (From Bartlett RH, et al. Studies on the pathogenesis and prevention of postoperative pulmonary complications. Surg Gynecol Obstet 1973; 137:926, with permission.)

has a stethoscope positioned on the chest. Some type of incentive spirometer is used for pulmonary prophylaxis in most hospitals in the United States. However, this is a waste of time and money if regular maximal inflation is not properly emphasized.

It is important to teach inspiratory exercise to surgical patients preoperatively. Maximal glottis–open inspiration is not a natural maneuver (except as occurs in yawning), and the technique does require some practice, which should be done before operation. In my opinion, preoperative teaching and postoperative pulmonary prophylaxis are the responsibilities of the

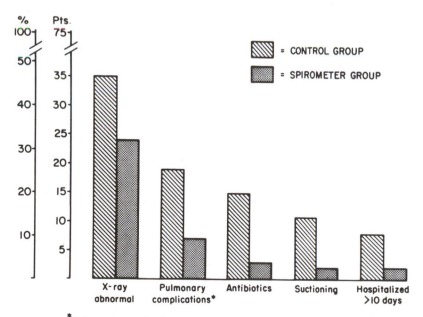

*Pulmonary complications = X-ray abnormality, Fever, Sputum, Physical findings

Figure 2   Pulmonary abnormalities in 150 postoperative patients treated with conventional nursing (control) and conventional nursing plus volumetric incentive spirometer ten times per hour (spirometer). The difference in the incidence of pulmonary complications is statistically significant. (From Bartlett RH, et al. Studies on the pathogenesis and prevention of postoperative pulmonary complications. Surg Gynecol Obstet 1973; 137:927, with permission.)

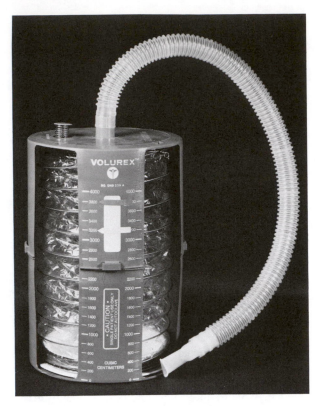

Figure 3 Volurex incentive spirometer.

surgeon and the surgical nurse. Respiratory therapists are needed for the care of high-risk patients, and they should not be expected to expend time on routine postoperative care. However, if surgeons and nurses abrogate this responsibility, respiratory therapists can certainly do it very well.

Suggested Reading

Bartlett RH. Respiratory therapy to prevent pulmonary complications of surgery. Resp Care 1984; 29:667–679.

Bartlett RH, Brennan ML, Gazzaniga AB, Hanson EL. Studies on the pathogenesis and prevention of postoperative pulmonary complications. Surg Gynecol Obstet 1973; 137:925–933.

Bartlett RH, Gazzaniga AB, Geraghty TR. Respiratory maneuvers to prevent postoperative pulmonary complications: a critical review. JAMA 1973; 224:1017–1021.

Craven JL, Evans GA, Davenport JL, Williams RHP. The evaluation of the incentive spirometer in the management of postoperative pulmonary complications. Br J Surg 1974; 61:793–797.

Ward RJ, Danziger F, Bonica JJ, Allen GD, Bowes J. An evaluation of postoperative respiratory maneuvers. Surg Gynecol Obstet 1966; 123:51–54.

Zikria BA, Spencer JL, Kinney JM, Broell JR. Alterations in ventilatory function and breathing patterns following surgical trauma. Ann Surg 1974; 179:1–7.

MUCOLYTICS

MARISSA SELIGMAN, Pharm. D.

Tracheobronchial secretions play an important role in the morbidity and mortality of pulmonary diseases, especially chronic obstructive pulmonary disease and bronchitis. The presence of thick, tenacious secretions in the airway may precipitate airway obstruction and impair gas exchange. Because these secretions are poorly cleared by cough, drugs have been developed that are used to facilitate their removal from the respiratory tree. Using these agents effectively requires a knowledge of the physiology of tracheobronchial secretions and the pharmacologic properties and clinical limitations of mucolytics and expectorants.

BASIC PRINCIPLES OF MUCUS PHYSIOLOGY

Mucus Production

Normally, the bronchi of the respiratory tract are covered with a thin, watery viscoelastic secretion that coats the epithelium in a changing and irregular fashion; this coat is generally about 5 μm deep. These secretions are produced primarily by the branching tracheobronchial glands of the respiratory tract (Fig. 1). A minor contribution to the tracheobronchial secretions comes from the goblet cells within the bronchial epithelium (see Fig. 1).

Submucosal glands secrete a fluid that is composed of both mucus and serous fluid, produced by the mucus and serous cells of the gland, respectively. The submucosal glands are directly innervated by the parasympathetic nervous system and are therefore affected by changes in vagus nerve activity. In contrast to the submucosal glands, goblet cells secrete only mucus. Also, mucus production by the goblet cells is stimulated primarily by direct contact with irritants such as ammonia and cigarette smoke.

Animal studies suggest that the volume of secretions produced by the lungs is about 100 ml per day, although human studies estimate the volume at as little as 10 ml per day.

Composition of Mucus

Tracheobronchial secretions can be resolved into several molecular substances that are dispersed into two phases: gel and sol. The gel phase is the outermost layer of the mucus. It is semisolid, and because of its chemical composition, sticky. Foreign particles easily adhere to its surface. The sol phase is the innermost layer; it is thin, readily allowing unimpeded movement of the cilia.

The gel phase of tracheobronchial secretions is composed of several compounds (Table 1). For every 100 g of wet secretions, about 95 percent is water, 1 percent ash, 1 percent carbohydrates, 1 percent proteins, 1 percent lipids, and 0.025 percent deoxyribonucleic acid (DNA).

The protein component of mucus is predominantly long, randomly coiled chains of glycoproteins. However, mucus also contains a small amount of serum proteins, enzymes, and proteins secreted by the bronchial lining. Glycoproteins are composed of a protein backbone and glucose side chains. The glycoproteins found in mucus contain a protein backbone made up of about 800 amino acid residues. Of these residues, serine and threonine account for 40 percent of the total. Since threonine and serine are the only amino acids in the protein chain hydroxyl-containing groups, these two amino acids are the only residues that can form O-glycosidic links to glucose molecules. Depending on the type of glucose side chains that are attached to the amino acid residues, the glycoproteins are either acidic or neutral. The presence of glucose moieties increases the water solubility of the glycoprotein chain.

The protein backbone of the glycoproteins found in mucus also contains the amino acid cysteine. The sulfhydryl group within this amino acid residue is critical to the gel-like nature of mucus, for its presence permits disulfide bonds. Disulfide bonding creates bridges between or within glycopeptide chains, thereby leading to large macromolecules of glycoproteins. The inclusion of proline in the glycoprotein molecules allows for hydrogen bonding, which is responsible for the random formation of glycoproteins within tracheobronchial secretions.

Glycoproteins avidly bind water molecules by forming hydrogen bonds between the glucose residues and water molecules. When the glycoproteins become hydrated, they expand; it has been estimated that 1 g of glycoprotein will expand to a solution volume of 40 ml. When all the glycoproteins are maximally hydrated, a gel forms as a result of the development of extensive intra- and intermolecular bonding and entanglements. Therefore, in the lung, it is the presence both of water and of long, randomly coiled glycoproteins that provides a waterproof gel to coat, line, and protect the respiratory tree epithelium.

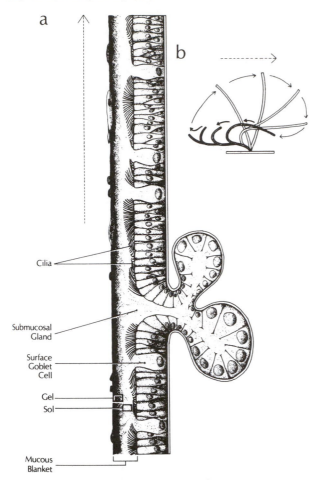

Figure 1 Structural representation of the tracheobronchial wall. From Shapiro BA, Harrison RA, Kacmarek RM, et al. Clinical application of respiratory care. 3rd ed. Chicago: Year Book, 1985.

Tracheobronchial secretions contain about 211 mEq per liter of sodium, 3 mEq per liter of calcium, 157 mEq per liter of chloride, and 17 mEq per liter of potassium (see Table 1). Normally, the pH of the secretions is slightly alkaline. This alkalinity, in addition to the loose inter- and intramolecular bonding of the glycoproteins, results in bronchial secretions of high fluidity, low viscosity, and high elasticity.

The sol phase tracheobronchial secretions contain a number of proteinaceous substances, including salivary amylase, lysozyme, lactoferrin, albumin, sialoglycoprotein, and salivary alpha, beta, and gamma globulins.

CHANGES IN TRACHEOBRONCHIAL SECRETIONS

In general, any disease or environmental stimulant that changes the character of tracheobronchial se-

cretions will subsequently change the rate of mucociliary clearance. As a result, airway caliber and the efficiency of gas exchange within the respiratory tract may be markedly affected.

Acute or chronic pulmonary disease usually increases mucus viscosity because of changes in the water content of mucus, increases in glycoprotein content, and/or changes in the chemical composition of mucus glycoproteins.

Investigators such as Yeager have reported that proper functioning of tracheobronchial secretions depends on the patient's state of hydration. Water deprivation causes thickening of the mucous blanket and impaired particle transport in the nasal mucosa and lower respiratory tract. Dehydrated patients with obstructive pulmonary disease have great difficulty clearing secretions. Although it is not clear whether excess hydration increases the output or improves the clearance of tracheobronchial secretions, I believe that dehydration is commonly neglected as a factor that may contribute to poor secretion clearance. Therefore, in patients who have difficulty clearing secretions or whose secretions are thick, tenacious, and inspissated, I suggest evaluating the patient's fluid status and administering adequate fluid via the oral, parenteral, or aerosol route (Table 2). Hydration before starting drug therapy will enhance the clearance effects of subsequent drug administration.

Environment can have marked effects on respiratory secretion clearance. Dry air exposure and minor trauma to the trachea have been shown to adversely affect tracheobronchial secretion flow as well as to impair function. In addition, lowering the pH below 6.5 causes ciliary activity to stop in vitro.

After exposure to irritants—e.g., smog, cigarette smoke—tracheobronchial secretion production and mucociliary clearance initially rise and then fall. A similar sequence occurs after exposure to bacteria and other infectious agents. Once an infection develops, a great deal of tissue destruction occurs. This, in turn, initiates various inflammatory and immunologic processes. As a result, the infectious process often evolves into a condition that is associated with markedly increased, purulent tracheobronchial secretions and their decreased clearance.

Pulmonary patients may respond differently and some not at all to mucolytic and expectorant drug therapy. This variability in response reflects the heterogeneity of patients who present with thick, tenacious bronchial secretions. For example, the mucus produced in states of chronic bronchitis and cystic fibrosis contains an increased number of acid glycoproteins, which reduce mucus fluidity and compromise ciliary function in these patients. In any inflammatory pulmonary disease, the numbers of both submucosal tracheobronchial glands and goblet cells increase. The increased production of secretions may

TABLE 1 Chemical Composition of Mucus in Sputum

Component	Approximate % per 100 g wet weight	mEq/Liter
Water	95	
Ash	1	
Carbohydrates	1	
Protein (glycoproteins, serum, secretory)	1	
Lipid	1	
DNA	0.025	
Electrolytes		
Sodium		211
Potassium		17
Calcium		3
Chloride		157

result in a mucus layer up to 100 μm thick. Chronic inflammatory diseases also reduce the population of ciliated epithelium, thereby decreasing mucociliary clearance.

If the viscosity of mucus is increased, the cilia of the respiratory epithelium poorly propel secretions toward the laryngopharynx, resulting in mucostasis. Secretions may become trapped in the bronchi, leading to obstruction and bronchospasm. Secretions trapped in the airway may become infiltrated with bacteria, inflammatory cells, and serum. This bolus of mucus and cells not only may impair gas exchange and stimulate a local inflammatory reaction but also may interfere with the normal clearance of secretions that are constantly being produced by the submucosal glands and goblet cells.

To reduce the development of mucostasis, the physiochemical properties of the mucus gel must be changed to decrease its viscosity. In addition, pulmonary secretions must be removed. These goals can best be accomplished by the use of hydration and by decreasing patient exposure to irritants and to extremes in environmental temperature and humidity. The use of mucolytic and expectorant drugs is common, but because this therapy is not without risk or toxicity, these drugs should not be used routinely. In addition, it remains unclear whether mucolytics and expectorants prevent airway obstruction by tenacious secretions any more effectively than simply increasing hydration and limiting exposure to irritants. Therefore the use of these drugs should be limited to patients in whom hydration, change of environment,

TABLE 2 Mucolytic and Expectorant Drugs

Drug Class	Agent (Trade Name)	Route of Administration	Dose
Hydration	Water	Oral	1.5–3 L/24 hr
		Intravenous	2–3 L/24 hr
		Aerosol	8–12 L/24 hr
Mucolytic	N-Acetylcysteine† (Mucomyst)	Nebulization	6–10 ml 10% 3–4 times/day
			3–5 ml 20%* 3–4 times/day
		Instillation	2–20 ml 10% every 2–6 hr
			1–10 ml 20%* every 1–6 hr
			1–2 ml 10% or 20% every 1–4 hr
Expectorant	Guaifenesin (Robitussin)	Oral	Adult: 200–400 mg every 4 hr
			Ages: 6–11: 100–200 mg every 4 hr
			2–5: 50–100 mg every 4 hr
	Potassium iodide	Oral	Adult: 300–650 mg 3–4 times/day
	Hydroidic acid	Oral	Adult: 70 mg 3–4 times/day
	Iodinated glycerol (Iophen, Organidin)	Oral	Adult: 60 mg 4 times/day
			Child: 30 mg 4 times/day
	Terpin hydrate elixir (alcohol content 42.5%)	Oral	Adult: 170 mg 3–4 times/day
			Ages: 10–12: 85 mg 3–4 times/day
			5–9: 40–45 mg 3–4 times/day
			1–4: 20–24 mg 3–4 times/day

* Diluted with an equal volume of sterile water or saline.

† Always use concurrently or immediately following administration of a nebulized or inhaled beta$_2$-adrenergic agonist (eg., isoetharine, metaproterenol).

Adapted from Hirsch SR. The pharmacotherapeutics of bronchial secretions. Hosp Form 1979; 14:419–428.

and postural drainage techniques have been unsuccessful in mobilizing secretions.

BASIC PRINCIPLES OF MUCOLYTIC AND EXPECTORANT THERAPY

The desired effect of mucolytic and expectorant drugs on tracheobronchial secretions is a change in the volume or physiochemical properties or both; they do not directly improve pulmonary function. Because thick and tenacious secretions can precipitate bronchospasm and inflammation, most attention should be focused on reducing their viscosity. However, the thinning of secretions is accomplished at the cost of increasing sputum volume. This may be hazardous to individuals who are unable to effectively clear secretions because of impaired ciliary function (e.g., as occurs in chronic bronchitis) or altered mental status (e.g., as in coma, oversedation from drugs). In addition, it should be noted that the use of these drugs does not restore the physiochemical properties of mucus to normal. Rather, they are agents that may be useful only to temporarily minimize the role of viscous secretions in airway obstruction, infection, and impaired gas exchange.

Patients who may benefit from using a mucolytic or expectorant are those with persistent and copious viscous, purulent secretions. Although clinical data are lacking, mucolytics and expectorants may be reasonable interventions, especially if the patient has failed a vigorous 4- to 6-day trial of bland aerosols. Another group that may benefit is composed of patients who are unable to effectively clear secretions following cardiothoracic procedures, such as thoracotomy and pneumonectomy. These patients may have impaired cough reflexes due to incisional pain and/or the use of opiates and sedatives postoperatively. Therefore, mucolytics and expectorants may facilitate the clearance of bloody secretions trapped in the airways. Theoretically, mobilization of these secretions should reduce the risk of the patient's developing postoperative pulmonary infections, although, again, no well-controlled studies demonstrating the efficacy of mucolytic and expectorant therapy in preventing pulmonary complications exist.

Acetylcysteine

Acetylcysteine (Mucomyst), the only commercially manufactured mucolytic, is the *N*-acetyl derivative of the amino acid L-cysteine. The mucolytic effect of acetylcysteine is dependent on the free sulfhydryl group contained within the drug; by reducing the disulfide bonds of the mucus glycoproteins, acetylcysteine reduces the viscosity of mucus. Acetylcysteine is most effective when bronchial secretions are between pH 7 and 9. The drug has no effect on protein or live tissue.

For treatment of pulmonary diseases, acetylcysteine must be administered via the airway. The majority of the administered dose interacts with mucus. However, some of the drug is absorbed through the respiratory epithelium and is deacetylated in the liver to cysteine.

Acetylcysteine is part of the management approach to patients with abnormal, viscous, or inspissated secretions. It is also used to facilitate bronchial lavage of secretions and in tracheostomy care to prevent endotracheal crusting with secretions.

The efficacy of acetylcysteine in the treatment of mucostasis is difficult to objectively assess and is highly variable from patient to patient and treatment to treatment. Few clinical trials have attempted to evaluate its usefulness as a mucolytic, and available studies have been flawed. For example, few of the available reports assessed effects on pulmonary function or clinical status, and difficulties in assessing sputum rheology have caused the studies to examine only crude measures of drug efficacy, such as sputum volume. Unfortunately, none of the available clinical trials conclusively documents that acetylcysteine is effective for patients with asthma, bronchiectasis, or those recovering from cardiothoracic surgery. Thus, when acetylcysteine is used, each patient's therapy must be individualized, and therapy should be monitored by ease of secretion mobilization and decreased secretion viscosity.

Acetylcysteine is reported to be a safe and relatively innocuous drug. However, based on my observation that the drug can precipitate bronchospasm or produce bronchorrhea or both, I feel that it is very irritating to bronchial epithelium. Acetylcysteine-induced bronchospasm is reported to occur primarily in patients with asthma or asthmatic bronchitis. To reduce the incidence of bronchospasm, a beta-adrenergic bronchodilator (e.g., isoetharine [Bronkosol] or metaproterenol [Alupent]) should always precede the use of acetylcysteine. Other unusual side effects of acetylcysteine include stomatitis, severe rhinorrhea, and generalized urticaria.

Acetylcysteine has a disagreeable odor and taste, which may lead to nausea or vomiting following a nebulization treatment. This unpalatableness makes the drug unpopular with patients and hampers compliance with nebulization protocols.

Because acetylcysteine is a reducing agent, it is incompatible with rubber and some metals (e.g., iron, copper). Therefore the drug can only be administered through equipment made of plastic, glass, or aluminum. Acetylcysteine is also physically incompatible with a number of antibiotics, including amphotericin B, tetracyclines, erythromycin, and ampicillin. In rare instances when these antibiotics are to be administered via nebulization, they need to be given separately from acetylcysteine.

In general, given the inherent toxicities of acetylcysteine, the difficulties in administering the drug, and the wide variation in clinical efficacy, I feel that it should be reserved for those patients who are adequately hydrated but have documented airway obstruction and impaired ventilation due to thick, tenacious, inspissated secretions. Acetylcysteine should be used cautiously in patients with a history of bronchospasm and those with severe respiratory insufficiency who will be unlikely to tolerate an increased volume of liquefied respiratory secretions.

For administration by nebulization, 10 percent and 20 percent solutions of acetylcysteine are available (see Table 2). The 20 percent solution should be diluted with normal saline or sterile water for injection. The 10 percent solution may be used undiluted. The usual dosage is 6 to 10 ml of the 10 percent solution or 3 to 5 ml of the 20 percent solution administered three to four times a day. Alternatively, 2 to 20 ml of the 10 percent or 1 to 10 ml of the 20 percent solution may be nebulized every 2 to 6 hours.

When acetylcysteine is used for routine care of tracheostomies, 1 to 2 ml of the 10 percent or 20 percent solution may be instilled into the tracheostomy every 1 to 4 hours. Prior to bronchial lavage, 2 to 4 ml of the 10 percent and 1 to 2 ml of the 20 percent solution may be administered by either nebulization or direct instillation into the airway.

Studies report the use of other mucolytic agents: mercaptoethanol sulfate, bromhexine hydrochloride, deoxyribonuclease (pancreatic dornase), proteolytic enzymes such as trypsin, chymotrypsin, and streptokinase, and L-arginine. However, because clinical studies with these agents have failed to show efficacy but do report significant local and systemic toxicity, use of these compounds as mucolytics in humans should be strongly discouraged.

Expectorants

The primary mechanism for expectorants is to stimulate the flow of secretions within the respiratory tract. This stimulation will theoretically increase ciliary activity and promote coughing, thereby propelling the loosened material toward the laryngopharynx.

The most commonly used expectorant is guaifenesin, previously termed glyceryl guaicolate. Many over-the-counter cough and cold preparations contain this drug. Although clinical data supporting the use of guaifenesin are lacking, many physicians and patients report that it is effective in improving secretion clearance. Fortunately, guaifenesin is well tolerated; nausea and drowsiness may occur but are rare.

Guafenesin can only be administered orally. The usual dose of the drug in adults and children older than 12 years is 200 to 400 mg every 4 hours, as needed. For children 6 to 12 years, the dose is 100 to 200 mg every 4 hours, as needed. Children between the ages of 2 to 6 years should be given 50 to 100 mg every 4 hours.

Another group of commonly used expectorants is the iodides: potassium iodide (including strong iodide [Lugol's] solution), hydroiodic acid, and iodinated glycerol. The iodides are believed to act as expectorants, and they liquefy thick sputum by directly stimulating the respiratory tract epithelium, but their exact mechanism of action is unclear. Because iodide is excreted by the bronchial glands, iodide administration may lead to increased production of secretions. In contrast to guaifenesin, there is some clinical evidence (although minimal) that iodides may be effective in treating chronic respiratory disorders (e.g., chronic bronchitis, bronchiectasis, and bronchial asthma) but not in treating acute respiratory infection.

Although the iodides may have some beneficial effects, their use may be associated with significant toxicities. Iodides may precipitate hypersensitivity reactions, which may be manifested by mucosal hemorrhage, angioedema, and the signs and symptoms of serum sickness (fever, arthralgia, lymph node enlargement). Also, chronic use of iodides may cause iodism, with symptoms such as irritation of the eyes, periorbital swelling, burning of the mouth and throat, and a metallic taste in the mouth. Other side effects include urticaria and gastrointestinal irritation with diarrhea. Patients given iodides are also at risk for developing thyroid gland hyperplasia, goiter, and severe hypothyroidism.

Because of the lack of controlled clinical trials clearly demonstrating efficacy of iodides and the high incidence of adverse reactions associated with their use, I feel that iodides should only be used in those patients with chronic bronchitis and bronchiectasis who are unresponsive to adequate hydration and safer expectorants such as guaifenesin.

Terpin hydrate is a drug formed by the action of nitric acid on rectified oil of terpentine in the presence of alcohol. Commercially, the drug is formulated as an elixir. Terpin hydrate is often used as an adjunct in treating chronic bronchitis and bronchial asthma because it is reported to have expectorant activity. However, clinical studies demonstrating this effect are lacking.

Terpin hydrate is most commonly used in combination with a cough suppressant such as codeine or dextromethorphan. The rationale for this combination is presumably to decrease the incidence of cough secondary to both the irritant effects of terpin hydrate and the underlying condition, while maintaining terpin hydrate's effects of stimulating lower respiratory tract secretion production. However, the efficacy of any combination of an expectorant and antitussive is unproved. Because the cough suppressant can impair secretion clearance and possibly lead to secretion impaction in the respiratory tree, I believe it is ill-advised to use such a medication in any patient with thick, tenacious secretions.

Suggested Reading

Alderson SH, Warren RH. Pediatric aerosol therapy guidelines. Clin Pediatr 1983; 84:553–557.

Barton AD. Aerosolized detergents and mucolytic agents in the treatment of stable chronic obstructive pulmonary disease. Am Rev Resp Dis 1974; 110:104–110.

Hirsch SR. The pharmacotherapeutics of bronchial secretions. Hosp Form 1979; 14:419–428.

Kory RC, Hirsch SR, Giraldo J. Nebulization of N-acetylcysteine combined with a bronchodilator in patients with chronic bronchitis. Dis Chest 1968; 54:18–21.

Lourenco RV, Cotromanes E. Clinical aerosols. II. Therapeutic aerosols. Arch Intern Med 1982; 142:2299–2309.

Marriott C. The effect of drugs on the structure and secretion of mucus. Pharm Int 1983; 47:320–323.

Miller WF. Aerosol therapy in acute and chronic respiratory disease. Arch Intern Med 1973; 131:148–155.

Yeager H Jr. Tracheobronchial secretions. Am J Med 1972; 50:493–508.

SYMPATHOMIMETIC BRONCHODILATORS, ANTICHOLINERGICS, AND CROMOLYN SODIUM

RICHARD M. SCHWARTZSTEIN, M.D.
SCOTT T. WEISS, M.D., M.S.

Approximately 16 million Americans suffer from obstructive airways disease. Half of these individuals are classified as asthmatic, whereas the other half fall into the category of chronic obstructive pulmonary disease (COPD), a term that includes the pathologic and clinical entities emphysema and chronic bronchitis. Obstructive airways disease produces significant disability in over a million people in the United States and interferes with the lives of millions more.

When approaching a patient with obstructive airways disease, one attempts to construct a therapeutic regimen that meets three main objectives: (1) to maximize the functional capabilities of the patient; (2) to minimize the side effects of the drugs utilized in the regimen; and (3) to avoid systemic steroids. The sympathomimetic and anticholinergic bronchodilators, along with cromolyn sodium, are the primary pharmacologic agents utilized in the treatment of obstructive airways disease. Used in the appropriate setting, these drugs diminish symptoms and permit the therapeutic objectives outlined above to be fulfilled. We will discuss the use of these drugs primarily within the context of an approach to the patient with asthma. Individuals with COPD pose a number of unique problems which are addressed separately.

MECHANISMS OF ACTION

Asthma is a condition characterized by reversible airflow obstruction. Airways obstruction is secondary to a combination of bronchospasm and mucosal inflammation. In patients with extrinsic asthma, an inhaled allergen forms a complex with immunoglobulin E. This formation leads to the degranulation of mast cells and to the release of mediators, which produce mucosal edema, inflammation, and bronchoconstriction. On the other hand, in patients with intrinsic asthma the stimulus that leads to airways obstruction is often less well defined. Loss of heat and water vapor from the bronchial mucosa may result in degranulation of mast cells. Viral respiratory infections may cause the bronchial mucosa to slough, thereby exposing receptors, which, when stimulated, induce bronchospasm. Activity of the parasympathetic nervous system, triggered either by neurohumoral or mechanical stimuli, e.g., gastroesophageal reflex, may also lead to bronchospasm. The nonsteroidal agents used to treat patients with airways obstruction impede several of these pathways by (1) stabilizing mast cells and preventing the release of mediators of bronchospasm, (2) relaxing bronchial smooth muscle cells, and (3) blocking normal activity in the parasympathetic nervous system.

Cromolyn Sodium

Cromolyn sodium appears to act primarily by stabilizing the membrane of the mast cell. More recent data suggest that cromolyn sodium may also have a role in suppressing activity of vagal nerve endings in the lung. Cromolyn acts to *prevent* bronchospasm. It has little, if any, activity as a bronchodilator.

Sympathomimetics

The sympathomimetics, a class of drugs that includes both beta-adrenergic agonists and methylxanthines, induce relaxation of bronchial smooth muscle cells. The concentration of cyclic adenosine monophosphate (cAMP) in bronchial muscle cells in part determines the tone of the muscle; high levels lead to decreased tone or relaxation of the muscle. Beta agonists stimulate receptors on the cell surface of bronchial smooth muscle, thereby activating the enzyme adenyl cyclase and increasing the intracellular concentration of cAMP. Continued use of beta agonists, however, may lead to down-regulation of these receptors, which results in less bronchodilation.

Methylxanthines inhibit the enzyme phosphodiesterase, which leads to an increase in the intracellular concentration of cAMP. However, recent data suggest that this may not be the primary mechanism of action for these drugs. Rather, the methylxanthines are now believed to act by binding to adenosine receptors. Blockage of the adenosine receptors may modulate the activity of the beta-adrenergic receptors and thus alter concentrations of cAMP.

Anticholinergics

The lung is innervated by both the sympathetic and parasympathetic autonomic neural systems. Efferent fibers from the vagus nerve innervate the muscles of the larger airways and neural impulses along these fibers are responsible for much of the tone of the muscles surrounding these airways. Blockage of these pathways with the anticholinergic leads to bronchodilation.

Mucociliary Clearance

Mucosal inflammation and edema contribute to airways obstruction in patients with asthma. Methylxanthines and beta agonists appear to increase clearance of mucus from the airways by enhancing ciliary function. The data on anticholinergics is more mixed. Laboratory studies show that atropine slows ciliary beat frequency and increases sputum viscosity. The newer quaternary ammonium compounds (e.g., ipratroprium bromide) do not have this effect. Although the effect of bronchodilators on mucociliary clearance is of theoretical interest, it does not appear to be of major clinical importance.

TOXICITY

One of the goals of any therapeutic regimen is to minimize the side effects of the drugs administered to the patient. The sympathomimetic bronchodilators have a relatively low toxic to therapeutic ratio, i.e., the drug levels associated with clinical toxicity are not much greater than the levels associated with a therapeutic effect. As a result, combinations of drugs at relatively low doses may need to be used in place of a single drug prescribed at a high dose.

Cromolyn Sodium

Cromolyn is now available in three forms: a powder administered with a spinhaler, a liquid delivered with a nebulizer, and in a metered dose inhaler. The major side effect associated with cromolyn is cough and wheezing, which may occur following use of the powdered form of the drug. This problem does not occur with the liquid and the metered dose inhaler. A few cases of allergic reactions to the medication have been described, but none was fatal. We generally prescribe cromolyn as a metered dose inhaler because it is well tolerated and easily used.

Beta Agonists

In the last 10 years a number of beta agonists have been developed that act primarily on the beta-2 receptors, i.e., those receptors found in bronchial smooth muscle. Consequently, these agents have relatively minor central nervous system and cardiovascular toxicity. Tremor is the side effect most likely to occur and to limit the use of these drugs. Restless-

ness, anxiety, palpitations, tachycardia, and headache may also be present. Significantly, arrhythmias and angina are rare with the inhaled beta agonists but can occur when the medications are administered parenterally, either intravenously or subcutaneously.

Methylxanthines

As we noted above, the methylxanthines have a low toxic to therapeutic ratio. Even patients who have "therapeutic levels" of these medications may experience distressing symptoms related to the toxicity of the drugs. This is particularly true in elderly patients. Side effects of the methylxanthines may involve the central nervous system (restlessness, insomnia, seizures), the cardiovascular system (flushing, ventricular and atrial arrhythmias), and the gastrointestinal system (nausea, vomiting, and diarrhea).

Anticholinergics

The use of inhaled atropine has been associated with a number of side effects including dry mouth, blurred vision, and palpitations. In older patients with prostatic hypertrophy, urinary retention may be a serious complication of atropine. The newer quaternary ammonium compounds appear to have fewer side effects than atropine, although a dry mouth may still be noted by some patients.

APPROACH TO THE OUTPATIENT WITH ASTHMA

The patient with mild to moderate asthma is often a young, active person who does not want to think of himself as "sick" and does not like the idea of taking medications on a regular basis. Compliance with a medical program, especially if there are any side effects from the drugs prescribed, is frequently poor. These factors must be considered if one is to treat successfully the patient with asthma.

The beta agonists are the most potent bronchodilators available. Since the beta-2 specific drugs are relatively free of side effects, they are our first choice when initiating therapy. The efficacy of these drugs is greater when administered via the inhalational route than when taken orally. Therefore, we usually start our patients on a metered dose inhaler of salbutamol (Ventolin, Proventil) or metaproterenol (Alupent). If the patient's symptoms are sporadic, e.g., associated only with exercise or cold air, we advise the patient to use his inhaler on an "as needed" basis with emphasis on the potential prophylactic effect of the drug if taken prior to the activity or exposure that is known to induce bronchospasm. If exercise is the primary precipitant of the patient's symptoms or if the patient has a significant history of atopy we may add cromolyn sodium (Intal) in the metered dose inhaler formulation to the regimen in an effort to provide better protection against bronchospasm. We advise patients to use cromolyn after they use the beta agonist. This facilitates the deposition of cromolyn throughout the bronchial tree. In the patient with persistent symptoms, the beta agonist should be used at least four times a day. During periods of more severe bronchospasm, the beta agonist may be used every 3 hours.

The patient with moderately severe asthma may have persistent bronchospasm, in spite of the use of the beta agonists. It is at this point that a theophylline preparation is added to the regimen. Although there are studies suggesting that theophylline adds little bronchodilation if beta agonists have been pushed to maximal doses, most patients experience tremors or a sense of "jitteriness" at these doses. Therefore, we proceed to moderately high levels of beta agonists, e.g., 2 puffs every 3 to 4 hours of a metered dose inhaler of Ventolin, and then add theophylline (Table 1). The longer-acting formulations of theophylline provide smoother levels of the drug and enhance compliance because they do not need to be taken as often. On a monthly basis, the 12-hour preparations are no more expensive than the generic aminophylline, which must be administered four times a day. Some patients prefer taking their medication only once a day. However, the 24-hour preparations of theophylline (e.g., Theo 24, Uniphyl), in our experience, are often associated with increasing bronchospasm toward the end of the dosing interval and appear to be more effective

when used on a twice a day schedule. It is important to remember that persistent use of the beta agonists may lead to down-regulation of the beta receptors and diminished bronchodilation. The addition of a theophylline compound may allow a temporary cessation of the beta agonists and restoration of normal receptor function.

We reserve the use of anticholinergic bronchodilators in patients with asthma to three clinical situations. First, the patient with persistent nocturnal bronchospasm who has symptoms consistent with gastroesophageal reflux may benefit from an anticholinergic inhaler. When the patient is recumbent, acid may reflux from the stomach to the esophagus and trigger a reflex mediated by the vagus nerve, thereby producing bronchospasm. Theophylline, to the extent that it causes relaxation of the lower esophageal sphincter, may exacerbate nocturnal asthma. Ipratroprium bromide (Atrovent), on the other hand, may block the reflex arc in the vagus and prevent bronchospasm. The second clinical indication for anticholinergic bronchodilators is psychogenic asthma. There is a growing body of literature on the use of ipratroprium in patients in whom emotional stress is a major precipitant of bronchospasm. Third, the patient with severe asthma who has worsening bronchospasm whenever steroids are withdrawn from the therapeutic regimen may be placed on an anticholinergic in an effort to reduce the dependency on steroids. Unfortunately, in this setting, atropine does not usually provide additional bronchodilation beyond that which results from the combination of beta agonists and theophylline.

TABLE 1 Formulations and Doses of Commonly Used Sympathomimetics, Anticholinergics, and Cromolyn Sodium

	Formulation	Dose
Sympathomimetics.		
Isoetharine	MDI	2 puffs q.i.d. (10 mg/puff)
(Bronkosol)	Liquid	0.25–0.5 cc via nebulizer
Metaproterenol	MDI	2 puffs q.i.d. (0.65 mg/puff)
(Alupent)	Liquid	0.3 ml of 5% solution via nebulizer
Albuterol	MDI	2 puffs q.i.d.
(Ventolin, Proventil)	Oral	2–4 mg po q.i.d.
Methylxanthines		
Theo-Dur	Oral	300 mg b.i.d.
Slo-Phyllin	Oral	200 mg t.i.d.
Theo-24	Oral	400–600 mg q.d.
Anticholinergics		
Atropine sulfate	Liquid	0.025–0.075 mg/kg via nebulizer
Ipratroprium bromide		
(Atrovent)	MDI	2 puffs q.i.d. (20 mg/puff)
Cromolyn sodium		
(Intal)	Powder (Spinhaler)	20 mg q.i.d.
	Liquid	20 mg q.i.d. via nebulizer
	MDI	2 puffs q.i.d. (1 mg/puff)

APPROACH TO THE PATIENT WITH STATUS ASTHMATICUS

In spite of the progress made in the treatment of asthma in recent years, status asthmaticus remains a potentially life-threatening condition. We make several modifications in our use of the sympathomimetic and anticholinergic bronchodilators in an effort to prevent respiratory failure.

Aggressive use of sympathomimetics is essential in status asthmaticus. First, we administer an inhaled beta agonist using a hand-held compressed air nebulizer. Patients with severe respiratory distress often have difficulty coordinating their hand and breathing movements sufficiently to use a metered dose nebulizer. In the critically ill patient we administer the rapidly acting drug isoetharine (Bronkosol) via the nebulizer every 20 minutes for the first hour, thereafter switching to treatments on an hourly basis. Second, we generally administer beta agonists parenterally to supplement the inhalation treatments. In a young patient with no history of hypertension or coronary artery disease, subcutaneous epinephrine is the drug of choice. In older patients, the beta-2 specific agent terbutaline, is preferred. Third, intravenous steroids, either methylprednisolone or hydrocortisone, are essential for the management of most patients with status asthmaticus. Fourth, aminophylline is administered intravenously to insure continuous therapeutic levels of the medication.

If, in spite of these measures, the patient's respiratory status continues to decline, aerosolized atropine may be added to the regimen. In rare circumstances, in a critically ill young patient we have given intravenous isoproterenol by continuous infusion in an effort to forestall endotracheal intubation. However, the risks of tachyarrhythmias and myocardial ischemia are considerable with isoproterenol, and the drug must be used with great caution. Fortunately, early aggressive use of sympathomimetics generally makes it unnecessary to resort to parenteral isoproterenol.

CHRONIC OBSTRUCTIVE PULMONARY DISEASE

Many patients with COPD have both fixed and reversible airways obstruction. The latter component is amenable to treatment with bronchodilators. While most of the principles outlined above, for the management of patients with asthma, apply to patients with COPD, there are several differences between the two patient groups which need to be considered. First, patients with COPD frequently have associated cardiovascular disease. The presence of significant coronary artery disease may limit the use of the sympatho-

mimetics. Second, ventilatory muscle fatigue is now felt to contribute to dyspnea and to respiratory failure in patients with COPD. This has led to an increased use of theophylline, even in the presence of toxicity, because of the potential beneficial effects of methylxanthines on diaphragmatic function. However, there are insufficient data demonstrating a clear clinical benefit to support this approach. Third, cholinergic hyperactivity appears to play a larger role in COPD than in asthma. Thus, anticholinergics may be more useful in the patient with COPD. Finally, cromolyn sodium is not indicated in patients with COPD.

Our general philosophy is to begin with aerosolized beta agonists in patients with COPD who demonstrate an element of reversible airways disease. Methylxanthines are used sparingly if at all. With the recent release of ipratroprium bromide, we are using the anticholinergics as our second-line agent and, based on clinical studies, this approach has proven efficacy.

ASSESSING RESPONSE TO THERAPY

There are two major end points to be kept clearly in mind when evaluating a response to a bronchodilator regimen: relief of symptoms and improvement in pulmonary function. For patients with mild asthma, who experience symptoms only in association with specific activities, relief of bronchospasm with a given exercise task is important. Subjective assessment of symptoms has been shown to correlate with pulmonary function. In managing any patient with obstructive lung disease, knowledge of the patient's baseline spirometry (forced expiratory volume in 1 second, i.e., FEV_1) is helpful in assessing therapy. The change in FEV_1 following a bronchodilator treatment should be at least 15 percent of the baseline value before one can claim a true physiologic response in patients with COPD. Finally, when caring for patients during an acute exacerbation of asthma or COPD, changes in FEV_1 with therapy help determine whether a patient requires hospitalization for more intensive treatment.

Judicious use of the sympathomimetic and anticholinergic bronchodilators and of cromolyn sodium in patients with obstructive lung disease allow the therapist to maximize the functional capabilities of the patient, minimize side effects of the drugs, and avoid systemic steroids.

Suggested Reading

Belman MJ, Sieck GS, Mazar A. Aminophylline and its influence on ventilatory endurance in humans. Am Rev Respir Dis 1986; 131:226–229.

Bergovsky EH, ed. Cholinergic pathway in obstructive airways disease. Am J Med 1986; 81(5A):1–102.

Bukowskyj M, Nakatsu K, Munt PW. Theophylline reassessed. Ann Intern Med 1984; 101:63–73.

Kemp JP. Adrenergic bronchodilators, old and new. J Asthma 1983; 20:445–453.

Newhouse MT, Dolovich MB. Control of asthma by aerosols. N Engl J Med 1986; 315:870–874.

Paterson JW, Woolcock AJ, Shenfield GM. Bronchodilator drugs. Am Rev Respir Dis 1979; 120:1149–1188.

Weinberger M, Hendeles L. Slow-release theophylline: rationale and basis for product selection. N Engl J Med 1983; 308:760–764.

Ziment I, Popa V, eds. Respiratory pharmacology. Clin Chest Med 1986; 7(3).

METHYLXANTHINES

MERI BUKOWSKYJ, B.Sc., M.Sc., M.D., F.R.C.P.(C), F.C.C.P.

Methylxanthines have played a major role in the management of airway obstruction for at least 50 years. Theophylline, the most common methylxanthine in therapeutic use, remains important as a bronchodilator, but, in recent years, has been shown to have other important benefits for patients with chronic obstructive pulmonary disease (COPD). Because of its narrow therapeutic range (10 to 20 μg per milliliter; 55 to 110 μmol per liter) and its hepatic metabolism, extensive research has been done on theophylline pharmacokinetics. This research has provided a great deal of information both about the drug itself and its interactions with other medications.

MECHANISM OF ACTION

The mechanism of action of theophylline has for many years been ascribed to phosphodiesterase inhibition. Although theophylline does inhibit phosphodiesterase, its effects at therapeutic concentrations are minimal and certainly not adequate to explain bronchodilation. A variety of other mechanisms have been proposed, including translocation of intracellular calcium, prostaglandin antagonism, stimulation of endogenous catecholamine release, beta-agonist activity, inhibition of cyclic guanosine monophosphate metabolism, and adenosine receptor antagonism. The most likely explanation for bronchodilation is the latter; adenosine has been shown to induce bronchoconstriction in asthmatic patients. Adenosine and theophylline are structurally similar, and theophylline competitively inhibits adenosine receptors in a variety of tissues at therapeutic concentrations. Unfortunately, a new xanthine, enprofylline, which is more potent than theophylline as a bronchodilator, is ineffective as an adenosine antagonist. Thus, the mechanism of action of theophylline has still not been established after 20 years of research on the subject.

INDICATIONS FOR USE

Theophylline remains a mainstay of therapy in the management of airway obstruction, both acute and chronic. Intravenous theophylline, in the form of aminophylline, is one of the drugs of choice in the management of an acute asthmatic attack or an acute exacerbation of COPD. Its oral use is usually extended for at least a few weeks after the initial event for an asthmatic and indefinitely for a COPD patient. Theophylline's bronchodilating abilities were initially reported to increase with increasing serum concentrations, but in recent years these abilities have been questioned. Some authors believe that maximal bronchodilation is achieved at low therapeutic concentrations, e.g., 10 to 12 μg per milliliter. Optimal bronchodilation at relatively low therapeutic concentrations decreases adverse side-effects, which tend to increase, even within the therapeutic range, as theophylline concentration rises. Patients with asthma that is classified as "more than mild" often require ongoing theophylline therapy in order to optimize their respiratory status. The addition of a theophylline derivative may make the difference between waking nightly with dyspnea and sleeping soundly. Similarly, it may allow the asthmatic to increase physical activity without the need to increase the use of beta agonists. In fact, many patients find that the addition of a theophylline derivative allows them to function normally while using only a beta agonist when necessary rather than regularly throughout the day.

For the patient with significant COPD, theophylline plays an even more important role. In this group, theophylline is one of the drugs that is used in conjunction with other bronchodilators often for the duration of the patient's life. Theophylline is important even in those patients without "reversible" airway obstruction. It is felt by some to actually improve pulmonary function when given chronically in this group of patients. Even if it does not improve lung function with prolonged therapy, theophylline has been shown to improve exercise tolerance and sense of well-being. In my own experience, most patients do, in fact, benefit from this kind of therapy; they feel symptomatically better and are often able to walk further distances after initiation of therapy. Whether this improvement is related to theophylline's bronchodilating effects, or to its more recently defined role as a respiratory muscle stimulant, is uncertain. In any case, it is of benefit.

NEWER ROLES

Theophylline has been known for years to function as more than a bronchodilator. It is a mild diuretic, a mild inotrope, and also a central respiratory stimulant. Though the latter effect is minor, theophylline is used as a central respiratory stimulant in pre-term infants to decrease both frequency and duration of episodes of apnea, and it has also been used to restore normal ventilatory pattern in patients with Cheynes-Stokes respirations. In the patient with acute respiratory failure, the role of theophylline as a central respiratory stimulant is certainly not large, but even a minor degree of stimulation may be of benefit.

The patient with acute respiratory failure, best illustrates the numerous roles that theophylline can play. In this type of patient, diaphragmatic and respiratory muscle fatigue play a major role, along with hypoxemia and cor pulmonale. Theophylline increases diaphragmatic contractility and decreases diaphragmatic fatigue, but it also provides some central respiratory stimulation, acts as a mild diuretic, is a mild inotrope, functions as a bronchodilator, and augments the ventilatory response to hypoxemia. Many of these roles are equally important in the patient with severe chronic lung disease and, hence, chronic respiratory muscle fatigue.

SIDE EFFECTS

Theophylline has a number of minor side effects including nausea, heartburn, diarrhea, irritability, insomnia, and tremor. Although gastrointestinal side effects are not life threatening, they can be unpleasant enough for patients to discontinue the drug. Therefore, it is important to have a regimen available to deal with these problem patients who are very much in need of this medication. This will be discussed more fully and is summarized in Table 1.

More serious adverse effects include seizures and cardiac arrhythmias. Seizures are the most worrisome of all the toxic side effects of theophylline because there is a 50 percent mortality rate associated with them. They can occur without warning signs of toxicity and are often refractory to usual anticonvulsant therapy. Seizures occur with increasing frequency when serum theophylline concentrations are greater than 40 μg per milliliter. Interestingly, this level in the face of chronic toxicity often induces a seizure, but in acute toxicity a concentration of 100 μg per milliliter may be required before seizures ensue. Also, younger patients tolerate higher concentrations of theophylline prior to the onset of seizures than do elderly patients.

Cardiac arrhythmias occur with increased frequency in the presence of theophylline toxicity. In particular, life-threatening arrhythmias can occur at concentrations of theophylline greater than 35 μg per milliliter. There have been anecdotal reports of atrial arrhythmias with theophylline concentrations within the accepted therapeutic range. A physician should therefore have a high index of suspicion for theophylline toxicity if a patient presents with a new atrial arrhythmia while being treated with a theophylline derivative. However, one must bear in mind that atrial arrhythmias are very common in patients with severe lung disease.

FACTORS AFFECTING METABOLISM

Since theophylline is metabolised in the liver, there are numerous factors that affect its clearance. These factors must be borne in mind when prescribing theophylline in both acute and chronic situations. The most important thing to remember is that a change in the clinical situation warrants a check on the patient's theophylline concentration in order to rule out a change in clearance.

Infancy and old age both result in decreased clearance of the drug, whereas children (older than 1 year) into early adolescence have very rapid clearances. Nonsmoking adults have clearances between these two extremes. Congestive heart failure causes a decrease in clearance, as does cor pulmonale.

Liver disease can result in markedly decreased theophylline metabolism and dosing in these patients should be done very carefully. Dosages should be very small and relatively infrequent owing to the markedly decreased clearance of the drug. Theophylline levels should be monitored daily in the initial week or so of therapy.

Infections are said to result in a decrease in theophylline clearance. However, there is insufficient information in the literature to validate this commonly-held belief.

The tars of cigarette smoke result in stimulation of hepatic metabolism and hence rapid clearance of theophylline. Of interest is the fact that smoking often overrides other factors that might contribute to alterations in theophylline clearance. In particular, an adult with a heavy smoking history and congestive heart failure may not need to have dosage adjusted down.

Drug Interactions

Since theophylline is a common drug, it is often given concomitantly with other drugs, some of which may alter theophylline metabolism. The following drugs have been shown to decrease theophylline clearance and hence require a decrease in the theophylline dosage in order to avoid toxicity: erythromycin,

TABLE 1 Side Effects of Methylxanthines

Minor	Major
Nausea	Seizures (50 percent mortality)
Heartburn	Cardiac arrhythmias
Diarrhea	
Irritability	
Insomnia	
Tremor	

cimetidine, high dose allopurinol, and oral contraceptives. Drugs that result in an increased clearance and, therefore, a dose adjustment upwards for theophylline include phenobarbital, phenytoin, furosemide, and enoxacin.

Drugs for which no dose adjustment in theophylline is required include co-trimoxazole (trimethoprim-sulphamethoxazole), cefaclor, tetracycline, cephalexin, ampicillin, rifampin, and ranitidine.

With the addition of any new drug to a patient's regimen, drug interaction and, therefore, possible theophylline toxicity, should be considered. As stated earlier, a theophylline level quickly allows the physician to determine whether the problem is related to drug interaction or to side effects of the additive agent.

APPROACH TO MANAGEMENT

The day-to-day management of patients needing chronic therapy with theophylline requires a certain degree of patience on the part of both physician and patient. In my experience, the most common side effects have been related to gastrointestinal upset, e.g., nausea, heartburn, eructation, and flatulence, and to the central nervous system, e.g., sleeplessness, tremulousness, and agitation. Gastric problems can be minimized in a number of ways, e.g., the use of sustained release formulations starting at a low dose—200 mg twice a day. I also advise patients that, if they develop nausea or other unpleasant gastrointestinal problems, they take their pills with meals or, at a minimum, with milk. Not all theophylline formulations are identical, however, with the absorption of some being adversely affected by the presence of food in the stomach or by gastrointestinal pH. Theodur is my drug of choice because of its consistent absorption, which is not affected by food or pH.

After patients have been taking theophylline for 1 week, I check their serum theophylline concentration and increase the dose in increments of only 200 mg per day, e.g., from 200 mg twice a day to 300 mg twice a day. The theophylline level is then checked again in another week's time and the dosage once again adjusted upward as necessary. The aim is to achieve a low therapeutic range, i.e., 10 to 12 µg per milliliter or 55 to 80 µmol per liter. This allows adequate, and some authorities believe maximal, bronchodilation. At the same time, this concentration minimizes gastrointestinal and central nervous system side effects, which appear to increase with increasing concentration of theophylline and may appear even within the accepted therapeutic range. Although most patients become tolerant of both the gastrointestinal and central nervous system side effects with time, the low initial dose and slow increase in dose minimizes these unpleasant problems for the patients.

If a patient is inordinately sensitive to theophylline derivatives, even when taken with food, I start at a very low dose, e.g., 100 mg twice a day. In this situation, I adjust the dose only after 1 month and increase the dosage in the same small increments, but at monthly rather than weekly intervals. Dietary intake is also important. If patients drink large quantities of tea or coffee, they are at increased risk for developing signs of theophylline toxicity since the former two substrates contain caffeine and hence compete with theophylline at the hepatic level. I therefore advise these patients to cut back on their caffeine intake.

There is a small subgroup of patients, however, who seem to be very intolerant to theophylline even at very low dosages. In this group, it is worth trying different product formulations just in case part of the problem is not related to theophylline, but to the matrix in which it is embedded.

There are many different oral preparations of theophylline available. Conventional tablets have consisted of various soluble salt forms of the drug, which are generally well absorbed with maximal plasma concentrations within 2 hours of ingestion. The major drawback is the frequency with which preparations must be given to maintain adequate serum concentrations. They are usually given every 6 hours—for smokers or children this interval may have to be shortened to every 3 or 4 hours. Although conventional tablets may still be used for patients with decreased clearance, most clinicians prefer the newer sustained-release formulations.

Early in the development of sustained-release formulations, many products had significantly different rates or degrees of absorption, but more recent formulations have improved. There are still products on the market that produce marked fluctuations in serum concentrations, but other preparations are consistent. These products provide the ability to treat patients more effectively since they do not have the wide fluctuations in predose and postdose concentrations seen with conventional tablets. One of the big advantages is that they can provide a sustained therapeutic concentration for a prolonged time and may therefore allow the difficult asthmatic to sleep at night rather than waking as a result of dyspnea. In fact, if nighttime dyspnea is a problem, a slight increase in the evening dose may be enough to provide improved bronchodilation and, hence, better sleep.

The timing of blood samples for theophylline concentration was more important in the past with conventional tablets, where peaks and troughs were often markedly different. The newer formulations tend to provide such smooth serum concentrations that one need only know the timing of the last dose to be able to determine dose adjustments.

In an attempt to improve patient compliance by decreasing dosing intervals, once-a-day formulations have been developed. Unfortunately, they tend to produce wide fluctuations in their peak and trough concentrations, often with peaks either in the high therapeutic or frankly toxic range. In addition, certain formulations have a dose-dumping effect if taken with a substantial meal. These drugs may have a place in the future but, at present, satisfactory control of theophylline concentration can be achieved with the currently available twice-daily dosage formulations.

The management of acute exacerbations of either chronic obstructive pulmonary disease or asthma with theophylline is well established. The intravenous loading dose of aminophylline in a patient not receiving theophylline is 5.6 mg per kilogram. Maintenance doses should be given according to clinical status (Table 2) and subsequently adjusted according to the serum theophylline concentrations. Patients who have been taking theophylline chronically should not be given a loading dose, but rather switched to a regimen of intravenous aminophylline equivalent to the previous maintenance dose (for example 800 mg per 24 hours of sustained release theophylline equals approximately 40 mg per hour of aminophylline). This rate should be maintained until a serum theophylline concentration is available to allow accurate dose adjustment. If a patient exhibits signs of toxicity, withhold aminophylline until the serum concentration is available. Most centers should be able to provide rapid assays for serum concentrations in order to improve patient management.

When switching a patient from intravenous aminophylline to one of the long-acting oral preparations, the conversion ought to be the reverse of oral to intravenous. Unfortunately, with the sustained release products, this theoretical consideration does not seem to work. If the dosages are switched (i.e., 40 mg per hour of aminophylline to 400 mg twice a day of sustained release theophylline), more often than not the serum concentration a few days to a week later will be in the high therapeutic or toxic range. This conversion is better done then with a slightly lower oral dose, e.g., 300 mg twice a day. Further adjustments can then be made gradually since the patient will presumably be clinically stable at that time.

THEOPHYLLINE OVERDOSE

Theophylline overdose, whether inadvertent or deliberate, poses a real threat to the patient. With the 50 percent mortality associated with theophylline-induced seizures it behooves the physician to be able to deal with this situation rapidly and effectively. Until recently the mainstay of therapy of major theophylline toxicity was hemoperfusion, but now there is clear evidence that the use of activated charcoal (30 g immediately, followed by 30 g every 2 hours, for a total of 120 g) increases theophylline clearance dramatically. This method works well for both orally and intravenously administered theophylline and may be life saving. Its onset of action is rapid and can be used as initial therapy for severe overdose that requires hemoperfusion as well. Less severe overdose can be treated with gastric lavage and activated charcoal alone.

Theophylline remains one of the mainstays of therapy for patients with asthma or chronic obstructive pulmonary disease, not just for its bronchodilating affects, but also for its more recently defined role in decreasing respiratory muscle fatigue. The rapid and reliable assays for serum theophylline concentrations are widely available and, together with more convenient dosage forms, have allowed improved patient management.

TABLE 2   Recommended Dosage of Intravenous Aminophylline According to the Clinical Status of the Patient

Patient Characteristics	Maintenance dose* mg/kg Body Weight·h
Healthy smoking adults	0.9
Healthy nonsmoking adults	0.5
Older patients (>60 yrs)	0.3
Patients with	
Cor pulmonale	0.3
Congestive heart failure	0.2
Liver disease	0.2

*Based on lean body weight in obese patients. A loading dose of 5.6 mg/kg is based on the actual body weights.

Suggested Reading

Bukowskyj M, Nakatsu K, Munt PW. Theophylline reassessed. Ann Int Med 1984; 101:63–73.

Hendeles L, Massanari M, Weinberger M. Update on pharmacodynamics and pharmacokinetics of theophylline. Chest 1985; 88:103S–111S.

Hendeles L, Weinberger M. Theophylline. A state of the art review. Pharmacotherapy 1983; 3:2–44.

Mahutte CK, True RJ, Michiels TM, et al. Enhancement of theophylline clearance by oral activated charcoal. Clin Pharmacol Ther 1983; 33:351–354.

Murciano D, Aubier M, Lecocguic Y, et al. Effects of theophylline on diaphragmatic strength and fatigue in patients with chronic obstructive pulmonary disease. N Engl J Med 1984; 311:349–353.

Weinberger M, Hendeles L. Slow-release theophylline: rationale and basis for product selection. N Engl J Med 1983; 308:760–764.

AEROSOLIZED DRUG DELIVERY: TECHNICAL ASPECTS

DEAN HESS, M.Ed., RRT

Therapeutic aerosols are commonly used in the treatment of patients with asthma and with chronic airway obstruction. These aerosols include beta-2 sympathomimetics such as metaproterenol (Alupent), albuterol (Ventolin, Proventil), terbutaline (Brethaire), bitolterol (Tornalate), and isoetharine (Bronkosol); steroids such as beclomethasone (Vanceril, Beclovent), triamcinolone (Azmacort), and flunisolide (AeroBid); anticholinergics such as atropine, and ipratropium (Atrovent); and prophylactic antihistamines such as cromolyn sodium (Intal). Inhalation of therapeutic aerosols has been shown to treat effectively reversible airway obstruction by topical deposition of the drug in the lungs. Systemic side effects are not produced to the same degree as with oral or parenteral administration of the drug. Use of sympathomimetic aerosols also tends to produce a greater and a more rapid bronchodilation than with oral administration of these drugs. Thus, the use of therapeutic aerosols may produce an ideal therapeutic ratio: optimal therapy with minimal side effects. Therapeutic aerosols may be administered by metered dose inhaler, by gas-powered nebulizer, or by intermittent positive pressure breathing (IPPB).

PENETRATION AND DEPOSITION OF THERAPEUTIC AEROSOLS WITHIN THE LUNG

The effectiveness of therapeutic aerosol administration depends upon the amount of the drug that is deposited in the lungs. For example, little bronchodilation occurs from deposition of aerosol in the buccal cavity or from intestinal absorption, if swallowed. Aerosol particles are deposited within the lungs as a result of sedimentation, of inertial impaction, and of diffusion. Penetration of aerosols into the lungs depends upon the aerodynamic size of the aerosol particles, the pattern of inhalation, and the extent of airway obstruction.

Sedimentation is the deposition of aerosol in the lung owing to the effect of gravity. Sedimentation is affected by the size and the density of the aerosol particles. Inertial impaction refers to the tendency of aerosol particles to be deposited when the air stream changes direction. Thus, aerosol particles tend to be deposited in the lung where airways divide. Diffusion is the deposition of extremely small aerosol particles because of the brownian movement of surrounding gas molecules.

An important determinant of aerosol penetration is the size of the aerosol particles. Large particles (those with aerodynamic diameter greater than 5 microns) do not penetrate the upper airway. The upper airway serves as a formidable barrier to the delivery of aerosol to the lower respiratory tract. The nose is a particularly effective barrier against aerosol penetration. Thus, therapeutic aerosols should be administered through the mouth. Most commercial nebulizers deliver aerosols in the 1 to 5 micron diameter range. Particles less than 1 micron in diameter may penetrate the lung more effectively. However, extremely small particles are stable (remain suspended in the gas stream) and thus are exhaled, rather than deposited in the airway.

Most of the aerosol delivered from an aerosol generator is not deposited in the lungs. The majority of the aerosol (about 80 percent) is deposited in the upper respiratory tract. Only about 10 percent is deposited in the lung, and the remaining 10 percent is exhaled.

The penetration and the deposition of aerosol in the lung is affected by the pattern of inhalation. Aerosol penetration and deposition improves significantly if slow, rather than fast, inspiratory flow rates are used. The volume of aerosol deposited in the lung can also be improved by increasing the volume of inhalation (tidal volume). An inspiratory breath hold is also important in improving aerosol deposition in the lungs. The optimal inspiratory pattern during therapeutic aerosol administration is a maximal slow inspiration of 5 to 6 seconds followed by an inspiratory hold of 10 seconds.

Pathologic airway obstruction decreases the penetration of aerosols in the lungs. For a given aerosol dose, the amount of aerosol deposited in the lung decreases with an increase in airway obstruction. Thus, during periods of increased airway obstruction patients may require an increase in dosage or an increase in the frequency of administration. The effectiveness of therapeutic aerosol administration may be limited during acute exacerbations of a patient's lung disease.

METERED DOSE INHALERS

A metered dose inhaler (MDI) is a convenient means of therapeutic aerosol administration (Fig. 1).

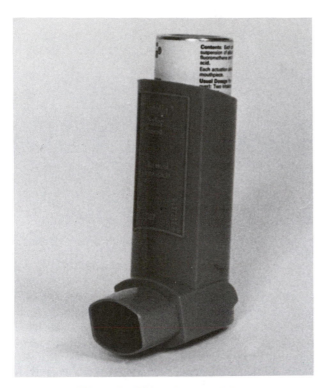

Figure 1 Metered dose inhaler.

The MDI is commonly used by stable outpatients, but is less commonly used for hospitalized patients. These devices became unpopular after a report in the late 1960s that related increased asthma deaths in England to increased use of sympathomimetics administered by MDIs. However, MDIs are again gaining popularity. The MDI consists of a drug-filled canister that is fitted to a mouthpiece actuator. Activation by compression of the canister into the mouthpiece results in release of a unit dose of medication.

Correct use of an MDI requires patient coordination and practice. It is usually necessary for the practitioner to teach the patient the correct method of use because most patients have difficulty learning to use an MDI correctly by reading the package insert. Before activation, the cap is removed from the mouthpiece and the MDI is shaken. The canister must be held upright for activation. The MDI is activated near the beginning of a slow (ideally, 5 to 6 seconds) deep inspiration through the mouth. The patient should be encouraged not to forcibly exhale before beginning the deep breath during which the MDI is activated. At the end of the deep breath, the patient should hold his or her breath for up to 10 seconds and should then exhale slowly. The MDI is activated only once for each deep breath. If more than one puff of aerosol is prescribed, the patient should wait several minutes before administering the next puff. The tongue should be positioned so that it does not obstruct the flow of aerosol through the mouth. There is some controversy regarding the position of the MDI with respect to the lips. Although some practitioners often recommend that the MDI be placed in the mouth with the lips closed around the mouthpiece, others recommend that the MDI be held 4 cm from a wide open mouth.

Patients with arthritic hands may have difficulty activating the MDI. There are many patients who have difficulty coordinating activation of the MDI with the deep breath. If the open mouth technique is used, the patient may have difficulty aiming the aerosol into the mouth. Another problem associated with the use of MDIs is pharyngeal deposition of the drug. When aerosolized steroids are used, oral candidiasis can result. Pharyngeal deposition of sympathomimetics can result in the drug's being swallowed with resulting gastrointestinal absorption and systemic side effects. The patient should be encouraged to rinse his or her mouth after using an MDI in order to prevent problems associated with the pharyngeal deposition of aerosolized steroids.

For patients with arthritic hands, a device is available that aids in activation of the MDI (Vent-Ease) (Fig. 2). A variety of MDI auxiliary devices have been introduced to overcome problems related to patient coordination and to pharyngeal deposition. These include large conical or pear-shaped devices such as Inhal-Aid and Nebuhaler (Fig. 3), extension tubes such as Azmacort (Fig. 4), collapsible bags such as InspirEase (Fig. 5), and rigid valved chambers such

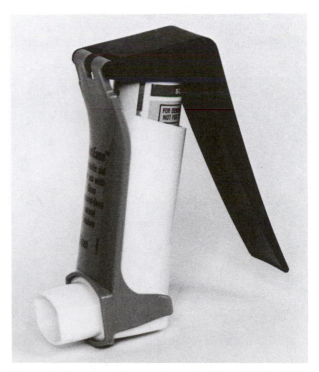

Figure 2 VentEase (Glaxo, Research Triangle Park, NC).

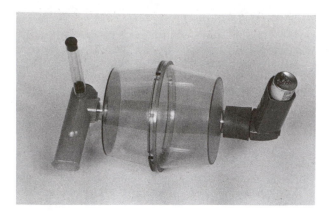

Figure 3 Inhal-Aid and Nebuhaler (Key Pharmaceuticals, Inc., Miami, FL).

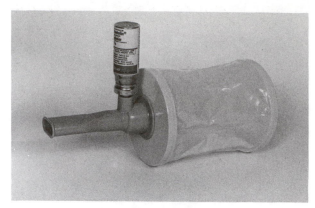

Figure 5 InspirEase (Key Pharmaceuticals, Inc., Miami, FL).

as Aerochamber (Fig. 6). In each of these devices, the aerosol is dispersed from the MDI into a holding chamber. The patient then inhales the aerosol from the holding chamber, rather than from the MDI directly. Thus, coordination between patient inhalation and MDI activation becomes less critical. Activation of the MDI results in impaction of large aerosol particles in the holding chamber, rather than the pharynx. Use of these auxiliary devices results in considerably less pharyngeal deposition and slightly greater pulmonary deposition of the aerosol, as compared to use of an MDI alone. Two of these devices (InspirEase and Aerochamber) provide auditory feedback to achieve a slow inspiratory flow rate, and one of these devices (InspirEase) also provides visual and tactile feedback

to assist the patient in achieving a targeted volume. For administration of sympathomimetics, MDI auxiliary devices are recommended for patients who have difficulty coordinating use of the MDI alone. For administration of aerosolized steroids, auxiliary devices are recommended, not only for patients with difficulty coordinating use of the MDI, but also to decrease the occurrence of oral candidiasis attributable to pharyngeal deposition of the drug.

GAS-POWERED HAND-HELD NEBULIZERS

Some patients cannot use an MDI effectively, even when used with an auxiliary device. This fact is particularly true in acutely ill hospitalized patients. In these patients, a gas-powered hand-held nebulizer (Fig. 7) is often used for therapeutic aerosol administration. These devices consist of a disposable or reusable nebulizer, a mouthpiece or facemask, and a pressurized gas source (pressurized air or oxygen). The solution to be nebulized is placed into the nebulizer chamber

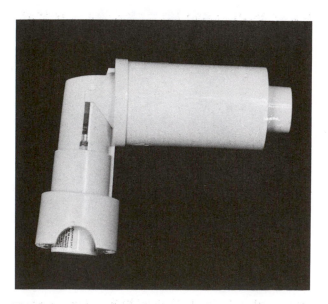

Figure 4 Azmacort (William H. Rorer, Inc., Fort Washington, PA).

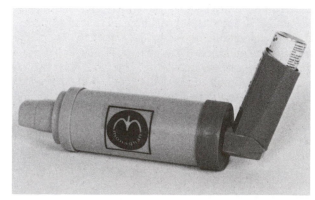

Figure 6 Aerochamber (Monaghan Medical Corp., Plattsburgh, NY).

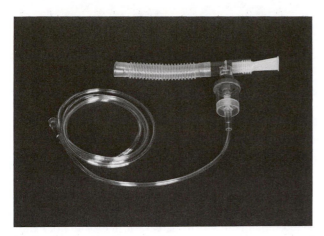

Figure 7 Hand-held nebulizer (Intec Medical, Inc., Blue Springs, MO).

for aerosolization. Use of these devices tends to be more expensive than use of an MDI because the devices themselves are more complex and expensive and because professional supervision is usually required to prepare the drug solution and to supervise the patient during aerosol administration.

To maximize aerosol delivery into the lung, a hand-held nebulizer should be used with a mouthpiece, rather than with a facemask. The patient should be coached to breathe slowly and deeply through the mouth. A breath hold should also be encouraged to promote aerosol deposition in the lungs.

The drug solutions placed into a hand-held nebulizer are more concentrated than those delivered by an MDI. This higher concentration is necessary for several reasons. Only 50 to 75 percent of the solution that is placed into the hand-held nebulizer is aerosolized, with the remainder being trapped in the nebulizer. Most hand-held nebulizers produce an aerosol continuously, so that the aerosol produced during exhalation is wasted. Thus, only a fraction of the solution nebulized is inspired by the patient, and a significant amount of this is not deposited in the lungs, but impacted in the upper airway or lost in the exhaled gas. For therapeutic aerosol administration with a hand-held nebulizer, the volume of drug solution should be about 4 ml, and the nebulizer should be powered by a gas flow of 6 to 8 L per minute.

With therapeutic aerosol administration using a hand-held nebulizer, the active drug is normally diluted with saline or with a mucolytic agent such as acetylcysteine (Mucomyst) or sodium bicarbonate. Usually, saline diluents are recommended, rather than mucolytics. There is little evidence that enough mucolytic is deposited in the lungs to affect mucus viscosity when mucolytics are used with a hand-held nebulizer.

Hand-held nebulizers can be used in the hospital or in the home. Commercially available compressor-powered hand-held nebulizers are available for home use. Before home use, the patient or caregiver must be instructed in the proper use of the hand-held nebulizer, the cleaning and infection control, and the preparation of medications. This instruction is usually best provided by a respiratory therapist or a pulmonary nurse specialist.

INTERMITTENT POSITIVE PRESSURE BREATHING (IPPB)

For many years, the principal means of therapeutic aerosol administration was by use of IPPB. Over the past 10 years, it has become increasingly recognized that IPPB is often unnecessary and undesirable as a means of aerosol administration. IPPB requires professional supervision (respiratory therapist) and sophisticated equipment, thereby making it the most expensive means of aerosol delivery.

Although it is not correct to use IPPB for all therapeutic aerosol treatments, it may be equally incorrect to never use IPPB. IPPB has limited indications, but can be an effective means of aerosol delivery when indicated. In patients who can voluntarily take a deep breath, aerosol penetration and deposition may actually be less with IPPB than with an MDI or a hand-held nebulizer. However, in patients who cannot voluntarily deep breathe (e.g., vital capacity less than 1 L), IPPB use is beneficial if the volume delivered by IPPB is greater than the inspired volume that the patient can generate spontaneously. Volumes must be measured during IPPB administration because the emphasis of IPPB is the delivery of an adequately deep breath (>1 to 1.5 L). The determination of patients who can benefit by use of IPPB thus requires measurement of the patient's inspiratory capacity (or vital capacity) and comparison of this measurement to the volume delivered during IPPB.

IPPB is indicated as a means of therapeutic aerosol administration in acutely ill patients who are not capable of spontaneously deep breathing. However, in patients with chronic obstructive pulmonary disease (COPD) who are stable and at home, there is no benefit of IPPB use over the use of a hand-held nebulizer or MDI.

AEROSOL DELIVERY IN INTUBATED PATIENTS RECEIVING MECHANICAL VENTILATION

In-line delivery of aerosolized medications is commonly used with intubated mechanically ventilated patients. Delivery of aerosolized drugs in these patients is accomplished by placing a hand-held nebulizer or an MDI in the inspiratory limb of the venti-

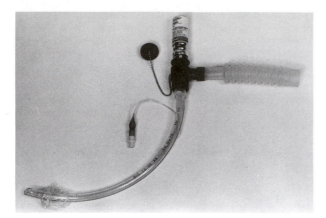

Figure 8 Bronchodilator Tee (Boehringer Laboratories, Wynnewood, PA).

lator circuit near the endotracheal tube (Fig. 8). Compared to spontaneously breathing nonintubated patients, aerosol deposition in the lungs is significantly reduced in intubated mechanically ventilated patients. This reduction is probably the result of the combination of a suboptimal breathing pattern, intrinsic airway disease, and the endotracheal tube serving as a site of aerosol deposition owing to inertial impaction. Thus, therapeutic aerosol administration in intubated mechanically ventilated patients may be less effective than aerosol therapy in spontaneously breathing patients.

SELECTION OF THERAPEUTIC AEROSOL ADMINISTRATION TECHNIQUE

The decision of whether a therapeutic aerosol should be delivered by MDI, by hand-held nebulizer, or by IPPB is often based on personal experience or on institutional policy. Unfortunately, this decision is not often made in an objective manner. An MDI should be used whenever the patient can demonstrate an acceptable technique with this device. IPPB should be reserved for those patients who are unable to use a hand-held nebulizer or an MDI effectively. A hand-held nebulizer should be used when IPPB or MDI use is not indicated. Traditionally, options regarding the device used for therapeutic aerosol administration were limited. Today, however, the practitioner is better able to match the delivery device to the patient's needs. Ideally, the selection of the administration technique should be a shared decision between the physician and the respiratory therapist.

EVALUATION OF AEROSOL BRONCHODILATOR THERAPY

Although aerosol bronchodilator therapy is commonly prescribed for hospitalized patients with pul-

monary disease, there is often little objective evaluation of the effectiveness and the appropriateness of this therapy. The Joint Commission for the Accreditation of Hospitals requires respiratory therapy departments to have a planned and a systematic process for monitoring the quality and the appropriateness of patient care, including therapeutic aerosol administration. Bedside assessment by a respiratory therapist should be part of aerosol bronchodilator administration. The benefit of this therapy is evaluated by the assessment of the pulse rate, the expiratory flow rate, the vital capacity, the breath sounds, and sputum production. Pulse rate should be evaluated because tachycardia is a potentially deleterious side effect of sympathomimetics. An increase in the expiratory flow rate or the vital capacity of 15 percent or greater supports the use of an aerosol bronchodilator. Benefit is also indicated by an improvement in breath sounds or in sputum production. Expiratory flow rates can be evaluated at the bedside by measuring FEV_1 or peak expiratory flow rate (PEFR). Bedside devices to measure PEFR are less expensive and easier to use than devices to measure FEV_1, although FEV_1 may be a better indicator of airflow obstruction than PEFR. Devices to measure PEFR can also be used by patients in the home.

COMBINATION THERAPY

Commonly, a patient may require the use of several therapeutic aerosols (e.g., sympathomimetic and steroid, sympathomimetic and cromolyn sodium, etc.). These patients also frequently require other forms of respiratory therapy, such as bland aerosol or chest physiotherapy. When a patient is receiving multiple respiratory therapies, it is usually recommended that the sympathomimetic be administered before the other therapy for several reasons. First, the onset of action of the sympathomimetics is rapid. Second, the sympathomimetics may prevent a potential bronchoconstrictive effect of other therapy.

Suggested Reading

Brain JD, Valberg PA. Deposition of aerosol in the respiratory tract. Am Rev Respir Dis 1979; 120:1325–1373.

Dolovich MB, Killian D, Wolff RK, Obminski G, Newhouse MT. Pulmonary aerosol deposition in chronic bronchitis: intermittent positive pressure breathing versus quiet breathing. Am Rev Respir Dis 1977; 115:397–402.

Konig P. Spacer devices used with metered-dose inhalers. Breakthrough or gimmick? Chest 1985; 88:276–284.

MacIntyre NR, Silver RM, Miller CW, Schuler F, Coleman E. Aerosol delivery in intubated, mechanically ventilated patients. Crit Care Med 1985; 13:81–84.

Newhouse MT, Dolovich MB. Control of asthma by aerosols. N Engl J Med 1986; 315:870–874.

Newman SP. Aerosol deposition considerations in inhalation ther-apy. Chest 1985; 88:152S–160S.

Newman SP, Pavia D, Moren F, Sheahan NF, Clarke SW. De-position of pressurized aerosols in the human respiratory tract. Thorax 1981; 36:52–55.

Popa V. Beta-adrenergic drugs. Clin Chest Med 1986; 7:313–329.

Sackner MA, Kim CS. Auxiliary MDI aerosol delivery systems. Chest 1985; 88:161S–170S.

Smoker JM, Tangen MI, Ferree SM, Hess D, Rexrode WO. A protocol to assess and administer aerosol bronchodilator ther-apy. Respir Care 1986; 31:780–785.

CORTICOSTEROIDS

PAUL HASSOUN, M.D.*
CHARLES A. HALES, M.D.

Corticosteroids have been used in the treatment of asthma since 1950 when the first synthetic analogues of the natural adrenal cortical hormone hydrocortisone (cortisol) became available. Although our understanding of their mechanism of action remains poor after more than 3 decades, corticosteroids are now widely used in the treatment of other chronic obstructive lung diseases, as well.

Because corticosteroids are potent drugs that may carry significant morbidity when used for lengthy periods of time, the physician who undertakes the treatment of lung diseases with these drugs should be well aware of the indications of therapy and the goals to be achieved by such therapy. Both the physician and the patient submitted to prolonged therapy should be aware of the potential side effects of corticosteroids. Invaluable drugs in the treatment of a reversible disease, such as acute asthma, they may be useless and harmful in a particular patient with chronic obstructive lung disease with no evidence of objective improvement on therapy.

MECHANISM OF ACTION

Corticosteroids are clearly different from beta agonists, methylxanthines, or anticholinergics. Nevertheless, corticosteroids do reduce airway obstruction. The main beneficial effect of steroids is attributable to their anti-inflammatory properties. Indeed, glucocorticoids suppress acute and chronic inflammation, irrespective of the cause, by inhibiting every step in the inflammatory process. These drugs reduce the leakage of fluids and cells into the inflammatory locus, inhibit the migration of macrophages and of leukocytes to the site of inflammation, and possibly block the response to some mediators of inflammation. In the lung, anti-inflammatory and decongestive effects of these drugs on bronchial mucous membranes alleviate airway obstruction. Therefore, glucocorticoids are theoretically active in both allergic and in nonallergic asthma, as well as in other lung conditions where inflammation may be a predominant feature, such as chronic bronchitis and emphysema.

Another major property of corticosteroids is their action on the beta-adrenergic system. Corticosteroids increase the density of adrenergic receptors by increasing their synthesis. Corticosteroids enhance the receptor affinity and coupling to adenylcyclase. These drugs interfere with the extraneuronal uptake and the inactivation of catecholamines. As a result, corticosteroids prolong the action of endogenous catecholamines and potentiate the responses to exogenous sympathomimetics and methylxanthines.

At a cellular level, all synthetic analogues of cortisol used for therapeutic purposes are capable of binding to glucocorticoid receptors, but have wide variations in their intrinsic potency owing to modifications in molecular structure. As for other hormones, the biochemical mechanism involves the binding of the steroid molecule to a specific intracellular receptor in order to form a complex. This activated steroid-receptor complex is rapidly translocated to the nucleus, where a messenger-RNA is synthesized. This property leads to subsequent synthesis of proteins that mediate the effect of the steroids. The translocation of the activated complex to the nucleus and the initiation of RNA synthesis begin within minutes after exposure of the cell to the steroid. However, the subsequent synthesis of specific proteins starts only about 1 hour later, which partly explains the delayed onset of action of steroids when used clinically.

INDICATIONS IN SPECIFIC LUNG DISEASES

Asthma

In the spectrum of chronic obstructive lung diseases, asthma is the only disease where the effectiveness of steroid therapy is well established for both the acute and the stable conditions. Although the treatment of asthma in the United States relies mainly upon the use of beta-adrenergics and of methylxanthines, corticosteroids—both inhaled and given systemically—have an invaluable role.

In the acute setting, there is increasing evidence that corticosteroids (e.g., intravenous methylprednisolone) given early in the treatment of moderate to severe asthmatic attacks, along with other routinely used drugs, such as intravenous theophylline and inhaled beta-adrenergics, reduce the number of hospitalizations and decrease health costs, even though ob-

* Acknowledgment: Work done during tenure of a fellowship from NIH Research Training Grant HL 07354.

jective spirometric data may not be affected. There is a lag between the time the steroid is given and the onset of a clinical response. Thus, we start steroids early in the course of the asthma attack, unless early and dramatic reversal occurs with the use of other agents. The dose of intravenous steroid to be given in an acute asthmatic attack is arbitrary. A study comparing doses of intravenous methylprednisolone, ranging from 20 mg to 125 mg every 6 hours, has shown no difference in the rate of improvement in patients' pulmonary function. However, other studies have shown a slower improvement when patients are treated with smaller doses (15 mg of methylprednisolone every 6 hours). Since few adverse effects are associated with large doses given for short periods, our own approach has been to use an initial intravenous bolus of 1 to 2 mg per kilogram of methylprednisolone sodium succinate (Solu-Medrol), followed by repeat doses of 1 to 2 mg per kilogram every 6 hours, until there is a clinical improvement. This initial dose should be followed by oral steroid therapy (prednisone 0.5 mg to 1 mg per kilogram per day) for at least 1 week in the case of a severe attack to allow good resolution of airway inflammation and edema. Prednisone can then be rapidly tapered and discontinued if the patient's clinical status allows. Aside from routine serial spirometric evaluations, a total eosinophilic blood count may be helpful in assessing the activity of the disease and in monitoring the response to steroid therapy. Indeed, sputum, and particularly peripheral eosinophilia, in the setting of airway obstruction, generally indicates a reversible component to the obstruction, whether this obstruction is allergic or nonallergic in origin. Aside from this qualitative association, there is a quantitative linear relationship between the level of peripheral eosinophilia and the measurement of airway obstruction in patients with asthma. In general, a total eosinophil count (TEC) greater than 1,000 per cubic millimeter is associated with forced expiratory volumes in 1 second (FEV_1) of 50 percent or less of the patient's best values. In addition to reflecting the severity of reversible obstruction, the TEC helps assess the adequacy of corticosteroid therapy. When a patient with an acute attack of asthma is treated with corticosteroids, one should expect a lowering of the TEC in parallel with an improvement in airway obstruction. An appropriate eosinopenic response (TEC < 85 per cubic millimeter [Note that TEC may vary from one laboratory to the other]) unaccompanied by a clinical response suggests superimposed infection or irreversible disease. Inadequate steroid dosage, patient noncompliance, drug interaction (e.g., phenytoin), or hyperthyroidism may explain a poor clinical response associated with persistent eosinophilia (TEC > 85 per cubic millimeter). If an acute asthmatic fails to respond to therapy within 48 hours of steroid initiation, we check a TEC, and if the TEC is not markedly suppressed (<85 per cubic millimeter) we double the steroid dose.

In chronic stable asthma, maintenance treatment also relies on theophylline preparations and on inhaled beta-adrenergics. However, some patients are not adequately controlled on such a regimen, and steroids are often used intermittently or for long periods of time. In these patients, steroids have been effective in reducing the severity of symptoms and the frequency of acute episodes. This benefit is at the cost of increased side effects from long-term steroid therapy. A logical approach is to administer the minimum dose that provides reasonable control of symptoms. If a daily dose is to be administered, we recommend giving the entire dose as a single dose, rather than divided doses, to reduce steroid-related side effects. An alternate-day schedule is even more preferable, if it is also effective in controlling the asthma. Unfortunately, we find that this is often not the case. Inhaled steroids are often the first line drugs used for chronic stable asthma in Europe and are becoming increasingly so in the U.S. The main advantage of inhaled steroids is that they allow substantial reduction of the systemic steroid doses and, therefore, reduction of the side effects. Inhaled steroids should not be used in the treatment of acute asthma, since they are topical agents and are unable to spread distally in an asthmatic with tight lungs. These drugs will be discussed in more detail later.

Emphysema and Chronic Bronchitis

The use of steroids in emphysema and chronic bronchitis is not as well defined as in asthma. A distinction must be made between acute and chronic stable disease. In acute disease, efforts should be made to identify and to treat the precipitating factor(s). The addition of steroid therapy to the main therapeutic regimen (intravenous theophylline, antibiotics, etc.) is beneficial, particularly in those patients whose bronchospasm seems to be a predominant clinical feature, although no single factor has been really useful in predicting the effect of steroid therapy in acutely decompensated COPD. Aside from the treatment of bronchospasm, corticosteroids in acute chronic obstructive lung disease are expected to decrease the volume of secretions and to reduce inflammation and edema, thereby alleviating airway obstruction. Corticosteroids may be particularly useful in exacerbations of chronic bronchitis, in which plugging of mucus is a prominent feature. Indeed, high dose methylprednisolone has been shown to hasten the improvement of respiratory flow rates in patients suffering an exacerbation of COPD, even when all patients with eosinophilia are excluded. As for asthma, treatment should be instituted early in the course of the decompensation, or the dose should be increased if the patient is already on steroids. Treatment should preferably be given intravenously and at generous doses (1 to 2 mg per kilogram of methylprednisolone given intravenously, followed by 0.5 mg per kilogram at 4 to 6 hour intervals). An infectious process should be carefully searched for in the initial evaluation, since infection may be masked later on by steroid therapy. When an objective clinical improvement has occurred (improvement in expiratory flows, improvement in CO_2 retention or hypoxia), prednisone can be given orally (40 mg in one daily dose) and intravenous methylprednisolone can be discontinued. Oral prednisone therapy can then be tapered slowly over the next 2 to 3 weeks.

The use of steroids in stable chronic obstructive lung disease has been disappointing. Some improvement in arterial oxygenation, attributed to either decreased ventilation-perfusion mismatching and/or increased diffusing capacity, has been found by some investigators, but not by others. Steroids may increase expiratory flows in a subgroup of patients who show some response to inhaled sympathomimetics. In other words, steroids may be helpful in patients with a bronchospastic component (evidence of reversible airway obstruction). Steroids have been shown not to affect minute ventilation ($\dot{V}E$) or maximum O_2 consumption ($\dot{V}O_2$ maximum) during exercise in patients with stable COPD, when compared to placebo. In spite of the contrary data, steroids continue to be widely used in stable COPD. We believe steroids are not indicated in most patients with stable COPD. We recommend that if these drugs are to be used in a particular patient, then the efficacy of treatment should be objectively assessed before and after drug administration. For example, a patient with severe COPD ($FEV_1 < 900$ ml), who is not well-controlled with oral theophylline and inhaled and/or oral beta-adrenergic agonists, may be given a short trial of oral corticosteroids (3 to 4 weeks). Arterial blood gases, as well as respiratory mechanics and work capacity, should be assessed before and while the patient is on a steroid trial. If no objective improvement is seen (an increase in FEV_1 of at least 20 percent, an increase in FVC of 20 percent, and an increase in arterial PO_2) then therapy should be tapered. Often the patient shows no objective response to the steroid trial, but reports an increased sense of well-being. This response is probably attributable to a central nervous system euphoric effect of the drug and should not be an indication for the continued use of steroids. If there is an objective improvement in a particular patient, an alternate-day regimen of steroids may be as effective as a daily regimen, but carries less side effects (e.g., depression of the pituitary-adrenal axis, obesity, growth retardation, and Cushingoid appearance). As in the case of asthma, inhaled steroids can be used in stable chronic obstructive lung disease and help to reduce or to alleviate the need for oral steroid therapy. In extremely severe COPD ($FEV_1 < 900$ ml) the inhaled aerosol may not spread far enough to have any impact on airway function.

Adult Respiratory Distress Syndrome

The use of steroids in the treatment of the adult respiratory distress syndrome (ARDS) is still debated. Steroids block complement aggregation of leukocytes and may decrease alveolar capillary permeability. Steroids do help in some animal studies of acute lung injury when given prior to or shortly after the injurious insult. In man, the injury is unfortunately usually not recognized at this time, and we only see the resulting sequelae of ARDS. Theoretically, steroids would be effective in ARDS if used early in the course of the disease. Experimental data, however, are conflicting, and since this syndrome represents a spectrum of several diseases, clinical studies are often difficult to interpret. At best, corticosteroids show no effect when given early in patients at a high risk of developing ARDS. At worst, steroids may increase the risk of pulmonary infections. Therefore, we do not recommend their use in ARDS.

Aspiration Pneumonia

Pulmonary aspiration of gastric contents is a common and a potentially fatal clinical problem. The injury to the lungs is at least twofold: injury to the airways and alveoli, and injury to the capillary vasculature. This injury results in capillary leakage of fluid and of protein into the perivascular and the peribronchial spaces, bronchoconstriction, atelectasis, etc. Hypoxia and hypovolemic shock usually precede the patient's demise. The use of corticosteroids in aspiration pneumonia remains controversial. The rationale for steroid use is based on the fact that corticosteroids are able to decrease inflammation, stabilize alveolar cell membranes, prevent lysosomal enzyme release, and possibly diminish alveolar capillary membrane permeability. Aerosolized corticosteroids sound like an appealing form of therapy because the initial lesion is airway-mediated. However, there are no available data on aerosolized corticosteroids for aspiration, and no convincing study has demonstrated any beneficial effect of systemic corticosteroids on microscopic changes or on survival rates in animal experimentation, unless steroids are given prior to the acid injury. Therefore, we cannot recommend the use of corticosteroids in aspiration, except in the unusual case where the aspiration event is witnessed and therapy is instituted immediately. Methylprednisolone (1 g) may be given intravenously, followed by 40 mg at 4- to 6-hour intervals. If there is no objective improvement within 24 to 48 hours, steroids should be discontinued to minimize the secondary risk of bacterial infection.

Pulmonary Sarcoidosis

It is not clear whether corticosteroids affect long-term outcome in sarcoidosis by limiting fibrosis. However, corticosteroids remain the drug of choice in this disease. The decision to treat depends on the stage of the disease (as assessed radiologically and physiologically) and on the progression of the disease (as assessed on serial pulmonary function tests). Three markers of disease activity are commonly used clinically: serum angiotensin converting enzyme (SACE), 67 gallium lung scan, and cellular contents of bronchoalveolar lavage (BAL). The results of these markers may not always correspond, since they may each reflect a different facet of the cellular sarcoid reaction. In Stage 1, when the patient is usually asymptomatic, we recommend observation alone, since spontaneous improvement occurs in more than 80 percent of the cases. For Stage 2 or 3, when lung impairment includes dyspnea, wheezing, a reduction in total lung capacity (TLC), a widened arteriolar-alveolar gradient on exercise, and a reduction in diffusing capacity for carbon monoxide (DLCO), steroid treatment should be strongly considered if there is evidence of continued progression or of continued activity of the sarcoid. Establishing ongoing activity or physiologic deterioration is important, as one otherwise gets into a bind of not knowing if steroids stopped progression of the sarcoid, or if the sarcoid had become inactive on its own. Treatment should be started at high doses (30 to 40 mg of prednisone per day) with tapered dosages over 6 months or more, as determined by a lack of evidence of renewed sarcoid activity. For practical purposes, we rely mainly on lung volumes, on serial single breath DLCO, on rest and exercise arterial blood gases, and on SACE levels to assess improvement on therapy and to assess continued stability during steroid tapering. A 67 Gallium lung scan and BAL may also be useful, but are expensive. Also, BAL is invasive and gallium scanning may involve a significant radiation dose. Therapy should be continued as long as there is evidence of active disease. The dose of corticosteroids should be tapered to the lowest effective dose that maintains remission. Along with corticosteroid therapy, isoniazid (INH) prophylaxis has been recommended in the case of a patient with a positive PPD or with complete anergy, as tuberculosis may coexist with sarcoidosis and can possibly reactivate with therapy. In Stage 3 pulmonary sarcoidosis, when diffuse fibrosis is established and little is gained from corticosteroids, therapy should be avoided in order to limit the incidence of long-term steroid complications.

Idiopathic Interstitial Pneumonitis

Interstitial fibrosis is a common pathologic response of the lungs to a wide variety of insults. It is not within the scope of this chapter to discuss the various etiologic conditions and their specific treatment. However, immunosuppressive agents, and steroids in particular, often remain the only therapeutic options left for the clinician dealing with this disorder. Some physicians feel that a patient who has a lung biopsy showing fibrosis, but little inflammation (e.g., usual interstitial pneumonitis), should not be given steroids. However, we feel that, because there is enough trouble with sampling error and because cases of usual interstitial pneumonitis with a high lymphocyte count in the bronchoalveolar lavage have responded to steroids, most cases of progressive interstitial fibrosis deserve a steroid trial. The clinician often has to decide when to treat with corticosteroids and for how long. The answers to both questions remain uncertain because our understanding of pathophysiology is incomplete and because there is no uniform opinion on how to best assess the activity of the disease. For example, the values of 67 Gallium lung scan or bronchoalveolar lavage (BAL) are still being debated. Nevertheless, it is possible to develop a strategy that hopefully benefits the patient and limits the complications of long-term therapy. Patients to be treated should be carefully selected on the basis of objective criteria, e.g., a widened alveolar-capillary oxygen tension difference at rest or on exercise, a decreased single-breath DLCO less than 70 percent predicted, an abnormal 67 Gallium lung scan, and/or an "active" cell population on BAL. However, a normal gallium scan or BAL should not exclude patients from a therapeutic trial. Treatment should be initiated at high doses (prednisone 1.5 mg per kilogram per day). Patients should be reassessed at the end of a 4-week period. If there is mild or significant improvement in rest or exercise arterial blood gases, in single breath DLCO, in 67 Gallium lung scan, or in BAL, treatment should be continued for at least 5 to 6 months; but the prednisone should be slowly tapered down to a maintenance dose of 25 mg to 20 mg every day, if possible. Initially, treatment should be monitored at 3- to 4-week intervals, with at least serial arterial blood gases (rest and exercise), pulmonary function tests (PFT), and single breath DLCO. We believe that these tests are reliable enough and are certainly less invasive and less expensive than the gallium lung scan or the BAL. However, if in doubt about flare of the disease as steroids are tapered a repeat 67 Gallium lung scan can be helpful. Doses of prednisone can be adjusted accordingly. After 6 months of therapy, efforts should be made to taper the patient off corticosteroids. Unfortunately, some patients remain dependent on corticosteroids, and the same recommendations given for long-term therapy of asthma or COPD apply.

MODE OF ADMINISTRATION

For the treatment of pulmonary diseases, steroids may be administered systemically (oral or intravenous) or topically (inhalation). Only systemic administration is of value in the treatment of acute lung diseases. Inhaled corticosteroids should be reserved for the treatment of stable chronic lung disease.

Systemic Corticosteroids

Biologic responses to the steroid preparations depend on the innate potency of the steroid analogue, its bioavailability and distribution into various body compartments, its rate of bioinactivation, and various host factors (metabolic state, patient's liver function, concomitant administration of other drugs). Although all routes of administration lead to systemic absorption and distribution, the penetration into certain body compartments varies; for example, systemically administered methylprednisolone (Solu-Medrol) penetrates bronchial lavage fluid much better than prednisone. We have no preference as to what steroid preparation to use in the acute situation. Table 1 lists the corticosteroids most commonly used for systemic administration, along with their approximate anti-inflammatory potency and their biologic half-life. It should be noted that some oral preparations have extremely long half-lives (36 to 54 hours for Celestone, Decadron, Haldrone) and could cause inhibition of the adrenal gland, even when given on an alternate-day basis.

There is some interaction between theophylline and corticosteroid metabolism. At low theophylline serum levels this interaction is of no clinical importance, but at high serum theophylline levels, corticosteroids may alter theophylline metabolism and thus result in either a higher or a lower theophylline serum level. Therefore, we recommend that theophylline serum levels be monitored when corticosteroids are added to the therapeutic regimen of a patient with chronic obstructive lung disease. Intravenous corticosteroids can usually be given at the same venous site as intravenous theophylline. The two drugs, however, should not be mixed in the same bottle because the pH of the solutions may not be compatible.

Side Effects of Systemic Corticosteroids

Two categories of toxic effects are encountered when using corticosteroids. The first category is related to sudden withdrawal of therapy after prolonged use; acute adrenal insufficiency is the most common and potentially the most lethal complication. Other complications include the recurrence of symptoms (such as bronchospasm). The second category of side effects is seen with prolonged use of large doses of steroids and includes fluid and electrolyte imbalances (hypokalemic alkalosis), hyperglycemia and glycosuria, increased susceptibility to infection (e.g., reactivation of tuberculosis), osteoporosis with vertebral compressions in patients of all ages, myopathy, psychosis, Cushingoid habitus, and glaucoma. Femoral head necrosis is a devastating complication and may

TABLE 1 Preparation of Adrenocortical Steroids and Their Synthetic Analogues for Systemic Administration

Corticosteroid (Example)	Glucocorticoid Dose (mg)	Approximate Anti-Inflammatory Activity	Oral Form Available?	Injectable? (IV, IM)	Biological Half-Life in Tissue (hr)
Short-Acting					
Cortisone					
(Cortone)	25	0.8	+	+	8–12
Hydrocortisone					
(Cortef)	20	1	+	+	8–12
Intermediate-Acting					
Methylprednisolone					
(Solu-Medrol, Medrol)	4	5	+	+	18–36
Prednisolone					
(Delta-Cortef)	5	4	+	+	18–36
Prednisone	5	4	+	—	18–36
Triamcinolone					
(Aristocort, Aristopan)	4	5	+	+	18–36
Long-Acting					
Betamethasone					
(Celestone)	0.6	20–30	+	—	36–54
Dexamethasone					
(Decadron)	0.5–0.75	20–30	+	+	36–54
Paramethasone					
(Haldrone)	2	10	+	—	36–54

TABLE 2 Corticosteroid Aerosols

Drug	μg/puff Inhalation	Recommended Dosage*
Beclomethasone dipropionate (Beclovent, Vanceril)	250 μg	2 inhalations t.i.d. or q.i.d.
Triamcinolone acetonide (Azmacort)	200 μg	2 inhalations t.i.d.
Funisolide (AeroBid)	250 μg	2 inhalations t.i.d.

* Doubling the dose does cause a decrease in adrenal response to ACTH, but does not alter circulating cortisol levels. Even twice the aerosol dose may then be expected to result in fewer side effects than oral steroids.

occur after even short exposure to moderate dose steroids (e.g., 30 to 40 mg of prednisone per day).

Inhaled Corticosteroids

Unfortunately, a number of patients with chronic asthma, and some patients with COPD, remain dependent on steroid therapy for maintenance treatment. These are the patients who cannot be controlled on oral theophylline and sympathomimetics and who show objective improvement with steroids. Inhaled corticosteroids should always be tried in these patients, the goal being to attempt to reduce the dose of oral steroids as much as possible. Certain inhaled corticosteroids are highly active topically and are poorly soluble in water, so that they have little systemic activity. Several clinical trials looking at the effectiveness of inhaled corticosteroids in steroid-dependent asthmatics have shown that 50 to 75 percent of the patients were able to taper their oral steroid dose and more than one-third were able to discontinue oral steroids altogether.

Three corticosteroid aerosols that are poorly soluble are currently available in the U.S.A. (Table 2): beclomethasone dipropionate (Vanceril, Beclovent), triamcinolone acetonide (Azmacort), and flunisolide (AeroBid). Although these drugs have all been shown to be much more effective than placebos in steroid-dependent asthmatics, there is no study comparing one to each other. Inhaled corticosteroids are all relatively free of systemic effects in doses of less than 1,500 to 2,000 μg per day. Flunisolide (AeroBid) can be administered twice a day, but treatment with flunisolide is twice as expensive as with Azmacort for the same doses. Azmacort is provided with a spacer device that theoretically delivers more corticosteroid to the bronchi and deposits less in the oropharyngeal cavity, thereby reducing the incidence of fungal colonization.

We recommend using aerosolized corticosteroids 10 to 15 minutes after the administration of inhaled beta-adrenergics. This ensures deeper inhalation of the steroid particles. A common cause of poor response to aerosol therapy is poor inhalation technique. Therefore, we advise physicians to personally observe the

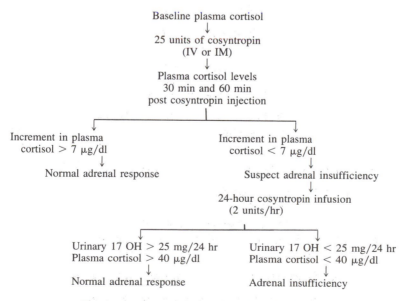

Figure 1 Screening for adrenal insufficiency.

patient's administration technique, especially when the patient is a child. This reveals the patients who do not inhale adequately and who require repeated instruction.

Side Effects of Inhaled Corticosteroids

The side effects of inhaled corticosteroids are similar for all three inhalants. Slight adrenal suppression is rare and has only been reported at extremely high doses. The most common problems are hoarseness, sore throat, and oropharyngeal candidiasis. Although up to 50 percent of the patients may be colonized with candida, oral thrush causes symptoms in only 5 percent of the patients. Discontinuation of inhaled corticosteroids is not required, and patients can be treated with topical antifungal drugs. Because of the problem of halitosis with nystatin (Mycostatin) tablets, we recommend using nystatin (Mycostatin) oral suspension 500,000 units (5 cc) three times a day to swish and swallow, rather than tablets (500,000 units three times a day), although tablets are more effective in treating oral candidiasis. If the oral suspension is ineffective, then tablet therapy is warranted.

Hoarseness may sometimes be attributable to an adductor vocal cord deformity (localized steroid myopathy). Patients should be advised to rinse their mouths with water or with a mouthwash after each inhalation dose to limit side effects. Caution should be applied when switching a patient from oral to inhaled steroids, since sudden adrenal insufficiency may supervene. Slow tapering of the oral dose may be indicated. When in doubt, the patient's adrenal response can be easily assessed by an adrenal stimulation test; serum cortisol levels are obtained before and after administration of 25 units of cosyntropin (Cortrosyn) and compared (Fig. 1).

Suggested Reading

Albert RK, Martin TR, Lewis SW. Controlled clinical trial of methylprednisolone in patients with chronic bronchitis and acute respiratory insufficiency. Ann Intern Med 1980; 92:753–758.

Bynum LJ, Pierce AK. Pulmonary aspiration of gastric contents. Am Rev Respir Dis 1976; 114:1129–1136.

Corticosteriod aerosols for asthma. The Medical Letter 1985; 27:679.

Crystal RG, Gadek JE, Hunninghake GW, et al. Interstitial lung disease: current concepts of pathogenesis, staging and therapy. Am J Med 1981; 70:543–568.

Fanta CH, Rossing TH, McFadden R Jr. Glucocorticoids in acute asthma: a critical controlled trial. Am J Med 1983; 74:845–851.

Fiel SB, Swartz MA, Glanz K, Francis ME. Efficacy of short-term corticosteroid therapy in outpatient treatment of acute bronchial asthma. Am J Med 1983; 75:259–262.

Littenberg B, Gluck EH. A controlled trial of methylprednisolone in the emergency treatment of acute asthma. N Engl J Med 1986; 314:150–152.

Mendella LA, Manfreda J, Warren CPW, Anthonisen NR. Steroid response in stable chronic obstructive pulmonary disease. Ann Intern Med 1982; 96:17–21.

Morris HG. Mechanisms of action and therapeutic role of corticosteroids in asthma. J Allergy Clin Immunol 1985; 75:1–14.

Schatz M, Wasserman S, Patterson R. The eosinophil and the lung. Arch Intern Med 1982; 142:1515–1519.

OTHER DRUGS ADMINISTERED VIA THE RESPIRATORY TRACT

HAROLD J. DEMONACO, M.S.

The absorption of nonvolatile drugs from the respiratory tract has been of considerable interest in the past few years. The reason for this renewed enthusiasm is unclear, but is undoubtedly based on the assumption that drug absorption from the respiratory tract is a rapid and complete process. However, until recently, little quantitative information has existed to substantiate this belief.

Since Claude Bernard first described the pharmacologic effects of endotracheally administered curare in the dog, the world's literature has been replete with anecdotal reports of the efficacy of this route of administration. Pulmonary absorption of a variety of pharmacologic agents has been demonstrated on the basis of both pharmacologic effect and the presence of drugs in the blood stream. However, the pharmacokinetics of drug administration via the respiratory tract are, at this late date, unclear and still to be elucidated. This lack of knowledge is especially true of the endotracheally administered emergency medications.

In this chapter I will discuss the pharmacokinetic principles of the administration of drugs via the respiratory tract. I will specifically discuss drugs administered in three clinical settings: during cardiopulmonary resuscitation; in the management of upper airway obstruction, including post-bronchoscopy; and the instillation and/or aerosolization of antibiotics in the treatment of pulmonary infections.

PHARMACOKINETIC PRINCIPLES

Most of our pharmacokinetic knowledge about drugs administered via the respiratory tract is based on animal studies and on uncontrolled clinical anecdotes. The few well-designed human studies have been conducted with relatively healthy individuals. The effects of chronic or acute pulmonary disease and of cardiovascular compromise on the pharmacokinetics of drugs administered via an endotracheal tube are unknown. As a result, many gaps in our understanding exist, especially regarding factors that alter both the rate and the extent of drug absorption, but several generalizations can be made.

The lungs provide a large surface area available for drug absorption. Moreover, they receive all of the cardiac output, thus assuring the rapid distribution of an absorbed drug. Drugs are probably absorbed throughout the respiratory tract, with the greatest absorption occurring at the alveolar-capillary interface.

Like all biologic membranes, the capillary membrane is not permeable to all drugs. There is speculation that a lung-blood barrier, much akin to the blood-brain barrier, exists and is responsible for alveolar integrity. While the absorption of lipid soluble drugs from the respiratory tract is consistent with the presence of a lipid-pore type membrane, a large number of lipid insoluble drugs have been shown to be rapidly absorbed. Data from experimental studies suggest that the rate of absorption of lipid insoluble compounds is dependent on molecular size. The rate of absorption of many of these compounds exceeds that of gastrointestinal absorption, at least in several animal species.

The absorption of drugs across the alveolar-capillary membrane appears to be by passive diffusion. The rate and the extent of absorption is related to the drug's lipid and/or water coefficient and the degree of ionization at a pH of 7.4. The greater the coefficient, the more rapid the absorption rate. The completeness of absorption remains speculative at this time. At least one radionuclide study using Technetium-99m (Tc-99m) diethylenetriamine pentaacetic acid in mechanically ventilated patients suggests that as little as 3 percent of the administered dose may reach the pulmonary circulation. This may be a result of the existing pulmonary disease, the suboptimal breathing pattern obtained, or the drug deposition on the endotracheal tube.

Curiously, drugs administered via the respiratory route may exhibit a longer duration of action than if administered intravenously. The exact reason for this "depot effect" is unclear.

Higher sputum antibiotic concentrations are achieved with drug instillation than with aerosolization. This discrepancy and apparent contradiction to common wisdom has been identified only with antibiotics. Other classes of drugs, such as locally administered bronchodilators, have not been studied to any extent. It is unknown whether drug aerosolization or instillation is the preferred method of providing optimal drug sputum or serum concentrations.

ENDOTRACHEAL ADMINISTRATION OF DRUGS IN CARDIOPULMONARY RESUSCITATION

Venous access, especially central, is highly desirable during emergency situations. The respiratory route has been employed in those instances where venous access may not be obtained quickly. It cannot be overstated, however, that, with the exception of epinephrine, drug administration via the respiratory route during cardiopulmonary resuscitation should not be considered routine.

Although a considerable body of data exists, these data are nearly all anecdotal and merely looks at crude outcome measures in uncontrolled settings. The unknown risks of this route of administration must be weighed against the potential benefit to the patient. Table 1 summarizes the drugs and the guidelines for their administration by endotracheal instillation that appear to me to be relatively safe and efficacious.

Epinephrine

Endotracheally administered epinephrine appears to be absorbed as rapidly as the intravenous route, but with a lower and a delayed peak serum concentration. In addition to the dose administered, the concentration, the diluent used, and the location of the endotracheal tube affect the pharmacologic response of epinephrine.

The appropriate dose of epinephrine for instillation via an endotracheal tube is debated. Several animal studies have suggested that endotracheal doses of up to 10 times the intravenous dose are required to produce the same hemodynamic effects. This dose difference would appear to be species-dependent, thus further complicating the question of appropriate dose. Data from a recent primate study suggest the endotracheal dose to be equal to the normally prescribed intravenous dose.

Controlled studies in dogs indicate that undiluted epinephrine (1 mg per milliliter) appears to be inferior to a dilute solution in 0.9 percent sodium chloride solution or in water (1 mg per 10 ml). Epinephrine absorption appears to be enhanced when drug instillation via an endotracheal tube is followed by positive pressure ventilation, or when a catheter is introduced down the endotracheal tube to serve as a drug introducer. Based on the anecdotal reports in the literature and on recent primate studies, the dose of epinephrine administered endotracheally should be equal to the intravenously administered dose. The cardiovascular side effects of epinephrine administered via an endotracheal tube mirror those side effects of the intravenous route. Curiously, at least in the dog model, a temporal difference may exist, with tachycardia appearing earlier with endotracheal administration than with intravenous administration at identical doses.

Atropine Sulfate

The first reported case of the endotracheal instillation of atropine during cardiopulmonary resuscitation appeared in 1982. Animal data derived in anesthetized dogs and subsequent data derived in clinical studies have suggested that the onset of action of atropine, when administered via an endotracheal tube, is more rapid than when a corresponding dose is administered intravenously. Additionally, the duration of action appears to be longer with endotracheal administration. As with epinephrine, the reasons for the prolongation of duration are unknown. Local vasoconstriction does not appear to be a cause because of the relative lack of cholinergic innervation of most vascular beds.

It is important to remember that dilution of atropine prior to endotracheal administration and subsequent positive pressure ventilation are both mandatory if the desired effect is to be expected in a reasonable length of time. Although no standards exist for dilution, it appears reasonable to provide a 0.1 mg per milliliter concentration in either sterile water for injection or 0.9 percent sodium chloride injection. Standard intravenous doses may be given when the endotracheal route is used. Side effects are similar to those seen with intravenous administration, namely tachycardia, elevated intraocular pressure, drying of mucous membranes, and urinary retention. Significant cardiac effects are uncommon when atropine is used in the management of bronchospasm or of chronic

TABLE 1   Drugs Instilled Endotracheally During Cardiac Arrest

Drug	Initial Adult Dose	Initial Pediatric Dose	Volume*	Comments
Atropine	0.5–1 mg	0.01 mg/kg	10 ml	May be required less frequently than IV dose
Lidocaine	50–100 mg	1 mg/kg	5–10 ml	
Epinephrine	1 mg	0.01 mg/kg	10 mls	May be required less frequently than IV dose
Naloxone	0.4–2.0 mg	0.01 mg/kg	10 mls	Has been administered in successful resuscitation without further dilution of commercial solution

* Recommended total volume in adult patients

obstructive pulmonary disease in otherwise healthy patients.

Lidocaine Hydrochloride

The endotracheal instillation of lidocaine has been shown to be an effective way of preventing the elevation in blood pressure and in heart rate that normally accompany laryngoscopy. As with atropine, animal data derived in anesthetized dogs suggest that the onset of action of endotracheally administered lidocaine is more rapid than the onset after intravenous injection.

The duration of action is prolonged twofold when compared to the same intravenous dose. However, data derived in humans do not confirm this dramatic difference. Only a limited number of patients have been studied in controlled settings. Preliminary results suggest that the onset of action is slower and the duration of action is more prolonged when lidocaine is administered endotracheally. Several anecdotal reports suggest that endotracheally administered lidocaine is effective in treating ventricular arrhythmias.

The recommended dose of lidocaine when administered by this route is unclear, as is the appropriate volume of diluent. It appears prudent to use the usual intravenous dose as a 10 mg per milliliter concentration if the respiratory route is to be used at all, although doses of up to 3 mg per kilogram have been recommended in the literature. The toxicities of endotracheally instilled lidocaine are identical to those associated with the intravenous route, e.g., nausea, seizures, and myocardial depression.

Naloxone

The endotracheal administration of naloxone to reverse narcotic-induced respiratory depression has been reported. Based on limited data, the onset of action and the duration of action of endotracheally administered naloxone resemble those obtained by the intravenous route. The doses reportedly used are the same as those for intravenous administration and have been administered undiluted. However, it seems prudent to dilute the desired dose to a final volume of 10 ml, using either sterile water or 0.9 percent sodium chloride, and to provide positive pressure ventilation immediately after instillation of the drug.

Isoproterenol Hydrochloride

Aerosolized isoproterenol is widely accepted for treating bronchospasm, and its use is based on the drug's local, rather than systemic, effects. Clinical experience with endotracheal instillation of isoproterenol for its systemic effects is limited. Animal data

derived from both rats and dogs suggest that isoproterenol is well absorbed when administered endotracheally, but there are no data in humans. However attractive, endotracheal instillation of isoproterenol for either cardiac or hemodynamic effects should not be considered.

Bretylium Tosylate

Little evidence is available to suggest that bretylium tosylate is effective when administered endotracheally. Limited animal data indicate poor absorption in anesthetized dogs. Given the paucity of information, this route of administration cannot be recommended at this time.

Diazepam

Although at least one animal study suggests that diazepam is well absorbed when administered endotracheally, the solution used was not the commercially available one. The commercially available solution has a relatively high pH and contains propylene glycol and alcohol. This route of administration cannot be recommended for diazepam until such time as more clinical information becomes available.

The drugs outlined in Table 1 represent a small number of the agents used in cardiopulmonary emergencies. Antiarrhythmics, beta-adrenergic blocking agents, and alpha-adrenergic agents are but a few of the agents that deserve further study. With the exception of atropine and epinephrine, none of the drugs discussed have been administered on a chronic basis. As such, the endotracheal route should only be used as a temporizing method until venous access can be obtained.

ENDOTRACHEALLY ADMINISTERED DRUGS IN THE MANAGEMENT OF AIRWAY OBSTRUCTION

A discussion of the various etiologies of airway obstruction is beyond the scope of this chapter. I shall limit my discussion to the pharmacologic management of acute airway obstruction associated with extubation.

The underlying causes of acute airway obstruction immediately following extubation may be categorized as either edema and/or spasm or mechanical obstruction attributable to secretions. While many other causes can be found, most are not amenable to pharmacologic management. Edema and laryngospasm may be caused by surgical trauma, by trauma associated with a difficult intubation, or by endotracheal tube movement. Inspiratory or expiratory stridor may not become apparent for several hours after extubation.

The absence of an airleak when the balloon is deflated is commonly taken as a sign of tracheal edema. The absence of an airleak strongly suggests edema, whereas the presence of an airleak may or may not exclude the presence of edema or its subsequent appearance (i.e., several hours after the endotracheal tube is removed).

Epinephrine and corticosteroids remain the mainstays of pharmacologic management, along with the humidification of inspired oxygen. Racemic epinephrine administered by inhalation has historically been the preferred drug, although the racemic form has no distinct advantages over the levorotatory isomer. Epinephrine is traditionally administered therapeutically, rather than prophylactically. Although no controlled studies exist to support the prophylactic use of epinephrine, this use would appear to be a prudent maneuver in high risk patients or in patients who have previously developed clinically significant laryngotracheal edema.

The use of corticosteroids to prevent laryngotracheal edema remains a controversial issue. Animal studies, using subglottic pressure measurements as a marker, have suggested a lesser degree of edema and a more prompt resolution of edema when dexamethasone is administered intravenously at the time of extubation. The only available randomized human study examined the efficacy of dexamethasone in the prevention of laryngotracheal edema following bronchoscopy for foreign body removal in pediatric patients. No difference was found between the dexamethasone-treated group and the controls. However, the number of patients examined was small, and no attempt was made to examine other factors, such as the type of foreign body removed.

The use of corticosteroids is reasonable when clinically significant edema is suspected, even though confirmatory controlled data are not available. The short-term use of corticosteroids carries little risk, but promises potential benefit. I recommend using dexamethasone 4 mg intravenously prior to extubation and every 6 hours for two additional doses after removing the endotracheal tube. It is prudent to administer the first dose 4 to 6 hours prior to extubation since steroids may take up to 12 hours for maximal anti-inflammatory effect.

AEROSOLIZED AND ENDOTRACHEALLY INSTILLED ANTIBIOTICS

Antibiotics, administered either by instillation or by aerosolization, have been used in treating established gram-negative respiratory tract infections and as prophylaxis in high-risk mechanically ventilated patients. Although a selective form of drug delivery to the site of infection is theoretically attractive, this route is not without risk and remains controversial.

The theoretic advantages of endotracheally administered antibiotics are obvious and include a lower dose with fewer and less severe side effects (both locally and systemically) and higher antibiotic levels in infected tissue. Several clinical studies have shown that endotracheally instilled antibiotics combined with systemic antibiotics are effective for gram-negative respiratory tract infections.

Differences in efficacy between aerosolized and endotracheally instilled antibiotics have been claimed by some investigators, but no direct comparison between aerosolization and instillation has been conducted to my knowledge. Sputum antibiotic levels have been reported to be consistently higher after instillation than after aerosolization. In addition, several studies comparing intravenous administration of gentamycin to endotracheal instillation have shown higher levels of gentamycin in bronchial secretions with intravenous administration than with instillation. However, the clinical significance of these levels has not been established.

Prolonged administration of aerosolized antibiotics has also been used to prevent gram-negative infections in high-risk, mechanically ventilated patients. However, prophylactic aerosolization of antibiotics in high-risk patients should be strongly discouraged until additional data supporting its efficacy become available because prolonged application may result in the development of resistant strains of organisms.

The ideal agent for endotracheal administration should be nonirritating, nontoxic, and nonallergenic. The drug should be poorly absorbed into the systemic circulation, and tissue antibiotic levels sufficient to exceed the minimum inhibitory concentration for the infecting organism should be achievable. Table 2 lists the antibiotics that have been administered by both aerosolization and instillation in treating gram-negative respiratory tract infections. None of the agents listed possesses the ideal qualities for this mode of administration.

Experimentally induced gram-negative infections in mice have been successfully treated. However, clinical trials have not shown an enhanced efficacy of aerosolized antibiotic over either intravenous administration or the combination of the two modalities. This lack of clinical response may be related to the poor penetration of aerosolized antibiotic to the site of infection or to inactivation by mucosal enzymes. Available clinical data suggest that serious gram-negative infections are best treated with systemically administered antibiotics.

In summary, although the direct aerosolization and instillation of antibiotics for the treatment of respiratory tract infections remains a theoretically attractive mode of therapy, both alone and in combination with systemic treatment, no substantial data exist to support their widespread application. The endotra-

TABLE 2   Instilled and Aerosolized Antibiotics Used in Treating Gram-Negative Infections

Drug	Dose	Comments
Gentamicin	20–80 mg four times a day	Systemic therapy recommended, 20–40% decrease in FEV_1 reported in asthmatics
Colistin	500,000–1,500,000 units three to four times a day	Systemic therapy recommended
Carbenicillin	1.0 g four times a day along with probenecid	Systemic therapy recommended

cheal instillation of antibiotics may be attempted in selected patients who fail to respond to appropriate systemic therapy, but given the paucity of information, such use should still be considered experimental and the risk of toxicity must be kept in mind.

Suggested Reading

Biller HF, Harvey JE, Bone RC, Ogura JH. Laryngeal edema, an experimental study. Ann Otol Rhinol Laryngol 1970; 75:1084–1087.

Ghorayeb DY, Shikani AH. The use of dexamethasone in pediatric bronchoscopy. J Laryngol Otol 1985; 99:1127–1129.

Gough PA, Schuddekopf-Jordan N. A review of the therapeutic efficacy of aerosolized and endotracheally instilled antibiotics. Pharmacotherapy 1982; 2:367–377.

Hasegawa AJ. The endotracheal use of emergency drugs. Heart Lung 1986; 15:60–63.

Melby MJ, Raehl CL, Kreul JF. Pharmacokinetics of endotracheally administered lidocaine. Clin Pharm 1986; 5:228–231.

Raehl CL. Endotracheal drug therapy in cardiopulmonary resuscitation. Clin Pharm 1986; 5:572–579.

CHEST PHYSICAL THERAPY

COLLEEN M. KIGIN, M.S., RPT

Techniques of chest physical therapy, such as positioning to clear retained secretions and breathing exercises to optimize lung function, were first described in the late 1800s. In the early 1900s, MacMahon described a treatment program for war victims with chest injuries that included optimizing the breathing pattern, removing excess secretions, optimizing rib cage mobility, and general conditioning. These same goals remain the mainstays of modern chest physical therapy, and the methods used to achieve these goals have remained remarkably stable.

BASIC PRINCIPLES OF CHEST PHYSICAL THERAPY

Maximizing Ventilation

Maximizing ventilation consists of the following two activities: (1) preventing or reversing hypoventilation and (2) preventing or reversing respiratory muscle fatigue or failure (Table 1). Hypoventilation occurs commonly in the immediate postoperative period. Treatment is directed at maximizing inspired volume at regular intervals (e.g., every hour). The simple maneuver of a self-initiated maximal inspiration is the optimal treatment and is as effective as intermittent positive-pressure breathing (IPPB) or incentive spirometry. Success in maximizing inspiration is determined by the clinician's ability to decrease thoracic or abdominal splinting after surgery.

The same principles used to train skeletal or striated muscles are used in chest physical therapy to improve respiratory muscle strength and endurance. Maximizing the resting position and applying overload or graded resistance according to muscle tolerance can be achieved by using weights (e.g., sand bags), other resistance to the muscle belly (e.g., hand resistance over the diaphragm), or general conditioning. The most recent use of techniques, such as resistive breathing and hyperpnea, are discussed elsewhere in this text.

Facilitating Clearance of Secretions

Postural drainage, percussion, and vibration techniques are generally used to facilitate secretion re-moval (see Table 1). Positioning (e.g., postural drainage) can facilitate secretion flow in individuals with abnormal mucus clearance. The use of dramatic positioning, such as Trendelenburg, has caused some clinicians to be wary of these techniques, feeling that their patients would be adversely affected. Concerns regarding desaturation during Trendelenburg positioning are generally unfounded and can usually be easily averted with brief periods of supplemental oxygen. Also, modified positions to promote drainage of secretions are available for patients who do not tolerate the Trendelenburg position.

Positioning not only facilitates secretion clearance but can also be used to optimize oxygenation. Placing the "good" lung in the dependent position can cause oxygenation to improve significantly, as well as promote secretion clearance from the "bad" or affected lung.

Thick tenacious secretions can be cleared with greater ease by using manual techniques (e.g., percussion, vibration, shaking, and chest compression). Though these techniques have been widely used for a long time, the optimum force, duration, and frequency of delivery remain unclear.

Traditionally, clinicians have been taught to focus on percussion and have also been told to use a towel to protect the rib cage during percussion. The percussive force should be adequate to dislodge secretions in the lung, but should in no way damage the rib cage or thoracic musculature. When percussion is properly performed, the cupped hand is comfortable on the rib cage. Using towels to increase comfort should therefore be reserved for cachectic patients, who may lack adequate tissue to protect the ribs.

Vibration is an expiratory technique that calls upon the therapist's motor skills and which may be more effective because it is even more comfortable for the patient. The technique can also accompany or follow stretch and resistance to maximize ventilation. Optimizing ventilation while also dislodging secretions is the ideal combination to maximize the benefits of chest physical therapy.

Shaking is a more vigorous form of vibration, which has also been called rib springing. The basic premise is that shaking dislodges resistant or thick secretions not moved by vibration. Also, it is felt that combining shaking and vibration can improve thoracic mobility, particularly in the patient who experiences rib cage stiffening as the result of the underlying disease, such as emphysema.

Secretion clearance requires expectoration by a cough or a huff or by means of a suction catheter.

TABLE 1   Chest Physical Therapy Techniques

Techniques	*Goals*
Breathing exercises	Optimize inspiratory volume to prevent, reverse atelectasis
Maximal inspiratory volume	Optimize muscle function, including optimizing resting position of diaphragm
Diaphragmatic stretch/resistance	to decrease work of breathing
Pursed-lip breathing	Train respiratory muscles for strength and/or endurance
Positioning	Optimize secretion clearance
Full positioning for gravity	Optimize oxygenation
assistance	
Modified	
Manual techniques	Mobilize excess, retained secretions
Percussion	
Vibration	
Shaking	
Secretion clearance	Clear retained secretions
Cough, huff, suction	
General conditioning/training	Maximize joint mobility including upper extremity motion post thoracotomy
	Maximize functional activity

Cough is the traditional approach, which is optimized by maximal inspiration and a fast forced expulsion while the patient is upright or sitting. However, many patients with retained secretions are not able to cough effectively either because of muscle weakness or paralysis (e.g., in spinal cord-injury), pain, or structural changes of the lung (e.g., in emphysema). Patients with abdominal or thoracic muscle paralysis need external support to clear secretions adequately, either through abdominal compression or, if this fails, use of a suction catheter. Patients with pain or structural changes of the lung may find forced exhalation with an open glottis (or huffing) to be very effective.

Promoting General Conditioning, Optimizing Functional Capacity

The concept of rehabilitation is not a separate entity but in fact is integral to chest physical therapy (see Table 1). General conditioning is covered in the chapter entitled *Exercise Techniques During Pulmonary Rehabilitation*.

TREATMENT APPROACHES TO SPECIFIC DISEASES

Postoperative Pulmonary Complications

Like most medical interventions, the best approach to postoperative pulmonary complications is prevention. Preoperative therapy sessions have been shown to significantly decrease postoperative complications, because the patient is able to understand the importance of maximizing inspiratory volumes and to practice deep breathing without fear of postoperative pain (Table 2). Learning about normal thoracic and abdominal movement during inspiration also helps the patient to minimize splinting after surgery. In addition to preoperative sessions, postoperative treatment is essential and focuses on maximizing inspiration (including stretch and resistance applied to the rib cage to minimize splinting) and instruction in frequent position change. Patients are encouraged to breathe deeply every hour. Manual techniques are employed if atelectasis is accompanied by retained secretions. In our experience, the first postoperative treatment for the thoracic, cardiac, or upper abdominal patient includes positioning from side to side and using manual techniques along with maximal inspiration.

For the high-risk patient, treatment sessions should be given by well-trained therapists twice a day for the first few postoperative days. Treatment is discontinued once the patient is ambulatory and able to ventilate without splinting. In thoracic patients, attention to the upper extremity range of motion, as well as general posture while ambulating, is also necessary to prevent future musculoskeletal problems.

Treating the patient who already has atelectasis, whether intubated or not, requires a more aggressive approach. This patient may have a segmental or lobar collapse, frequently caused by retained secretions and plugging. The preferred strategy is to define the site of atelectasis carefully, to position the patient so that the atelectic lung can drain, and to use manual techniques to loosen or dislodge the secretions. As the obstructing secretions are mobilized, clinical signs of decreased or absent breath sounds can change dramatically, followed by improvements in oxygenation and in chest film.

Pneumonia

Although the value of chest physical therapy for accelerating recovery from pneumonia has been recently questioned, doubts have stemmed from the indiscriminate use of chest physical therapy techniques.

TABLE 2 Treatment Goals and Techniques for Acute Disease Entities

Disease Entity	Goals	Techniques and Considerations
Atelectasis	Prevent/reverse collapse	Thoracic stretch/resistance to maximize inspiration
		Therapist intervention twice/day to *prevent* atelectasis; more frequent intervention for patient with documented atelectasis
		Use of manual techniques if needed for secretion clearance
		Patient compliance to do hourly maximal inspirations between therapy sessions, with or without use of incentive spirometry
Pneumonia	Remove excess secretions	Use of positioning to maximize oxygenation, clear secretions (good lung down)
	Prevent/reverse atelectasis	Intervention of accompanying manual techniques when patient is unable to clear own secretions (nonambulatory, poor cough debilitated)
ARDS	Maximize oxygenation, mobilize retained secretions	Use positioning to optimize oxygenation (good lung down if unifocal/or use of prone)
		Use of positioning to optimize secretion clearance often requiring modified positioning

The goal of treatment is to help clear sputum or debris from the pneumonia as it collects in the airway (see Table 2). A secondary goal is to reverse or prevent atelectasis that accompanies hypoventilation during bed rest and immobility. For patients whose pneumonia does not require intubation, chest physical therapy techniques to clear secretions are only necessary when the patient cannot clear his or her own secretions.

Treating the mechanically ventilated patient presents a different problem. This person has a severely compromised respiratory system with abnormal mucociliary clearance. Whether or not the pneumonia has precipitated the intubation, the ability to clear secretions is greatly diminished. The patient should undergo frequent changes of position, with the "good" lung down as much as possible. This optimizes oxygenation as well as secretion clearance. The patient should also receive manual techniques to further remove secretions. Even clearing small amounts of secretions (e.g., 1 to 3 cc) has been accompanied by dramatic improvements in oxygenation. Treatments should be offered between every 2 and 6 hours, depending on the severity of the underlying problem.

Acute Respiratory Distress Syndrome and Thoracic Trauma

Acute respiratory distress syndrome can pose numerous problems in management. The patient requiring ventilation with high inspired oxygen levels, large amounts of positive end-expiratory pressure (PEEP), or high-frequency ventilation may seem too frail to be repositioned or to receive manual techniques. However, like hardier patients, these patients can respond dramatically to being positioned with a "good" lung down, if the process is primarily unifocal, or to being turned prone (see Table 2). Rolling the patient

from supine to prone may require a number of personnel, but can produce dramatic rises in arterial oxygenation.

The patient with adult respiratory distress syndrome (ARDS), whether supine, side-lying, or prone, can also benefit greatly from manual techniques, even when only small amounts of secretions are mobilized. When possible, the approach is to remove the patient from the ventilator and to bag the patient manually, using 100 percent oxygen administered through an Ambu bag. In this way, sustained inspiration can be used, the respiratory rate can be varied, and the patient can be allowed to cough between breaths. Using the Ambu bag also allows the therapist to coordinate vibration with exhalation.

Instilling 3 to 5 cc of saline before suctioning may stimulate a cough and provide a moist medium for removing secretions. Also, vibrating during suctioning can greatly facilitate secretion removal.

The patient who is on high-frequency ventilation or high levels of PEEP may not tolerate being removed from the ventilator, even for short periods of time. This patient is therefore treated while on the ventilator and suctioned with appropriate support at the end of the vibration or percussion. Patients with rib fractures or flail chests traditionally have been spared chest physical therapy for fear of worsening the injury. However, no patient is more prone to atelectasis than the one splinting due to rib fractures or the one with disrupted asynchronous thoracic motion. Treating the patient with simple rib fractures is fairly basic, with the patient instructed in maximal inspiration and minimal splinting of the fracture site. If retained secretions are a problem, then the patient can be safely rolled or repositioned appropriately, and percussion or vibration can be done to a site distal to the fracture. Contrary to common belief, vibration can be applied remarkably close to the fracture site without disrupting the fracture. Overall, the risk of disrupting the fracture is lower during controlled vibration than it is during a cough.

The patient with a severe anterior flail, such as from a steering-wheel injury, may be kept supine, and dramatic rolling may be discouraged. This patient is acutely ill, with major ventilatory impairment attributable to the flail, and is usually mechanically ventilated. The potential for retained secretions in the dependent regions of the lung is great. Though limited, effective positioning may still be possible with a partial roll. Vibrating by placing the hands under the posterior portion of the rib cage, while the patient is kept supine, can also improve secretion clearance.

Emphysema and Chronic Bronchitis

Patients with emphysema have an inefficient breathing pattern, resulting from alveolar hyperinflation and subsequent flattening of the diaphragm, as well as distortion of the rib cage. The work of breathing can be decreased by restoring the diaphragm's resting position; this restoration can be accomplished by stretching the diaphragm during exhalation (Table 3). It is also possible to improve diaphragmatic strength by applying gentle pressure over the upper abdomen during inspiration. Both the stretch and resistance can be provided and adjusted according to tolerance and need. Another helpful maneuver is pursed-lip breathing, which not only provides PEEP (thereby decreasing premature airway collapse), but also appears to optimize diaphragm position by causing the abdominal muscles to contract.

Classically, the patient with emphysema does not have retained secretions. However, many patients with emphysema also have chronic bronchitis, which is associated with excess secretions. Under usual circumstances, chronic bronchitics are able to clear excess secretions well, often by using bronchodilators, which enhance mucociliary clearance (see Table 3). However, if the volume of secretions is large or if the patient is acutely distressed by infection, then chest physical therapy techniques can be beneficial. Optimal positioning, including the Trendelenburg position, is employed. The patient is also instructed to huff during treatment; this seems to clear secretions with less energy expenditure.

The patient with emphysema and respiratory muscle insufficiency is frequently viewed as too dyspneic to tolerate any intervention. However, this patient can optimize diaphragmatic function and subsequently feel less dyspneic, as well as be able to subsequently increase general activity. Although the value of drainage and percussion is difficult to assess, chronic bronchitics often feel less dyspneic and congested after such treatment. Such patients can also be put on a home program of self-drainage and condi-

tioning and can clear secretions adequately without formal supervision or treatment. However, acute exacerbations may still require the therapist's attention. Like the patient with emphysema, the chronic bronchitic can also benefit from general conditioning, which is often incorporated into a pulmonary rehabilitation program. Though pulmonary function values do not change with this intervention, the increased exercise capacity and the decreased need for hospitalization are valuable benefits.

Bronchiectasis

The constant production of large amounts of mucopurulent secretions in bronchiectasis requires aggressive treatment. Postural drainage, huffing, and percussion are essential components of routine care and can often be performed by the patient with minimal help from family members (see Table 3). Clearing secretions early in the morning often allows the patient with bronchiectasis to participate in routine activities without becoming embarrassed by constant coughing to clear secretions. The required frequency of treatments and the need for help from the therapist are evident from the volume of secretions and the success at self-treatment. During an exacerbation, even the most self-reliant patient requires a therapist's attention to clear secretions while minimizing energy expenditure. Finally, the vigorous coughing with bronchiectasis and the inflammation itself may result in hemoptysis. Blood-streaked sputum should not cause alarm, but treatment should be discontinued if frank hemoptysis occurs and resumed once the hemoptysis has resolved.

Cystic Fibrosis

Patients with cystic fibrosis may experience even more secretions than patients with bronchiectasis. It is useful to initiate chest physical therapy at the initial diagnosis, when the treatment goal is routine clearance of excess retained secretions, thereby minimizing the potential for infection and secondary processes, such as bronchiectasis (see Table 3). Self-treatment has received increased attention and is especially valuable for the college-aged patient and for others responsible for more self-care. General conditioning and upper extremity activity may greatly decrease the need for actual drainage sessions.

Aggressive drainage is essential for the patient hospitalized with a secondary infection, and such patients should be instructed in periodic maximal inspirations, in addition to controlled coughing or huffing during the treatment period. Once stable, patients should also be instructed in a conditioning program, including instructions for home conditioning after discharge.

TABLE 3 Treatment Goals and Techniques for Chronic Disease Entities

Disease Entity	Goals	Techniques and Considerations
Emphysema	Decrease work of breathing, maximize activity	Maximize resting position and contraction of diaphragm through stretch/resistance/pursed-lip breathing Maximize general conditioning
Chronic bronchitis	Mobilize secretions, maximize activity	Self-treatment/activity for secretion clearance Manual techniques to mobilize excess secretions Maximize general conditioning
Bronchiectasis	Mobilize secretions, maximize activity	Frequent use of manual techniques (incorporate self-treatment) to clear large volume of secretions Maximize general conditioning
Cystic fibrosis	Mobilize secretions, maximize strength/endurance	Frequent clearance of secretions throughout lifetime; promotion of self-treatment in conjunction with therapist/family treatment General exercise conditioning potentially including respiratory muscle training, or upper extremity training
Asthma	Decrease anxiety, work of breathing, mobilize secretions	Positioning, tactile stimuli to decrease work of breathing; modified positionings, manual techniques to tolerance to facilitate secretion removal (skill of therapist imperative)
Restrictive lung disease	Maximize thoracic mobility/activity	Maintain mobility of thorax through thoracic muscle training Minimize sensation of dyspnea, maintain functional activity Manual techniques to mobilize secretions, even with small amounts of secretions
Rib fracture/flail chest	Prevent/reverse atelectasis, mobilize retained secretions	Maximizing inspiratory volume may be sufficient for the noncomplicated rib fracture Positioning to optimize oxygen and secretion flow may be contraindicated with unstable flail; use a partial roll or treat supine Percussion and vibration performed distal to site of fracture without fracture disruption (skill of therapist imperative) Vibration to the posterior chest with the flail patient supine
Abscess	Mobilize secretions	Manual techniques/full positioning to mobilize secretions Attention to potential of "flooding" with quick clearance of abscess
Spinal cord injury	Maximize ventilation, mobilize secretions	Inspiratory muscle training (e.g., weights) Manual techniques followed by abdominal support during coughing/suctioning ("quad cough")

Although patients with cystic fibrosis are prone to hemoptysis, slight blood-streaked or blood-tinged sputum does not warrant discontinuing therapy. On the other hand, frank hemoptysis is potentially life threatening and therapy should be discontinued until the hemoptysis subsides. At our institution, therapy is begun 12 to 24 hours after frank hemoptysis with close observation of patient response.

Asthma

The treatment of asthma addresses the major physiologic causes of airflow obstruction, which include smooth muscle constriction, edema, and excess mucus production, including peripheral plugging. Although many clinicians recommend avoiding chest physical therapy in asthma for fear of exacerbating bronchoconstriction, the fact that peripheral plugging is a major problem with status asthmaticus leads us to favor the use of chest physical therapy in this setting.

Treatment should focus on decreasing the anxiety, and therefore the work of breathing and modified positioning, thereby minimizing dyspnea while mobilizing secretions (see Table 3). In the patient who presents to the emergency ward in acute distress, creating a quiet, controlled environment is a primary step after the patient has received fluids and bronchodilators. I have found that these patients can then respond better to verbal and tactile stimuli to establish a more controlled breathing pattern. This allows the patient to assume a modified drainage position, in which gentle percussion or vibration is used. Carefully evaluating breath sounds at the onset and during treatment allows the clinician to monitor wheezing or bronchoconstriction. If there is evidence of increased wheezing during treatment, the treatment is discontinued. Treatment may move out only a few mucus plugs, but there may be dramatic improvement, both in terms of perceived dyspnea and in arterial blood gas values. Short, frequent treatments are often best tolerated and most beneficial.

Attention to the mechanism of cough is also essential. A vigorous, uncontrolled cough often leads to a cough-like spasm with increased wheezing and no secretion clearance. A controlled cough using the huff technique is preferred.

Lung Abscess

The goal of treating the patient with an abscess is controlled drainage of fluid from the lung (see Table 3). Frequently, the bronchial airway near the abscess is edematous because of the infection, and the abscess may actually have little or no communication with the bronchial tree. As the edema subsides, prompted by appropriate drug therapy, the abscess fluid may be cleared. The patient is repositioned to allow specific drainage of the abscess, and the treatment proceeds with the usual evaluation and use of manual techniques to facilitate secretion clearance. Chest radiograms (to locate the abscess) may also be helpful for exact positioning and drainage. Clinical and radiographic assessment (e.g., change in the air-fluid level) allow clinicians to monitor the success of the drug and drainage treatment.

The abscess may suddenly communicate with the bronchial tree and drain a large amount of fluid in the airway. Although this is rare, recognition is important and patients should be immediately positioned so that the abscess is in a gravity-dependent position. This localizes drainage into one area of the lung and allows adequate ventilation to the remaining areas.

Restrictive Lung Disease

The patient with restrictive lung disease may have either chest-wall deformity or interstitial lung disease. With chest-wall deformity, chest physical therapy should begin early in the course, with the goals of minimizing musculoskeletal deformity by mobilizing the chest and strengthening the trunk muscles (see Table 3).

Patients with interstitial lung disease (e.g., pneumoconiosis) do not generally retain large amounts of secretions but have extreme dyspnea as the disease process progresses. Training the patient to gain some control over the sensation of dyspnea, through relaxation and optimal breathing patterns, and to maintain activity may be the best available therapy.

Spinal Cord Injuries

A spinal cord injury results in a decrease in respiratory capacity, as well as a marked decrease in the expulsive force in a cough. Maximizing inspiratory volumes from the outset and mobilizing retained secretions, including abdominal support during cough, can minimize respiratory complications (see Table 3). Training the inspiratory muscles can increase the vital capacity and can decrease hospitalization time (as compared to patients not offered inspiratory muscle training).

Suggested Reading

Kigin CM. Advances in chest physical therapy. In: O'Donohue WJ Jr, ed. Current advances in respiratory care. Park Ridge, IL: American College of Chest Physicians, 1984:37.

Mackenzie CF, Ciesla N, Imle PC, Klemic N. Chest physiotherapy in the intensive care unit. Baltimore: Williams & Wilkins, 1981.

Zadai CC. Physical therapy for the acutely ill medical patient. Phys Ther 1981; 61(12):1746–1754.

AIRWAY APPLIANCES AND MANAGEMENT

DONNA J. WILSON, R.N., RRT

Airway management is an essential part of respiratory care. Although the importance of airway management has been recognized for several decades, many health care practitioners are unfamiliar with many of the appliances available. This chapter describes the appliances and techniques commonly used in acute and chronic airway management. The variety of tube styles available for individualized patient selection, as well as the assessment and ongoing evaluation of the airway, are addressed. Several problems such as air leak, stomal infection, and tracheal pathology are also described and suggestions are made for their management.

ENDOTRACHEAL AIRWAYS

Endotracheal intubation is performed by either the oral or the nasal route. The indications for endotracheal intubation are (1) to provide access for positive pressure ventilation, (2) to protect the airway from aspiration, (3) to remove tracheobronchial secretions, and (4) to relieve airway obstruction. Adult endotracheal tubes are available in full and half sizes ranging from 6 to 10 mm internal diameter (ID). Single-use polyvinyl chloride tubes are adequate for most purposes as long as they have a high-volume, low-pressure cuff. For oral intubation, an 8, 8.5, or 9 mm ID tube is used for men and a 7, 7.5, or 8 mm ID tube is used for women. One-half-size smaller tubes are usually used for nasal intubations. With the difficult-to-intubate patient, the endotrol tube (National Catheter, Argyle, NY) is extremely useful. It has a ring loop at the operator end, which moves the tip of the tube anteriorly when the loop is pulled. I have found this tube useful in blind nasal intubations, especially when the neck cannot be manipulated.

There are clear advantages and disadvantages to both oral and nasal intubation, which are summarized in Table 1. Tube selection is generally based on patient assessment and the relative advantages and disadvantages in each case.

In emergency situations, oral endotracheal tubes are normally used because of the speed and ease of their placement. In addition, a larger tube can be placed orally so that suctioning and access for bronchoscopy are not limited. The primary disadvantage of oral endotracheal tubes is patient intolerance, due to stimulation of the gag reflex. They also stimulate the production of more saliva and make it more difficult for patients to swallow than do nasal tubes. Thus, self-extubation is observed more frequently with oral than with nasal tubes.

When nasal tubes can be placed blindly, complications of direct laryngoscopy can be avoided. When using a nasal tube it is suggested that the softest and smallest-bore nasogastric tube possible be used to prevent a tracheoesophageal fistula. With a nasal tube in place, oral hygiene can be done more effectively and patients can communicate by mouthing words. If drainage is observed from the nose, a culture should be performed. When patients complain of an earache, sinusitis or otitis should be suspected and the nasal tube should be replaced by an oral tube, or a tracheostomy tube should be considered.

Many of the complications of oral or nasal endotracheal tubes can be avoided by careful observation and assessment by respiratory care personnel. One should understand and be able to recognize the following problems quickly: (1) esophageal intubation, (2) right main stem bronchus intubation, (3) kinking or obstruction of the tube, and (4) altered position of the tube. If the tube is high, the cuff may extrude through the vocal cords, requiring large volumes for cuff seal, or if the tip of the tube is at the carina, the patient may buck with each positive-pressure breath.

INDICATIONS FOR TRACHEOSTOMY TUBES

Tracheostomy was first performed by the ancient Egyptians (3,000 B.C.) and is a surgical procedure for placement of a metal or plastic tube into the trachea. A tracheostomy tube is the airway of choice for long-term airway maintenance, airway protection, pulmonary toilet, and positive-pressure ventilation.

When should an endotracheal tube be replaced with a tracheostomy tube? A frequent response to this question is, after 12 to 14 days of endotracheal intubation. However, I have observed various clinical circumstances in which longer periods of endotracheal intubation were required without incident. In one patient, a tracheostomy was contraindicated because of radiation therapy to the neck region. Endotracheal intubation lasted $2\frac{1}{2}$ months. In a second case, a burn patient required nasotracheal intubation for 3 months. At the time of extubation neither patient experienced any complications of long-term endotracheal intubation. Thus, the decision to perform a tracheostomy

TABLE 1 **Advantages and Disadvantages of Various Airway Appliances**

Type	Advantages	Disadvantages
Oral endotracheal tube	Easy to insert Large bore; work of breathing less Shorter length; easier to suction Less acute angle; less likely to kink	Requires laryngoscopy Easily dislodged Poorly tolerated by some patients Patients require more sedation Occluded by patient biting tube Oral hygiene difficult Patient has difficulty swallowing Unable to communicate Lip laceration Difficult to stabilize Inadvertent extubation common Laryngeal pathology
Nasal endotracheal tube	Easily secured Tolerated better by patient Insert blindly when neck motion or visualization is limited Allow for oral hygiene Able to swallow Requires less sedation Communication; mouthing of words	Skilled personnel for placement Nasal passageway limits size of tube Tube kinking due to curvature Inability to drain sinuses; sinusitis Obstruction of eustachian tube; otitis media Nasal soft tissue injury Laryngeal pathology

Tracheostomy tube	Most comfortable
	Easiest to suction
	Communication; mouthing words, talking
	    or fenestrated tracheostomy tubes
	Ability to swallow
	Reinsertion of trach tube relatively easy
	    with mature stoma
	No laryngeal injury
		Surgical procedure
		Complications postsurgery
		    bleeding
		    pneumothorax
		    subcutaneous emphysema
		    infection
		Posterior tracheal wall rupture during
		    insertion
		False passage in subcutaneous tissue
		Stenosis, stoma; cuff
		Granulation tissue formation
		Innominate artery erosion

should be individualized. Factors to be considered include tolerance of the endotracheal tube, the need for a long-term artificial airway or mechanical ventilation, bronchial hygiene, and the complications of either airway.

My general approach in patients who are intubated for longer than 10 days is to begin evaluation for tracheostomy tube placement, assessing all the advantages and disadvantages of each airway in view of the patient's present illness. I am not reluctant, however, to maintain an endotracheal tube if at each assessment it appears that the airway will be required for only a few more days.

I particularly believe that a tracheostomy tube is the preferred airway in patients who are difficult to wean from mechanical ventilation. The tracheostomy tube is more comfortable, is shorter, and has a less acute curvature than an endotracheal tube. Therefore, it creates less resistance to airflow and the passage of a suction catheter. Patients can communicate by mouthing words and may even talk with a "talking" tracheostomy tube or with a fenestrated tracheostomy tube. Most patients have the ability to swallow. Rein-

sertion of a tracheostomy tube is relatively easy once a permanent track has been established. However, accidental extubation of an endotracheal tube normally creates a clinical emergency. Today, we are sending more patients home with permanent tracheostomy tubes than ever before. These airways are well tolerated for months to years and do not require the services of an acute care facility.

The disadvantages of tracheostomy tube placement include hemorrhage, pneumothorax, incisional infection, and subcutaneous emphysema. The morbidity and mortality of this procedure increase if it is done on an emergency basis, whereas severe complications of endotracheal intubation are unusual.

ANATOMY OF THE TRACHEOSTOMY TUBE

Presently, tracheostomy tubes come in a wide variety of types. They differ in their rigidity, neck flange (plate), tube length, internal and external diameter, the angle from the neck flange to the tip of the tube, and cuff design.

Rigidity

The rigidity of the tube is determined by its composition. The metal tubes are stainless steel or sterling silver and thus inflexible; the former are more common. Most tubes are made of a thermoplastic polymer, polyvinyl chloride (PVC), and their stiffness ranges from hard to soft, depending on the composition of the PVC. There are also Silastic and silicone tracheostomy tubes, which are very soft, flexible, and least irritating to the tracheal tissue. The rigidity of a tube is important, because the more rigid the tube, the greater its tendency to cause mucosal trauma and increase the risk of tracheal wall perforation both during insertion and while the tube is in place. The soft, pliable, and flexible tubes conform easily to extreme neck shapes and positions.

Neck Flange

There are several designs of neck flanges. The most common is a small solid-surface flange with openings for trach ties. Shiley (Irvine, CA) makes a swivel neck plate that allows conformity to the individual's neck anatomy. A wing flange provided by Portex, Inc. (Wilmington, MA) maintains stability of the tube by holding the flange flush with the neck, preventing excessive movement of the tube. There are adjustable flanges available by National Catheter Mallinckrodt Inc. (Argyle, NY) and Rüsch, Inc. (New York, NY) that allow the length of the tracheostomy tube to be varied. Neck plate type desired is normally a matter of personal preference. I believe that the small, rigid, solid flanges can cut into the patient's neck, causing irritation around the stomal area. Occasionally, adjustable flanges are difficult to secure and very large flanges may also cause irritation. Flange type should be individualized to the patient based on anatomy.

Size

Sizes of various tracheostomy tubes are listed in Table 1. The ID of tracheostomy tubes is identical to that of endotracheal tubes and ranges from 5 to 10 mm in adults. The wall thickness of most tubes is 3 mm. The size of each tracheostomy tube is located on its neck flange. The Shiley and Jackson (Pilling, Fort Washington, PA) tracheostomy tubes are sized by the English method as well as the internal and external diameters; for example, a Shiley No. 6 tracheostomy tube has a 7 mm ID.

Length

Another important aspect of tracheostomy tube design is the length of the tube. Most do not realize that the smaller the ID of a tube, the shorter its length; also, tube lengths vary among companies. The lengths of standard 7 to 10 mm ID tubes are given in Table 2. For years, if a long tube was necessary, one had to use a tube with a larger internal diameter or make one from an endotracheal tube and an adjustable flange. Presently, various companies make extra-long tubes in sizes 7 to 10 mm ID. The Portex extra-long tracheostomy tube has an increased distance from the flange to the bend and then drops fairly vertically. This tube is used in patients with a short bull neck, obese patients, or those with tumors of the neck. The Shiley single-cannula long tracheostomy tube has a shorter distance from the flange to its circular, less vertical bend. The need for this tube is normally determined during surgery or when problems exist in sealing a standard tube because of anatomic variation.

Cuff

Most of the currently used tubes have thin-walled, soft, and compliant cuffs that are cylindrical or sausage shaped, of high volume, applying low pressure to the tracheal wall if properly used. However, design does not ensure that low pressure is maintained if cuffs are overinflated. A general clinical rule is to maintain the cuff seal at the lowest possible volume and pressure required (minimal occlusive volume or minimal leak volume). Cuff volumes and pressures larger than necessary can cause a wide spectrum of tracheal damage that is well documented in the literature. I believe that the cuff pressure should be maintained less than 25 mm Hg in order to ensure that the blood flow is maintained to the tracheal mucosa. The tracheal ar-

TABLE 2   Sizes of Tracheostomy Tubes

Cuffless tubes (Shiley/Jackson)		Cuffed tubes (Portex/Shiley/Rusch/NCC/Bivona)— internal diameter	Olympic buttons—Outer diameter of cuffed tube
4	4	5 mm	8.5 mm
	5	6 mm	9.0 mm
6	6	7 mm	10.0 mm
	7	8 mm	11.0 mm
8	8	9 mm	12.0 mm
	9	10 mm	13.3 mm

terial tissue perfusion pressure in a normotensive patient has been estimated at about 30 mm Hg.

Most tracheostomy tubes come with an obturator for insertion unless the tracheostomy tube has a Magill tip. Single and double cannula tubes have a 15-mm adapter for connection to respiratory care equipment. Most single cannula tubes do not have permanent inner cannulas. Occasionally, some have disposable inner cannulas. The double-cannula tracheostomy tube has an inner cannula with a 15-mm adapter. Normally, a swivel adapter is attached to the cannula to facilitate attachment to respiratory care equipment and minimize torque on the airway.

MODIFIED TRACHEOSTOMY TUBES

Several modifications of standard tracheostomy tubes are available. Bivona Surgical Inc. (Gary, IN) makes the Kamen-Wilkinson fome cuf tracheostomy tube, which is also longer than the standard tube. The foam cuff, which is covered with silicone, spontaneously expands when exposed to atmospheric pressure. To insert the tube, air is removed from the cuff (about 35 ml). Notably, a cuff leak often occurs in patients on mechanical ventilation with peak inspiratory pressures greater than 45 cm H_2O. Air can be added to maintain a seal, but the low pressure advantage may be lost; thus, the cuff pressure should be monitored. Cuff rupture from overinflation releases foam into the airway, generally requiring bronchoscopy for retrieval.

Rüsch makes a tracheostomy tube similar to the armored endotracheal tube employed by anesthetists in head and neck surgery. This tube works particularly well in patients with short, fat necks or abnormal anatomy. The length of this tube can be changed with the adjustable flange. The tube is secured by tightening the adjustable flange; however, care must be taken not to compress and obstruct the inflation line of the pilot balloon as the flange is secured. Compression of the pilot balloon inflation line may also cause a falsely high intracuff pressure to be recorded. If the flange is insufficiently tightened, the tube may slide backward and forward; therefore, the tube should be marked just exterior to the flange to note any displacement.

TALKING AND FENESTRATED TRACHEOSTOMY TUBES

Talking tracheal appliances, such as fenestrated and "talking" tracheostomy tubes, are used to allow chronically ventilated patients to speak. Although many of these appliances are now available, most health care practitioners are unfamiliar with them. As a result, chronically ventilated patients who are candidates for talking appliances may go without them.

Talking Tubes

Portex and National Catheter manufacture cuffed talking tracheostomy tubes in sizes 7, 8, and 9 mm ID (Fig. 1). These tubes allow patients, with practice, to speak while keeping the cuff sealed and positive airway pressure maintained. Thus, ventilation and speaking are independent. A small tube (separate from the cuff inflation tube) is set into the outer wall of the airway, ending with an opening just above the cuff. At the proximal end, there is a two-way connector that is attached to a gas source at a flow rate of 4 to 8 L per minute. This flow exits from the opening above the cuff in the trachea when the two-way connector is occluded and forces gas through the vocal cords, allowing vocalization. Each patient is evaluated to see what liter flow is needed to make the voice audible. It is important to explain to the patient that the voice will sound different from normal, usually lower pitched. If the flow is too high, patients may find it irritating and complain of a sore throat. Instruct patients to speak in short sentences because with long sentences the voice will drift off to a whisper, owing to the continuous flow of gas through the vocal cords. It is critical to distinguish the cuff port from the talking (gas flow) port (they are clearly marked by the manufacturer) because if gas flow enters the cuff it will rupture, making an emergency tracheostomy tube change necessary. If the gas flow port becomes occluded with secretions it can be cleaned with a 50–50 solution of saline and acetylcysteine (Mucomyst).

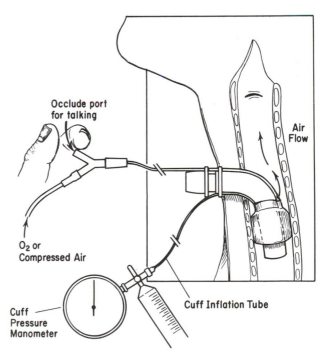

Figure 1 Talking tracheostomy tube.

Once this tube is placed, wait 2 days before instructing the patient in its use so that the stoma track can close down around the tube, preventing the flow of gas from the talk port from extruding into the pretracheal tissue or out the stoma. If this continues to happen after a few days, a larger tube is indicated. Because the larger tube is also a longer tube, the internal tip of the talking port may now be located below the anterior tracheal stoma to allow the patient to speak better.

If there is a history of aspiration, it can be evaluated by suctioning from the talking port, thus removing secretions sitting on the cuff. To monitor this closely, give the patient ice chips with five to six drops of methylene blue by mouth with the tracheostomy tube cuff inflated. (Use only a small quantity of methylene blue; it is very bitter.) Suction via the talk port. Collecting the contents in a sputum trap will help predict the degree of potential aspiration.

Fenestrated Tubes

Shiley and Portex produce a cuffed fenestrated tracheostomy tube in sizes 5, 7, 8, and 9 mm ID (Fig. 2). This is a standard cuffed tracheostomy tube with a precut fenestration, inner cannula, and plug. The fenestration is a window cut into the outer cannula. When the fenestration is open (removal of inner cannula, plugged outer cannula) and the cuff deflated, the patient may breathe spontaneously, cough, and phonate via the upper airway. This tube does not allow the patient to speak if positive pressure is applied to the airway. When the fenestration is closed (inner cannula in place and plug removed) and the cuff is inflated, mechanical ventilation and airway protection is provided. Patients must be able to protect their airway whenever a fenestrated tube is employed. The administration of methylene blue with the cuff deflated is used to determine the patient's ability to protect the airway. If methylene blue can be suctioned from the lower airway after swallowing, a fenestrated tube should not be placed.

If it is determined that airway protection is adequate and a fenestrated tube is to be employed, it is critical to ensure that the fenestration lies entirely within the lumen of the trachea, that is, it does not touch the tracheal wall. One method of determining this is an overexposed x-ray film of the lateral neck. The location of the fenestration is determined by measuring the distance between the tracheal air column and skin. At the bedside, measurements with sterile pipe cleaners can determine proper location of the fenestration (Figs. 3 and 4). Measurements from skin to the anterior and posterior tracheal wall are made. These measurements determine where on the tracheostomy tube the area of the fenestration should lie. Before inserting the fenestrated tube, cover the stoma with

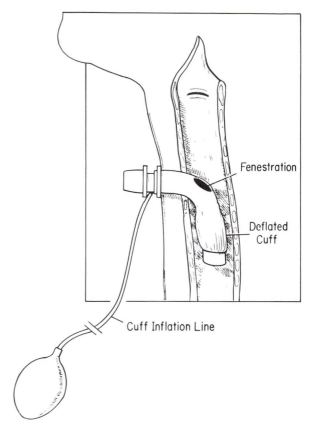

Figure 2 Proper positioning of a cuffed fenestrated tracheostomy tube in the trachea. The tube is plugged with the fenestration open and the cuff deflated to allow the patient to breathe and speak normally.

gauze to evaluate the upper airway. Assess the patient's breathing pattern, voice, and cough. If any stridor is heard the fenestrated tube should not be placed and the patient's upper airway should be evaluated by otolaryngology or by thoracic surgery. If the fenestration is not in proper position, granulation tissue can grow into the fenestration causing bleeding during placement and removal of the inner cannula and possible airway obstruction.

During use of the fenestration, the inner cannula is removed and the cuff is deflated. Deflation yields a greater cross-sectional area for airflow, thereby decreasing airway resistance. The tube is plugged to allow vocalization by forcing gas flow past the vocal cords. If respiratory distress occurs, the inner cannula is reinserted and the cuff inflated to allow positive-pressure ventilation to be applied.

In the literature and from my clinical experience, factory precut fenestrated tubes fit only 50 percent of the time. If the distance between skin and anterior tracheal wall is greater than 34 mm, precut tubes generally do not fit correctly. If this occurs, the fenestration would be located in the pretracheal tissue. Thus,

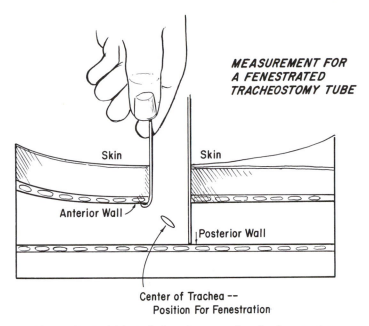

Figure 3 Bedside technique in measuring for fenestration.

a customized fenestrated tube is required. Fenestrated tubes may be made of plastic or metal. Metal has the advantage of being less structurally weakened by the placement of the fenestration. However, metal tubes are generally cuffless. Plastic tubes are normally used for custom fenestration because they can be cut at the bedside or by the medical engineering department. If plastic tubes are customized, it is important to ensure a smooth surface and structural integrity. Generally, the size of the fenestration should not be larger than the lumen of the tracheostomy tube, or approximately 8 to 10 mm in length and 6 to 8 mm in width. The tube is placed and then examined by bronchoscopy or by direct vision with a light source.

OTHER AIRWAY APPLIANCES

Olympic Trach Button

The purpose of a trach button (Olympic Medical, Seattle, WA) is to maintain the patency of the tracheostomy stoma (Fig. 5). It allows for tracheal suction-

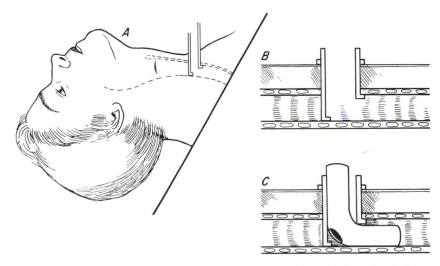

Figure 4 Measurement for fenestration. *A*, Hyperextend head for good visualization. *B*, Bedside measurements with sterile pipe cleaners, anterior and posterior wall to skin measurement. *C*, Measurements determine location of fenestration on tracheostomy tube.

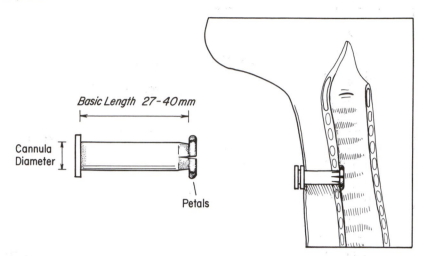

Figure 5 Olympic trach button. Cannula length is available in two sizes to be adapted to fit most patients. The button maintains stoma patency and allows access for suctioning and normal respiration.

ing and access for emergency ventilation. The closure plug on the button allows for normal respiration and phonation. The Olympic button comes in both a 27 mm and a 40 mm length and therefore can be adapted to fit almost any patient. The cannula length within the stoma track can be reduced by adding spacer rings. Outer diameters of 9, 10, 11, 12, and 13 mm are available. Before a tracheostomy button is placed, the methylene blue swallowing test should be performed. In addition, the chest x-ray film should show no progressive infiltrates and less than 40 percent oxygen should be required.

To place the Olympic tracheostomy button, remove the tracheostomy tube. Then measure the stoma length by placing a small hooked pipe cleaner into the stoma. Pull the pipe cleaner back until the hook is against the anterior tracheal wall. Mark the pipe cleaner at the skin surface (Fig. 6). The length of the cannula is then determined by holding the pipe cleaner next to the cannula. The cannula length must not exceed that of the stoma track; otherwise the cannula can slip backward into the trachea, causing obstruction of the airway. The button is lubricated and placed into the stoma. The closure plug is then inserted. The closure plug causes the petals of the button to flare and locks the button against the anterior wall of the trachea. Once the button is in place, rotate it 180 degrees to make sure that it does not adhere to tissue. Then remove the closure plug and with a light source ensure that no obstruction exists around the pedicles of the button. If resistance to rotation is encountered, the button may be malpositioned. If the button appears to be protruding, remove the closure plug and apply gentle pressure to the outer cannula to reposition the button flush with the neck. Improper positioning may limit function and increase the risk that the trach button will inadvertently come out of the stoma.

Once the button is inserted, patients should be encouraged to cough and deep-breathe to mobilize secretions. If difficulty mobilizing secretions is encountered, suction through the Olympic button. Preoxygenate, remove the closure plug, and suction normally. Between passes of the catheter, instruct the patient to breathe deeply from an oxygen mask while you occlude the button.

The Olympic button may be left in place for sev-

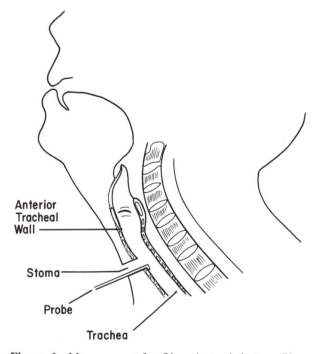

Figure 6 Measurement for Olympic trach button. Place probe through stoma and hook onto anterior tracheal wall, then mark at skin to determine length of stoma track.

eral days to several weeks. I have a large series of patients who have used the button with minimal complications. Many patients go home with the button in place.

Montgomery Silicone Tracheal Cannula

The tracheal cannula (Boston Medical Products, Waltham, MA) is also used to maintain stoma patency (Fig. 7). As with the Olympic button, it does not project into the trachea but extends only from the anterior tracheal wall to the skin. The cannula is flexible and is constructed of silicone, so it does not cause tissue irritation. The cannula comes only in an 8 mm ID size. Its components are the cannula, closure plug, flange, and ring washers to adjust cannula length. The cannula is normally placed with a curved hemostat, either in the operating room or at the bedside. After insertion, the cannula is pulled anteriorly until the inner flange fits snugly against the anterior tracheal wall. If the cannula protrudes from the skin it can be cut, followed by insertion of the closure plug.

The Montgomery tracheal cannula also comes with a one-way speaking valve. This valve is very easy to clean and is durable.

T-Tube

The T-tube (Hood Laboratories, Pembroke, MA) is made of silicone and used to maintain dilatation of the trachea (Fig. 8). It can serve both as a stent and as a tracheostomy tube. Its ends are tapered to prevent

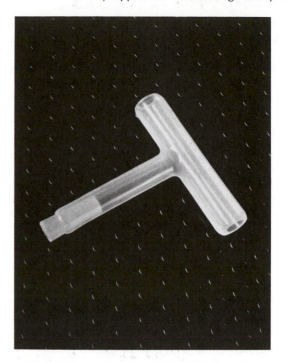

Figure 8 T-tube serves as a tracheal stent.

mucosal injury and mucus does not readily adhere to its smooth silicone surface. Frequent changing of the T-tube is not necessary, and it allows the patient to have normal respiration and phonation. The T-tube does not protect against aspiration, nor is it routinely used with positive-pressure ventilation.

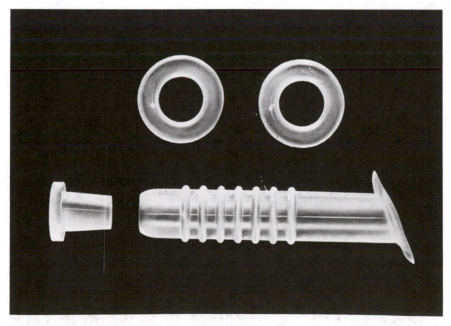

Figure 7 Montgomery long-term silicone tracheal cannula. Consists of outer cannula, closure plug, and washer to adjust cannula length; this maintains stoma patency.

Patients who are not candidates for tracheal reconstruction are primary users of this tube. It is often used as a palliative measure for patients with unresectable carcinomas of the trachea or in patients with temporary tracheal inflammation. The T-tube extends from just below the vocal cords to just above the carina, with an extension exiting the stoma that may be plugged for phonation.

The T-tube is placed in the operating room and requires constant humidification for the first week postoperatively. After the first week the T-tube is plugged, allowing normal respiration via the upper airway. Patients at home with T-tubes must regularly clean them with acetylcysteine (Mucomyst) and normal saline (Table 3).

COMMON PROBLEMS AND THEIR MANAGEMENT

Air Leak

In our experience, the most common cause of air leak in the patient with a tracheostomy tube is a crack or slow leak in the housing of the one-way inflation valve. If a visible crack is seen in the housing, cut off the valve and insert a butterfly or 20-gauge Intracath into the cut-off tubing and attach to a three-way stopcock. This will allow cuff inflation until the tube can be replaced.

When a tracheostomy is performed, it is important immediately to ensure a proper cuff inflation with appropriate gas volume. This normally ensures that the tube is of correct size and properly placed. Inability initially to seal a previously tested cuff may indicate that the tube is outside the trachea or is too small for the patient.

Rupture of a cuff is fairly uncommon. Lack of normal resistance to inflation of the cuff and an inability to feel the inflating cuff in the suprasternal notch normally are indicative of a rupture, which may be confirmed by absence of an inflated cuff on radiographic or bronchoscopic examination. If a cuff is necessary, the tube must be changed.

As previously described, longer tubes may be required for correct fit and to seal with normal cuff pressures. I have found that the Bivona foam cuff has a large surface area and may provide a seal when other tubes fail. If the Bivona foam cuff tube is not adequate, overinflating a standard cuff with 40 ml of air for 20 minutes prior to placement may provide a proper seal. This changes the compliance of the cuff, maintaining a low pressure in spite of a larger inflating volume.

Before changing a tube because of a leak, thoroughly examine the cuff volume and pressure and the tube position. For example, tubes are frequently pulled to one side by ventilator tubings, causing them to sit eccentrically within the trachea, preventing the cuff from sealing. An x-ray examination can determine the tube position as well as the presence and size of the cuff. Persistent leaks may indicate tracheomalacia or tracheoesophageal fistula and require further consultation.

Malposition

Malposition is difficult to separate from an air leak, because the former commonly causes the latter. As noted, a tube that is too small in diameter or too short may result in an air leak. Measurement of the distance to the anterior tracheal wall with the pipecleaner method described may help to determine whether one of the extra long tubes is required. A swivel attachment on tracheostomy tubes connected to ventilator tubing should decrease sideways pull on the tube. In addition to air leak, pulling on the tracheostomy tube can cause obstruction if the tip of the tube touches the posterior tracheal wall. Obstruction can also be caused by a tube that is grossly short or partially pulled out so that the tip falls on the back wall of the trachea. Notably, tracheostomy tubes do not have Murphy eyes, which are the side-facing holes at the tips of standard endotracheal tubes. Malposition may also contribute to unnecessary tracheal mucosal damage at the tube tip.

Peristomal Inflammation and Bleeding

I have found the following approach to peristomal inflammation to be useful. First, a bacterial culture of the area is performed. If the area is infected, wet-to-dry gauze dressings with povidone-iodine (Betadine) are applied every 4 hours. If the area is not infected, wet-to-dry dressings with saline are applied.

If bleeding occurs postoperatively, the area should be packed, coagulation rechecked, and the surgeon

TABLE 3   Length of Tracheostomy Tubes

	Portex Standard		*Portex Extra Long*	*Shiley Single Cannula*
Size				
7 mm ID	75 mm		84 mm	80 mm
8 mm ID	82 mm		95 mm	89 mm
9 mm ID	87 mm		106 mm	99 mm
10 mm ID	98 mm		—	105 mm

notified. Reexploration may be required. If bleeding occurs after the perioperative period, the surgeon should be notified immediately. It could be a result of erosion into the innominate artery, causing life-threatening hemorrhage.

Tube Replacement

It is my policy that the first tracheostomy tube change be performed by a physician. Equipment for ventilation, reintubation, and resuscitation should be at hand. Within the first postoperative week, the stomal tract may not be well established and the airway can be lost when the tracheostomy tube is removed. Some surgeons secure a flap of trachea anteriorly to secure a tract before it forms anatomically. Although this is probably helpful in the case of accidental extubation, I feel it does not ensure a patent stoma in the first postoperative week. If a tube is accidentally dislodged during the first week, one may gently attempt to replace it, but the effort should stop if resistance is encountered, because a false passageway can easily be created. The tube should be replaced as soon as possible because the stoma begins to heal and shrink with unpredictable speed.

After caring for many home mechanically ventilated patients, I have found that changes of cuffed tracheostomy tubes are normally not necessary more often than once every 3 to 4 weeks. During change, the tracheostomy tube should be inserted carefully to prevent laceration of the posterior tracheal wall. If the tube has been chronically deviated by ventilator tubing, the track may also be deviated, requiring a specific angle for insertion. Granulomas forming above and below the stoma or flaps of trachea may make recannulation difficult and necessitate use of a smaller diameter tube. If this is noticed, bronchoscopy may be required to evaluate airway patency and the integrity of the anterior tracheal wall. Finally, the string that secures the flange should be snug but allow a finger to pass easily underneath to prevent vascular compression.

Tracheomalacia

Tracheomalacia should be suspected if the cuff volume required for sealing progressively increases or if the cuff diameter is 1.5 times the tracheal diameter determined by anteroposterior x-ray examination. As a result, a larger tube may be required to maintain a low-pressure seal. When the patient is weaned from positive-pressure ventilation, surgical consultation should evaluate the need for stenting with a T-tube.

Tracheal Stenosis

Tracheal stenosis is most common at the site of the stoma and should not cause airway obstruction if a functioning tube is present. Tracheal stenosis or laryngeal obstruction from previous endotracheal intubation should also be kept in mind when the patient is being fitted with a stomal button or removal of the tracheostomy tube. In both cases the stoma should be occluded to ensure that the patient has a patent airway before a tube is permanently removed.

Tracheal Damage

Granulomas, either at the tracheostomy site or at the site of erosion by the tube tip, may be easily managed by bronchoscopic removal. Anterior, U-shaped stenosis at the stomal site or circumferential stenosis at the cuff site requires surgical excision with end-to-end tracheal anastomosis for definitive treatment.

A rare complication of tracheostomy is persistence of the stoma. This results from extensive local damage, unusually prolonged maintenance of a tracheostomy tube, or disease or treatment with depressed potential healing. The technique of closure consists of using the already healed tracheocutaneous junction and circumferentially inverting a small margin of skin around the persistent stoma to provide at once a fully epithelialized surface inside the trachea.

Suggested Reading

Harris RB. National survey of aseptic tracheostomy care techniques in hospitals with head and neck/ENT surgical departments. Cancer Nurs 1984; February: 23–32.

Heffner IE, Miller KS, Sahn SA. Tracheostomy in the intensive care unit, part 1: indications, technique, management. Chest 1986; 90:269–274.

Heffner JE, Miller KS, Sahn SA. Tracheostomy in the intensive care unit, part 2: complications. Chest 1986; 90:430–436.

Lewis FR, Schlobolm RN, Thomas AN. Prevention of complications from prolonged tracheal intubation. Am J Surg 1978; 135:452–457.

Long J, West G. Evaluation of the Olympic trach button as a precursor to tracheostomy tube removal. Respir Care 1980; 25:1242–1243.

Safar P, Grenvik A. Speaking cuffed tracheostomy tube. Crit Care Med 1975; 3(1):23–26.

Selecky PA. Tracheostomy: a review of present day indications, complications, and care. Heart Lung 1974; 3:272–283.

Snyder GM. Individualized placement of tracheostomy tube fenestration and in-situ examination with the fiberoptic laryngoscope. Respir Care 1983; 28:1294–1298.

Stauffer JL, Olsen DE, Petty TL. Complications and consequences of endotracheal intubation and tracheostomy. Am J Med 1981; 70:65–76.

Weber AL, Grillo HC. Tracheal stenosis: an analysis of 151 cases. Radiol Clin North Am 1978; 39:291–308.

SUCTIONING AND AIRWAY CARE

ROBERT L. WILKINS, M.A., RRT

Critically ill patients usually have one or more factors present that promote the retention of airway secretions. For example, artificial airways can interfere with the patient's ability to cough and contribute to the need for assistance in the removal of sputum. If proper airway care is not provided, secretions may be retained and result in atelectasis, hypoxemia, and pneumonia. Retained secretions may also increase airways resistance, increasing the work of breathing (WOB). This increase in the WOB can place added stress on an already compromised cardiopulmonary system. Providing proper airway care is a crucial part of respiratory care that must be performed by qualified individuals who understand its potential effects on the cardiopulmonary system.

SUCTIONING

Indications

It is our practice to suction patients only when clinically indicated. Suctioning according to a time schedule is inappropriate in most cases, except with neonates, because it exposes the patient to unnecessary risks. In neonates, routine suctioning is necessary to maintain the artificial airway patent. Because the airway in these patients has such a small diameter, it can easily and rapidly be obstructed by even a small accumulation of secretions.

Suctioning is normally indicated when coarse rales (crackles) are identified, with or without the aid of a stethoscope. Visible secretions near the opening of the artificial airway, coughing, and dyspnea also indicate that airway secretions have accumulated and need to be removed by suctioning. In mechanically ventilated patients, sudden unexplained increases in the peak inspiratory airway pressure may indicate that excessive airway secretions are present.

In certain situations, attempting to pass a suction catheter is of value in checking airway patency. In patients suddenly demonstrating signs of severe dyspnea and labored breathing, obstruction of the artificial airway should be considered. Attempting to pass a catheter can rapidly assess the patency of the arti-

ficial airway. If the catheter does not pass easily or at all, the airway has become obstructed by a herniated cuff, mucous plugs, a foreign body, or kinking of the airway. If continued attempts to pass the catheter, deflate the cuff, and reposition the airway fail to relieve the obstruction, the artificial airway should be removed and ventilation provided by bag and mask.

Suctioning should not be performed within 15 to 20 minutes prior to a scheduled blood gas sampling. In addition, suctioning should be avoided during periods of hemodynamic instability. Of course, the problems with retaining secretions must be weighed against the potential harm of suctioning in all cases.

Catheter Selection

Routine suctioning for the removal of airway secretions requires careful consideration of the catheter type and size. Numerous catheter designs are commercially available. Ideally, the best catheter is one that is effective in removal of secretions while minimizing tissue trauma. Conventional end-hole and side-hole catheters (Fig. 1A) pose the risk of tissue trauma, because they allow the bronchial mucosa to invaginate into the holes when the catheter tip contacts the airway wall. They are, however, effective at removing sputum.

The Argyle Aero-Flo (Fig. 1B) was designed with an end hole and numerous small side holes proximal to a flared ring to minimize tissue trauma. Although tissue trauma may be less with this catheter, the catheter appears to be less efficient than conventionally designed catheters in removing bronchial secretions. In addition, the distal ring adds significantly to the diameter of the catheter at the tip, making it more difficult and traumatic to insert.

For patients whose cardiovascular system is unstable, or for those on high levels of positive end-expiratory pressure (PEEP), the Trach-Care suction catheter system (Fig. 2) may be useful in minimizing the potential side effects of suctioning. This system is a self-contained device that is maintained in the ventilator circuit and used for 24 hours. It contains a catheter in a sealed plastic envelope with external suction controls that allows aspiration of the patient's airway without interrupting ventilation. Use of gloves is not necessary because the catheter is advanced into the patient's airway using the external plastic envelope.

Use of the Coudé angle-tipped catheter (Fig. 1C) increases the success rate of selective cannulation of the left main stem bronchus. This also can be accomplished by turning the patient's head to the right dur-

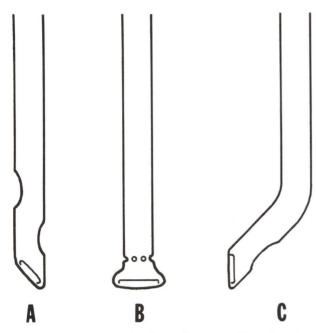

Figure 1 *A*, Conventional end-hole and side-hole catheter; *B*, Argyle Aero-Flo cathether; *C*, Coudé angle-tipped catheter.

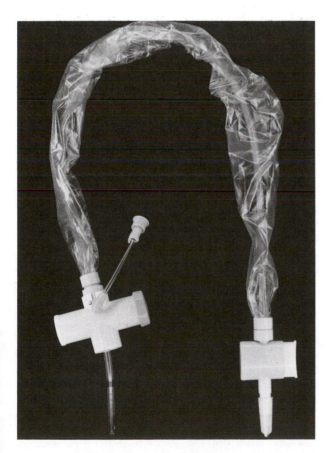

Figure 2 Trach-Care catheter.

ing insertion of the Coudé catheter. In infants and children, the angle of the main stem bronchi is more symmetrical than in adults and cannulation of the left bronchus should be no more difficult than entering the right bronchus.

The diameter of any suction catheter should not exceed one-half the internal diameter of the artificial airway. Catheters that exceed this optimal size promote evacuation of the gas distal to the catheter tip during aspiration and may increase the incidence of atelectasis. If the catheter diameter is too small, the efficiency of secretion removal is diminished, especially if secretions are thick. When sputum removal is difficult and of primary concern, it is my practice to use a larger catheter, up to two-thirds the internal diameter of the airway, for selective suctioning attempts.

Most suction catheters are sized in French units based on the outside catheter circumference in millimeters, whereas artificial airways are sized by internal diameter in millimeters. To determine the maximum size suction catheter to use safely, multiply the internal diameter of the airway in millimeters by 3 and divide the total by 2. For example, in a patient with an 8 mm airway:

$$\frac{(8 \times 3)}{(2)} = 12 \text{ F catheter}$$

Technique

Suctioning should always be performed as a sterile technique to prevent contamination of the patient's airway. This requires the use of sterile gloves and catheter. In addition, the suction catheter should be used only once and then discarded. Other equipment required includes sterile rinsing solutions and container, vacuum source, a hand resuscitator with 100 percent oxygen, and 5 to 10 ml syringe for injection of lavage solutions.

The vacuum pressure should be checked and adjusted, if necessary, prior to each suctioning procedure. If the vacuum is set too low, secretion removal is diminished, and if it is set too high, tissue trauma is likely. General guidelines are provided in Table 1. I recommend starting at the lower end of the range and making adjustments, if needed, according to the results.

TABLE 1 Vacuum Settings for Suctioning Patients Based on Age

Setting	Patients
60–80 mm Hg	Infants
80–120 mm Hg	Children
120–150 mm Hg	Adults

Once the equipment is at the bedside, good hand-washing technique with an appropriate antimicrobial preparation is important before suctioning. This simple step is helpful in reducing contamination of the patient's airways. It should be omitted only during emergency suctioning.

Prior to suctioning, the patient must be adequately preoxygenated because it is likely that oxygenation will decrease during the application of vacuum. If the patient's oxygenation status is already marginal, preoxygenation may avoid severe hypoxemia and its consequences. Preoxygenation can be achieved with either a hand resuscitator or with the ventilator if the patient is being mechanically ventilated.

If the ventilator is utilized to preoxygenate, ventilator washout time must be considered and may take as long as 2 minutes before an F_{IO_2} of 1.0 can be delivered. Hand resuscitators should always be set up to deliver 100 percent O_2. That is, sufficient gas reservoirs should be attached and liter flow set above 10 L per minute. The mechanical ventilator offers the advantage of delivering larger tidal volumes during preoxygenation than the volumes achieved with hand resuscitators. This can result in better oxygenation and help minimize suction-induced hypoxemia.

Practitioners using hand resuscitators must ensure that their technique is suitable for delivering adequate tidal volumes. In many cases, hyperinflation may not be achieved during use of the hand resuscitator. The hand resuscitator does allow a "feel" for the resistance to airflow and the presence of secretions.

Once the patient is preoxygenated, insert the catheter without vacuum until it is past the distal tip of the artificial airway and resistance is felt. At this point, pull the catheter back slightly prior to applying suction to prevent occlusion of a bronchus and collapse of a lobe or segment. Then apply intermittent suction while rotating the catheter during withdrawal. Rotating the catheter may help minimize airway damage while enhancing secretion removal.

The catheter should never be in the airway for more than 10 to 15 seconds during any suction attempt. In addition, the entire procedure should not result in the patient's ventilation and oxygenation being interrupted for more than 20 seconds.

Suctioning through a swivel adapter may result in smaller decreases in PaO_2 than suctioning with the gas delivery tubing removed from the airway, especially if the patient is on high levels of PEEP. In critically ill patients who are hemodynamically unstable, this technique may be especially useful in minimizing hypoxemia.

After the catheter is removed, immediately reoxygenate and hyperinflate the patient by ventilating with an elevated F_{IO_2} for at least six to ten breaths. Observe the patient's vital signs and electrocardiograph (ECG) monitor to identify the patient's status before repeating the suctioning process. If dysrhythmias or other signs of distress are present, discontinue the suctioning process and monitor the patient closely while ensuring adequate oxygenation.

If complications are not identified, the procedure is repeated until the airway is clear of secretions. Once the trachea has been cleared, the same catheter can be used to remove secretions in the patient's oropharynx and nose. After clearing the upper airway the catheter should be disposed of and never reused to suction the trachea.

After suctioning, it is important to take a minute to ensure that the patient is returned to the appropriate F_{IO_2} and ventilator settings. Once this is done, the vacuum and supplemental oxygen sources should be turned off and the results of the procedure documented. The color, consistency, and quantity of sputum suctioned are especially important to note. Changes in the color or increases in the quantity of sputum may indicate the presence of infection.

Use of Lavage Solutions

When pulmonary secretions are thick and difficult to remove, instillation of a lavage solution into the artificial airway prior to suctioning may be helpful. In the adult patient, 5 to 10 ml of normal saline injected into the airway seems to aid in the removal of secretions. In infants, only a few drops are necessary. It is my opinion that use of 100 percent humidified gas at body temperature is the most effective way to maintain thin secretions and assist in their removal. If 100 percent humidification is provided, instillation of lavage solutions is rarely required.

Nasotracheal Suctioning

Nasotracheal suctioning is technically more difficult to perform and has the potential for greater hazards than suctioning via an artificial airway. For these reasons I do not recommend this technique as a routine procedure for clearing the airway. There are occasions, however, when an artificial airway is not in place and retained secretions exist. If the patient is stable, nasotracheal suctioning is of benefit because it stimulates a strong cough and helps to mobilize secretions into the upper airway for removal. A nasopharyngeal airway may be helpful in patients requiring frequent suctioning.

The equipment needed is similar to that of other types of airway suctioning. A water-soluble lubricant to facilitate passage of the catheter through the patient's nasal passages is also helpful. The patient must be well oxygenated and should be placed in a Fowler's position prior to suctioning. With the catheter disconnected from the vacuum source, advance it through the nares to a point just above the larynx.

Airflow sounds can be identified from the proximal end of the catheter as it is advanced. If the sounds stop, the catheter has probably entered the esophagus. Slowly withdrawing the catheter until airflow sounds return should place it back just above the larynx.

Advancing the catheter during inspiration helps to place the distal tip into the larynx. As the catheter enters the larynx, the patient normally coughs and is unable to talk in a normal tone. After passing the vocal cords, reoxygenating the patient is helpful. If the patient appears stable at this point, connect the catheter to a vacuum source and suction the trachea. The instillation of a lavage solution into the trachea through the catheter can facilitate a good cough and thin retained secretions. After the trachea has been cleared, reoxygenate and monitor the patient.

Nasotracheal suctioning has the same complications noted with artificial airway suctioning, with the addition of laryngospasm, nasal irritation, and bleeding. Laryngospasm may be life threatening. If it develops, remove the catheter, seek assistance, and ventilate with bag and mask.

Adjuncts

Proper humidification of the inhaled gases is an essential part of airway care. It makes airway secretions less viscous and increases the ease of their removal. Frequent turning is also helpful in promoting the clearance of sputum. Rotating beds or chest physical therapy in bedridden patients with retained secretions assists movement of secretions toward the upper airway where they can more easily be removed. Positioning the patient not only aids in secretion clearance, but also improves the matching of ventilation and perfusion in the bedridden patient.

Complications

Hypoxemia

Aspiration of secretions from the airways results in the evacuation of oxygen-enriched gases and diminished oxygenation of the arterial blood. As hypoxemia occurs, other complications may surface, including tachycardia, premature ventricular contractions, or bradycardia. Watching the cardiac monitor during suctioning is helpful in identifying the potential consequences of hypoxemia. If arrhythmias do occur, the suctioning procedure should be discontinued and ventilation reestablished. The incidence of hypoxia is minimized by proper preoxygenation and by limiting the procedure to 15 seconds or less.

Tissue Trauma

Frequent suctioning can lead to irritation and trauma of the mucous membranes. Almost all patients who are suctioned have some tissue trauma owing to the catheter's rubbing against airway walls or the invagination of the mucosa into catheter holes when the vacuum is applied. In most cases, blood can be identified in the secretions when tissue trauma occurs. Damage to the mucous membranes can be minimized by using catheters made with softer material and by using an appropriate vacuum setting. The incidence of tissue trauma is increased if suctioning is done when excessive airway secretions are not present. Perhaps the absence of secretions allows more direct contact of the catheter with airway walls.

Atelectasis

The application of the vacuum to the patient's airway can result in removal of gas distal to the catheter tip, especially if the catheter is too large. Atelectasis may be difficult to detect when the degree of lung tissue involved is small; however, careful auscultation before and after the suctioning procedure may be useful. Persistent hypoxemia may be a sign that significant atelectasis has occurred. Careful selection of the appropriate-size catheter reduces the incidence of atelectasis and hyperinflation after the procedure helps to reinflate lung segments that are atelectatic.

Hypotension

Vagal stimulation, coughing, and hypoxemia are possible side effects of suctioning, and each can result in hypotension. Vagal stimulation causes bradycardia, coughing reduces venous return, and hypoxemia causes arrhythmias and peripheral vasodilation. Hypotension is easy to detect in patients with arterial lines in place. If an arterial line is not in place, measurement of blood pressure before and after suctioning is useful, especially in patients who are not tolerating the procedure well.

Although systemic blood pressure can drop during suctioning, intracranial pressure (ICP) usually increases. In patients with head trauma, this can lead to further compromise of cerebrovascular status. The elevation of ICP seems to be transient, with a return to baseline following the suctioning procedure. Adequate preoxygenation, hyperventilation, and hyperinflation that raises PaO_2 and lowers $PaCO_2$ may be helpful in minimizing increases in ICP.

Airway Constriction

Suctioning may cause direct mechanical stimulation of the respiratory mucosa and lead to constriction of the airway. During nasotracheal suctioning, laryngospasm may occur. If labored breathing with stridor occurs, an artificial airway may need to be placed to ventilate the patient. Suctioning can also cause bronchoconstriction, resulting in wheezes. Bronchodilator therapy should be used if this occurs.

AIRWAY CARE

Endotracheal Tubes

Once the endotracheal tube has been inserted, the patient's breath sounds should be identified to assure that bronchial or esophageal intubation has not occurred. If bronchial intubation has occurred, the tube usually enters the right main-stem bronchus, resulting in absent breath sounds over the left lung. A chest roentgenogram can demonstrate the exact position of the tube. The tip of the tube should be about 1 inch above the carina.

When the tube is correctly positioned, it should be secured to the patient's face to prevent movement and accidental extubation. The tube should not be secured in such a manner that it compresses tightly against oral or nasal structures, thereby increasing the chance of tissue breakdown. If the patient is orally intubated, movement of the tube from one side to the other on a regular basis helps to minimize tissue damage to either side of the mouth. With nasal tubes, care should be taken to guard against necrosis of the external nares. The factors influencing tracheal damage from endotracheal tubes are listed in Table 2.

A common clinical question with endotracheal tubes is, how long should they be left in place prior to tracheostomy? It is our practice to consider each case separately. Any time between 5 days and 2 weeks may be appropriate to consider tracheostomy. Factors such as prognosis, predicted length of mechanical ventilation, and ease of secretion removal influence the decision to do a tracheostomy. If, at the end of 5 to 10 days, the patient's need for mechanical ventilation is expected to be lengthy, a tracheostomy should be performed. If the prognosis is good and weaning is imminent, endotracheal tube usage should continue. When secretions are thick and difficult to remove, tracheostomy affords easier removal.

Cuff Inflation Techniques

The purpose of cuff inflation is to provide an adequate airway seal that allows positive pressure ventilation while preventing aspiration. At the same time cuff inflation should not cause excessive pressure on the tracheal mucosa that may lead to ischemia. Two techniques are frequently used to assure optimum cuff

TABLE 2   Factors that Increase Tracheal Damage from Endotracheal Tubes

High cuff pressure
Low blood pressure
Movement by patient
Long-term intubation
Infection in airways
Use of tube that is too large or too small

inflation: minimal occluding volume (MOV), and minimal leak technique (MLT).

MOV is achieved by slowly inserting air into the cuff until no leak is heard while auscultating the neck during peak inspiratory pressure. At this point an airtight seal is present. This technique is especially useful in patients who are being ventilated with high positive pressures. When MOV is reached, the volume of air in the cuff should always be noted.

MLT is achieved in a similar manner to that of MOV, except that once MOV is reached small amounts of air are removed from the cuff until a small leak can be heard at peak inspiratory pressure. This technique, along with high-volume, low-pressure cuffs, is very useful in minimizing the incidence of tracheal damage. The small leak may need to be compensated for by an increase in the ventilator tidal volume setting. MLT should be checked regularly and whenever the patient changes position, or with significant changes in the ventilatory pressure levels.

It is my practice to deflate the cuff every 8 hours and reestablish MLT or MOV. The cuff volume needed to achieve MLT/MOV is carefully noted and documented. If increasing volumes are needed, tracheal dilatation or cuff herniation is considered. Periodic cuff deflation probably does little to reduce tracheal ischemia but allows removal of stagnated secretions around or above the cuff that may promote infection. When the cuff is deflated, the airway below the cuff must be suctioned immediately.

Serial measurement of intracuff pressure can provide data regarding cuff and tracheal wall status. This requires no special equipment; however, a manometer or mercury column and three-way stopcock are needed. Cuff pressures kept below tracheal arterial-end capillary pressure help to minimize tracheal wall ischemia. In general, cuff pressure is maintained at 20 cm H_2O, or lower if possible, and should be monitored and recorded along with cuff volumes every 8 hours. Increases in cuff pressure with consistent cuff volumes represent edema at the cuff site. As with the use of MOV, cuff pressure may need to be increased in the presence of high PEEP or peak inspiratory airway pressure levels.

I feel that measuring intracuff pressure does not usually result in a decision to reduce cuff volumes, because I frequently use MLT. If intracuff pressures are high and MLT has been established, reducing intracuff volume may jeopardize effective ventilation and airway protection.

Tracheostomy Care

The wound of the tracheostomy must be kept clean and dry. It should be cleaned with a 3 percent hydrogen peroxide solution and rinsed with normal saline routinely. If the wound is not kept clean and secretions are allowed to build up around the tracheostomy, infection is likely to occur.

The tracheostomy tube should be secured with "ties" to prevent extubation and trauma to the wound. The tube must not be secured too tightly against the patient's neck to avoid excessive pressure on the wound.

The tracheostomy tube should be cleaned every shift and changed weekly to monthly, depending on the length of cannulation and patient's clinical status. The initial change of the tracheostomy tube should be performed by a physician who is trained in this procedure, because the fresh stoma may be difficult to recannulate when the tube is removed.

Suggested Reading

Baker PO, Baker JP, Koen PA. Endotracheal suctioning techniques in hypoxemia patients. Respir Care 1983; 28:1563–1568.

Chapman GA, Kim CS, Frankel J, Gazeroglu HB, Sackner MA. Evaluation of the safety and efficiency of a new suction catheter design. Respir Care 1986; 31:889–895.

Lomholt N. Design and function of tracheal suction catheters. Acta Anaesthesiol Scand 1982; 26:1–3.

Off D, Braun SR, Tompkins B, Bush G. Efficacy of the minimal leak technique of cuff inflation in maintaining proper intracuff pressures for patients with cuffed artificial airways. Respir Care 1983; 28:1115–1120.

Shapiro BA, Harrison RA, Kacmarek RM, Cane RD. Clinical application of respiratory care. 3rd ed. Chicago: Year Book, 1985.

THERAPEUTIC BRONCHOSCOPY

MUZAFFAR AHMAD, M.D.

In the past decade the fiberoptic bronchoscope (FOB) has emerged as the premiere diagnostic and therapeutic tool in the management of tracheobronchial disorders. With few notable exceptions it has replaced the rigid bronchoscope as the instrument of choice because of ease of insertion, better patient tolerance, and ever-improving flexibility enabling exploration of segmental and subsegmental bronchi, even of the upper lobes. This discussion concerns the role of therapeutic bronchoscopy using fiberoptic and rigid bronchoscopes, and therapeutic bronchoscopy in patients on mechanical ventilation.

INDICATIONS, TECHNIQUE, AND COMPLICATIONS

The indications for therapeutic bronchoscopy are summarized in Table 1. With the exception of foreign body aspiration and possibly massive hemoptysis, the instrument of choice is the FOB. Several models by different companies are commercially available in the United States. Differences are in degree of mobility, suction capabilities, outside diameters, and torsion characteristics. There are also subtle differences in fiber bundles and optics. All models prove adequate for therapeutic bronchoscopy when the size of the patient, mode of insertion, and outside diameter are taken into consideration.

Patients are premedicated with 50 to 75 mg meperidine, 50 to 75 mg hydroxyzine, and 0.25 mg atropine by intramuscular injection half an hour before the procedure. Lidocaine jelly and 4 percent lidocaine solution are used to anesthetize the upper airway. Methods of insertion include transnasal, transoral, and insertion through an endotracheal tube or a rigid bronchoscope. The transnasal approach is used most often; it is tolerated extremely well by most patients. To reduce potential for exposure to infection, the operator and assistants should take precautions to avoid contact with body fluids. These precautions should include wearing gowns, goggles, and gloves.

The incidence of complications associated with FOB is quite small. The incidence of minor complications is 0.2 percent; major complications 0.08 percent; and mortality, 0.01 percent. The complications are listed in Table 2. Reaction to the topical anesthetic agent, trauma due to insertion of the bronchoscope, hemorrhage from biopsy procedures, and hypoxemia due to occlusion of bronchi, bronchospasm, or instillation of solution are possible complications. In patients with pulmonary disease, FOB decreases the PaO_2 by 10 mm Hg or more. The use of supplemental oxygen is therefore recommended throughout and following the procedure.

PLACEMENT OF ENDOTRACHEAL BRONCHIAL TUBES

FOB is very helpful in difficult intubation. Factors associated with difficult intubation include obesity, short thick necks, cervical spine disease or deformity, head trauma, oropharyngeal tumors, and previous history of difficult intubation. The endotracheal tube is advanced over the FOB to its proximal end. After visualization of vocal cords, the scope is advanced to the mid-trachea and the tube is then inserted over the bronchoscope in the trachea. I use an 8-mm tube for nasal intubation and an 8.5-mm tube for the oral route. A bite block is used during oral intubation to prevent damage to the bronchoscope. Elective and emergency nasotracheal intubation can also be carried out in children. A 3.2-mm bronchoscope (with 4.5-mm tube) in small children and a 5.8-mm bronchoscope (with a 6.5-mm tube) in older children can be used safely.

FOB is also used for endobronchial isolation and ventilation of each lung. The technique can be extended to insertion of a double-lumen tube. A pediatric bronchoscope is inserted through the bronchial lumen for placement in the appropriate main stem bronchus. The scope is then inserted through the tracheal lumen to ensure proper location of the endobronchial balloon cuff and orientation of the tracheal lumen orifice. In critically ill patients, the FOB can be used to change endotracheal tubes safely. This is done by placing the replacement tube over the proximal end of the bronchoscope, which is then used to visualize the position of the original tube through the vocal cords. The original tube is then removed and the replacement one advanced into the trachea.

ATELECTASIS

A major indication for therapeutic bronchoscopy is acute lobar or whole lung atelectasis. Numerous studies have shown improvement in ventilation and

TABLE 1   Indications for Therapeutic Bronchoscopy

Difficult intubation
One-lung isolation
Change of endotracheal tubes
Insertion of double-lumen tubes
Lobar or whole lung atelectasis
Removal of secretions and mucous plugs (status asthmaticus, cystic fibrosis)
Massive hemoptysis (tamponade bleeding site)
Foreign body removal*
Biopsy excision of endobronchial tumors
Bronchoscopic cryotherapy*
Placement of after-loading catheter for brachytherapy

* Rigid bronchoscope is the instrument of choice.

blood gas levels after removal of mucous plugs and secretions with the aid of bronchoscopy. Improvement follows partial to complete reexpansion of the collapsed lobe or lung as evidenced radiographically. FOB is the instrument of choice in most cases; rigid bronchoscopy is rarely needed. It should be stated however, that no controlled study comparing the efficacy of bronchoscopy with intensive respiratory therapy has shown significant difference in the outcome at 24 and at 48 hours. It is therefore my recommendation that bronchoscopy be performed when respiratory therapy is ineffective or cannot be given because of individual patient factors. Occasionally, bronchoscopy should be the initial intervention if underlying pathology is suspected. Endobronchial tumors, aspirated foreign material, and granulomatous disorders have been diagnosed in this fashion with obvious therapeutic impact. Early bronchoscopy is also

TABLE 2   Complications of Bronchoscopy

Fiberoptic bronchoscopy
Secondary to premedication
    Respiratory depression
    Syncope
    Hyperexcitable state
    Hypotension
Secondary to local anesthetic
    Seizures
    Arrhythmias
    Cardiovascular collapse
    Laryngospasm
Secondary to procedure
    Laryngospasm
    Bronchospasm
    Arrhythmias
    Vasovagal reactions and syncope
    Hemorrhage (following biopsy or introduction trauma)
    Fever
    Hypoxemia
    Respiratory failure (rare)
    Pneumonia (rare)
Rigid Scope
Same as for fiberoptic bronchoscopy
Subglottic edema
Higher incidence of mechanical trauma

advisable if prompt improvement in ventilation and oxygenation is desired. These exceptions underscore the importance of clinical judgment in individual cases.

Flexible FOB can also be used in infants and young children for management of atelectasis. Atelectasis successfully resolves after direct visualization, washing, and removal of mucous plugs. This is accompanied by improvement in arterial blood gas levels.

REMOVAL OF SECRETIONS AND MUCOUS PLUGS

Bronchoscopy has been recommended for evacuation of copious secretions and for suctioning of the left tracheobronchial airways, which are difficult to do blindly. Although there is no clinical evidence that bronchoscopy is superior to respiratory therapy in these conditions, there are some clinical situations in which bronchoscopy is of significant benefit. In severe asthma, when conventional therapy has been ineffective and thick mucous plugs are a significant problem, bronchoscopy and lavage often mobilize secretions from the more peripheral portions of the tracheobronchial tree. Some patients may even expectorate branching casts of the bronchial tree following the procedure. A lavage solution consisting of normal saline (250 to 500 ml), 10 percent N-acetylcysteine (20 to 30 ml) and isoetharine mesylate (2.0 ml) can be used. Acetylesteine reduces the viscosity of pulmonary secretions and isoetharine acts as a bronchodilator at the site. It must be emphasized that bronchoscopy should be considered along with intensive, conventional therapy, including high-dose corticosteroids; it has a role in a small subset of asthmatic patients. The procedure is not without risk and may itself aggravate bronchospasm. Bronchoscopy should be performed by experienced operators under controlled conditions. Selected cystic fibrosis and allergic bronchopulmonary aspergillosis patients may also benefit from therapeutic bronchoscopy for evacuation of copious and tenacious secretions.

BRONCHOPULMONARY HEMORRHAGE

Bronchoscopy not only is useful for identifying the site of bleeding, but also has therapeutic potential. Epinephrine at 1:20,000 mg per milliliter dilution can be instilled at the bleeding site. I have found it useful in controlling bleeding after endobronchial and even transbronchial biopsy. Iced saline lavage through the bronchoscope has also been successful for controlling massive hemoptysis (greater than 600 ml in 24 hours). The definitive medical or surgical treatment can then be initiated after respite from hemorrhage has been achieved with this technique. The technique for iced saline lavage requires a rigid bronchoscope, which is positioned in the bronchus over the region of bleeding. Irrigation is then performed with normal saline at 4° C in 50 ml aliquots for 30 to 60 seconds. Fluid is then removed by gentle suction. Reduction in bleeding facilitates localization of the exact source of bleeding, following which the involved lobe is lavaged until bleeding ceases. Early resectional surgery is advocated in most cases of massive hemoptysis to reduce the high mortality.

Tamponade of the bleeding lobar or segmental bronchus by a balloon-tipped catheter introduced through the FOB can also be used to control bleeding. A modified Fogarty catheter (Balloon Retrieval Catheter, 8.5 mm OD, 200 cm long, Microvasive) is inserted into the bleeding lobar or segmental branches under direct vision through the FOB. After inflation of the balloon the scope is removed by slipping it over the Fogarty catheter. The catheter may be removed at surgery or left in place for up to 24 hours. The same technique can be used to control bleeding from a biopsy site and for long-term control of severe hemoptysis in otherwise inoperable conditions. The technique can also be applied through the rigid bronchoscope. Whether an FOB or a rigid bronchoscope is used as the initial instrument in massive hemoptysis is a matter of availability, personal preference, and most importantly, expertise. With the new larger fiberoptic bronchoscopes and ever-improving suction capabilities, my preference is to use the FOB as the initial instrument and use the Fogarty catheter technique for tamponade if necessary. However, good comparative studies are needed before the question of rigid versus flexible bronchoscopy in massive hemoptysis can be answered definitively.

OTHER INDICATIONS OF THERAPEUTIC BRONCHOSCOPY

The rigid bronchoscope remains the instrument of choice for removal of foreign bodies from tracheobronchial airways, but FOB often helps to establish the diagnosis. The development of large forceps, wire baskets, and claws have increased the role of FOB so that its increased range can be optimally used not only in identification but also occasionally in removal of foreign bodies. Still, its role for this purpose remains to be elucidated.

Bronchoscopic biopsy excision through the rigid scope has been used successfully for many years. Both benign and malignant tracheobronchial tumors have been treated by use of endoscopic punch forceps and snares. This use has now been extended to the FOB, with the use of large alligator, cup, or rat-tooth forceps and flexible scissors. Local anesthesia can be used. Lesions most amenable to this treatment are relatively less vascular, especially following radiation therapy. In properly selected patients, bronchoscopic biopsy excision is a safe, effective palliation of airway obstruction. Bronchoscopic cryotherapy of localized endobronchial tumors can also be used in selected patients. A closed liquid nitrogen system and a long insulated probe are manipulated through an open ventilating bronchoscope. The procedure results in local tumor control, decreased bleeding, and improved airway patency. Probe tip temperatures of −160° C or less are important for good results. The procedure can be tried in patients who are not candidates for conventional therapy. FOB is also used for placement of an after-loading catheter for the purpose of delivering endobronchial radiation by placing a radioactive source near the tumor (brachytherapy). Only a small volume of tissue receives the therapeutic dose (usually 1,000 cGy), thus reducing normal tissue damage. This technique can be used as an adjunct to bronchoscopic laser therapy to treat the submucosal part of neoplasms, for optimum palliation (see also chapter on *Laser Applications in Respiratory Care*).

BRONCHOSCOPY IN PATIENTS ON MECHANICAL VENTILATION

FOB has made it possible to perform bronchoscopy in intubated and mechanically ventilated patients. The therapeutic indications include tracheobronchial toilet (to remove copious, tenacious secretions), reexpansion of atelectatic lung, removal of mucous plugs in status asthmaticus, and confirmation of proper placement of endotracheal tubes. The bronchoscope is inserted through a T-piece mounted on the end of an endotracheal tube. To minimize air leaks, the open end of the T-piece is sealed with a rubber diaphragm (Fig. 1). The FOB is introduced through a slit in the diaphragm and controlled ventilation is continued uninterrupted throughout the procedure. The bronchoscope is lubricated to allow free movement through the adapter and endotracheal tube. The optimal patient endotracheal tube size for fiberoptic bronchoscopy is 8.5 mm internal diameter, but patients with smaller tubes can also be examined. Table 3 provides guidelines for introducing 5 and 6 mm (outside diameter) bronchoscopes through different sized endotracheal tubes. However, whenever possible, patients with tubes of less than 8 mm internal diameter should not undergo bronchoscopy, because of a resulting significant increase in peak inspiratory pressure. In some of these patients, obstruction of the tube can be avoided by inserting the FOB transnasally and passing it into the tracheobronchial tree alongside the smaller endotracheal tube.

Introduction of the bronchoscope during mechanical ventilation causes a decrease in tidal volume and in PaO_2 and an increase in $PaCO_2$. The incidence of barotrauma may be increased in the presence of positive end-expiratory pressure (PEEP). Repeated and

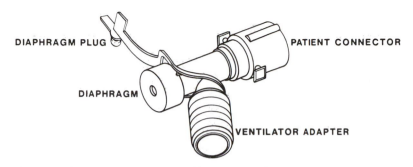

Figure 1 Tracheostomy adapter with diaphragm for bronchoscope insertion.

prolonged suction further decreases tidal volume and reduces functional residual capacity, resulting in further worsening of hypoxemia. To minimize complications, it is prudent to use an endotracheal tube of optimum size, discontinue PEEP, use 100 percent oxygen, and use suction for short periods only. Bronchoscopy time, of course, should be minimized as much as possible, and as with any other intervention, the risk:benefit ratio should be carefully examined.

TABLE 3 Acceptable Endotracheal Tube and Bronchoscope Tube Sizes for Bronchoscopy

Endotracheal Tube Inside Diameter (mm)	Bronchoscope Tube Size Outside Diameter	
	6 mm	*5 mm*
9.5	Yes	Yes
9.0	Yes	Yes
8.5	Yes	Yes
8.0	Yes	Yes
7.5	No	Yes
7.0	No	Yes
6.0	No	No

Suggested Reading

Ahmad M, Livingston DR, Golish JA, et al. The safety of outpatient transbronchial biopsy. Chest 1986; 90:403–405.

Conlan AA, Hurwitz SS. Management of massive hemoptysis with the rigid bronchoscope and cold saline lavage. Thorax 1980; 35:901–904.

Feldman NT, Huber GL. Fiberoptic bronchoscopy in the intensive care unit. Int Anesthesiol Clin 1976; 14:31–42.

Gottlieb LS, Hillberg R. Endobronchial tamponade therapy for intractable hemoptysis. Chest 1975; 67:482–483.

Lindholm CE, Ollman B, Snyder JV, et al. Cardiorespiratory effects of flexible fiberoptic bronchoscopy in critically ill patients. Chest 1978; 74:362–368.

Mahajan VK, Catron PW, Huber GL. The value of fiberoptic bronchoscopy in the management of pulmonary collapse. Chest 1978; 73:817–820.

Marini JJ, Pierson DJ, Hudson LD. Acute lobar atelectasis: a prospective comparison of fiberoptic bronchoscopy and respiratory therapy. Am Rev Respir Dis 1979; 119:971–978.

Mehta AC, Livingston DR. Biopsy excision through a fiberoptic bronchoscope in the palliative management of airway obstruction. Chest 1987; 91:774–775.

Sackner MA. Bronchofiberoscopy. Am Rev Respir Dis 1975; III:62–88.

Saunderson DR, Neel HB, Fontana RS. Bronchoscopic cryotherapy. Ann Otol 1981; 90:354–358.

LASER APPLICATIONS IN RESPIRATORY CARE

ATUL C. MEHTA, M.D.

Laser technology was introduced into the field of medicine almost a quarter-century ago, and over the years its role has been acknowledged in a majority of the subspecialities. Application of lasers in pulmonary medicine, however, is rather new and is possible mainly because of the invention of powerful laser lights with wavelengths short enough to be transmitted through a flexible quartz filament and thus to be easily delivered to the lower airways. The carbon dioxide laser, a widely used medical laser, operates at a wavelength of 10.6 μm and requires rigid, bulky, mirrored, articulated arms to change the direction of its beam. Hence, its role is limited to easily reached structures such as skin, larynx, cervix, or open surgical wounds. On the contrary, the neodymium-yttrium-aluminum garnet (Nd-YAG) laser operates at much shorter wavelength of 1.06 μm and, using a flexible quartz filament through an endoscope, its light can be easily aimed at lesions involving either the gastrointestinal tract or endobronchial tree without requiring surgical exploration. Similarly, argon (Ar), krypton (Kr), and rhodamine B dye laser lights with even shorter wavelengths can be applied to such deeper structures without much difficulty. Furthermore, the noninvasive nature of fiberoptic endoscopic techniques has simplified the use of lasers in gastroenterology and pulmonary medicine.

The laser produces tissue effects by three different mechanisms: thermal effect, photochemical effect, and electromagnetic effect. While the latter still remains a matter of research, the former two are currently used in the management of lesions involving the endobronchial tree. Indications for their use are listed in Table 1.

THERMAL EFFECT

The most common use of lasers in pulmonary medicine is in management of symptomatic but surgically unresectable benign or malignant major airway lesions. Resection is indicated primarily for exophytic lesions; it has little value in treating submucosal processes or airway obstruction caused by extrinsic compression.

Patients usually present with intractable cough, hemoptysis, dyspnea, partial or complete collapse of the lung, or postobstructive pneumonia, and occasionally with asphyxiation or septicemia related to postoperative pneumonia.

Thermal energy produced by the laser beam is used to coagulate and then excise the lesion; this can be done using endoscopic instruments without significant bleeding. When necessary, especially while dealing with excessively hemorrhagic lesions, actual vaporization of the lesion can also be produced by using higher power settings. The Nd-YAG laser, being a very powerful system, is most commonly used for this purpose, while the relatively low-powered Ar laser device is now seldom used. Nd-YAG laser light is also poorly absorbed by both water and hemoglobin and thus penetrates the tissue deeper than other lights. As a result, it affects a much greater mass of the tissue and disperses adequate energy for effective coagulation (Fig. 1). The procedure can be performed under either local or general anesthesia. Maintenance of adequate ventilation during the photoresection is challenging and requires coordination between the surgeon and the anesthesia team. The detailed description of the procedure is beyond the scope of this chapter; readers are referred to prior publications.

Even though some authors feel strongly that the procedure should be carried out only through the rigid bronchoscope, I believe it can also be performed safely using the flexible bronchoscope. Selection of the appropriate endoscope for the procedure depends on several factors (Table 2). A major deciding factor is the operator's technical expertise. The methodology of the Nd-YAG laser photoresection was developed by French physicians with vast experience at rigid bronchoscopy. Physicians with similar backgrounds can of course perform the procedure with great confidence using a rigid scope. However, pulmonologists who are interested in adopting the procedure may have little experience with a rigid scope but be expert at fiberoptic bronchoscopy. For them, it would be more practical to get acquainted with laser use through fiberoptic bronchoscopy. Of course the procedure is much more time consuming when performed through the fiberoptic bronchoscope, because much smaller pieces of tumor tissue can be excised using flexible forceps. However, use of flexible scissors, Dormia baskets, and Fogarty catheters can help to reduce the time requirement significantly.

In some patients, general anesthesia is contraindicated because of their underlying cardiopulmonary status. In these patients, use of the rigid bronchoscope under local anesthesia would be hazardous. Even though laser photoresection is mainly indicated for lesions involving the trachea and major bronchi, often treatment of lesions of lobar bronchi becomes necessary. Under the circumstances, aiming the laser beam is much easier through the fiberoptic scope than the rigid scope. For dealing with excessively vascular lesions, the rigid scope is probably superior, because the body of the scope can be used to tamponade the bleeding site, and suctioning of the blood and photocoagulation can be performed simultaneously. In case of massive bleeding, a safe airway can be easily es-

TABLE 1 Role of Laser in Respiratory Care

By Thermal Effects (Nd-YAG, Ar Laser)	By Photochemical Effects

Photoresection of airway lesions
  Malignant: Bronchogenic
    carcinoma, metastatic lesions
  Benign: Tracheal stenosis or
    stricture, granulomas,
    neoplasms, amyloidosis
Photocoagulation
  Management of epistaxis
  Bleeding cavitary lesions
	Diagnostic usage (Kr laser)
	  Carcinoma in situ
	  Superficial bronchogenic carcinoma
	Therapeutic usage (rhodamine B dye
	  laser)
	  Palliative resection of malignant
	    airway lesions
	  Curative therapy for carcinoma in
	    situ and superficial bronchogenic
	    carcinoma

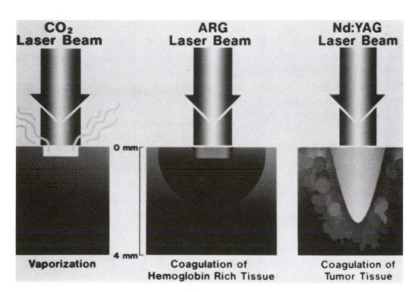

Figure 1 Schematic diagram of depth of penetration and related tissue effects of different therapeutic lasers.

TABLE 2 Factors Determining Use of Rigid Versus Flexible Bronchoscope for Nd-YAG Laser Therapy

Factor	Rigid	Fiberoptic
Expertise	Thoracic surgeon, otolaryngologist	Pulmonologist
Time Commitment	Short	Long
Anesthesia	General only	General or local
Lesion		
Location	Trachea, major bronchi	Also lobar bronchi
Vascularity	Highly vascular	Less vascular
Epistaxis	No	Yes
Bleeding cavity	No	Yes
Cervical Spine Abnormalities	No	Yes
Endobronchial Ignition	Less likely	Possible

tablished using the rigid scope. However, in my experience with more than 150 procedures performed through the flexible bronchoscope, such a need has never been encountered. I have been successful in controlling moderate amounts of bleeding with endobronchial instillation of epinephrine and laser photocoagulation. In the event of major vessel perforation there are no reports, at least to my knowledge, of the rigid bronchoscope's changing the overall outcome for the patient, because the majority of the patients undergoing the laser procedure have limited pulmonary reserve and are not candidates for major thoracic surgical intervention. Photocoagulation of arterio-venous (A-V) malformations involving the nasal cavity or bleeding cavitary lesions involving the lung can be exclusively performed through the flexible bronchoscope. Obviously use of the rigid scope is contraindicated in patients with abnormalities of the cervical spine such as ankylosing spondylitis or rheumatoid arthritis.

The most feared complication of Nd-YAG laser photocoagulation is endobronchial ignition. Chances of this complication are increased when the procedure is performed through the fiberoptic bronchoscope, because commonly used endotracheal tubes and even the bronchoscope are made of combustible material. However, by keeping the tips of the laser fiber and the bronchoscope meticulously clean and maintaining both the lowest possible FIO_2 during actual use of the laser and maximum distance between the treatment site and distal end of the endotracheal tube, such a complication can be avoided.

Finally, any conventional fiberoptic bronchoscope with a working channel of at least 2.3 mm in diameter can be used, but one has to select one of the several specially designed rigid bronchoscopes for laser photoresection.

In my opinion, both instruments are complementary to each other and working knowledge of both types of scopes is highly preferred.

Treatment of Malignant Lesions

Bronchogenic Carcinoma

Nd-YAG laser photoresection has been used in the palliative management of airway obstruction caused by unresectable bronchogenic carcinoma. Laser therapy is usually used after a conventional means of palliation, i.e., radiation therapy or chemotherapy (in case of small cell carcinoma), has been tried, unless the patient's clinical status warrants immediate palliation. It must be emphasized that laser photoresection in these patients is strictly for palliation of the symptoms caused by the obstructing lesion and is not a substitute for curative surgery.

I have achieved immediate palliation in more than 90 percent of my patients, and in two-thirds of these patients I have also demonstrated significant objective improvement in the patient's pulmonary status. Whether this treatment prolongs the survival of these patients, however, is not yet known. Unfortunately, owing to the clinical status of the majority of the patients qualifying for laser photoresection, a randomized trial to answer the above question is neither practical nor ethical. In comparison with historical controls, Nd-YAG laser therapy has been shown to prolong the overall survival of this group of patients by a few weeks; however, the validity of such comparisons is questionable. In my opinion, in selected cases (e.g., in a patient with a large tracheal obstruction by a radioresistant or recurrent non-small cell bronchogenic carcinoma), Nd-YAG laser therapy has great potential in prolonging survival. However, because these unresectable malignancies often have systemic effects, in the remaining patients such local measures are unlikely to change the overall outcome of bronchogenic carcinoma.

Synergism of Nd-YAG laser therapy with yet newer modalities such as endobronchial radiation or photodynamic therapy in patients with bronchogenic carcinoma remains to be studied.

Metastatic Lesions Involving the Airways

Lesions metastatic to the airways, especially from renal cell, breast, or colon carcinoma, are not uncommon. Involvement of the airways can also occur by contiguous spread from thyroid or head and neck malignancies. On occasion, both Hodgkin's and non-Hodgkin's lymphoma can also involve the airways. If these lesions are exophytic, Nd-YAG laser photoresection can be performed in a fashion similar to that described earlier and equally good palliation can be established (Fig. 2). A word of caution is that if carcinoma of the esophagus involves the airways contiguously, photoresection is contraindicated because it greatly increases the chances of tracheoesophageal fistula.

Treatment of Benign Lesions

Major airway obstruction caused by benign processes can also be ablated using thermal energy of Nd-YAG laser light. Tracheal strictures related to prolonged intubation or healed infection such as endobronchial tuberculosis may be successfully treated in this fashion. Treatment of web or diaphragmatic-type strictures is most likely to be successful, but bottleneck-type strictures are difficult to treat because tracheomalacia is usually the major component of such obstruction and alternative methods of repair are necessary. Idiopathic or inflammatory papillomatosis and large areas of granulation tissue related to tracheos-

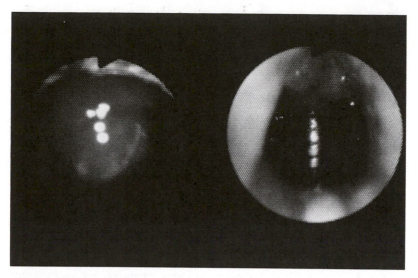

Figure 2 Metastatic thyroid carcinoma producing subtotal obstruction of subglottic trachea before (*left*) and after (*right*) Nd-YAG laser photoresection. A Norton endotracheal tube is placed through the tracheostomy stoma.

tomy can also be removed using this method. Removal of granulomas related to a foreign body, suture material, or broncholiths is also possible. When necessary, suture material can be vaporized and large broncholiths can be shattered using laser energy. Laser photoresection is usually not indicated for endobronchial carcinoid tumor unless unresectability of this lesion has been previously proven. I have also used this modality in the palliative treatment of endobronchial amyloidosis of the major airways in two patients; however, because of coexisting involvement of the smaller airways in both patients, the results of laser treatment were unsatisfactory. No significant improvement in either ventilation or perfusion scan was noticed following treatment. Long-term results following laser photoresection of benign lesions depend on the etiology of the lesion and the structural integrity of the involved airway.

Alternative Methods

Ablation of airway lesions similar to that produced by Nd-YAG laser can also be achieved using either cryoprobe or electrocautery. Both of these alternatives require a rigid bronchoscope for their application, because flexible cryoprobes or electroprobes are not yet available for general use. Besides, unlike laser photocoagulation, the cryoprobe does not establish the patency of the involved airway instantaneously. It requires several days for the frozen tissue to slough. This time factor could be crucial in some patients, especially those with postobstructive pneumonia or symptoms of asphyxiation.

Excessive smoke production is associated with electrocauterization. Tissue sticking to the tip of the

probe is also a problem, and use of the probe through long rigid metallic instruments increases the chances of electric shock to the operator. Excessive bleeding could occur with either of these modalities. However, further experience with these techniques is necessary before a fair comparison with laser therapy can be made.

Photocoagulation

Using appropriate laser energy, effective thermal coagulation of the bleeding lesion can be easily produced. This technique has been used in elective treatment of epistaxis from A-V malformations related to Osler-Rendu-Weber syndrome involving nasal cavities. The procedure is performed using general anesthesia and the flexible bronchoscope. Thermal coagulation of the area surrounding the malformation is produced, avoiding direct injury to the lesion. Attempts are made to achieve just the pale discoloration of the tissue while carbonization is avoided (Fig. 3). Results are temporary, and the procedure is repeated when necessary. In a study done at my institution, in 70 percent of the patients emergency room visits and blood transfusions for epistaxis were prevented for at least 3 months following laser treatment. The majority of these patients had had prior argon laser therapy, skin grafting, or electrocauterization of the lesions and these treatments had failed.

Photocoagulation of bleeding sites with the laser has also been found to be helpful in managing patients with bleeding in association with radiation necrosis of the bronchus, a rare complication of squamous cell carcinoma. Two of my patients with this complication presented with significant hemoptysis. The source of

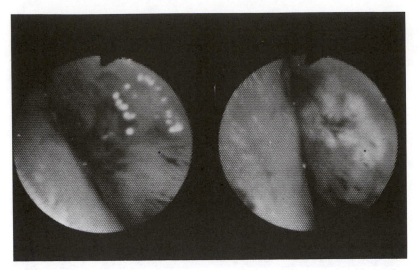

Figure 3 Nd-YAG laser photocoagulation of arterio-venous malformation involving the nasal septum, before (*left*) and after (*right*) the procedure. Note pale discoloration of the tissue encircling the vascular anomaly.

the bleeding was the necrotic walls of the resultant cavities. Nd-YAG laser photocoagulation of bleeding sites through the fiberoptic bronchoscope was successful in alleviating the bleeding.

PHOTOCHEMICAL EFFECT

Photosensitizers are chemicals that can be activated in situ by penetrating light of specific wavelengths, leading to fluorescence of different wavelengths, tissue necrosis, or both. Some of these photosensitizers are retained by most malignant and some premalignant tissues in higher concentration and for longer duration than by surrounding normal tissue. Usefulness of these properties of photosensitizers in early diagnosis and management of malignancies involving the endobronchial tree is currently being studied. Light of the specific wavelength required to precipitate these effects is derived using an appropriate laser system.

Of all the available photosensitizers, hematoporphyrin derivative (Hpd) has received most attention. Recently, it was learned that its photosensitization characteristics are mainly due to its major constituent, dihematoporphyrin ether (DHE). Forty-eight hours following intravenous administration of Hpd or DHE, it is mainly retained by tumor tissue, while it has been cleared by most normal tissues. At this time, such tumor tissue can be exposed to appropriate laser light for fluorescence or tissue necrosis.

Diagnostic Use

When tumor tissue retaining Hpd or DHE is exposed to violet light as a wavelength of 405 nm, it emits a salmon red-colored fluorescence at 630 and 690 nm. The applicability of this photochemical reaction is currently being studied in localizing the site of lesions in patients with occult lung carcinoma. The violet light required for the purpose is usually obtained from a krypton ion laser.

Patients with positive sputum cytologic findings but normal chest radiographs and no apparent abnormality of the head and neck region or endobronchial tree are usually encountered during mass screening for lung cancer or on presentation with hemoptysis as the only symptom. Localization of the source of malignant cells can be accomplished using this fluorescent technique. Forty-eight hours following intravenous administration of Hpd or DHE, the search for the red fluorescence is carried out while suspected areas of the endobronchial tree are exposed to the violet light. Such lesions are usually very small and retain miniscule amounts of photosensitizing substances. Also, significant optical losses of fluorescent signals occur when using the fiberoptic bronchoscope. Hence, some form of detector, such as an image intensifier or an ultrasensitive camera is required to increase the fluorescence gain. Once the tumor size is localized, multiple biopsy specimens are obtained for histological confirmation. Kato and Cortese used this method in 36 patients who were already known to have bronchogenic carcinoma. It was effective in detecting the malignancy in 33 patients. False-negative results occurred in three patients in whom disease tissue was either submucosal or covered by blood or necrotic tissue. Also, false-positive readings were obtained from areas of severe metaplasia in three examinations.

Using the same principle, the tumor site was correctly localized in eight of 11 patients with truly oc-

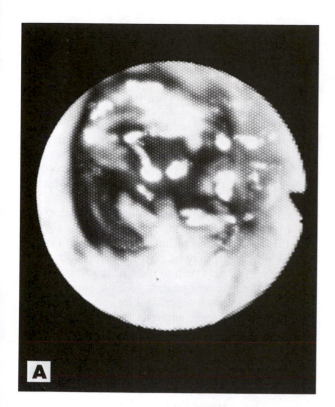

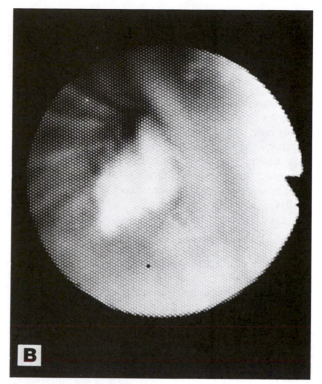

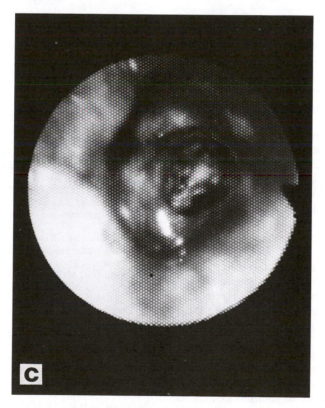

Figure 4 *A*, Exophytic, hemorrhagic tumor mass producing total occlusion of the left lower lobe bronchus. *B*, Tumor mass 48 hours following photodynamic therapy. Note pale discoloration suggesting the necrotic changes. *C*, Patent left lower lobe bronchus (same patient) following clean-up bronchoscopy.

cult lung cancer identified from the Mayo Clinic lung cancer screening project. In two of the remaining three in whom no fluorescence was detected, the lesions were eventually found beyond the range of fiberoptic bronchoscope; thus there was only one false-negative result.

Because lung cancer screening projects have been found to be of limited practical value, patients with occult lung cancer are difficult to find. However, this technology has great potential in early detection of lung cancer and may revitalize interest in similar screening programs. Research is in progress to find more tumor-specific photosensitizers to minimize false-positives and false-negatives.

Therapeutic Use

When tumor tissue retaining Hpd or DHE is exposed to the red light of 630 nm, cytocidal effects of these chemicals occur, mainly by the production of singlet oxygen. This red light is derived from the argon-pumped rhodamine B dye laser and is delivered via a flexible quartz filament. It takes 48 hours for tissue necrosis to develop, after which clean-up bronchoscopy is needed to remove sloughed tissue. This form of therapy is often referred to as photodynamic therapy (PDT).

A study by Hayata and co-workers of a subgroup of eight patients with superficial and stage 1 unresectable squamous cell carcinoma showed complete remission in all following PDT during 13 to 64 months' follow-up. One patient was still alive at 64 months. In a similar study at the Mayo Clinic, 8 of 19 patients had complete remission during 8 to 59 months of follow-up.

Balchum and Doiron used PDT as a palliative modality in selected patients with surgically unresectable primary and secondary malignancies involving the endobronchial tree. Unlike the instantaneous results obtained with Nd-YAG laser photoresection, it required 48 hours to establish the patency of the lumen, but successful palliation was achieved in all 72 patients without complication (Fig. 4, A through C).

Studies have also demonstrated the role of PDT in reducing, from pneumonectomy to lobectomy, the extent of lung resection for bronchogenic carcinoma. In selected patients, it has helped to reduce the local extent of the malignancy and thus to convert unresectable to resectable disease. Overall outcome of these patients remains to be studied.

The only side effect associated with the use of Hpd and DHE is skin photosensitization. It is necessary to avoid direct exposure to sunlight as long as these chemicals are retained by the skin, which could be anywhere from 4 to 8 weeks following their intravenous administration.

The photochemical effects of laser light have great diagnostic and therapeutic potentials. Although investigational at present, these modalities are not far from being a reality.

CONCLUSIONS

The laser has become a powerful addition to the pulmonologist's armamentarium in various areas of clinical medicine. It has added new dimensions to using the bronchoscope not only as a diagnostic tool but also as a potent therapeutic device. Airway obstruction by an endobronchial lesion can be alleviated to provide immediate palliation without surgical exploration, and bleeding lesions can be effectively coagulated. Early diagnosis of lung cancer, while it is still resectable in most, may be possible using fluorescent techniques; PDT may help to reduce the extent of lung resection in lung cancer patients who have limited lung function or may cure superficial lesions without surgery. Methods of laser angioplasty in various different organ systems are currently being studied and significant progress has been reported in the development of pulmonary angioscopy. Combinations of these two technologies could begin a new era in respiratory care.

Suggested Reading

Balchum O, Doiron DR. Photoradiation therapy of endobronchial lung cancer. Clin Chest Med 1985; 6:255–275.

Brutinel WM, Cortese DA, McDougall JC, Gillio RG, Bergstralh EJ. A two-year experience with neodymium-YAG laser in endobronchial obstruction. Chest 1987; 86:159–165.

Dougherty TJ. Photosensitizers of malignant tumors. Semin Surg Oncol 1986; 2:24–37.

Dumon JF, Shapshay S, Bourcereau J, Cavaliere S, Meric B, Garbi N, et al. Principles for safety in application of neodymium-YAG laser in bronchology. Chest 1984; 86:163–168.

Edell ES, Cortese DA. Bronchoscopic phototherapy with Hpd for treatment of localized bronchogenic Ca: a 5-year experience. Mayo Clin Proc 1987; 62:8–14.

Hayata Y, Kato H, Konaka C, et al. PDT with Hpd in early stage lung cancer. Chest 1984; 86:169–177.

Kato H, Cortese DA. Early detection of lung cancer by means of Hpd fluorescence and laser photoradiation. Clin Chest Med 1985; 6:237–254.

Kato H, Konaka C, Kawate N, et al. 5-Year disease free survival of lung cancer patient treated only by PDT. Chest 1986; 90:768–770.

Livingston DR, Mehta AC, Golish JA, Ahmad M, Deboer G, Tomaszewski MZ. Palliation of malignant tracheobronchial obstruction by Nd-YAG laser: an updated experience at the Cleveland Clinic Foundation. JAOA 1987; 3:226/61–234/69.

Mehta AC, Livingston DR, et al. Ventilatory management during Nd-YAG photoresection of subglottic lesions. Trans ABEA 1987; 148–153.

Mehta AC, Livingston DR, Crisostomo A, Golish JA, Ahmad M. Radiation necrosis of bronchus and its palliative management using Nd-YAG laser (abstract). Am Rev Respir Dis 1987; 135(4):A243.

Mehta AC, Livingston DR, Levine HL. Fiberoptic bronchoscope and Nd-YAG laser in the treatment of severe epistaxis from nasal hereditary hemorrhagic telangiectasia and hemangioma. Chest 1987; 91:791–792.

SMOKING CESSATION TECHNIQUES

LOUISE M. NETT, R.N., RRT
SANDRA M. DINGUS, M.A.

There are over a billion physician-patient encounters each year in the United States, and this offers health professionals a unique opportunity to intervene with their smoking patients. Only 10 percent of smokers who want to quit smoking take the initiative to attend smoking cessation classes, so the physician and health professional's initiative to intervene can be an important factor in encouraging and supporting the 90 percent who do not attend classes.

For the health professional, knowing how best to help the smoker quit comes from knowing where the individual is in the process of quitting. There are four, and possibly six, stages through which each "quitter" must pass. These are (1) precontemplation, (2) contemplation, (3) action, and (4) maintenance. Stages 5 and 6, through which many smokers pass, are relapse and renewed action.

In this discussion, techniques for smoking cessation are described according to the stage of cessation at which the technique is most effectively used. Each of the stages is easily identified, including the distinction between precontemplation and contemplation. In the precontemplative stage, the individual says that he has never considered quitting. The person who is in the contemplative stage answers affirmatively when asked, "Have you ever considered quitting?" Helping the smoker to move from the precontemplation stage to the contemplation stage can be both as difficult and rewarding as it is to help him move from the contemplation to the action stage.

PRECONTEMPLATION STAGE

In the precontemplation stage, it is important to guide the smoker to a personalized reason to quit. This can be accomplished by examining with him his attitudes about health and about smoking, as well as possible health symptoms and problems resulting from his cigarette habit.

Examine the Smoker's Smoking-Related Symptoms

Relate for the smoker any health symptoms and problems to his cigarette habit. There are many opportunities to do this. The symptoms of headache, sinus congestion, indigestion, nervousness, and irritability may all be related to smoking. Identify the role smoking plays in high blood pressure, palpitations, and difficulty in healing an ulcer.

Biologic Tests

Smokers who have not considered quitting need health information personalized, and abnormal biologic tests are a way to get the attention of the smoker. Use of biologic testing to measure the effects of tobacco, followed by interpretation of the smoker's data as compared to that of a nonsmoker, may help the smoker to consider stopping.

Pulmonary function tests can be used as a motivator, whether or not their results are positive. A person with a normal pulmonary function test may be relieved to discover there is no airway damage. An abnormal pulmonary function test may get the attention of other individuals. Interpreting the test in light of the expected normal values may be a frightening but effective method of getting a smoker's attention.

Dr. James Morris uses the technique of interpreting these test results in terms of lung age. A 6-foot tall, 35-year-old man with expected vital capacity of 5.35 L and FEV_1 of 4.2 L who has half that value will be shocked to know his lung age is over 80 years old. Using a pulmonary function paper graph to display predicted versus actual values helps the patient to see, as well as hear, about his abnormality (Fig. 1).

Exhaled carbon monoxide testing is simple, safe, and inexpensive. The carbon monoxide level of an inhaling daily smoker is always elevated, so the smoker with normal pulmonary function can always be shown the effect smoking has on his body. In general, the public is concerned about elevated levels of carbon monoxide in the ambient air, and a smoker can view his own air pollution by watching the meter on the carbon monoxide unit elevate. Nonsmokers register levels of eight parts per million or less. One-pack-a-day smokers often have levels of 25 parts per million, and some one-pack-a-day smokers have even higher levels, depending on the pattern of inhalation. Usually, the carbon monoxide level is directly related to

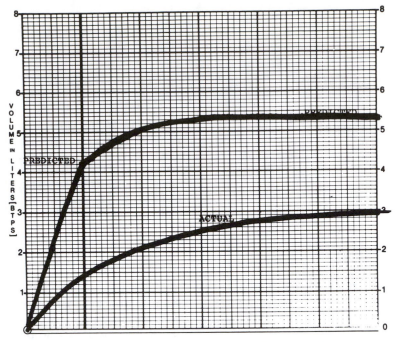

Figure 1 Predicted versus actual FVC. Visual demonstration of abnormality may help smokers realize the effect smoking has on their lung function.

consumption, and the best time to measure levels is in the afternoon.

Researchers are using other biologic tests to assess tobacco consumption. Although these tests are not yet common in clinical medicine, they may be available soon, because the involvement of health professionals in the smoking cessation problem will necessitate better monitoring of compliance or participation with therapy. Combustion of the cigarette releases hydrogen cyanide. Hydrogen cyanide is metabolized by the liver to thiocyanate. Thiocyanate has a half-life of 14 days, so it is useful for measuring tobacco consumption. It takes a chronic smoker 3 to 6 weeks to clear thiocyanate levels after cessation. Levels of 85 to 100 micromoles per liter have been suggested as a cut-off for smokers versus nonsmokers. However, one must be cautious in interpreting these values if the patient is a vegetarian or consumes large amounts of leafy vegetables or nuts. Thiocyanate is typically measured in the serum or plasma, but it can also be measured in saliva. Salivary measurements are the more common way to measure in the outpatient setting.

Blood concentrations of nicotine can be measured by gas chromatography or radioimmunoassay. Clinical measurement has been difficult in the past, but new techniques may make it less problematic. Careful handling of the samples is important in obtaining meaningful results.

Cotinine is a metabolite of nicotine that can be measured in blood, saliva, and urine, although it is fairly costly to do. The half-life of cotinine is around 19 hours. Nonsmokers have blood values below 10 ng per milliliter. The radioimmunoassay or gas chromatography required to measure cotinine is probably too costly for routine clinical use, but these tests provide an important measurement for smoking cessation research.

Focus on the Smoker's Health Attitudes and Attitudes about Smoking

In the precontemplation stage, it is useful to explore other health habits. Does the smoker do regular exercise, avoid cholesterol, use seat belts, or do monthly self-examination of breasts or testicles? If the smoker does any of these, he has already made the decision to participate in health and to take personal control. This is obvious to the health professional, but the smoker may need to have his controlling role pointed out.

Many smokers say they are aware of the health risks, but "you have to die of something." Pointing out the very real risk of smoking may best be done by a written, signed contract. The contract or informed risk letter may serve two purposes. The smoker is asked to sign the form (Fig. 2) and is given one copy. The original is placed in the chart to avoid possible future litigation. The physician or health profes-

Dear Patient _____

   As your physician I am concerned about your smoking habit and addiction. I want to be sure that you are aware of the facts about smoking and the health risks you are incurring by continuing to smoke.

RISKS OF SMOKING	BENEFITS OF QUITTING	RELATIVE RISKS: FILTER-TIPPED, LOW T/N BRANDS	RISKS OF SMOKING	BENEFITS OF QUITTING	RELATIVE RISKS: FILTER-TIPPED LOW T/N BRANDS
Risk: Shortened life expectancy. 25-year-old 2-pack-a-day smokers have life expectancy 8.3 years shorter than nonsmoking contemporaries. Other smoking levels: proportional risk.	**Benefit: Reduces risk of premature death cumulatively.** After 10–15 years, ex-smokers' risk approaches that of those who've never smoked.	Reduced risk of death from certain diseases (see below) implies increased life expectancy.	**Risk: Coronary heart disease.** Cigarette smoking is major factor; responsible for 120,000 excess U.S. deaths from coronary heart disease (CHD) each year.	**Benefit: Sharply decreases risk after one year.** After 10 years ex-smokers' risk is same as that of those who never smoked.	Low T/N male smokers had 12 percent lower CHD rate, female low T/N smokers 19 percent lower than high T/N smokers.
Risk: Lung cancer. Smoking cigarettes "major cause in both men and women." [SG 1979]	**Benefit: Gradual decrease in risk. After 10–15 years, risk approaches that of those who never smoked.**	Filter tips reduce risk, but it is still 5 times that of nonsmokers. Low T/N brands reduce male risk by 20%, female risk by 40%.	**Risks: Chronic bronchitis and pulmonary emphysema.** Cigarette smokers have 4–25 times risk of death from these diseases as nonsmokers. Damage seen in lungs of even young smokers.	**Benefit: Cough and sputum disappear** during first few weeks. **Lung function may improve** and rate of deterioration slow down.	No identified benefit.
Risk: Larynx cancer. In all smokers (including pipe and cigar) it's 2.9 to 17.7 times that of nonsmokers.	**Benefit: Gradual reduction of risk after smoking cessation. Reaches normal after 10 years.**	Filter tips reduce risk 24 to 49 percent.	**Risks: Stillbirth and low birthweight.** Smoking mothers have more stillbirths and babies of low birthweight— more vulnerable to disease and death	**Benefit: Women** who stop smoking before 4th month of pregnancy **eliminate risk of stillbirth and low birthweight** caused by smoking.	No identified benefit.
Risk: Mouth cancer. Cigarette smokers have 3 to 10 times as many oral cancers as nonsmokers. Pipes, cigars, chewing tobacco also major risk factors. Alcohol seems synergistic carcinogen with smoking.	**Benefit: Reducing or eliminating smoking/drinking reduces risk in first few years; risk drops to level of nonsmokers in 10–15 years.**	No identified benefit.	**Risks: Children of smoking mothers** smaller, underdeveloped physically and socially, seven years after birth.	**Benefit: Since** children of nonsmoking mothers are bigger and more advanced socially, inference is that **not smoking during pregnancy might avoid such underdeveloped children.**	No identified benefit.

Figure 2   This informed risk letter highlights for the patient the risks of continued smoking and the benefits of quitting.

RISKS OF SMOKING	BENEFITS OF QUITTING	RELATIVE RISKS: FILTER-TIPPED, LOW T/N BRANDS	RISKS OF SMOKING	BENEFITS OF QUITTING	RELATIVE RISKS: FILTER-TIPPED LOW T/N BRANDS
Risk: Cancer of esophagus. Cigarettes, pipes and cigars increase risk of dying of esophageal cancer about 2 to 9 times. Synergistic relationship between smoking and alcohol.	**Benefit:** Since risks are dose related, reducing or eliminating smoking/drinking **should have risk-reducing effect.**	No identified benefit.	**Risk: Peptic ulcer.** Cigarette smokers get more peptic ulcers and die more often of them; cure is more difficult in smokers.	**Benefit:** Ex-smokers get ulcers but these are **more likely to heal rapidly and completely** than those of smokers.	No identified benefit.
Risk: Cancer of bladder. Cigarette smokers have 7 to 10 times risk of bladder cancer as nonsmokers. Also synergistic with certain exposed occupations: dyestuffs, etc.	**Benefit:** Risk decreases **gradually to that of nonsmokers over 7 years.**	No identified benefit.	**Risk: Allergy and impairment of immune system.**	**Benefit:** Since these are direct, immediate effects of smoking, they are obviously **avoidable by not smoking.**	No identified benefit.
Risk: Cancer of pancreas. Cigarette smokers have 2 to 5 times risk of dying of pancreatic cancer as nonsmokers.	**Benefit:** Since there is evidence of dose-related risk, reducing or eliminating smoking should have risk-reducing effect.	No identified benefit.	**Risks: Alters pharmacologic effects of many medicines, diagnostic tests and greatly increases risk of thrombosis with oral contraceptives.**	**Benefit: Majority of blood components elevated by return to normal after cessation.** Nonsmokers on Pill have much lower risks of thrombosis.	

DATE _____ DOCTOR _____

Acknowledge by signing below that you have read the above information, that you understand the risks you are taking by continuing to smoke and the benefits of quitting, and that you have been advised by me to quit smoking.

DATE _____ PATIENT _____

Figure 2 Continued. (Data from Dangers of smoking. Benefits of quitting. American Cancer Society. Used with permission.)

sional has informed the patient that smoking is risky and should be avoided.

A second useful written document is a prescription, prescribing that the patient stop smoking. All this may sound melodramatic, but it serves notice to the smoker who does not take seriously advice to quit smoking.

During the health history, one should identify any relatives of the patient who have died of a tobacco-related disease. The patient in precontemplation often says something like, "Why should I quit, when my Uncle Henry smoked every day until he was 92 and died in a car accident?" A careful history often uncovers two or three other relatives who smoked and

died young of a smoking-related disease. Again, the health professional is trying to uncover the facts and point out the true risks to the smoker.

A quiz developed by Daniel Horn when he was the Director of the National Clearinghouse for Smoking and Health may help the smoker at this stage (Fig. 3). The quiz on the effects of smoking is scored for importance, personal relevance, value of stopping, and capability of stopping. The smoker who scores low for importance needs additional education about the health hazards and true risks of smoking. Pamphlets that contain data related to health risks may help this smoker. A person who has a low score in personal relevance may be impressed by the carbon monoxide

WHAT DO YOU THINK THE EFFECTS OF SMOKING ARE?

For each statement, circle the number that shows how you feel about it. Do you strongly agree, mildly agree, mildly disagree, or strongly disagree?

Important: Answer every question.

	Strongly agree	Mildly agree	Mildly disagree	Strongly disagree
A. Cigarette smoking is not nearly as dangerous as many other health hazards.	1	2	3	4
B. I don't smoke enough to get any of the diseases that cigarette smoking is supposed to cause.	1	2	3	4
C. If a person has already smoked for many years, it probably won't do him much good to stop.	1	2	3	4
D. It would be hard for me to give up smoking cigarettes.	1	2	3	4
E. Cigarette smoking is enough of a health hazard for something to be done about it.	1	2	3	4
F. The kind of cigarette I smoke is much less likely than other kinds to give me any of the diseases that smoking is supposed to cause.	1	2	3	4
G. As soon as a person quits smoking cigarettes he begins to recover from much of the damage that smoking has caused.	1	2	3	4
H. It would be hard for me to cut down to half the number of cigarettes I now smoke.	1	2	3	4
I. The whole problem of cigarette smoking and health is a very minor one.	1	2	3	4
J. I haven't smoked long enough to worry about the diseases that cigarette smoking is supposed to cause.	1	2	3	4
K. Quitting smoking helps a person to live longer.	1	2	3	4
L. It would be difficult for me to make any substantial change in my smoking habits.	1	2	3	4

HOW TO SCORE:

1. Enter the numbers you have circled in the spaces below, putting the number you have circled to Question A over line A, to Question B over line B, etc.
2. Total the 3 scores across on each line to get your totals. For example, the sum of your scores over lines A, E, and I gives you your score on *Importance*—lines B, F, and J give the score on *Personal Relevance*, etc.

Totals

$$\frac{\quad}{A} + \frac{\quad}{E} + \frac{\quad}{I} = \frac{\quad}{\text{Importance}}$$

$$\frac{\quad}{B} + \frac{\quad}{F} + \frac{\quad}{J} = \frac{\quad}{\text{Personal Relevance}}$$

$$\frac{\quad}{C} + \frac{\quad}{G} + \frac{\quad}{K} = \frac{\quad}{\text{Value of Stopping}}$$

$$\frac{\quad}{D} + \frac{\quad}{H} + \frac{\quad}{L} = \frac{\quad}{\text{Capability for Stopping}}$$

Scores can vary from 3 to 12. Any score 9 and above is *high*; any score 6 and below is *low*.

Figure 3 Quiz developed by Daniel Horn. Used to determine the importance, personal relevance, and value of stopping and the capability of an individual to stop smoking.

or other biologic tests that measure consumption. There is value to stopping smoking no matter what the patient's age. Elderly patients may be impressed that they will have increased brain blood flow or decreased mortality risk if they quit. Younger patients could be given the American Cancer Society's booklet, "Dangers of Smoking and Benefits of Quitting." This booklet was written for the health professional, so it would be better to condense the information to a one- or two-page information sheet written at the reading level of patients served in the office or hospital. Another technique is writing the information in the form of the risk letter (see Fig. 2). The individual who feels it would be difficult to stop may be the addicted smoker. It may be reassuring for that patient to know there are pharmacologic agents available to help with withdrawal symptoms.

CONTEMPLATION STAGE

It may take weeks or months, and occasionally years, to move the smoker to the contemplation stage. However, when the person admits to thinking about quitting, it is important to move him to a decision about a quit date. The person who says, "Yes, I know I should quit, I'm going to do it one of these days" needs special encouragement and some homework assignments. During this stage, the smoker needs to learn some details about his habit and addiction. Recording, tracking, or diary forms are useful during this stage. The usual things to record are time of day, intensity of need, and reason for a cigarette (Table 1). After one or two weeks of recording, the smoker knows what his main triggers are for smoking. This information is useful for planning coping strategies as a nonsmoker. Developing coping strategies early will help prevent relapse after cessation. The smoker who always has a cigarette during phone calls will have the same desire for a cigarette after cessation. A planned coping response could be a lollipop, doodling, deep breaths, or standing instead of sitting while using the telephone.

Another tool developed by Daniel Horn is the "Why Do You Smoke?" quiz (Fig. 4). This quiz helps smokers to identify their main reasons for smoking. It scores the smoker for stimulation, handling, relaxation and tension reduction, craving and psychological addiction, and habit. Smokers who score high for stimulation use cigarettes in place of healthy stimulation. Often these individuals are sedentary and need to adopt a new health habit: exercise. Isometrics, walking, and stair climbing are better alternatives. Handling is easily replaced by a pen, pencil, lollipop, toothpick, swizzle stick, worry stone, or prayer beads. Using cigarettes for relaxation and tension reduction is more complicated. Some smokers can use visualization or meditation. For others, just getting up and moving around helps. Total body tensing and relaxing, or stretches and ten deep breaths are also alternatives. Deep breaths probably are more important during cessation than we realize. Most smokers take ten deep inhalations with each cigarette. The person who scores high for craving and psychological addiction may be physically addicted. Use the Fagerstrom test to investigate further the smoker's addiction. Remember, all smokers have the habit. It will take 5 to 6 weeks to disassociate or replace the habit.

Other homework during contemplation is using reverse-hand smoking, relocating cigarettes from their usual place, restricting smoking to certain areas, and timing the urges. Developing a negative image is valuable to the young, health-conscious smoker. A friend can help by taking a roll of film while the smoker is inhaling a cigarette. Displaying these pictures in prominent places at work and at home will emphasize the negative during the contemplation stage.

ACTION STAGE

Pharmacologic Support

The action stage begins when the smoker has made the decision to quit. Now is the time to determine whether the patient is a candidate for pharmacologic assistance. Nicotine-polacrilex (Nicorette) gum is most useful in the drug-dependent smoker. Nicotine-dependent smokers occasionally smoke in the middle of the night, smoke first thing in the morning, enjoy the

TABLE 1   Form Used to Record Daily Smoking Activity

Time	Intensity of need 0 (least)–5 (greatest)	Why are you smoking cigarettes?

WHY DO YOU SMOKE?

Here are some statements made by people to describe what they get out of smoking cigarettes. How *often* do you feel this way when smoking them? Circle one number for each statement.

Important: Answer every question.

	Always	Fre-quently	Occa-sionally	Seldom	Never
A. I smoke cigarettes in order to keep myself from slowing down.	5	4	3	2	1
B. Handling a cigarette is part of the enjoyment of smoking it.	5	4	3	2	1
C. Smoking cigarettes is pleasant and relaxing.	5	4	3	2	1
D. I light up a cigarette when I feel angry about something.	5	4	3	2	1
E. When I have run out of cigarettes I find it almost unbearable until I can get them.	5	4	3	2	1
F. I smoke cigarettes automatically without even being aware of it.	5	4	3	2	1
G. I smoke cigarettes to stimulate me, to perk myself up.	5	4	3	2	1
H. Part of the enjoyment of smoking a cigarette comes from the steps I take to light up.	5	4	3	2	1
I. I find cigarettes pleasurable.	5	4	3	2	1
J. When I feel uncomfortable or upset about something, I light up a cigarette.	5	4	3	2	1
K. I am very much aware of the fact when I am not smoking a cigarette.	5	4	3	2	1
L. I light up a cigarette without realizing I still have one burning in the ashtray.	5	4	3	2	1
M. I smoke cigarettes to give me a "lift."	5	4	3	2	1
N. When I smoke a cigarette, part of the enjoyment is watching the smoke as I exhale it.	5	4	3	2	1
O. I want a cigarette most when I am comfortable and relaxed.	5	4	3	2	1
P. When I feel "blue" or want to take my mind off cares and worries, I smoke cigarettes.	5	4	3	2	1
Q. I get a real gnawing hunger for a cigarette when I haven't smoked for a while.	5	4	3	2	1
R. I've found a cigarette in my mouth and didn't remember putting it there.	5	4	3	2	1

HOW TO SCORE:

1. Enter the numbers you have circled in the spaces below, putting the number you have circled to Question A over line A, to Question B over line B, etc.
2. Total the 3 scores on each line to get your totals. For example, the sum of your scores over lines A, G, and M gives you your score on *Stimulation*—lines B, H, and N give the score on *Handling,* etc.

Totals

```
___  +  ___  +  ___  =  _____
 A        G        M        Stimulation

___  +  ___  +  ___  =  _____
 B        H        N        Handling

___  +  ___  +  ___  =  _____
 C        I        O        Pleasurable Relaxation

___  +  ___  +  ___  =  _____
 D        J        P        Crutch: Tension Reduction

___  +  ___  +  ___  =  _____
 E        K        Q        Craving: Psychological Addiction

___  +  ___  +  ___  =  _____
 F        L        R        Habit
```

Scores can vary from 3 to 15. Any score 11 and above is *high;* any score 7 and below is *low.*

Figure 4   Quiz developed by Daniel Horn. Used to identify reason why people smoke.

first cigarette the most, smoke a pack or more per day, have difficulty refraining from cigarettes in places where it is prohibited, smoke when ill, and inhale the cigarette smoke.

Success with the gum depends on patient understanding and education. The keys to successful gum use are listed briefly in Table 2. Commitment to quitting is 50 percent of the battle in conquering the habit and addiction of smoking. A support person is most important in the first 3 months, when relapse is highest.

The smoker should practice with a piece of gum during a patient visit so that the physician or health professional can observe the technique. Proper use is as follows: (1) Warm the gum in the mouth; (2) chew until a peppery sensation is noticed; (3) park the gum in the mouth; (4) take a deep, slow breath through the mouth; (5) chew, park, and take a deep breath; (6) repeat this technique for up to 30 minutes. It is also best to use the gum when there is something in the stomach. We suggest that the patient eat wheat biscuits, rye crisp, or a handful of bran flakes prior to chewing the gum. If gum chewing encourages saliva production, the patient is encouraged to expectorate into tissue, and discard. Swallowing the gum saliva on an empty stomach may lead to hiccups and even nausea. Avoid coffee or pop intake while using the medication gum. The nicotine in the gum base is not absorbed in an acid environment.

The dosage is one piece of gum for every cigarette smoked. Although a one-pack-a-day smoker should be relieved of withdrawal symptoms by using 10 to 12 pieces of gum a day, we suggest using the one-to-one ratio during the first 2 weeks of cessation, when withdrawal symptoms are most intense. The best success is with smokers who use it long enough—at least 3 months. Because relapse is highest in the first three months, it seems obvious that this would be the case. Smokers should be educated that it takes approximately 30 minutes to increase the morning blood level of nicotine. Therefore, smokers who previously smoked a cigarette on arising should not wait until they desire a cigarette but should use the gum prophylactically.

The smoker should be educated that the gum relieves withdrawal symptoms such as lack of concentration, nervousness, and irritability. It does not re-

TABLE 2 Key Elements to Successful Use of Nicorette Gum

Ready to commit to quitting
Support person
Practice with gum
Instructed in use
Know behavior skills
Use enough (1 stick per 2 cigarettes)
Use long enough (≥3 months)
Educated

TABLE 3 Ten Behavioral Techniques to Cope with Cravings

1. Relocate—move away from the urge.
2. Take slow deep breaths through the mouth, hold, and exhale through pursed lips.
3. "Ping" wrist or ankle with a rubber band.
4. Draw a self-portrait.
5. Walk up three flights of stairs.
6. Make a chain of 25 paper clips.
7. Pound 25 nails into a board.
8. Stand up and stretch and twist and turn torso for 3 minutes.
9. Do three words in a crossword puzzle.
10. Do a mental silent scream.

lieve the craving sensation. Behavioral techniques are required to interrupt the cravings. See Table 3 for a list of behavioral techniques to cope with cravings. The gum user should anticipate situations in which cigarettes were always used. The gum should be chewed prior to a high-risk situation. Use of the gum should precede a coffee break or meeting by 10 or 15 minutes. Always caution that Nicorette is a medication, not just a gum. After 3 months of cigarette abstinence, tapering from the gum should be started. One technique is illustrated in Table 4. Dependency on the gum occurs in 7 to 10 percent of users.

Behavior Support

Smokers should start the quit date as a nonsmoker rather than quit in the middle of the day. Planned activities for the first day and first week help to fill up the time. The smoker should avoid typical smoking situations such as coffee breaks or after-work drinks with smoking friends for a couple of weeks. Once the smoker quits, it is best to tell friends so that they understand if the smoker is irritable and short-tempered.

Smoking cessation is best done when the job pressures are not unusual. Accountants who try to quit on April 1 may not be realistic about this quit date. Extra physical activity should be encouraged the first day to 2 weeks for a new ex-smoker. Taking short walks or climbing a flight of stairs each hour can help decrease anxiety and agitation. Preparations that can help for the quit date are removing ash trays from car, home, and office and getting rid of other reminders of smoking, such as lighters and cigarette cases; posting No Smoking or clean air notes; and placing low- or no-calorie substitutes where cigarettes were usually stored. These could include sugarless lollipops and gum, toothpicks, swizzle sticks, lip gloss, word puzzles, and paper clips and safety pins to make chains.

Switching to lightly caffeinated or decaffeinated drinks may be a help the first several weeks. Nonsmokers get more effect from caffeine than do smokers.

Smokers may need help with stimulation the first week or two. Some nonchemical stimulants that can

TABLE 4 Suggested Reducing Formula from Nicorette Gum (For a 14-piece-per-day user)

	Time of day	Day 1	2	3	4	5	6	7	8	9	10	11	12	13	14
1st Dosage		N*	N	N	N	N	N	N	N	N	N	N	N	N	R
2nd		N	N	N	N	N	N	N							
3rd		N	N	N	N	N	N		N	N			N		
4th		N	½	N	N	N	N	N			N				
5th		N	N		N				N		N				
6th		½	½	N				N		N					
7th		N	N		N	N	N		N						
8th		N	N	N	N	N		N			N				
9th		N	N	N			N			N					
10th		N	½	N		N		N	N						
11th		N	N		N		N								
12th		½	½	N	N	N		N	N	N	N	N			
13th		N	N	N			N								
14th		N	N	N	N	N									
Reduced by Total Nicorette		13	12	11	10	9	8	7	6	5	4	3	2	1	0

N = 1 piece of Nicorette.

be used at work are complete body stretches, ice or hot water compresses to the face and neck, or rubber band "pings" to ankle or wrist.

MAINTENANCE STAGE

Preparation Helps Maintenance

Maintenance of nonsmoking is enhanced by education during the contemplation stage. Individuals who understand their smoking habit and addiction may be better prepared to handle potential relapse situations. Smokers who have filled out a daily diary of cigarette usage may have an understanding of when and why they smoked. This information can be used to prepare for coping responses in high-risk situations as a nonsmoker.

Maintenance of nonsmoking is tested every time the new ex-smoker encounters a situation for the first time. Mental rehearsal prior to the event should be helpful. By visualizing the situation and the participants, the new ex-smoker can plan coping strategies so that the temptation to smoke is reduced. Coping strategies are behavioral and cognitive. Behavioral strategies include any activity designed to reduce the urge to smoke (Table 3). Cognitive strategies are thoughts or self-conversations that the ex-smoker uses to maintain nonsmoking. Some examples of self-talk are, "I'm stronger than the cigarettes" and "That little weed can't get the best of me, I'm not smoking today."

The reasons that the smoker wanted to quit smoking in the first place may be helpful in maintaining quitting. There are usually multiple reasons for quitting smoking, among them personal health and financial and social reasons. A handwritten list may serve as a personal contract. Rereading the list may be a potent biofeedback technique for some in sustaining efforts at cessation.

The Role of the Support Person

A support person can be of special help during the first 3 months of maintenance. Support can be given verbally and by actions. Thank-you notes sent to the work place or home, a flower, an invitation to dinner, a back rub, and words of endearment help ease the discomfort in the early stages. Smokers who are able to identify one special person who will help them are best positioned to ask for help when faced with a crisis that may lead to relapse.

Physical Discomforts and Maintenance

The physical discomforts of weight gain and constipation may plague some new ex-smokers. Both may be helped by adequate exercise and increases in fluid and fiber intake. A recent study by Angela Hofstetter reported in the *New England Journal of Medicine,* found that smoking 24 cigarettes per day increases overall energy expenditure by 10 percent. This means that new ex-smokers need to increase activity to burn more calories or reduce intake in order to avoid weight gain.

Constipation occurs in about 40 percent of new ex-smokers. The smoker who always smoked a cigarette during a bowel movement is a prime candidate for constipation problems. We suggest that this individual start a daily program of increased fiber and water intake to avoid problems.

RELAPSE

Lapse Occurs First

Relapse is preceded by a lapse. Sometimes the lapse is planned as a self-testing game, and this is especially true with the first-time quitter. The smoker talks himself into testing whether he can be the unusual smoker who has "just an occasional cigarette." Usually, that one cigarette leads to two, three, and a whole pack, and the smoker is "rehooked." The health professional can help the smoker to avoid this situation by asking the smoker whether he plans to test himself after cessation. It is surprising how many answer yes. Guide them away from this risky thought.

Usually a relapse occurs when the ex-smoker is unprepared to handle a crisis. Most relapses are related to negative emotional situations. Interpersonal conflicts and social pressure situations also contribute to relapse (Table 5). Interestingly, urges and temptations account for only 5 percent of relapses, according to researcher C. Alan Marlatt. He describes the "Abstinence Violation Effect" as playing a major role in relapse. Simply stated, the new nonsmoker who

TABLE 5   Factors That Influence Smoking Relapse

A response to cues such as alcohol or coffee
The partner continues to smoke
Best friends continue to smoke
Response to stress
Negative emotional situations

has a lapse (one cigarette) feels so guilty for breaking his personal commitment to be a nonsmoker that it contributes to a full-blown relapse. Advising the new ex-smoker that he should be kind, considerate, and forgiving toward himself if a lapse does occur may help the ex-smoker to stay on track. Those not informed about this effect may react so harshly to a slip that a relapse occurs. Looking at smoking cessation as a black-white, either-or situation may be too harsh for some new ex-smokers. The new ex-smoker who does relapse should be given praise for trying and not criticized for failure. By using a positive attitude, the health professional can help bring the smoker back to renewed action.

RENEWED ACTION

Renewed action is a stage 80 percent of smokers will cycle through. The long-term quit rate is 20 percent for first time quitters who are not involved in intensive cessation programs. The long-term quit rate improves, however, each time a smoker attempts to quit. Seventh-time quitters can expect to be successful 83 percent of the time, according to a U.S. Department of Health, Education and Welfare 1975 citation. Accordingly, it is important for the health professional to develop a positive attitude and encourage the smoker to try again.

Suggested Reading

American Cancer Society. Dangers of smoking: benefits of quitting. New York: American Cancer Society, 1980.

Grabowski J, Bell CS. Measurement in the analysis and treatment of smoking behavior, Rockville, MD: US Department of Health and Human Services, NIDA Research Monograph 48, 1983.

Grabowski J, Hall SM. Pharmacological adjuncts in smoking cessation. Rockville, MD: US Department of Health and Human Services, NIDA Research Monograph 53, 1985.

Krasnegar N. The behavioral aspects of smoking. Rockville, MD: US Department of Health, Education, and Welfare, Research Monograph 26, 1979.

Marlatt GA. Relapse prevention: a self-control program for the treatment of addictive behaviors. In: Stuart RB, ed. Adherence, compliance and generalization in behavioral medicine. New York: Brunner/Mazel, 1982.

Marlatt GA, Gordon JR. Relapse prevention. New York: Guilford, 1985.

Proceedings of the national working conference on smoking relapse in health psychology. Vol. 5 Supplement. Hillsdale, NJ: Lawrence Erlbaum Associates, 1986.

Schwartz J. Review and evaluation of smoking cessation methods: the US and Canada, 1978–1985. Bethesda, MD: NIH Publication No. 87-2940, 1987.

RESPIRATORY CARE QUALITY ASSURANCE PROGRAM

KATHRYN W. HARRIS, RRT

To receive accreditation by the Joint Commission on Accreditation of Hospitals (JCAH), hospitals must have active quality assurance programs that meet specified criteria. In this chapter I give background on development of hospital quality assurance programs, present the current respiratory care standards, and describe the quality assurance program of the Respiratory Care Department at the Massachusetts General Hospital.

Beginning in the early twentieth century, a small group of physicians from the American College of Surgeons began surveying hospitals and granting accreditation based on compliance with a one-page list of required standards of care. In 1952, the JCAH took over this function of surveying hospitals. Today, the JCAH has a staff of over 400, a multimillion dollar budget, and 300 pages of accreditation standards. The JCAH has five parenting bodies: the American College of Physicians, the American College of Surgeons, the American Dental Society, the American Hospital Association, and the American Medical Association. For many years accreditation was truly voluntary; however, hospitals viewed accreditation as a stamp of approval from a national organization with experience and skill in evaluating standards of care. Although technically accreditation is still voluntary, the 1968 federal Medicare legislation requires accreditation by the JCAH or by local health authorities to be eligible for federally supported hospital care.

A hospital that meets JCAH standards is awarded accreditation for 3 years. At the end of the 3 years, the hospital must undergo and pass another survey in order to maintain accreditation.

The JCAH standards are delineated in an Accreditation Manual for Hospitals. Included in this manual are standards for hospital administration, building and ground safety, sanitation, medical staff, nursing services, infection control, laboratories, quality assurance, and support services.

Since its founding in 1951, the JCAH has stressed the review, evaluation, and analysis of the quality of clinical practice. The initial requirements for effective quality assurance were the establishment of objective evaluation criteria and the development of systematic review.

In 1974, the JCAH required review of the quality and appropriateness of patient care by support services, including respiratory therapy. At this time, the JCAH stressed the review of medical records for clinical indications for therapy and documentation of all departmental patient procedures.

Under these guidelines, respiratory care departments began auditing medical records. On a quarterly basis, medical records were examined to see if respiratory therapy orders included the following:

1. Diagnosis related to therapy
2. Indication for treatment based on established criteria
3. Oxygen concentration, frequency and duration of treatment, dosage of drug, and amount of diluent
4. Therapeutic objective: evaluation of the effectiveness of the treatment by a physician

A report of the results of the audit would be submitted to the quality assurance committee. Compliance to the established guidelines was often difficult to enforce. Frequently, nothing was done to alter inappropriate care and subsequent audits would reveal the same problems. A respiratory care order sheet that requires essential information before treatment is given (Fig. 1) has been used by some as a solution to this problem. However, the trouble with this approach is that the focus is on physicians and how to change their practice, and not on problems occurring within the respiratory care departments.

REVISED QUALITY ASSURANCE STANDARDS

In 1984 the JCAH introduced new standards for support services in their Accreditation Manual for Hospitals. These new standards required the continuous monitoring and evaluation of clinical aspects of patient care. The emphasis of quality assurance changed from retrospective audits to prospective ongoing monitoring of clinical activities with the goal of improving patient care. The audits could still be used; however, ongoing evaluation of patient care was required.

The current required characteristics of a quality assurance program are the following:

1. The quality and appropriateness of patient care is monitored systematically as part of a written quality assurance plan.
2. All major clinical functions of the department are to be evaluated, using objective criteria reflecting current standards of care.
3. The physician director of the respiratory care de-

PLEASE STATE
DIAGNOSIS RELATING TO THERAPY:_____

UNIT CLERK _____ TIME CALLED _____

THERAPIST _____ TIME REC'D _____

_____ _____
DATE   PHYSICIAN

PHYSICIAN'S RETROSPECTIVE EVALUATION
[TO BE PERFORMED EVERY 72 HRS.]

- RETROSPECTIVE EVALUATION TO BE COMPLETED BY PHYSICIAN AFTER 72 HRS. AND PRIOR TO REORDER.
- UNLESS DURATION IS SPECIFIED, TREATMENTS WILL BE GIVEN FOR 24 HRS. ALL ORDERS TERMINATE AFTER 72 HRS.
- INDICATIONS AND OBJECTIVES TO BE COMPLETED BY PHYSICIAN **BEFORE** THERAPY IS INITIATED.

	Improved	Deteriorated	No Change
CHEST X-RAY	___	___	___
BREATH SOUNDS	___	___	___
OXYGENATION	___	___	___
COUGH	___	___	___

specify other
☐ OBJECTIVES ACHIEVED — D/C THERAPY
☐ OBJECTIVES NOT ACHIEVED — RENEW AS FOLLOWS

TREATMENTS

INCENTIVE SPIROMETRY [check one]
☐ **BEDSIDE** -Prevent post-op complications due to:
SPIROMETER   a. upper abdominal surgery
[circle indication]   b. thoracic surgery
c. documented acute or chronic lung disease
Frequency **Only one pre & post-op instruction**

☐ **SPIROCARE** - Treatment of **documented** acute pulmonary disease (atelectasis)
Frequency: _____ Duration: _____

IPPB [check indication]
☐ Atelectasis unresponsive to simpler therapy
☐ Inspiratory capacity less than 1 liter
☐ Ineffective cough mechanism
☐ Severe hypoventilation/avoid mechanical vent
☐ **STANDING ORDER:**   ☐ **CHANGE STANDING**
Frequency: QID   **ORDER TO:**
Duration of 24 Hrs.
O_2 Conc. At pt's FIO_2
Pressure 20-25 cmH$_2$O
ADMINISTER WITH: [check one]
☐ Normal Saline ☐ Medication (See meds section)

NEBULIZATION THERAPY
☐ MEDICATION NEBULIZER
☐ ULTRASONIC NEBULIZER
☐ SPUTUM INDUCTION AFB ____ CYTOLOGY ____
PYOGENS ____ FUNGUS ____
THERAPY OBJECTIVES
☐ Hydration of dried, retained secretions
☐ Administration of pharmacological agent
Frequency _____ Duration:_____
Length of Tx _____ min
O_2 Conc _____ %
ADMINISTER WITH: [check one]
☐ Saline ☐ Medication (See meds section)

MEDICATIONS
☐ METAPROTERENOL (Alupent, 5% Sol.)
☐ ISOETHARINE (Bronkosol, 1% Sol.)
☐ ISOPROTERENOL (Isuprel, 1 200 Sol.)
☐ ACETYLCYSTEINE (Mucomyst, 20% Sol.)
☐ RACEMIC EPINEPHRINE (Vaponephrine, 2 25% Sol.)
☐ OTHER _____
specify
DOSE: _____ TO _____
quantity of drug   quantity of dilutent

HUMIDITY / OXYGEN

OXYGEN THERAPY
THERAPY OBJECTIVES
☐ Decrease work of breathing
☐ Decrease myocardial work
☐ Treat hypoxia
DEVICE
☐ NASAL CANNULA _____ 1/min
☐ SIMPLE MASK (35-55%) _____ 1/min
☐ VENTI MASK 24 26 28 30 35 40 50
☐ MASK WITH RESERVOIR (60-90%)
☐ CPAP MASK (30-100%) _____ %
5.0cmH$_2$O 7.5cmH$_2$O 10.0 cmH$_2$O 12.5 cmH$_2$O

HIGH HUMIDITY OXYGEN
☐ AEROSOL (35-100%) FIO_2 _____ %
Aerosol Mask ____ Face Tent
T-Piece ____ Tracheostomy Collar
☐ HEAD HOOD FIO_2 _____ %
☐ CROUP TENT FIO_2 _____ %

DIAGNOSTIC

☐ CARDIAC OUTPUT
☐ HEMODYNAMIC PROFILE
OTHER _____
SPECIFY

☐ PRE-OP PULMONARY SCREENING (FEV$_1$/FVC)
History of smoking
Occupational exposure
Pulmonary signs and symptoms
Other _____

☐ RESPIRATORY PARAMETERS
Vt/Vc/NIF Frequency _____
Peak Expiratory Flow

☐ OXIMETRY
Ear Oximeter
Oximetrix (Pulmonary artery catheter)

☐ RESPIRATORY CONSULTATION

ADDRESSOGRAPH:

MED RECORD NO: BIRTHDATE: SEX:

PATIENT NAME:

ADDRESS: ROOM:

CHART

Figure 1 A respiratory care order sheet to facilitate physician compliance to JCAH standards.

partment is responsible for assuring that the process is implemented.

4. There is ongoing collection of information.
5. There is periodic assessment of the information.
6. Problems are identified that have an impact on patient care.
7. Identified problems are resolved by appropriate action.
8. The effectiveness of the action is evaluated.
9. Patient care is improved.
10. Findings, conclusions, recommendations, action taken, and the results of action taken are documented and reported to the hospital quality assurance committee.
11. The quality assurance program is reviewed annually for effectiveness and compliance to established standards.

THE ONGOING MONITORS

Ongoing reports currently used to identify problems may act as monitors (Table 1). Examples include the following:

1. *Hospital incident reports:* This type of report is used in most hospitals. We use these reports in situations in which a patient's welfare has been affected.
2. *Infection control reports:* We receive reports from the infection control department that involve our equipment and/or personnel. For example, sporadic cases of *Acinetobacter* bacteremia were recently reported in patients in several intensive care units. We were alerted to the possibility that mercury manometers we use in calibrating transducers were a potential vector for transmission.

TABLE 1 Department of Respiratory Care Quality Assurance Ongoing Monitors

Monitor	Frequency
Incident reports/problem resolution forms	Daily
Categorized into	
Respiratory equipment mechanical failures	
Clinical errors	
Central processing equipment problems	
Systems: oxygen, air, electrical	
Equipment shortages	
Accidents	
Infection control	
Communication problems	
Outside services	
Complaints from staff, patients, other personnel	Daily
Supervisor's end-of-shift report	Daily
Assessment of all unusual occurrences	
Infection control reports	Daily
Documentation review	As generated
Supervisor assessment of charting	
Audits of appropriateness and effectiveness of therapy	Quarterly

3. *Shift reports:* We use an end-of-shift report to be certain that essential information is passed on to the next supervisor in charge. Any unusual situation or problem is recorded and the report is reviewed daily by the associate director.

4. *Documentation review:* Respiratory care documentation in patient charts by staff therapists is reviewed by supervisors on an ongoing basis to assure compliance with departmental and JCAH standards.

5. *Audits:* Audits review appropriateness and effectiveness of care. We continue to do audits of medical records. The new standards recommend that these audits be done on a prospective basis.

THE MASS GENERAL APPROACH: THE PROBLEM RESOLUTION FORM

At the Massachusetts General Hospital a problem resolution form is used, in addition to the above monitors, to identify and solve problems (Fig. 2). Anyone who experiences a clinically related problem is requested to use this form. The therapist making out the form is asked to state the problem and, if possible, identify reasons why the problem occurred. A space is also provided to list possible solutions to the problem. The forms are always available and completed forms are processed by the associate director. If a staff therapist fills out a problem form, he or she must notify the supervisor so that immediate action can be taken, if necessary. These forms are reviewed weekly at supervisors' meetings for group input, discussion, and problem resolution. Actions taken are documented and subsequently evaluated. The forms are then put into a large loose-leaf notebook, which is divided into the following categories by the type of problem addressed.

Respiratory Equipment Mechanical Failures

All ventilator failures are documented and kept in this section. The reports are then separated by type of ventilator (e.g., Emerson, Puritan-Bennett 7200, MA-2, Seimens Servo, Hamilton, Bear 1 and 2). The equipment section includes blender problems, regulators, tanks, and so forth. By organizing the me-

Your Name:	Date: Shift:
Patient's Name:	Supervisor Notified:
Room #:	
Equipment:	Incident Report:

Problem:

Cause (if known):

Possible Solutions:

Action Taken:

Figure 2 Quality assurance ongoing monitors problem resolution form: department of respiratory care

chanical failures in this manner, we can easily identify recurrent problems involving the same piece of equipment. Equipment performance can easily be evaluated, influencing maintenance schedules and purchasing decisions.

Examples

During an afternoon shift, black smoke suddenly filled the pediatric intensive care unit. The smoke came from a smoldering black rubber anesthesia bag used on a ventilator patient circuit. The cause was an overheated transformer inside the ventilator. The following action was taken:

1. The manufacturer was notified.
2. A report was filed with US Pharmacopeia via the Medical Device and Laboratory Product Reporting Program.
3. The Massachusetts General Hospital safety department was notified.
4. The ventilator was returned to the manufacturer.
5. The transformer was identified as the source of the problem. It had overheated owing to inappropriate equipment plugged into an electrical outlet on the ventilator.
6. The manufacturer agreed to put labels on all ventilators, warning of the possibility of overloading the transformer.
7. The staff was informed of the problems through in-service education.

Repeated malfunctions of a single ventilator resulted in its replacement. One particular ventilator was repeatedly returned to the department for service. Careful documentation of each problem was kept. At one time the ventilator was renumbered after it returned from service to avoid prejudice regarding its use. However, it again seriously malfunctioned. The manufacturer replaced the ventilator at no cost.

Clinical Errors

Clinical errors are documented and examined to determine the cause of each problem. If the problem results from lack of knowledge, additional training, reference materials, or increased supervision is provided. The JCAH requires that part of an in-service education program be based on findings from the monitoring and evaluation of clinical services. In-services that result from problem resolution forms are documented. When a knowledge deficiency is recurrent and involves several staff members, it may require a change in the overall orientation of new employees or the revision of policies or procedures.

Example

We found that some therapists were not filling humidifiers on ventilators as often as necessary. This was the result of a failure to follow procedure but also of difficulty in seeing the water level in some of the old humidifiers. The following action was taken:

1. Appropriate disciplinary action, if warranted
2. A change in our ventilator flow sheets to include a space for checking the humidifier
3. Replacement of the old humidifiers with new equipment

Equipment Processing Problems

Equipment failures that result from problems with the processing of equipment are identified. Because the processing of equipment is the responsibility of a central processing department, intra-departmental cooperation is required for problem resolution.

Example

We have had problems with central processing's improper assembly of resuscitator bags. Our equipment manager took the documentation of this problem to the director of central processing. Together, they worked out a system for tracking individuals processing the equipment and detailed in-service education was provided.

System Problems

Recorded in this section are general hospital system problems: air, oxygen, paging, telephone, electrical. Resolution of system problems requires clear, accurate documentation and intra-departmental cooperation.

Examples

Oxygen System. While in the process of renovating a patient room, a construction worker cut through an oxygen line. The following action was taken:

1. Respiratory care is now notified by maintenance prior to any construction that could potentially affect the oxygen and compressed air systems.
2. We reviewed the oxygen system and decided it was necessary to install a backup system of large cylinders to protect against failure of the cryostats or breaks in the main oxygen lines.

Communication System. Problems receiving pages in various areas of the hospital were impacting on our ability to deliver respiratory care services safely and appropriately. The following action was taken: With the help of the communications department, a new paging system was tested by our department. Because respiratory therapists cover every patient care building, any problems with the new system were rapidly identified. The new system proved to be very effective and our paging problems were eliminated.

Equipment Shortages

All equipment shortages that impact on the delivery of respiratory care services are recorded. This information is useful in determining inventory requirements and planning for the operating and capital budgets.

Example

Problem reports identified an insufficient number of resuscitator bags. We were unable to decrease the turnover time of the central processing department, not could we decrease the loss of manual resuscitators. To solve the problem, a supply of disposable resuscitator bags is maintained for use when deficiencies exist in nondisposable bags.

Accidents

This section records all accidents involving staff members. Accidents are evaluated to determine if action can be taken to prevent recurrence.

Example

While draining the ventilator circuits of water, staff members reported that condensate splashed in their faces. They were concerned because many patients had communicable infections. The following action was taken:

1. Water traps to collect tubing condensate were incorporated in ventilator circuits of all patients in isolation.
2. Plastic goggles were distributed to all staff members.

Communication Problems

Problems that impact on patient care are recorded in this section: problems with verbal orders, ventilator changes made by personnel other than respiratory care personnel, incomplete reports between shifts, and so on. The goal is to improve communication both within the department and between departments. The resolution of these types of problems often involves memos as well as meetings with head nurses and physicians to clarify roles and responsibilities.

Example

The therapist taking care of a woman with severe lung disease was concerned over a decision to make a patient DNR (do not resuscitate). The family wanted the DNR status. The therapist pointed out that it was documented in the patient's chart that the patient wanted everything possible done for her. The optimal care committee was called in to help resolve the conflict. The DNR status was altered to indicate the need for aggressive treatment of the patient's pulmonary process and cardiac arrhythmias.

Outside Services

The Massachusetts General Hospital Respiratory Care Department provides service to two institutions without a designated respiratory care department: the Shriners' Hospital for Crippled Children of Boston, and the Massachusetts Eye and Ear Infirmary. Ongoing monitoring, evaluation, and problem resolution of our services is required by the JCAH.

Example

We experienced a conflict over the role of the nurse and the role of the respiratory therapist in making ventilator changes in one of these institutions. A meeting took place between the management personnel of both departments. Specific guidelines were written that were agreed upon by both groups. We have had no further problems.

THE QUALITY ASSURANCE REPORT

The hospital quality assurance committee receives reports from every department. These reports must be clear, direct, and concise. Included in our reports are the following:

1. The ongoing monitor(s) that identify specific problems
2. The results of the assessment of the findings
3. Small photographs or diagrams, as necessary, to illustrate the findings
4. The action taken
5. The plan for follow-up

MAKING IT WORK

An effective quality assurance program requires active participation by staff members. Problems must be followed up as soon as possible. Action must be taken to resolve problems and keep the staff informed of progress toward resolution.

The new JCAH standards provide a framework for systematically reviewing patient care. In my experience, it has been an excellent mechanism for getting a handle on the extent of problems and often provides the documentation necessary to implement change.

The goal of a quality assurance program is improvement of patient care. It is not intended to be used as a mechanism for documenting administrative problems, such as staffing. Whether a department meets the JCAH quality assurance standards depends to a large extent on its ability to demonstrate improved patient care.

Suggested Reading

Burt J, Gill F. Complying with JCAH quality control standards. Respir Care 1977; 22:820–827.

Joint Commission on Accreditation of Hospitals (JCAH). Accreditation manual for hospitals 1987. Chicago: JCAH, 1986.

Joint Commission on Accreditation of Hospitals (JCAH). Advanced approaches. Chicago: JCAH, 1984.

Williamson J. Assessing and improving health care outcomes: the health accounting approach to quality assurance. Cambridge, MA: Ballinger, 1978.

MECHANICAL VENTILATION IN THE INTENSIVE CARE UNIT

APPROPRIATE VENTILATOR SELECTION

CHARLES B. SPEARMAN, B.S., RRT

Patients requiring mechanical ventilatory support in the intensive care unit (ICU) present with a wide variety of management problems. Lung compliance in adult patients can range from more than twice normal to one-tenth normal, airway resistance can range from normal to severely increased, and respiratory drive can range from absent to excessive. Although the vast majority of mechanically ventilated patients require simple methods of ventilation and monitoring, active ICUs should have ventilators available that can also meet the unusual needs. This chapter focuses on what I believe are the necessary or desirable features for adult mechanical ventilators intended for the ICU patient population.

BASIC CAPABILITIES

Volume Orientation

Ventilators that attempt to provide control over volume delivery tend to minimize the changes in tidal ventilation caused by changing airflow resistances or lung compliance. This can be accomplished by either volume-cycled or time-cycled ventilators. With time-cycled ventilators, flow or flow pattern must also be controlled in order to provide volume-limited ventilation.

As peak pressures change in response to changing airflow resistances or compliances, volumes delivered to the patient also change owing to the compressible volume of internal and external circuits. Generally the amount of tidal volume not delivered to the patient is around 10 to 20 percent of the set volume, although in severe conditions the difference can be greater. Still, larger changes in tidal volume occur with pressure-cycled ventilators than with volume-oriented ventilators. Ideally the ventilator's internal compressible volume should be kept to a min-

imum so that the primary source is the external tubing circuit.

Some newer-generation ventilators have systems that attempt to correct for compressed volume loss and maintain an even more consistent delivered tidal volume. Examples are the Puritan Bennett 7200a and the BEAR 5 ventilators. Although this is technically appealing, the real need for such fine control is unproved and it is probably not necessary for most patients.

The range of settable tidal volumes should be from about 200 to 2,000 ml. If the ventilator will also be used for small children, then settings down to 50 ml are desirable as long as internal compressible volume is negligible and smaller tubing circuits can be used.

Pressure-generated ventilation is useful for pediatric patients and may be desirable for selected adults under special circumstances, but in general the volume-oriented approach is preferred in adults and in children with cuffed endotracheal tubes.

Pressure Capabilities

Most patients can be adequately ventilated at peak pressures less than 60 cm H_2O. However, active ICUs with patients having severe lung disease often encounter the need to apply peak pressure up to 100 cm H_2O. Rarely have I seen patients requiring peak pressures above 100 cm H_2O and even more rarely have I seen such patients survive. Therefore I believe a practical maximum pressure for a ventilator to be 100 to 120 cm H_2O. The ventilator should be able to maintain its flow pattern at or near its maximum pressure capability, i.e., act as a flow generator. This helps prevent undue changes in inspiratory time and I:E ratio when pressure changes occur during volume ventilation.

Increased I:E ratio with a sustained pressure plateau is currently under investigation in the United States and Europe as an alternative method of ventilation that may reduce the need for such high maximum pressures.

Flow Capabilities

Flow generally either is controlled separately or is a function of volume and inspiratory time settings.

Peak flows of 10 to 120 L per minute are desirable to produce reasonable inspiratory times using tidal volumes from 50 to 2,000 ml. Typically flows over 100 L per minute are used only for the severely ill or patients with high ventilatory drives.

The work of breathing is clearly influenced by the flow set on the ventilator during patient-triggered assisted breaths. It is important that clinicians pay close attention to this variable.

An independent flow control system settable in known calibrations of liters per minute is preferable to a system that sets inspiratory time in seconds or as a percentage of total cycle time. The latter allows for other settings such as volume or rate to influence flow and, unless it is calculated, the flow is usually unknown. An alternative is for the ventilator to display the flow when inspiratory time or tidal volume settings are changed.

The range of flow for spontaneous breathing should be at least equal to that for mechanical breaths. Flows for spontaneous breaths can be given by continuous, demand, or continuous plus demand flow systems. Both laboratory and clinical evaluations have been performed comparing continuous flow and demand flow systems. Continuous flow systems showed the least level of work required in early studies, although the demand systems used for some of the new ventilators have fared well in the laboratory.

High continuous flows (40 L per minute or more) may reduce inspiratory work but can also contribute to both inspiratory and expiratory work if used with a circuit with significant resistance to flow. Monitoring is interfered with owing to the continuous flow. Because of these problems, demand flow systems with sufficiently low levels of added work are often preferred. Indeed, some of the newer ventilators cannot be readily used with externally applied continuous flow systems. Ventilators with a combination of continuous plus demand flow systems such as the 7200a and BEAR 5 ventilators look promising.

Oxygen Control System

Every ventilator designed for use in the ICU must be able to provide independent control of inspired oxygen from 21 to 100 percent. Incremental changes of 1 or 2 percent are desirable. Most systems used today provide an accuracy of within 3 percent oxygen from the setting or better. An ideal system would provide an accuracy of within 1 percent oxygen (or better) from the setting. The oxygen setting must not be influenced by pressure, flow, or changes in other parameters such as rate, I:E ratio, or tidal volume.

METHODS OF VENTILATION

It has become apparent that no one approach to ventilator support is clearly superior to another for all patients. Because of the variety of patient problems seen in an active ICU, I believe a choice of ventilator modes is desirable. Assist-control (A-C) mode and intermittent mandatory ventilation (IMV) or synchronized IMV (SIMV) are commonly employed in today's ICU. Pressure support ventilation (PSV) is a newer method consisting of patient-triggered, pressure-generated, flow-cycled breaths and is another form of assisted ventilation. It can be used alone or in combination with SIMV during the periods normally used for spontaneous breathing. This technical modification of pressure-limited ventilation is gaining widespread clinical interest and is available on most of the new-generation ventilators, although there have been no definitive studies to help discern its role as compared with other methods of ventilation.

I believe that the mechanical ventilator designed for ICU patients should have at least A-C and IMV and SIMV modes available and that positive end-expiratory pressure (PEEP) should be available in each mode.

All breaths that depend on patient triggering (such as mechanical "assist" or SIMV breaths and demand flow spontaneous breaths) should have an adjustable sensitivity system available. The sensitivity system should allow for use with the full range of PEEP levels available and should sense the patient's efforts as close to the proximal airway connection as possible.

Because PSV allows the patient control over more aspects of the ventilatory pattern than A-C and because various levels of this support can be set during "spontaneous" breaths, I believe PSV can be a useful adjunct to methods of ventilator support. In my view, PSV is a desirable, but not mandatory feature for the ICU ventilator.

With A-C, IMV and SIMV, PEEP and continuous positive airway pressure (CPAP) and possibly PSV on the ventilator, most ventilator approaches can be provided.

OTHER OPERATIONAL CHARACTERISTICS

Rate. Mechanical rates should be settable from less than one breath per minute (BPM) to at least 60 BPM. Some clinicians have found even higher rates (up to 120 BPM) useful while others rarely exceed 20 BPM for adults. Rate systems that are independent of inspiratory time and flow are preferred.

PEEP and CPAP. PEEP should be settable to at least 30 cm H_2O. The PEEP should be compatible with the trigger sensitivity mechanism so that A-C and CPAP modes are available with PEEP. Resistance to flow through the PEEP system should be low to provide a "threshold resistor" type of response. The flow resistance characteristics should not change with different levels of PEEP.

I:E Ratio. The mechanical ratio of inspiration

to expiration should be variable. Independent controls for tidal volume, flow, and rate are preferred to controls of inspiratory and expiratory times because the former allow less interaction of the primary ventilation pattern. When possible a display for I:E ratio or inspiratory and expiratory times is desirable.

Humidification System. A heated humidifier is a must for mechanical ventilation in the ICU. A bubbler (cascade style) or wick type is preferred. The heater must be adjustable and have a system to avoid overheating. Servo-controlled heater systems with appropriate safety systems and with a temperature display are desirable. The heated humidifier should be able to provide inspired gases with 100 percent relative humidity at 32 to 37° C at all inspiratory flow and for minute volumes of at least 30 L. If the ventilator senses pressure for patient triggering inside the ventilator (rather than at the proximal airway connection), then a low resistance humidifier such as a wick type is a must to minimize patients' work.

Nebulizer System. A pressurized system for aerosolized medications is best provided during ventilatory support when the system has the following characteristics: operates during mechanical or spontaneous breaths (inspiration only); does not influence O_2 percent, tidal volumes, or monitoring and alarm systems; has sufficient power (pressure); and is not detrimental to the ventilators operation. Even if a nebulizer system is not provided, the ventilator should be able to operate when aerosol is added to the patients' breathing circuit.

Inspiratory Hold (Inflation Hold, Inspiratory Pause). Adding a time of no flow following a volume-oriented inspiration and prior to active expiration can allow for estimates of so-called effective static compliance and can be useful as a monitoring tool. Generally an adjustable time of 0 to 2 seconds is sufficient. Some ventilators (e.g., those using continuous flow during expiration such as the BEAR 5) cannot safely have their exhalation valves manually occluded to provide this maneuver.

SAFETY AND ALARM SYSTEMS

Pressure Limit. Every volume ventilator must have at least one adjustable system that limits the peak airway pressure available. When the set pressure is reached, either the breath should be ended or the pressure should be held at that level until inspiration ends. Ending inspiration and activating an audible and visual alarm is the preferred method when the system is being used as a safety mechanism. When it is intended that the set pressure be reached and held throughout each inspiration (such as in pediatric ventilators), then no alarm should occur. When this approach is employed a secondary pressure limit should be added, preferably with an alarm. Sensing pressure

should be done as close to the proximal airways as possible or at least have an open pathway to the patient connection.

Low Pressure. All ventilators should have some system for detecting low pressures in the patient circuit. Low-pressure alarms with proper logic systems can detect circuit leaks, tubing disconnects, and inadequate flow. With a timer added, low rates can also be detected. Refinements of simple low-pressure detection include the separation of low pressure during a mechanical inspiration and the loss of PEEP and CPAP levels.

High Pressure. Although high-pressure alarms are usually associated with pressure limits during mechanical inspiration, there are other times when a high pressure in the circuit can occur. Ventilators with electronically controlled exhalation valves (e.g., Siemens 900C) or that use continuous flow (e.g., BEAR 5) are examples of those in which a high-pressure alarm may be needed for both inspiration and expiration.

Power Failure. Battery operated systems must be available as an alarm when electric power systems fail. If the power source is pneumatic only (e.g., Monaghan 225/SIMV) then a battery-operated pressure-sensing system (or equivalent) must be used. This may be the same as the low-pressure sensor or another, separate device.

Oxygen System. The preferred method is to monitor oxygen in the patient circuit with a calibrated analyzer with high and low alarms *and* have a gas pressure inlet alarm for oxygen (and air if applicable) for the oxygen blending system. In the absence of one of these systems, the other must be present.

Rate System. Ensuring that the patient receives a minimum number of breaths can be monitored by systems such as failure-to-cycle and apnea alarms. A system for counting and displaying respiratory rate can also provide useful information concerning the patient's status. Low rates can indicate patient fatigue or ventilator malfunction. If the low-pressure alarm system does not have a timing mechanism included to detect low rates, then some other system or apnea alarm is needed. Increasing rates can often be an early signal to patient stress or deteriorating lung function. High rates from the ventilator self-cycling due to leaks while PEEP is used occur before the leak can be detected by low-pressure systems.

Volume System. Volume-monitoring systems may be considered less essential than low pressure or disconnect alarms, but I believe they are important tools. Monitored volume can give insights into the patient's breathing pattern, adequacy of ventilator function, and amount of spontaneous ventilation and can often be more sensitive to leaks in the system than low-pressure alarms. In some ventilator systems, the low-volume alarm system is used to detect leaks, disconnections, and low rates while high-volume alarms are used to detect the results of high rates and some ventilator malfunctions.

Temperature of Inspired Gases. Whenever a heated humidification system is used, temperatures at or near the proximal airway need to be monitored. Ideally the temperature sensor should be associated with an alarm and be able to shut down the heater system if temperatures exceed a set level. Most systems alarm at about 41° C, and some are adjustable. Low temperatures are associated with reduced humidity levels. The accuracy of temperature sensors is best when placed in a continuous flow system, while with cyclic ventilation (i.e., A-C or SIMV with demand flow) the readings are averages and tend to be lower than the actual inspired gas temperature owing to cooling that occurs during expiratory phases. It may be wiser to set an adjustable high-temperature alarm level lower when using cyclic ventilation modes than when continuous flows are being used.

THE NEW GENERATION OF VENTILATORS

Since the early part of the 1980s, several new ventilators have been introduced to the United States market that use computer or microprocessor control systems, multiple modes of ventilation, computer-compatible monitoring, and extensive data collection capabilities. Examples include the Siemens Servo 900C, the Puritan-Bennett 7200a, the BEAR 5, and the Hamilton Veolar. They are proving to be very versatile, offering a variety of capabilities. None of the ventilators meets all criteria listed in this chapter, but each has additional features not discussed. In each case there are trade-offs, just as there have always been when attempting to choose one ventilator over another.

Of the four new ventilators mentioned, the 7200a and BEAR 5 take an "American" approach for establishing ventilator settings, while the Servo 900C and Veolar are a bit more "European." By this I mean that the 7200a and BEAR 5 offer single, independent settings for tidal volume, respiratory rate, and inspiratory flow, leaving inspiratory time and I:E ratio to be a result of these. The Servo 900C and Veolar use rate and inspiratory percent controls (percent of the total cycle as established by the rate setting) to determine actual inspiratory time and influence flow. The Servo 900C has minute volume and rate settings to establish tidal volume, while the Veolar has an independent tidal volume control. I prefer the approach taken by the 7200a and BEAR 5 because inspiratory flow is not influenced by changes in volume or rate as it is with the other approach. Inspiratory flow is the variable that I see abused most often, and it affects the patient's work of breathing significantly. Without knowledge of the flow value, clinicians tend to forget assessment of flow adequacy. It was initially common

in ICUs to see Servo 900Cs set for 33 percent inspiratory time to produce the textbook I:E ratio of 1:2 regardless of the patient's actual flow needs. Forcing the therapists to calculate the inspiratory flow also reminded them to assess its adequacy by observation of the patient and pressure manometer.

Recently the Veolar has added a display of peak inspiratory flow (for both mechanical and spontaneous breaths), and this should be helpful. Now when tidal volume, rate, or inspiratory time percent controls are changed, the resultant change in flow will also be obvious.

Many of the new ventilators, including those mentioned, can provide a wide variety of monitoring and patient data collection, both current and trend form. Most patients can be managed adequately without collection of mountains of this information. However, the versatility of these ventilators allows clinicians to decide what information is useful for each individual patient and to use the aspects of the ventilators that are thought to be useful. The increased amounts of monitoring can also allow us to learn more about the management approach being used and perhaps make modifications as necessary.

By providing several modes of ventilation, wide flow ranges, and selection of flow and pressure patterns, the new ventilators allow more individualization of ventilator support than ever before. It is hoped that future studies will help to determine which groups of patients benefit most from particular features. However, even in the absence of proof that these features change the ultimate outcome of patients, having the potential to individualize care, maximize patient comfort, and optimize physiological function because of ventilator versatility is worthwhile. The new ventilators with their multiple features should allow the art of ventilator management to improve. They provide additions to our armamentarium of ventilator support of the most challenging patients. Although the new-generation ventilators may not be necessary for all hospitals, I believe that centers with active ICUs should at least consider these devices and attempt to evaluate their possible benefits for the patient population receiving mechanical ventilation.

Patients with severe adult respiratory distress syndrome (ARDS) are often the respiratory care practitioner's greatest challenge. Severe decreases in compliance and increases in physiologic shunt, deadspace ventilation, and respiratory drive contribute to the management difficulties. These patients may benefit from the variety of approaches available on the new ventilators when individualized care is desired. Monitoring variables such as compliance, resistance, and mean airway pressure can be useful in setting and evaluating levels of tidal volume and PEEP, particularly when the patient's condition is changing. Changing pressure and flow waveforms may prove beneficial in individual patients, and the increased levels of monitoring available on the ventilators having these capabilities make the use of alternative approaches safer.

For patients that are difficult to wean, options such as the respiratory mechanics package with the 7200a ventilator offer a convenient method for gathering data for vital capacity and negative inspiratory pressure. Having the ability to change approaches to weaning (e.g., SIMV, CPAP, pressure support) on one ventilator is also a convenient advantage when dealing with these patients.

At times ventilators are chosen because they have specific features not available on other units. As an example, the Servo 900C can be used to provide inverse I:E ratio ventilation in its "pressure control" mode. This mode provides a pressure-limited time-cycled form of A-C ventilation.

Certainly clinical studies are needed to help delineate which patients benefit most from which management approaches, which ventilator features truly make a difference, and what amount of monitoring and data collection is prudent. Because of the sophistication provided by the new ventilators I believe the tools are available to help in this regard.

PERSPECTUS

No attempt is made in this chapter to describe an "ideal" ventilator. Instead, certain minimum requirements for ICU, adult ventilators are presented. Any description I could invent for the ideal ventilator would be too far from reality, because of course I would wish it to be state-of-the-art technologically but inexpensive; highly versatile with multiple capabilities, yet simple to understand and operate; powerful yet safe; and, naturally, maintenance-free.

Suggested Reading

Banner MJ. Expiratory positive-pressure valves: flow resistance and work of breathing. Respir Care 1987; 32:431–439.

Kacmarek RM, Venegas J. Mechanical ventilatory rates and tidal volumes. Respir Care 1987; 32:466–478.

Katz JA, Kraemer RW, Gjerde GE. Inspiratory work and airway pressure with continuous positive airway pressure delivery systems. Chest 1985; 88:519–526.

MacIntyre NR. Pressure support ventilation: effects on ventilatory reflexes and ventilatory-muscle workloads. Respir Care 1987; 32:447–457.

Marini JJ. The role of the inspiratory circuit in the work of breathing during mechanical ventilation. Respir Care 1987; 32:419–439.

Marini JJ, Rodriguez MR, Lamb VJ. The inspiratory workload of patient-initiated mechanical ventilation. Am Rev Respir Dis 1986; 134:902–909.

McPherson SP, Spearman CB. Respiratory therapy equipment. 3rd ed. St. Louis: CV Mosby, 1985.

Pierson DJ, Capps JS, Hudson JD. Maximum ventilatory capabilities of four current generation mechanical ventilators. Respir Care 1986; 31:1054–1058.

Spearman CB, Sanders HG. The new generation of mechanical ventilators. Respir Care 1987; 32:403–418.

Viale JP, Annat G, Bertrand O, Ing D, Godard J, Motin J. Additional inspiratory work in intubated patients breathing with continuous positive airway pressure systems. Anesthesiology 1985; 63:536–539.

MODES OF MECHANICAL VENTILATION

ROBERT R. KIRBY, M.D.

Ventilator design in the 1950s and 60s focused on mechanical features and on the limited methods of gas delivery. The available modes of support, assisted (patient-triggered) and controlled ventilation, limited the clinical application of these devices. Throughout the 1970s and into the 80s, techniques of support increased in an almost bewildering fashion. Clinicians now have a variety of modes from which to choose and a level of sophistication with respect to electromechanical flow mechanisms that was not even thought of 10 years ago. What is not clear is whether such capabilities enhance or improve patient care. I am a bit suspicious that ventilator design and development have fallen victims to the technological imperative: we do things because we can, not because we should.

Nevertheless, evaluations of any technique or therapeutic intervention require an understanding of what the therapy is intended to accomplish. In the subsequent pages, I will present my views on the merits of the five most commonly employed modes of ventilator support: control, assist-control, intermittent and synchronized intermittent mandatory ventilation, and mandatory minute ventilation. Other specialized methods are discussed in separate chapters. Little objective data exist to support the superiority of one technique over another. Therefore, in the absence of such information, my biases will be evident.

SUPPORT MODES

Controlled Mechanical Ventilation (CMV)

Historically, this technique predates all others. In terms of what the ventilator does, CMV is mechanically the simplest, and in a sense the most reliable mode of ventilatory support. Early development of CMV resulted from the application of positive pressure ventilation to victims of poliomyelitis who, in many cases, were incapable of any spontaneous respiratory effort. In such cases, the ventilator substituted for the inspiratory muscles and provided the entire work of breathing.

Such a technique works well for patients who are totally paralyzed and whose pulmonary parenchymal function is essentially normal (indeed, the mortality of acute bulbar poliomyelitis decreased from approx-

imately 80 percent to 40 percent in the early 1950s when mechanical ventilators were so employed). Now, however, this category represents a small minority of patients for whom ventilatory support is indicated. For the majority of the other patients, CMV is a poor choice as a stand-alone mode. The basic problem is that the patient's respiratory efforts must be overcome (induced hypocapnia), suppressed (heavy sedation), or eliminated (neuromuscular paralysis). Such pharmacologic intervention predisposes to the possibility of serious injury or death should an inadvertent disconnection or a loss of the airway occur. This risk is unacceptable in current medical practice in all but the rarest of circumstances.

A second problem relates to the fact that a paralyzed patient, or one who is sedated into a state of virtual unconsciousness, cannot give any meaningful indication of the adequacy of the support being rendered. It is a rare team of physicians and respiratory therapists that can arbitrarily set a pattern and a magnitude of ventilator therapy that is "just right." All other techniques can be modified, at least to some degree, by the patient's spontaneous effort.

For these reasons, I feel that CMV should be relegated to a category of historical interest and should *never* be used as a stand-alone mode. If a reasonable indication exists, CMV should be utilized only in the form of intermittent mandatory ventilation. Patients for whom such a combination of therapy is appropriate include those with central nervous system dysfunction in whom respiratory control mechanisms are damaged; those whose respiratory muscles are paralyzed by neuromuscular damage or by neuromuscular blocking drugs such as pancuronium (Pavulon), atracurium (Tracrium), vecuronium (Norcuron), etc.; and those who are recovering from the residual effects of anesthesia or of drug overdosage.

Assist-Control Ventilation

Assisted, or patient-triggered, ventilation was initially developed for intermittent positive pressure breathing (IPPB) devices, rather than for long-term ventilator support. However, the obvious disadvantages of CMV suggested the need for alternative modes, and the concept of ventilator support that could be initiated by the patient's spontaneous inspiratory effort had a certain logical appeal. Such therapy had one major disadvantage resulting from the inconsistency of the spontaneous breathing pattern associated with many forms of respiratory failure. A patient who became apneic for any reason obviously could not cycle a ventilator into its inspiratory phase. The concept of a backup control mechanism, generally set at a lower rate than the patient's spontaneous, assisted rate, was a natural solution. Should apnea ensue, or should the patient be unable to trigger the machine, the automatic control mechanism would take over.

In theory, assist-control ventilation has two primary advantages. First, the patient, to some extent, determines minute ventilation by setting the cycling frequency (tidal volume still is dependent on the same factors as in a CMV mode). Under these circumstances, one would expect that significant aberrations in $PaCO_2$ and in pHa would occur less frequently than with CMV, wherein minute ventilation is arbitrarily selected by a physician or a respiratory therapist. In fact, no scientifically valid data support this view, either in adult or in neonatal ventilation; several studies show the acid-base derangements to be just as great with assist-control modes as with CMV.

The second purported advantage is that use of the respiratory muscles to trigger the ventilator to the inspiratory phase maintains their conditioning and thereby prevents atrophy. Even less evidence supports this contention, and if any conditioning occurs, it must be minimal.

Recent work (1985) suggests that, even when the ventilator assist mechanism sensitivity is set as optimally as possible, the patient's spontaneous work of breathing often exceeds that generated by the ventilator as it delivers its tidal volume. This observation is explained by at least two mechanisms. First, the intrinsically poor designs of many ventilator circuits incorporate high resistance elements that necessitate an increase of inspiratory effort. Second, the patient continues efforts to inhale during the interval in which a spontaneous inspiration is initiated, the ventilator cycling mechanism responds, and a flow of gas is accelerated into the airway. Gas flow is delayed, however, and the result is wasted energy expenditure without any useful work in either the physical or the physiologic sense.

Experience suggests that assist-control modes work reasonably well in patients with normal or, at worst, mild to moderate respiratory insufficiency. Such therapy is rarely of value when the lungs have significantly reduced compliance and/or increased airway resistance, as in severe adult respiratory distress syndrome (ARDS) or chronic obstructive pulmonary disease (COPD). My personal viewpoint, challenged by many, is that this mode has little to recommend it and has no scientific documentation as to its efficacy.

Intermittent Mandatory Ventilation (IMV)

If ever a technique generated debate and created a polarization of viewpoints within the respiratory care community, IMV is a top contender (rivaled only,

perhaps, by high-frequency ventilation). I have never met an individual who professed even modest interest and knowledge concerning mechanical ventilation and who voiced neutrality. People either love IMV or hate it! There is no middle ground.

The technique evolved out of general dissatisfaction with the aforementioned problems of CMV and of assist-control techniques. In addition, it was readily apparent that not all patients with respiratory failure required total support of ventilation and of oxygenation. Many were capable of maintaining some, but not all, of their spontaneous ventilation. A technique that allowed individualization of the support rendered, and also permitted spontaneous breathing according to the patient's requirements, seemed to circumvent many of the problems of the time. Other advantages additionally suggested included lower mean airway and intrapleural pressures. These lower pressures lessened the impact of mechanical ventilation on cardiovascular function (i.e., decreased venous return, decreased cardiac output). Better control of acid-base status, primarily a decreased incidence of respiratory alkalemia, also was documented both by proponents and opponents of IMV. The latter individuals felt, however, that the improvement was not clinically relevant.

In recent years, it has become clear that the major problems with IMV are related, not to the concept, but to the equipment. This difficulty can be attributed, in large part, to several ventilator manufacturers. Unfortunately, the problem, in many cases, has been made worse with the newest and the most sophisticated microprocessor-controlled ventilators. We have documented 300 percent or greater increases in spontaneous work of breathing associated with inadequate circuit design. Patients in severe respiratory failure cannot reasonably be expected to maintain such effort for a long time. To argue that IMV is a poor mode of support, simply because one chooses inappropriately designed equipment, makes no more sense than to condemn the automobile because Ford once made the Edsel.

My personal feeling is that IMV and synchronized IMV have more evidence that supports their efficacy than does any other form of mechanical ventilation. This evidence has not convinced those individuals who do not favor the technique. Nevertheless, according to a recent survey of 3,000 U.S. hospital departments of respiratory therapy, over 1,000 of which responded, 72 percent used IMV and/or SIMV as their primary modes of mechanical ventilation, and 90 percent employed these techniques for weaning. In view of the extremely negative comments about IMV published in recent years, these figures are somewhat surprising. They suggest that user experience, perhaps, is a better guide to therapeutic efficacy than are the writings of experts in this field.

Synchronized Intermittent Mandatory Ventilation (SIMV)

Much of what I have written about IMV is also applicable to SIMV. A major worry of many clinicians employing IMV was the possibility that the ventilator might cycle and deliver a large, mechanical breath just as the patient completed a spontaneous inspiration. The resultant doubling or tripling of the total volume, it was argued, might predispose to circulatory embarrassment and to pulmonary barotrauma. In voicing this argument, they seemed to lose sight of the fact that for many years the deliberate administration of a tidal volume two to three times larger than normal (sighing) was considered a desirable goal in order to prevent miliary atelectasis. The sigh mechanism is still incorporated into the design of most mechanical ventilators. However, its utility in preventing the complication that it was designed to overcome (which actually never was demonstrated to occur anyway) is totally unsubstantiated.

Be that as it may, most manufacturers, ever mindful of the profit motive, incorporated SIMV into their designs. In essence, SIMV incorporates an assist mode that is superimposed upon the spontaneous breathing pattern. Depending upon the selected frequency, a "window" opens at certain intervals, during which a spontaneous inspiration triggers the delivery of a mechanical tidal volume.

The question to be answered, of course, is whether SIMV *prevents* the problems that *do not* occur with IMV. If this statement sounds as though it is straight out of Alice in Wonderland and Through the Looking Glass, I have succeeded in expressing my thoughts precisely as I planned. The few studies that have addressed the nonissue reported no differences in complications or in outcome between IMV and SIMV. The one clearly superior aspect of the latter is that it costs more and therefore increases the manufacturers' profit margin. That is hardly a recommendation for improved patient care.

Mandatory Minute Ventilation (MMV)

Minute ventilation with IMV and SIMV ventilators is variable, since only the ventilator rate and tidal volume are programmable. Wide variations occur, depending upon how much or how little spontaneous breathing occurs. In 1977 investigators from Great Britain proposed that a preselected minute ventilation might be more physiologic. The original concept incorporated a known constant flow of gas from which the patient could breathe spontaneously. Any gas over and above that breathed by the patient accumulated in a bellows and, when a certain volume was reached, the ventilator cycled, thereby delivering this volume to the patient. If spontaneous ventilation decreased, the bellows accumulated gas more rapidly, and more frequent ventilator breaths were delivered. Conversely, if the spontaneous component increased, gas collected in the bellows more slowly, and the number of mechanical breaths decreased. In both cases, however, minute ventilation remained constant; only the proportion breathed spontaneously by the patient or provided by the ventilator changed. Several microprocessor ventilators provide MMV, but use a different method in which the accumulating gas volume is continuously compared to the preset minute ventilation. Any deficit is supplemented by mechanical breaths.

The theoretic benefit to MMV, which originally also was claimed for CMV, is that a guaranteed minimal level of ventilation is supplied. Weaning presumably is automatic in that an increase in spontaneous breathing is accompanied simultaneously by a decrease in mechanical support. The major limitation, however, is the arbitrarily selected minute ventilation, which can be more or less than that needed or desired by the patient. An excess results in the continued delivery of mechanical breaths when they are no longer required; a deficit renders the patient hypercapnic, dyspneic, and tachypneic. Furthermore, a tachypneic individual may "use up" all of the gas flow with rapid, shallow, ineffectual breathing, thereby receiving no mechanical augmentation at a time when such assistance is most needed.

PERSPECTIVE

As should by now be obvious, very little objective evidence supports particular modes of mechanical ventilation. Certain conditions necessitate CMV (paralysis, severe respiratory depression), but, as I mentioned previously, this technique should only be used with an IMV system, so that if the patient begins to attempt spontaneous breathing, a fresh gas supply is available.

I recently had occasion to review the outcome of respiratory failure treatment for the past 20 years. Despite the development of new generations of mechanical ventilators, the introduction of new techniques, and improvements in patient monitoring, the mortality of ARDS is unchanged. The mortality averages 60 percent, but increases to as much as 100 percent with multiorgan system failure. The outlook for acute exacerbations of COPD is somewhat better. Mortality is 28 percent for the first episode of failure, but increases to 60 percent and 68 percent with the second and third episodes, respectively.

Of importance, however, is the fact that respiratory failure is the direct cause of death in a minority of cases. Dr. Leonard Hudson recently emphasized that patients die *of* ARDS and *with* ARDS. Sepsis and multiorgan failure are the principal culprits, and available evidence suggests that only 15 to 20 percent of patients with ARDS die of refractory hypoxemia. The conclusion to be drawn is that we are better at treating respiratory failure than other organ system dysfunctions. In years past, we did not see the other problems nearly as often, because patients did not survive their initial bouts of severe respiratory insufficiency long enough to develop the secondary complications.

With this information, I can argue that the wider variety of techniques available and the increasingly sophisticated ventilators with which they can be administered have, in fact, had a major impact on the outcome of respiratory failure. This favorable effect does not translate into improved survival, however, because ventilators cannot correct renal and hepatic insufficiency, CNS dysfunction, blood dyscrasias, and sepsis.

I doubt that any ventilator mode can be demonstrated to be clearly superior in adult respiratory disease. So far as I am aware, absolute efficacy has been demonstrated for only two positive airway pressure techniques. The first is the already mentioned use of CMV in the treatment of poliomyelitis, and the second is the application of continuous positive airway pressure (CPAP) to infants with hyaline membrane disease. These conditions share one characteristic: they primarily involve only pulmonary dysfunction (by admittedly different mechanisms). Most other types of respiratory failure are multifactorial and frequently are associated with other organ system dysfunction that is not amenable to tracheal intubation and mechanical ventilation.

The history of "advances" in this field is characterized by the introduction of support modes that were not investigated prospectively. In the case of IMV, this practice has been resoundingly (though sometimes unfairly) condemned. Even today, papers appear that criticize work originally published as early as 1973. One would suppose, then, that a lesson has been learned and that newer techniques are subjected

to more rigorous scrutiny before they are introduced. Such is not the case with MMV, nor with pressure support ventilation discussed elsewhere in this text. The latter was incorporated into popular ventilators before most clinicians were aware of its existence. Since that time, a concerted effort has been mounted to justify the use of pressure support ventilation without prospective, scientifically valid clinical studies. Only recently have competent investigators attempted to evaluate this technique objectively and to place it into perspective with other approaches. History has a way of repeating itself!

Suggested Reading

Avery EE, Mörch ET, Benson DW. Critically crushed chests: a new method of treatment with continuous hyperventilation to produce alkalotic apnea and internal pneumatic stabilization. J Thorac Surg 1956; 32:291–311.

Bushnell LS, Pontoppidan H, Hedley-Whyte J, et al. Efficiency of different types of ventilation in long-term respiratory care: mechanical versus spontaneous. Anesth Analg 1966; 45:696–703.

Cournand A, Motley HL, Werko L, et al. Physiological studies of effects of intermittent positive pressure breathing in cardiac output in man. Am J Physiol 1948; 152:162–174.

Downs JB, Klein EF, Desautels D, et al. Intermittent mandatory ventilation: a new approach to weaning patients from mechanical ventilators. Chest 1973; 64:331–335.

Engström CG. Treatment of severe cases of respiratory paralysis by the Engström universal respirator. Br Med J 1954; 2:666–669.

Hasten RW, Downs JB, Heenan TJ. A comparison of synchronized and nonsynchronized intermittent mandatory ventilation. Respir Care 1980; 25:554–557.

Hewlett AM, Platt AS, Terry VG. Mandatory minute volume. A new concept in weaning from mechanical ventilation. Anaesthesia 1977; 32:163–169.

Maloney JV, Derrick WS, Whittenberger JL. A device producing regulated assisted respiration. Surg Forum 1951; 588–595.

Mushin WW, Rendell-Baker L, Thompson PW, et al. Automatic ventilation of the lungs. 3rd ed. London: Blackwell Scientific Publications, 1980.

Nunn JF. Applied respiratory physiology. 2nd ed. London-Boston: Butterworths, 1977.

FiO₂ AND PEEP

S. DAVID REGISTER III, MAJOR, U.S.A.F.(M.C.)
JOHN B. DOWNS, M.D.

There are three primary pulmonary causes of clinically significant arterial hypoxemia: (1) alveolar hypoventilation, (2) impaired diffusion of oxygen (O_2) to pulmonary capillary blood, and (3) right-to-left intrapulmonary shunting of blood. Patients with arterial hypoxemia secondary to intrapulmonary shunting do not demonstrate a significant increase in arterial oxygen tension (PaO_2) when given supplemental inspired O_2. In contrast, patients with the other two abnormalities usually demonstrate a significant increase in PaO_2 with supplemental O_2. However, in spite of an increase in PaO_2, supplemental O_2 may not be the safest or most appropriate form of therapy. We do not consider such a maneuver therapeutic in such patients because the underlying pulmonary abnormality is not corrected. Instead, our approach to O_2 therapy, continuous positive airway pressure (CPAP), and mechanical ventilation is directed toward improvement in pulmonary function. This approach should be clearly distinguished from approaches that view O_2 and CPAP as mechanisms to produce adequate oxygenation while awaiting spontaneous improvement in pulmonary function.

ADVERSE EFFECTS OF O₂ THERAPY

In many cases, supplemental O_2 may worsen pre-existing pulmonary dysfunction. For example, an increased inspired O_2 concentration (FIO_2) may further decrease alveolar ventilation in patients with severe obstructive lung disease, chronic hypercapnia, and a "hypoxic drive to breathe." Even more commonly, the administration of O_2 may further decrease the ventilation-perfusion ratio in patients with pre-existing mismatching of ventilation ($\dot{V}$) and perfusion ($\dot{Q}$).

Briscoe and co-workers proposed that administration of a high FIO_2 might cause lung units with low $\dot{V}/\dot{Q}$ to collapse as a result of uptake of alveolar O_2 at a rate exceeding alveolar ventilation, thus resulting in absorption atelectasis. Briscoe proposed that the critical $\dot{V}/\dot{Q}$ is increased 100-fold as the FIO_2 is increased from 0.21 to 1.0.

Wagner and others measured continuous distributions of ventilation and perfusion based on the steady-state elimination of six inert gases of varying solu-bility in blood. None of the subjects studied had measurable intrapulmonary shunting of blood while breathing room air. However, after breathing 100 percent O_2 for only 30 minutes, three of the four younger patients and all five of the older patients developed measurable intrapulmonary shunting. This suggests that critically ill patients with a large percentage of alveolar units with a low $\dot{V}/\dot{Q}$ ratio may develop significant intrapulmonary shunting of blood as a result of absorption atelectasis after breathing supplemental inspired O_2. Thus, even though PaO_2 initially may increase, pulmonary function can be worsened.

Supplemental O_2 also may inhibit hypoxic pulmonary vasoconstriction (HPV). This can cause an increase in blood flow to poorly ventilated regions of the lung, further decreasing $\dot{V}/\dot{Q}$ and increasing the possibility of absorption atelectasis. Eiser and colleagues demonstrated that HPV is partially relieved by inhalation of only 30 percent oxygen in some patients with obstructive lung disease.

Thus, it is not yet clear what constitutes a clinically "safe" FIO_2. It is established that an FIO_2 of 0.6 or greater may result in O_2 toxicity. In common clinical usage, the term toxicity refers to the histopathologic lung parenchymal changes associated with hyperoxic exposure rather than to the pulmonary dysfunction that may occur in the absence of structural changes. Several investigations have demonstrated that O_2 tension in the conducting and gas-exchange regions of the lung, rather than the PO_2 of systemic blood, is the primary determinant of O_2 toxicity. The degree of injury is a function of both lung O_2 tension and time of exposure. Significant injury has not been demonstrated in animals or humans exposed to 40 percent O_2 at one atmosphere for several weeks. However, 100 percent O_2 at one atmosphere may be lethal within 7 days. Therefore, an FIO_2 of 0.21 to 0.4 should not be considered "toxic" in the classic sense but also must not be considered benign and devoid of harmful side effects.

An elevated FIO_2 is administered by many clinicians in an attempt to increase PaO_2 and provide a "margin of safety" in the event of sudden disaster. However, the arterial hemoglobin concentration and oxyhemoglobin saturation, not the PaO_2, are the major determinants of arterial O_2 content. Therefore, it is not surprising that there is no evidence of clinical benefit from increasing the FIO_2 to increase the PaO_2 above 60 mm Hg. It is also not surprising that an elevated FIO_2 does not provide a significant "margin of safety" in the event of unexpected deterioration of cardiopulmonary function. For example, a 20 percent increase in FiO$_2$ for a patient with a functional residual capacity (FRC) of 1,000 ml will increase pulmonary O$_2$ reserves by only 200 ml. In a normal adult this represents a safety margin of less than 60 seconds in the event of a catastrophic complication, such as a ventilator disconnection. Total blood O$_2$ content increases less than 100 ml when O$_2$ saturation is increased from 90 to 100 percent. In exchange for this small margin of safety, pulmonary gas exchange may be significantly impaired. We recently demonstrated residual impairment of pulmonary gas exchange following extubation of patients who had received 50 percent O$_2$ for 16 to 24 hours postoperatively, compared with similar patients who had received no more than 30 percent inspired O$_2$ for the same period of time. In addition, patients who received 50 percent oxygen demonstrated a progressive fall in PaO$_2$ prior to extubation, suggesting that they were experiencing progressive absorption atelectasis.

Douglas and co-workers analyzed pulmonary venous admixture as a function of FiO$_2$ in 30 patients requiring postoperative mechanical ventilation. In every patient, pulmonary venous admixture decreased as FiO$_2$ was increased from 0.21 to 0.40, and then remained unchanged as the FiO$_2$ was increased to 0.60. As the FiO$_2$ was increased from 0.60 to 1.0, pulmonary venous admixture increased, probably secondary to inhibition of hypoxic pulmonary vasoconstriction or absorption atelectasis or both. The decrease in venous admixture was thought to result from increasing alveolar O$_2$ tension in areas with low $\dot{V}/\dot{Q}$ or increasing O$_2$ diffusion across an alveolocapillary diffusion barrier. This demonstrated that the decreased PaO$_2$ and increased alveolar-arterial oxygen tension difference characteristic of low $\dot{V}/\dot{Q}$ is most readily diagnosed when the FiO$_2$ is low. Administration of an inappropriately elevated FiO$_2$ may delay diagnosis and appropriate therapy of an underlying pulmonary abnormality.

We believe that supplemental inspired O$_2$ often is utilized inappropriately, whereas CPAP is underutilized. Most clinicians regard O$_2$ therapy as benign as long as toxic FiO$_2$ is avoided. Meanwhile, CPAP is feared to have frequent and serious complications, limiting its clinical application. Also, a high FiO$_2$ can be delivered quickly and easily in nearly every clinical setting, whereas appropriate application of CPAP is limited by equipment availability and clinician experience and bias.

CPAP: COMMON MISCONCEPTIONS

CPAP may be underutilized for other reasons. For example, in postoperative patients with significantly decreased FRC, pulmonary compliance is decreased and the work of breathing is increased, perhaps to excessive and intolerable levels. Hypoxemia and respiratory muscle fatigue may necessitate therapeutic intervention. The clinician may inappropriately institute mechanical ventilation with high FiO$_2$. However, CPAP should be administered to restore normal FRC, thereby improving pulmonary compliance, decreasing the work of breathing, and improving $\dot{V}/\dot{Q}$ matching. PaO$_2$ usually will increase without increasing the FiO$_2$.

Many fail to appreciate the complex interaction between mechanical ventilation, CPAP, and O$_2$ therapy. For example, positive end-expiratory pressure (PEEP) was originally utilized only in conjunction with mechanical ventilation, even in patients who required only an increase in FRC without mechanical ventilator assistance. The observed complications of such combination therapy often were attributed to PEEP, without consideration of mechanical ventilation as the primary culprit.

Application of positive pressure to the airway has a variety of physiologic effects that vary according to methodology. In addition, confusing terminology has resulted in conflicting reports and contradictory recommendations for therapy. When an above-ambient, or positive, airway pressure is maintained at the termination of exhalation, a residual volume of gas is held within the lungs and FRC increases. Initially, this was done with positive pressure maintained at end expiration and was termed PEEP. Clearly, if a continuous positive pressure is maintained (CPAP), FRC will be increased even further, whether or not mechanical ventilation is applied.

Problems have arisen when CPAP has been applied to spontaneously breathing adults. In the absence of a continuous flow of gas, a resistance to exhalation could be applied that would cause expiratory airway pressure to increase; however, inspiratory airway pressure might decrease to ambient, unless some means is provided to pressurize the inspired gas. With such a circuit, FRC increases, but the work of breathing also increases, often to intolerable levels because of the fluctuations in airway pressure. The definitions of PEEP as a pattern used only with a mechanical ventilator and CPAP as a pattern used only during spontaneous ventilation are inaccurate and misleading. Since there is little clinical utility for allowing a decrease in inspiratory airway pressure to ambient, and since CPAP can adequately describe the airway pressure pattern used during most clinical circumstances, with or without a ventilator, we will use the term CPAP, without regard to the presence or absence of mechanical ventilation.

CPAP: INDICATIONS

With few exceptions, CPAP is indicated only when a restrictive ventilatory defect has resulted in a decrease in FRC. Such defects commonly are associated with arterial hypoxemia secondary to decreased

$\dot{V}/\dot{Q}$ or right-to-left intrapulmonary shunting of blood or both. Restrictive defects also are associated with a decrease in lung compliance. This can be depicted graphically as a rightward and/or downward shift of the lung pressure-volume curve. Very high expiratory airway pressures may be required in order to restore FRC to normal.

FRC may be quantified in the laboratory with gas dilutional techniques but is not readily measured with bedside techniques. Consequently, the presence of decreased FRC must be detected clinically by radiologic techniques, by demonstrating arterial hypoxemia, and by evidence of decreased lung compliance and increased work of breathing. Decreased lung compliance automatically results in lowered tidal volume and increased respiratory rate. Marked fluctuation in transduced central vascular pressures may suggest similar fluctuation in intrapleural pressure and also indicates increased work of breathing. Intercostal, subcostal, and suprasternal retractions may be observed in patients with significantly decreased lung compliance.

The correct amount of CPAP, applied with appropriate equipment, increases FRC within seconds, often resulting in improved arterial oxygenation and decreased work of breathing. It is imperative that the airway pressure remain positive throughout the respiratory cycle in order to minimize the work of breathing. Therefore, it is necessary that gas flow during both inhalation and exhalation be sufficient to prevent significant airway pressure fluctuation. Inspiratory and expiratory circuit resistance must be minimized to achieve appropriate CPAP therapy. Therefore, careful attention must be given to demand valve sensitivity, adequacy of inspiratory flow with continuous flow systems, humidifier resistance, and expiratory valve flow resistance. Airway pressure waveform may be analyzed to detect signs of inspiratory or expiratory flow retardation.

OPTIMAL CPAP

Many clinicians have attempted to define "optimal CPAP." In the 1970s, PEEP was applied in an attempt to obtain "adequate" PaO_2 while avoiding a toxic FiO_2 despite persistence of severe degrees of pulmonary dysfunction. Optimal CPAP was considered to be that level which provided an adequate PaO_2 at any FiO_2 not greater than 0.60. Other clinicians realized that mechanical ventilation, combined with high levels of CPAP, may improve PaO_2 but decrease oxygen delivery by decreasing cardiac output. Thus, they defined optimal CPAP in terms of maximizing oxygen delivery, without much concern for reversing the underlying pulmonary dysfunction. We believe that these approaches prolong the period of pulmonary dysfunction and increase morbidity secondary to complications of mechanical ventilation, infection, and cardiac dysfunction. If an increase in O_2 delivery were the primary goal, transfusion of blood to increase hemoglobin concentration would be a more efficacious form of therapy.

We define optimal CPAP as the airway pressure necessary to increase FRC to normal, thereby minimizing the mechanical work of spontaneous ventilation and improving the matching of ventilation and perfusion. Restoration of FRC with CPAP should provide adequate oxygenation at the lowest possible FiO_2. This approach promotes improvement of pulmonary function rather than maintenance of a tolerable level of pulmonary dysfunction. Thus, CPAP assumes an important supportive role while other therapy is administered simultaneously, such as antibiotics for patients with bacterial pneumonia. Unfortunately, many disease processes that severely decrease FRC have underlying etiologies for which there is no specific therapy, such as adult respiratory distress syndrome (ARDS). In these cases, CPAP is applied until normal healing permits its removal.

Optimal CPAP varies not only from patient to patient but also from day to day in the same patient. For example, a patient with ARDS may require much higher levels of CPAP than a patient with a small-volume gastric fluid aspiration. As acute respiratory distress syndrome resolves and pulmonary compliance returns to normal, it is possible to decrease the level of CPAP.

In order to quantitate $\dot{V}/\dot{Q}$ and allow objective evaluation of optimal CPAP, calculation of pulmonary venous admixture, or right-to-left intrapulmonary physiologic shunt fraction, has gained widespread clinical application. As with most clinical variables, it is the overall trend of values and not a single calculation that provides useful information regarding patient status and the adequacy of therapy. Although normal pulmonary venous admixture is calculated to be approximately 5 percent of the total cardiac output, critically ill patients may have physiologic shunting of blood exceeding 30 percent of their total cardiac output. Some authors have advocated increasing CPAP until the calculated venous admixture is decreased below an arbitrary limit of 15 percent of cardiac output. We believe that venous admixture should be minimized with the level of CPAP that can be applied without causing significant depression of cardiac output. Spontaneous ventilation is encouraged, since mechanical ventilation is much more prone to alter hemodynamic function. It is possible to continuously assess $\dot{V}/\dot{Q}$ by continuous monitoring of arterial oxyhemoglobin saturation with a pulse oximeter and mixed venous oxyhemoglobin saturation with a pulmonary artery oximetry catheter. It is important to use the lowest possible FiO_2 that will maintain arterial saturation above 90 percent. Equally important, however, is frequent physical examination of the patient. As CPAP is increased to the optimal level, lung compliance will increase. The work of breathing will decrease significantly, resulting in an increase in tidal volume and a decrease in respiratory rate. However, if the level of CPAP applied becomes either inadequate or excessive, lung compliance will again decrease. With a decrease in lung compliance the patient will develop tachypnea, shallow breathing, and retractions, indicating the need for readjustment of the CPAP. If excessive, CPAP may cause relative hyperinflation of the lungs, resulting in an increase in the expiratory work of breathing. Such a reversal of the normal inspiratory:expiratory work of the breathing pattern may be an indication to decrease the level of CPAP.

It is difficult to assess pulmonary mechanics during total mechanical ventilation. Calculation of lung-thorax compliance by dividing tidal volume by the change in airway pressure reflects changes in both lung and thoracic compliance. Changes in thoracic compliance may obscure changes in lung compliance.

SUPPORTIVE CPAP

The term "prophylactic CPAP" is a misnomer. CPAP is of no benefit and may even be harmful if administered to patients with normal or increased FRC. If FRC is decreased, for example, following upper abdominal surgery, and yet arterial oxygenation is satisfactory and the work of breathing is tolerable, CPAP may be considered "prophylactic" by some. Administration of low levels of CPAP to such patients increases FRC but may not markedly increase PaO$_2$. We regard this as a supportive, rather than a prophylactic, application of CPAP. The increased FRC improves lung compliance and decreases the work of breathing, as evidenced by a slight increase in tidal volume and a decrease in respiratory rate in such patients. This does not imply, however, that we believe that every patient with a decreased FRC must receive CPAP.

HAZARDS OF CPAP

Unfortunately, most clinicians confuse the hazards of CPAP with those of mechanical ventilation. Many of the complications attributed to CPAP are actually the result of mechanical ventilation with CPAP. However, CPAP has certain risks, even in the absence of mechanical ventilatory support. Although CPAP is applied in an attempt to decrease the mechanical work of breathing, the use of inappropriate or defective equipment may result in increased work of breathing. This is best detected by frequent physical examination of the patient and airway pressure monitoring.

Pulmonary barotrauma is one of the most feared hazards of CPAP. However, in spontaneously breathing patients with significantly decreased FRC, barotrauma is uncommon, even when high levels of CPAP are applied. Mechanical ventilation in conjunction with CPAP, however, increases the risk of barotrauma secondary to marked increases in peak airway pressure. Thus, the risk of barotrauma can be minimized by allowing spontaneous ventilation. Minimizing or withholding CPAP for fear of barotrauma may allow the FRC to decrease even further, making spontaneous ventilation inadequate. Mechanical ventilation with high peak airway pressures plus CPAP would then be required, increasing the risk of barotrauma.

Positive airway pressure may compromise hemodynamic function in a variety of ways. Excessive decreases in intrapleural pressure during spontaneous inspiration may increase left ventricular afterload. Therefore, some patients with pre-existing left ventricular dysfunction may not tolerate spontaneous ventilation, even with CPAP. In patients with otherwise normal cardiac function, significant hemodynamic compromise is rarely detectable unless CPAP exceeds 20 cm H$_2$O when patients breathe spontaneously. However, mechanical ventilation plus CPAP greatly increases intrathoracic pressure and significantly decreases venous return and cardiac output. The appropriate therapy in this situation is not necessarily to decrease the CPAP or to administer large volumes of intravenous fluids. Instead, an attempt should be made to increase cardiac output by allowing spontaneous breathing to occur.

Pulmonary vascular resistance, which is influenced by resting lung volume, may alter right ventricular function. In general, pulmonary vascular resistance is lowest when FRC is normal. If FRC is decreased, the extra-alveolar pulmonary vessels become tortuous, resulting in an increase in pulmonary vascular resistance. If FRC is increased well above normal, as it may be with excessive levels of CPAP, alveolar capillaries are compressed, resulting in an increase in pulmonary vascular resistance and right ventricular afterload. Thus, attempts to optimize right ventricular function should include normalization of FRC by titration of CPAP.

Mechanical ventilation with CPAP increases inferior and superior vena caval pressures. This may result in extrathoracic organ dysfunction. Renal, hepatic, and cerebral dysfunctions may occur during mechanical ventilation with CPAP but are very unlikely with spontaneous ventilation with CPAP less than 20 cm H$_2$O.

PERIODIC DISCONTINUANCE OF CPAP

CPAP increases FRC and may improve arterial oxygenation within minutes. Conversely, sudden interruption of CPAP results in an immediate reduction in FRC and a decrease in arterial oxygenation within seconds. Moreover, a higher level of CPAP then may be required to again increase FRC and improve oxygenation to the levels previously attained. Therefore, discontinuation of CPAP for transportation or bathing of the patient should be avoided whenever possible. Discontinuation of CPAP for tracheal suctioning is particularly hazardous and may cause a profound decrease in PaO_2. Therefore, tracheal suctioning should be performed only when required and not according to an arbitrary time schedule. Furthermore, we believe that such maneuvers should be monitored continuously by pulse oximetry since O_2 desaturation is likely to occur. We also avoid discontinuation of CPAP during central vascular pressure and cardiac output measurements. In addition to causing an abrupt decrease in FRC, such practice yields inaccurate and misleading data.

WEANING OF CPAP

Decreasing the rate of mechanical ventilation causes a decrease in mean airway pressure and may, therefore, cause FRC to decrease. For this reason, we recommend that CPAP not be decreased until the rate of mechanical ventilation has been decreased to two breaths per minute, or less, during intermittent mandatory ventilation. Meanwhile, the FiO_2 should be decreased to the lowest possible level, preferably 30 percent or less. Then, to avoid a rapid, marked, and potentially dangerous decrease in FRC and arterial oxygenation, CPAP should be decreased in 2 cm H_2O decrements. Following each decrement in CPAP, the patient's oxygenation and work of breathing must be re-evaluated. Since 90 percent of the alteration in oxygenation and lung mechanics will be complete within 3 minutes of a change in CPAP, re-evaluation should occur within 10 minutes or less.

Although the mechanism is not well understood, it appears that there are plateaus in weaning progress that occur at CPAP levels of approximately 20, 10,

and 5 cm H_2O. Weaning may proceed rapidly to these levels, but deterioration frequently occurs when CPAP is decreased further. Therefore, we pay particular attention to respiratory rate and PaO_2 when CPAP is decreased to 16 to 18 cm H_2O, 8 cm H_2O, and 5 cm H_2O. Many patients may discontinue CPAP once they have tolerated weaning to 5 cm H_2O CPAP.

The existence of "intrinsic PEEP," that is, PEEP created by exhalation against a partially closed glottis, remains controversial. However, it is clear that some patients who have been tracheally intubated for prolonged periods of time and all patients who have undergone tracheostomy have less ability to create intrinsic PEEP and may not tolerate abrupt discontinuation of CPAP.

Suggested Reading

Dantzker DR, Wagner PD, West JB. Instability of lung units with low V_A/Q ratios during O_2 breathing. J Appl Physiol 1975; 38:886–895.

Douglas ME, Downs JB, Dannemiller FJ, et al. Change in pulmonary venous admixture with varying inspired oxygen. Anesth Analg 1976; 55:688–695.

Downs JB, Modell JH. Patterns of respiratory support aimed at pathophysiologic conditions. ASA refresher courses in anesthesiology. Philadelphia: JB Lippincott, 1977; 5(6):71.

Eiser NM, Jones HA, Hughes JMB. Effect of 30% oxygen on local matching of perfusion and ventilation in chronic airways obstruction. Clin Sci Mol Med 1977; 53:387–395.

Kirby RR, Downs JB, Civetta JM, et al. High level positive end-expiratory pressure (PEEP) in acute respiratory insufficiency. Chest 1975; 67:156–163.

Kirby RR, Perry JC, Calderwood HW. Cardiorespiratory effects of high positive end-expiratory pressure. Anesthesiology 1975; 43:533–539.

Kirby RR, Taylor RW. An approach to mechanical ventilation. In: Kirby RR, Taylor RW, eds. Respiratory failure. Chicago: Year Book, 1986:530.

Register SD, Downs JB, Stock MC, et al. Is 50% oxygen harmful? Crit Care Med 1987; 15(6):598–601.

Wagner PD, Laravuso RB, Uhl RR, et al. Continuous distributions of ventilation-perfusion ratios in normal subjects breathing air and 100% O_2. J Clin Invest 1974; 54:54–68.

West JB. Respiratory physiology. Baltimore: Williams & Wilkins, 1985.

CLINICAL USE OF INSPIRATORY AND EXPIRATORY WAVEFORMS

MICHAEL J. BANNER, M.Ed, RRT
SAMSUN LAMPOTANG, M.E.

Patients with pulmonary parenchymal disease have increased airways resistance (Raw), decreased lung compliance, or both. Raw may be altered by decreased patency of the small airways, such as with asthma, chronic bronchitis, or emphysema. Lung compliance may be decreased by several factors, e.g., pneumonia or interstitial or alveolar edema. Regional changes in Raw and lung compliance precipitate maldistribution of ventilation, which disturbs the relationship between ventilation and perfusion ($\dot{V}_A/\dot{Q}$) in the lungs. Areas of increased $\dot{V}_A/\dot{Q}$ (more ventilation than perfusion) or decreased $\dot{V}_A/\dot{Q}$ (less ventilation than perfusion, or relative shunt) cause hypercapnia and hypoxemia. In addition, maldistribution of ventilation during mechanical positive pressure breathing can cause regional hyperinflation, which increases the risk of alveolar rupture and other forms of pulmonary barotrauma.

Distribution of ventilation in patients with compromised pulmonary function is influenced by the ventilator inspiratory flow waveform, time (T_I), pressure, and frequency (f) during mechanical positive pressure breathing. For example, certain inspiratory flow and pressure waveforms and ratios of inhalation-to-exhalation times (I:E) promote better distribution of ventilation according to some studies. Flow and pressure waveforms may also be manipulated during the exhalation phase. Retarding flow during exhalation, which prolongs the duration of exhalation, slows the rate of drop of the airway pressure waveform; these effects are thought to be salutary in chronic obstructive pulmonary disease (COPD). This chapter discusses these ventilatory considerations with emphasis on the effects of T_I and inspiratory flow waveform vis-à-vis the distribution of ventilation during mechanical positive pressure breathing.

INSPIRATORY FLOW WAVEFORMS

Sinusoidal, constant, decelerating, or accelerating inspiratory flow waveforms are available on many newer microprocessor-controlled mechanical ventilators (Fig. 1). Whether a particular type of flow waveform can improve the distribution of ventilation, $\dot{V}_A/\dot{Q}$ matching, and gas exchange is controversial. The discrepancy among some reports relates to a host of confounding variables. In some studies, altering the inspiratory flow waveform may have affected T_I, I:E ratio, peak inspiratory flow rate, tidal volume (V_T), and minute ventilation. Some investigators, using an end-inspiratory plateau, have compared various inspiratory flow waveforms and have found little difference in arterial blood gas values. However, the duration of T_I is increased by the presence of an end-inspiratory plateau, which suggests that the duration of T_I is as important in influencing the distribution of ventilation and gas exchange, if not more so, as the type of flow waveform.

Ventilation in mechanical lung models and patients has been studied to evaluate the effects of inspiratory flow waveform on gas distribution by altering the inspiratory flow waveform and by keeping other ventilator variables constant. Several studies of lung models with multiple compartments having different resistances have demonstrated that a decelerating inspiratory flow waveform distributes ventilation more evenly than other types of waveforms. These data may be relevant to treating patients with COPD who require ventilatory support. Clinical reports suggest similar findings. In one investigation in which V_T, T_I, I:E ratio, and f were held constant, peak inflation pressure (PIP), deadspace-to-tidal volume ratio (V_D/V_T), and alveolar-arterial gradient for oxygen were significantly lower with a decelerating inspiratory flow waveform than with a constant inspiratory flow waveform. However, with the decelerating flow waveform, mean airway pressure was greater, which may predispose a patient to adverse hemodynamic effects.

TIME CONSTANT, AND INSPIRATORY TIME

Temporal and spatial differences in V_T distribution in the lungs are related to local differences in resistance and compliance. The lungs are composed of elements that branch and are not all similar mechanically. Because of these mechanical differences, the elements operate asynchronously, even when subjected to the same driving force. Dr. Arthur B. Otis asserted that if T_I were long enough, partially obstructed areas would fill until volume were evenly distributed throughout the lung; the duration of T_I needed would depend on the resistance and the compliance of each alveolar compartment.

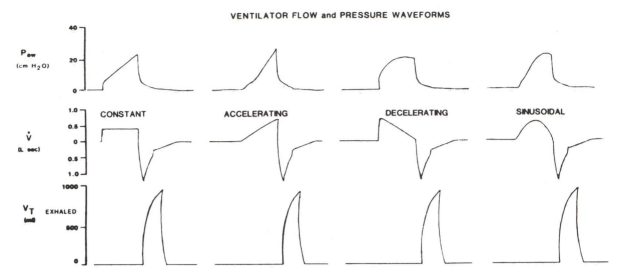

Figure 1 Airway pressure (Paw), flow rate ($\dot{V}$), and tidal volume (VT) are shown for constant, accelerating, decelerating, and sinusoidal inspiratory flow waveforms. Inspiratory time and VT were held constant during the measurements. Peak inflation pressure was highest with the accelerating waveform and lowest with the decelerating one; however, mean airway pressure was highest with the latter waveform.

The time constant (τ) of the total respiratory system is the product of Raw and dynamic lung-thorax (or total) compliance (CLT). τ represents the time required for the system to reach 63 percent of its equilibrium value and is an indication of the time required for adequate filling. When TI is less than τ of the alveolar compartment, no inspiratory flow waveform, in and of itself, can distribute ventilation evenly!

When pressure is applied to the airway opening, inflation of the lungs depends on Raw and CLT and on the pattern of the pressure waveform. If a pressure of constant magnitude is applied suddenly (a step-change in pressure), flow begins immediately and the flow rate attains a maximal value; the duration of time required for filling depends on both Raw and CLT (i.e., τ). Filling time is prolonged when Raw is increased because flow rate is decreased and when CLT is increased more gas is required to distend the lung to the point of equilibrium and vice versa. The rate at which alveolar pressure and volume increase and flow rate decreases after a step change in pressure at the airway opening is governed by τ (Fig. 2).

With $\dot{V}$A/$\dot{Q}$ mismatching, as in acute lung injury and COPD, a series of alveolar units may have altered time constants. Prolonging TI during mechanical inhalation improves the distribution of ventilation among lung units with different time constants. In one study, VD/VT and venous admixture were less when TI was increased than when TI was decreased.

Since the duration of TI affects gas distribution and alveolar ventilation, a systematic method of titrating TI to better match $\dot{V}$A/$\dot{Q}$ would be useful. The total τ of the respiratory system may be used as a basis for titrating TI. Engel has posited that when TI is greater than 3τ, the ratio of volume of gas to lung unit A and volume of gas to lung unit B is independent of TI, even when τ of lung unit A $\neq$ τ of lung unit B. When TI is less than 3τ, volume of gas to lung unit A and volume of gas to lung unit B varies with TI.

Ideally, when TI = 3τ, 95 percent filling is achieved. Since the total τ of the respiratory system can be calculated (τ = Raw $\times$ dynamic CLT), adjusting TI to greater than or equal to 3τ is a potentially better approach than setting TI to some arbitrary value. We have provided evidence to support this in a lung model with slow- and fast-filling compartments. System resistance and compliance were measured at 16 cm H_2O per liter per second and at 0.05 L per cm H_2O respectively; thus, the total system τ equalled 0.8 seconds. VT and f were held constant while sinusoidal, decelerating, accelerating, and constant inspiratory flow waveforms were applied at a TI of 0.8 seconds (1τ), 1.6 seconds (2τ), 2.4 seconds (3τ), 3.2 seconds (4τ), and 4 seconds (5τ). Longer TI improved the distribution of ventilation with *all flow waveforms*, as evidenced by decreases in end-tidal CO_2. The optimal duration of TI was equivalent to 3 to 4τ. Additionally, CO_2 elimination was greatest when a decelerating waveform was used. Ventilation was maldistributed (as indicated by higher regional and end-tidal CO_2 values) when TI was less than 3τ; this was most evident with an accelerating inspiratory flow waveform (Fig. 3). These data suggest that, in patients whose major disorder is increased Raw (e.g., COPD), using a TI greater than or equal to 3τ and a

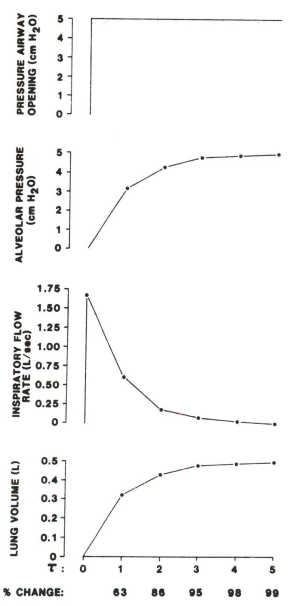

decelerating inspiratory flow waveform may result in more even distribution of ventilation.

Heretofore, much emphasis has been placed on manipulating the inspiratory flow waveform to promote better $\dot{V}_A/\dot{Q}$ matching, whereas less attention has been given to manipulating T_I. However, our data have shown that increasing T_I sufficiently (e.g., T_I greater than or equal to 3τ) and decreasing flow rate (to keep V_T constant) for the same inspiratory flow waveform promotes more uniform filling of the lung (compare Fig. 4A and 4B).

A caveat of increasing T_I is that mean airway and intrapleural pressures may be increased excessively, which precipitates decreases in thoracic venous blood inflow, preload, and cardiac output. Careful attention should be given to monitoring ventilatory and hemodynamic effects in patients when T_I is increased.

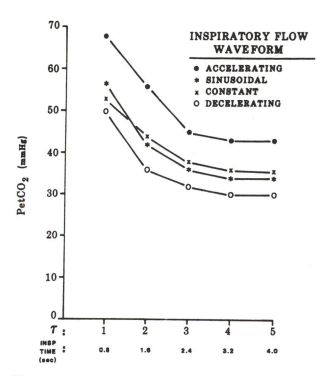

Figure 2 Exponential changes in pressure, flow rate, and volume after a step-change in pressure of 5 cm H₂O at the airway opening. Lung-thorax compliance (C_{LT}) is 0.1 L per cm H₂O, airways resistance (Raw) is 3 cm H₂O per liter per second (normal adult values), and the time constant (τ) (C_{LT} × Raw) is 0.3 seconds. When inspiratory time is equal to 1τ, a 63 percent change in pressure, flow rate, and volume occurs; at 2τ, 86 percent; at 3τ, 95 percent; and so on. The following equations are used to calculate the changes in alveolar pressure (Palv), inspiratory flow rate (V), and lung volume (V):

$$1. \quad \text{Palv} = \text{Pao}(1 - e^{-T_I/\tau})$$
$$2. \quad \dot{V} = (1/\tau)(V_O e^{-T_I/\tau})$$
$$3. \quad V = V_O(1 - e^{-T_I/\tau})$$

where Pao = step change in pressure at airway opening (5 cm H₂O), e = the base for natural logarithms (2.718), T_I = inspiratory time (sec), and V_O = volume limit of the system (V_O = total lung-thorax compliance × pressure, i.e., 0.5 L = 0.1 L per cm H₂O × 5 cm H₂O).

Figure 3 Carbon dioxide elimination, as measured by partial pressure of end-tidal carbon dioxide (PetCO₂), with different inspiratory flow waveforms and times in a lung model with slow- and fast-filling compartments. The time constant (τ) of the lung model was 0.8 sec (resistance = 16 cm H₂O per liter per second × compliance = 0.05 L per cm H₂O). When tidal volume and frequency were held constant, PetCO₂ decreased substantially when inspiratory time was increased; this effect was enhanced by a decelerating inspiratory flow waveform. At constant minute ventilation, PetCO₂ at inspiratory time = 1τ reflects hypoventilation for all flow waveforms; at inspiratory time = 3τ, ventilation is adequate with all flow waveforms except the accelerating type. Even at an inspiratory time = 5τ, PetCO₂ was abnormally high (reflecting hypoventilation) with an accelerating flow waveform. These data may be relevant in treating patients with chronic obstructive pulmonary disease. (All data are mean values.)

Inspiratory Flow Waveforms and Lung Compliance

With regional differences in Raw but uniform lung compliance, pressure *and* volume equilibrate in the lungs given sufficient TI during mechanical positive pressure ventilation. Conversely, with regional differences in lung compliance, relatively normal and uniform Raw, and sufficient TI, only pressure will equilibrate in the lungs, and VT will be unequally distributed because of the regional differences in compliance. If the inflating pressure is maintained for a sufficient TI, the mechanically delivered VT will be distributed according to the following relationship:

$$VT = \sum_{n=1}^{N} PCn$$

where P = sustained inflating pressure (cm H_2O), Cn = compliance of the nth lung compartment (ml per cm H_2O), and N = total number of lung compartments.

Consider that two lung units A and B have identical resistances, but B has half the compliance of A. The τ for unit B is also half that of A, and the time required to fill unit B is half that required to fill A. However, since the compliance of unit B is half that of A, the ultimate increase in volume of B can only

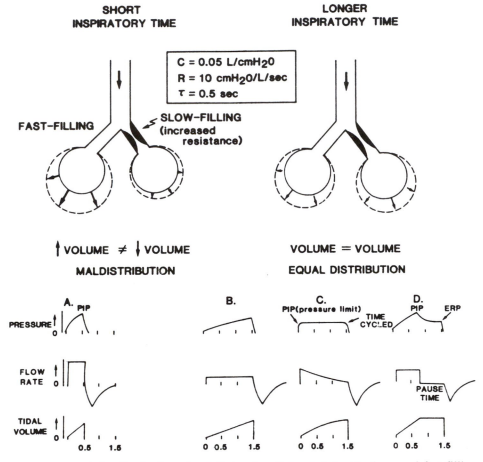

Figure 4 Inspiratory time and the distribution of ventilation in a lung model with slow- and fast-filling compartments. Compliance (C), resistance (R), and time constant (τ) are indicated. In *A*, when inspiratory time = 1τ and the inspiratory flow waveform is constant, maldistribution of tidal volume results in contrast to when inspiratory time = 3τ with the same flow waveform and tidal volume, which results in equal distribution *B*. In *C*, pressure-limited time-cycled ventilation, and *D*, end-inspiratory plateau (EIP), inspiratory time and tidal volume are the same as in *B* and equal distribution of ventilation results (adequate inspiratory time, as in *B*, *C*, and *D*, promotes equal distribution of ventilation, irrespective of the inspiratory pressure and flow waveform used). The peak inflation pressure (PIP) is greatest in *A* and lowest in *C*. In *C*, PIP is limited and the ventilator time-cycles "OFF" after a set inspiratory time. With EIP *D*, PIP is generated while gas flows from the ventilator; during the pause, no flow is delivered to the patient and airway pressure decreases to the level of the static elastic recoil pressure (ERP) or plateau pressure of the system; after the previously determined pause time, the exhalation valve opens, which allows passive exhalation.

be half that of A when T_I is prolonged indefinitely. The relative distribution of gas between the two units is not constant throughout inflation and depends on the duration of T_I. Pressure rises more rapidly in unit B (lower compliance), and if T_I is brief and followed by a postinflation hold, gas is redistributed from unit B to unit A until *pressure* equilibrates between the units, at which time the increase in *volume* of unit A is *twice* that of unit B.

Distribution of ventilation is related not only to the difference in compliance between lung units, but also to the difference in the rate of change of compliance between lung units during mechanical inflation. Mecca has noted that lung units that are highly compliant receive a disproportionately large volume of gas during the early phase of inhalation. At some point during inhalation these units reach the top of their pressure-volume curves and, thus, the compliance of these units becomes less than that of others that initially exhibit low compliance. As a result, gas flow is diverted to these initially underventilated alveoli as they become relatively more compliant.

The effect of the inspiratory flow waveform on the distribution of ventilation with regional differences in lung compliance has been studied. Bergman applied constant, sinusoidal, decelerating, and accelerating waveforms to a branched, resistive-capacitive electrical circuit lung analogue. At all values of regional compliance and with all waveforms, the branches received volumes proportional to their compliance—no inspiratory flow waveform provided superior uniform ventilation.

From studies of variations in compliance with various inspiratory flow waveforms, the decelerating flow waveform was found to give the highest compliance and the accelerating the lowest compliance (Johansson and Lofstrom; Baker). Jansson and Jonson speculated that an accelerating inspiratory flow waveform may be favorable in patients in whom compliance varied in different lung compartments. Also, the accelerating flow waveform has resulted in lower mean airway (see Fig. 1) and intrapleural pressures than have other waveforms, which may affect venous return and pulmonary capillary perfusion pressure. It has been hypothesized that the accelerating inspiratory flow waveform may thus be advantageous in patients with circulatory problems involving low pressure in the pulmonary capillary bed.

Inspiratory Flow Waveforms and Normal Lung Function

In a study of the effects of various types of inspiratory flow waveforms when lung compliance and Raw were normal, Watson noted that the various waveforms had no effect on V_D/V_T ratio and lung compliance of conscious, totally paralyzed patients with normal lung function. These findings were confirmed by Bergman in dogs and in anesthetized subjects with normal cardiopulmonary function and by Adams in normo-, hypo-, and hypervolemic dogs.

END-INSPIRATORY PLATEAU

Postinflation hold, end-inspiratory pause, or end-inspiratory plateau (EIP)—all terms for the same procedure—represents a period of time after mechanical inhalation when no flow is delivered from the ventilator, positive pressure is maintained in the lungs and the opening of the exhalation valve is delayed (Fig. 4D). EIP is considered a part, or extension, of the mechanical inspiratory phase because the ventilator does not initiate exhalation until after the EIP time has elapsed. The duration of EIP is designated in seconds or is expressed as a percentage of the total time of the respiratory cycle.

EIP has been advanced by several investigators as a method of enhancing distribution of inhaled V_T and, thus, of decreasing arterial carbon dioxide tension and V_D/V_T. This may be explained by the fact that T_I is increased during EIP, if T_I is long enough to exceed the τ of slow-filling spaces in the lung, distribution of ventilation is improved. Collateral ventilation and Pendeluft flow, also thought to enhance the distribution of ventilation, occur more readily when time is allowed for pressure to equalize throughout the lung during the EIP. Collateral ventilation occurs when gas enters alveoli through collateral channels; these may be channels in the alveolar walls (Kohn's pores) or communications between the bronchioles and alveoli (Lambert's canals). Pendeluft flow occurs when, during the EIP, surplus volume from fast-filling spaces redistributes and flows to slow-filling spaces. Gas flow between different regions of the lung is caused by instantaneous pressure gradients resulting from inequalities of time constants among these regions.

Elastic and resistive components of the peak inflation pressure (PIP) can be estimated by using EIP. Factors affecting PIP may be represented mathematically as follows:

$$PIP \propto (V_T/C_{DYN}) + (Raw \times \dot{V}_I)$$

where C_{DYN} is dynamic lung-thorax compliance (L per cm H_2O) and $\dot{V}_I$ is inspiratory flow rate (L per second). EIP may be used to differentiate C_{DYN} from static lung-thorax compliance (C_{ST}) and to determine Raw as follows:

$$C_{DYN} = V_T/(PIP - \text{baseline pressure})$$

where baseline pressure is atmospheric pressure or the positive end-expiratory pressure value, and

$C_{ST} = V_T/$(static elastic recoil pressure [ERP] or plateau pressure of the lung-thorax system
— the baseline pressure).

Finally,

$$Raw = (PIP - ERP)/\dot{V}_I \text{ (see Fig. 4D).}$$

PRESSURE-LIMITED, TIME-CYCLED MECHANICAL VENTILATION

The term "inflation hold" has been used incorrectly to refer to pressure-limited, time-cycled mechanical ventilation. With this form of mechanical inflation, a pressure limit is applied by presetting an overpressure governor to limit the PIP at a selected value. Once the pressure limit is reached, airway pressure is held at that level until the ventilator time-cycles off (mechanical inhalation terminates when a selected T_I is reached) (Fig. 4C). Gas actively flows from the ventilator during the pressure limit or at the inspiratory pressure plateau hold period. This is in contrast to EIP; when flow from the ventilator is interrupted during the hold period, gas is redistributed throughout the ventilator circuit and the patient's airways, and a characteristic decrease in airway pressure from PIP to ERP occurs (see Fig. 4D). The decrease in pressure is directly related to Raw.

Pressure-limited time-cycled mechanical ventilation is often used for infants with hyaline membrane disease. Limiting PIP may reduce the risk of barotrauma. Pressure-limited time-cycled ventilation has been advocated by Reynolds, who has posited that one factor in the pathogenesis of bronchopulmonary dysplasia is mechanical trauma caused by high airway pressures during mechanical ventilation. In terms of gas exchange, it is contended that, if alveoli are held open longer with mechanical inhalation, arterial oxygenation and distribution of ventilation may be improved.

RETARDATION OF FLOW DURING EXHALATION

It has been theorized that retardation of flow during exhalation (expiratory retard) enables uniform emptying of the lungs of patients with COPD. Patients with airway obstruction have difficulty exhaling because peripheral airways are constricted. Chronic emphysema attenuates the walls of the small airways, which, therefore, tend to collapse during exhalation. By attaching a flow-restricting device distal to the exhalation valve on the ventilator circuit, *rate* of flow and pressure decrease from the lungs are reduced. Retardation of flow during exhalation decreases the slope of the expiratory airway pressure curve, thereby maintaining back pressure in the small airways and, in effect, keeping them open. With this technique,

given sufficient time, airway pressure returns to zero at end-exhalation. Therefore, this is not the same as positive end-expiratory pressure, in which airway pressure is positive at end-exhalation. Pursed-lip breathing can accomplish the same effect, i.e., slower and more even emptying of the alveoli.

The equal-pressure point theory is used as a rationale for retarding flow, pressure, and volume during exhalation in patients with COPD. Alveolar pressure (Palv), which is the sum of the recoil pressure of the lung and the intrapleural pressure (Ppl), is normally zero. After positive pressure inhalation, however, Palv and Ppl are greater than atmospheric pressure. During exhalation, the rate of decrease of Palv is affected by Raw. Airway pressure decreases progressively from the alveoli to the airway opening, but at some point along the airway (the equal-pressure point), the intrabronchiolar pressure and the pressure surrounding the airways (the extrabronchiolar pressure or Ppl) are equal. Toward the airway opening, however, the transmural pressure (intrabronchiolar pressure − extrabronchiolar pressure) becomes negative—intrabronchiolar pressure less than extrabronchiolar pressure. As a result, the airways are subject to dynamic compression, which impedes exhalation, traps gas in the alveoli, and, thus, causes hypercapnia. By retarding flow and, consequently, the rate at which pressure decreases in the lungs during exhalation, intrabronchiolar pressure likely remains higher than extrabronchiolar pressure, thereby maintaining positive transmural pressure in the airways, which keeps them open and allows flow to continue throughout exhalation.

The exhalation τ of the total respiratory system (τexh) governs the rate of exhaled flow during exhalation. Since a 95 percent change in pressure, flow, and volume occurs when time equals three time constants, then, a priori, to allow sufficient time for emptying, exhalation time should be equal to at least $3\tau exh$ when flow is retarded. For example, consider a patient with COPD whose lung-thorax compliance is 0.1 L per cm H_2O and expiratory Raw is 15 cm H_2O per liter per second, the total τexh (compliance × resistance) is 1.5 seconds; exhalation should be prolonged to 4.5 seconds or more. When retarding flow, this approach may be more practical than prolonging exhalation time to some arbitrary value.

A potential disadvantage of retarding flow and decreasing pressure and volume during exhalation is that mean airway pressure is increased. This increases mean Ppl and, thus, decreases thoracic venous blood inflow, thereby making the cardiovascular system unstable. Thus, cardiac output and blood pressure should be monitored when exhalation is being retarded.

Acknowledgement: Lynn M. Carroll provided editorial assistance.

Suggested Reading

Adams AP, Economides AP, Finlay WEI, Sykes MK. The effects of variations of inspiratory flow waveform on cardiorespiratory function during controlled ventilation in normo-, hypo-, and hypervolemic dogs. Br J Anaesth 1970; 42:818–824.

Al-Saady N, Bennett ED. Decelerating inspiratory flow waveform improves lung mechanics and gas exchange in patients on intermittent positive-pressure ventilation. Intens Care Med 1985; 11:68–75.

Baker AB, Colliss JE, Cowie RW. Effects of varying inspiratory flow waveform and time in intermittent positive pressure ventilation. II. Various physiologic variables. Br J Anaesth 1977; 49:1221–1233.

Banner MJ, Boysen PG, Lampotang S, Jaeger MJ. End-tidal CO_2 affected by inspiratory time and flow waveform—time for a change. Crit Care Med 1986; 14:374.

Bergman NA. Effect of different pressure breathing patterns on alveolar-arterial gradients in dogs. J Appl Physiol 1963; 18:1049–1055.

Bergman NA. Fourier analysis of effects of varying pressure waveforms in electrical lung analogues. Acta Anaesthesiol Scand 1984; 28:174–181.

Engel LA. Dynamic distribution of gas flow. In: Macklem PT, Mead J, eds. Handbook of physiology. The respiratory system. Section 3, volume 3. Bethesda: American Physiologic Society, 1986:575.

Fulerham SF. Effect of mechanical ventilation with end-inspiratory pause on blood gas exchange. Anesth Analg 1976; 55:122–130.

Jansson L, Jonson B. A theoretical study of flow patterns of ventilators. Scand J Respir Dis 1972; 55:237–246.

Johansson H, Lofstrom JB. Effects on breathing mechanics and gas exchange of different inspiratory gas flow patterns during anaesthesia. Acta Anaesthesiol Scand 1975; 19:8–18.

Mecca RS. Pulmonary physiology. In Kirby RR, Taylor RW, eds. Respiratory Failure. Chicago: Year Book, 1986:22.

Nunn JF. Applied respiratory physiology. 2nd ed. Woburn, Massachusetts: Butterworths, 1977:238.

Otis A, McKerrow C, Bartlett R, Mead J, McIlroy M, Selverstone N, Radford E. Mechanical factors in distribution of pulmonary ventilation. J Appl Physiol 1956; 8:427–432.

Reynolds EOR. Pressure waveform and ventilator settings for mechanical ventilation in severe hyaline membrane disease. Bourns Educational Series ES1. Boston: Little, Brown, 1977:1.

Sykes MK, Lumley J. The effect of varying inspiratory:expiratory ratios on gas exchange during anaesthesia for open heart surgery. Br J Anaesth 1969; 41:374–380.

PRESSURE SUPPORT: INSPIRATORY ASSIST

NEIL R. MacINTYRE, M.D.

Pressure support ventilation (PSV) is a form of mechanical ventilatory support that assists an intubated patient's spontaneous inspiratory effort with a clinician-selected amount of positive airway pressure (Fig. 1). This pressure can range from 1 to 100 cm H_2O, is designed to be held constant through servo control of delivered flow, and is terminated when a certain inspiratory flow minimum is reached. This mode of ventilatory support clearly differs from conventional volume-cycled ventilation (VCV) in that with PSV the clinician selects only the inspiratory pressure level, whereas the patient is allowed to control ventilatory timing and to interact with the delivered pressure to set the inspiratory flow and tidal volume (V_T). PSV also differs from continuous positive airway pressure (CPAP) in that PSV is designed primarily as ventilatory support (i.e., through pressure applied only during inspiration), whereas CPAP is designed primarily as oxygenation support (i.e., through the alveolar stabilizing effects of positive expiratory pressure). PSV is, in fact, similar to older forms of pressure-assisted ventilatory support (e.g., intermittent positive pressure breathing [IPPB]), but differs from IPPB in that airway pressure is held constant throughout the inspiratory effort with PSV, and comprehensive alarm packages are available on modern ventilators equipped to deliver PSV.

PHYSIOLOGIC EFFECTS OF PSV

Pressure support of a spontaneous breath may have several effects on the respiratory system that are different from either unsupported spontaneous breaths or clinician-controlled VCV breaths. Two such effects that may have clinical relevance involve the interaction of PSV with ventilatory pattern reflexes and the interaction of pressure support with ventilatory muscle function.

To understand the potential effects of PSV on ventilatory pattern reflexes, it is important to realize that the lungs and thoracic cage have stretch and irritant receptors that supply input into the central nervous system regarding the mechanical aspects of ventilation. It is thought that the ventilatory control center

in the central nervous system utilizes these inputs, along with gas exchange input from arterial blood gas tensions, to set the ventilatory pattern (i.e., rate, tidal volume, and inspiratory flow), which results in the best gas exchange for the least amount of muscle work. Dyspnea occurs when these relationships are suboptimal. Ideal mechanical ventilatory support, therefore, should not only support gas exchange, but should do so in a manner that interacts properly with these mechanoreceptors to produce patient-ventilator "synchrony" and to minimize dyspnea. Since a PSV breath allows the patient more control over inspiratory flow, inspiratory time, and tidal volume than a VCV assisted breath, we might expect PSV to interact better with these mechanoreceptors in spontaneously breathing patients. Moreover, patient-ventilator synchrony might be further promoted when using PSV as a sole support mode since constant muscle work, intrapulmonary stretch, and gas exchange would result from every spontaneous inspiratory effort.

To understand the potential effects of PSV on ventilatory muscle function, it is important to realize that ventilatory muscle fatigue and failure are often the precipitating events of acute respiratory failure. Moreover, persistent ventilatory muscle dysfunction is thought to be a contributing factor in the inability to wean patients from prolonged mechanical ventilatory support. Despite these important roles, the mechanisms of ventilatory muscle fatigue and recovery are not well understood. However, indirect clinical evidence and extrapolation from other skeletal muscle data allow us to make several inferences about ventilatory muscle function under these circumstances. First, the primary ventilatory muscle, the diaphragm, performs work moving the required minute ventilation against the various components of respiratory system impedance (i.e., compliance, resistance, and inertance). Various disease states that increase minute ventilation demands, increase airway resistance, or reduce lung compliance will necessarily increase this work demand. Second, excessive workloads result in diaphragmatic fatigue and failure. This is manifest clinically as tachypnea, paradoxical abdominal motion, and an inability to remove CO_2. Third, fatigued muscles require a reduction in workload to subfatiguing levels for recovery. Prolonged, absolute rest, however, can result in muscle atrophy. Thus appropriate workloads need to be placed upon ventilatory muscles as they recover. Fourth, ventilatory muscle workloads can emphasize either strength or endurance muscle conditioning depending upon the pressure and volume change characteristics of that work (i.e., work = $\int$

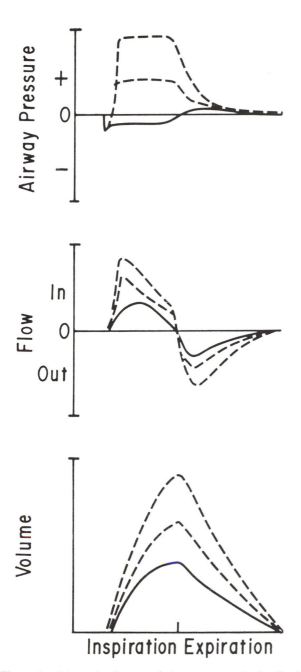

Figure 1 Schematic diagram of airway pressure in the distal endotracheal tube (top panel), air flow (middle panel), and lung volume changes (lower panel) in spontaneously breathing, intubated patients on a mechanical ventilator. The horizontal axis depicts time. The solid lines depict an unassisted breath; the dashed lines depict two levels of pressure-assisted breaths with PSV. Note that under all conditions, an initial negative airway pressure change is required by the patient to open demand valves and initiate flow. Thereafter, continued negative airway pressure is required by the unassisted patient to maintain flow and deliver a V_T. With PSV, however, a plateau of pressure is produced that augments the patient's inspiratory efforts to increase flow and V_T.

pressure × volume change [$\int P \times \Delta V$]). Specifically, high pressure-low volume change work tends to stimulate strength conditioning (through the development of increased sarcomeres), whereas low pressure-high volume change work tends to stimulate endurance conditioning (through the development of increased mitochondrial density).

All of these features of ventilatory muscles may have important implications when mechanical ventilatory support is delivered. Ideally, mechanical ventilation should initially rest fatigued muscles and then, during recovery, provide appropriate conditioning workloads (both in the quantity of work and in the pressure-volume change characteristics of that work) to prevent atrophy and to optimize ventilatory muscle reconditioning. Current practices with VCV, however, may not be ideal (Fig. 2). With these modes, ventilatory muscle work occurs by the patient's taking unsupported spontaneous breaths (either as "t tube" trials or as unassisted breaths interspersed with volume assisted or controlled breaths: intermittent mandatory ventilation [IMV]). The limitation to these approaches is that whereas the amount of work a patient performs is clinician-controlled (i.e., by adjusting the mandatory breath rate), the pressure-volume change characteristics of this spontaneous breathing work are fixed in a high $P/\Delta V$ pattern by the increased airway resistances and the reduced lung compliances that are characteristic of intubated patients in respiratory failure. In contrast, pressure supporting a spontaneous breath should allow clinician manipulation of both the total work per breath and the $P/\Delta V$ work characteristics of that breath (see Fig. 2). The more normal $P/\Delta V$ work relationship that can occur with a pressure-supported breath may contribute to patient comfort. Moreover, the emphasis on endurance conditioning that this type of work provides may be advantageous to the diaphragm, a primary endurance-oriented muscle with a capability for high power outputs. It must be pointed out, however, that this conditioning advantage is only theoretical and this hypothesis remains untested in clinical ventilatory muscle failure.

CURRENT APPROACHES TO THE CLINICAL APPLICATION OF PSV

Three basic approaches to PSV are currently being used: (1) low level PSV in conjunction with IMV; (2) low level PSV in patients intubated for nonventilatory support reasons; and (3) high level PSV as a stand-alone ventilatory support mode (Table 1).

PSV in conjunction with IMV employs 2 to 10 cm H_2O pressure during inspiration to overcome the resistive component of inspiratory work imposed by an endotracheal tube. The exact pressure requirement can actually be calculated by knowing the endotra-

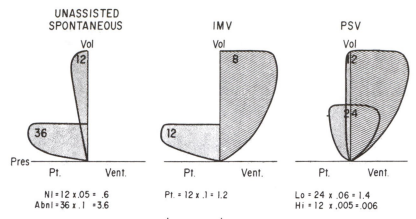

Figure 2 Schematic comparison of both the magnitude and the pressure-volume change characteristics of ventilatory muscle work during unassisted breathing, during IMV, and during PSV. Each panel plots ventilatory pressures (to the left for the patient, to the right for the ventilator) versus V_T. Work per breath is the area under this curve (stippled for patient work, hatched for ventilator work). Numbers inside each curve represent the respiratory rate required for a constant muscle ventilation using that V_T. At the bottom of each panel is the calculation for total work per minute (i.e., W = breathing frequency [min^{-1}] × work per breath [kg·m]). In the left panel is unassisted breathing in both the normal (nl) and the diseased (abnl) lung. The normal lung is represented by a normal work per minute and a low pressure-high volume change type of breath (this latter relationship can be expressed at the P/ΔV ratio for that breath). The diseased lung is characterized by a six-fold increase in total work and a marked increase in P/ΔV. In the middle panel, eight volume control breaths are being given to the diseased lung as IMV. To maintain the constant MV, the patient only has to take 12 breaths per minute. Patient work is thus reduced to only one-third of its unassisted level, but the P/ΔV characteristics remain constant. In the right panel, two levels of PSV assisting the diseased lung are depicted. With low levels of PSV (Lo), both patient work and the P/ΔV ratio are reduced moderately. With high levels of PSV (Hi), both patient work and the P/ΔV are near zero.

cheal tube diameter and the inspiratory flow characteristics. The rationale for this approach is that the air flow resistance associated with an endotracheal tube produces an undesirably high P/ΔV workload that may compromise comfort and ventilatory muscle function during the spontaneous breaths of IMV. This use of PSV may thus be indicated in any patient on IMV in whom tachypnea, dyspnea, or ventilator-patient asynchrony is felt to be at least partially due to the spontaneous ventilatory muscle work characteristics imposed by the endotracheal tube. The weaning approach using low level PSV with IMV remains that of a progressive reduction in mandatory breaths. The hazards

of this approach appear minimal although the elevation in mean intrathoracic pressure may compromise cardiovascular function in susceptible individuals.

PSV in patients intubated for nonventilatory support reasons (e.g., for airway protection or for alveolar stabilization with CPAP) also utilizes pressures of 2 to 10 cm H_2O. As with PSV during the spontaneous breaths of IMV, the rationale for this approach is to reduce (or eliminate) the resistive inspiratory work imposed by an endotracheal tube so as to improve comfort and ventilatory muscle function. This level of PSV may thus be indicated in any patient requiring an endotracheal tube for nonventilatory support rea-

TABLE 1   Clinical Applications of Pressure Support Ventilation

Application	Pressure Levels	Goals
Intermittent pressure assist (i.e., during spontaneous breaths of IMV)	2 to 10 cm H_2O	Reduce discomfort and high P/ΔV workloads imposed by high resistance endotracheal tubes
Pressure assist with every breath:		
Low levels in patients requiring endotracheal tubes only for airway protection or for application of CPAP to support oxygenation	2 to 10 cm H_2O	Reduce discomfort and high P/ΔV workloads imposed by high resistance endotracheal tubes
High levels in patients requiring substantial levels of ventilatory support	5 to 100 cm H_2O	Provide an alternate form of mechanical ventilatory support that may improve comfort and provide a more "physiologic" workload on the ventilatory muscles

sons in whom tachypnea or dyspnea is felt to be a consequence of the inspiratory workload related to that tube.

PSV as a stand-alone ventilatory support mode employs whatever level of inspiratory pressure is necessary for a desired tidal volume and minute ventilation. Pressure levels can thus range as high as 50 to 100 cm H_2O in patients with large minute ventilation demands and severely impaired ventilatory system mechanics. A useful initial setting for PSV under these circumstances is to provide whatever inspiratory pressure is necessary for a tidal volume of 10 to 12 ml per kilogram. This level of PSV has been termed PSVmax and, because it appears that this amount of inspiratory pressure can reduce patient work to near zero, this level of ventilatory support approaches that provided by conventional assist-control VCV. Weaning of PSV from this point is accomplished by reductions in the level of airway pressure and can generally be guided by the patient's alveolar ventilation (i.e., $PaCO_2$) and the respiratory rate. Abrupt elevations in either of these parameters indicate an excessive ventilatory muscle load. The rationale for using this approach is to provide patients requiring ventilatory support with an alternative mode to intermittent VCV that may be more comfortable and that may supply a more physiologic workload to the ventilatory muscles. It is important to note, however, that since patients have considerable control over ventilation with this form of PSV, only patients who have a reliable ventilatory drive and a measure of stability in their ventilatory requirements should be selected for its application. Thus, this approach to PSV should primarily be used in the recovery phase of respiratory failure. In this setting, it may be particularly useful in those patients who are difficult to make comfortable or who may require a lower $P/\Delta V$ workload to facilitate muscle conditioning and weaning. Hazards to this approach, as noted above, include potentially higher mean intrathoracic pressures and consequent cardiovascular compromise. In addition, there is the potential for suboptimal alveolar ventilation in a patient with unstable ventilatory drives or rapidly changing lung impedances.

Clearly clinician enthusiasm for PSV exists and manufacturers have responded to this by providing the PSV mode on most of the current generation of mechanical ventilators. However, specific questions need to be answered before the true role of PSV is determined. These questions include: (1) What advantage, if any, is there to allowing the patient more control over the ventilatory pattern? Will it significantly improve patient-ventilator synchrony, thereby reducing dyspnea and the need for sedation? Or, conversely, will it either yield too much clinician control or perhaps make patients more difficult to wean? Studies on ventilatory drive and various assist techniques are necessary to address these issues. (2) What is the optimal amount of work for a patient during mechanical ventilatory support? Moreover, how important is the pressure-volume change characteristic of that work in producing strength or endurance training effects? Answers to these require more specific measurements of ventilatory muscle function than are currently available. (3) What are the hemodynamic effects of pressure supporting every breath? Specifically, is the lack of negative pleural pressure (as one gets during unsupported spontaneous breaths) detrimental to cardiac filling? (4) In designing a pressure-supported breath, what is the optimal pressure pattern? Most systems today have a fixed rapid initial flow rate that may or may not provide optimal pressure-supporting effects. Perhaps adjustable flow rate systems are going to be required for maximal use of PSV.

Thus at the present time we have an interesting mode of ventilatory support that appears to make spontaneous breathing more comfortable for patients and, at the same time, offers a means to adjust both the magnitude and the characteristics of ventilatory work to these patients. Because of the theoretical advantages and the safety of the mode in appropriately monitored patients, it is unreasonable not to recommend using the mode until definitive studies become available. Rather, judicious clinical use, which is based upon a good understanding of the potential effects of pressure support on ventilatory drive and muscle work, seems appropriate for the present. At the same time, however, we need to further study the complex process of ventilatory reflexes and muscle reconditioning during mechanical ventilation to fully establish the proper role of PSV.

Suggested Reading

Braun NMT, Faulkner J, Hughes RL, Roussos C, Sahgal V. When should respiratory muscles be exercised? Chest 1983; 84:76–84.

Leith DE, Bradley M. Ventilatory muscle strength and endurance training. J Appl Physiol 1976; 41:508–516.

MacIntyre NR. Respiratory function during pressure support ventilation. Chest 1986; 89:677–683.

Marini JJ. The physiologic determinants of ventilator dependence. Respir Care 1986; 31:271–281.

Marini JJ, Capps JS, Culver BH. The inspiratory work of breathing during assisted mechanical ventilation. Chest 1985; 87:612–618.

Otis AB, Fenn WO, Rahn H. Mechanics of breathing in man. J Appl Physiol 1950; 2:592–607.

Proctor HJ, Woolson R. Prediction of respiratory muscle fatigue by measurements of the work of breathing. Surg Gynecol Obstet 1973; 136:367–370.

Rochester DF, Arora NS. Respiratory muscle failure. Med Clin North Am 1983; 67(3):573–597.

SELECTION OF THE INSPIRATORY:EXPIRATORY RATIO

MICHAEL J. GUREVITCH, M.D.

Selection of a specific inspiratory:expiratory ratio (I:E ratio) is usually not considered when ventilator orders are written. Responsibility for this parameter lies with the respiratory therapist who sets a flow rate or inspiratory time knob depending on which type of ventilator is used. For most ventilated patients, this may not be of vital importance; however, in some critically ill individuals, inhomogeneity of ventilation may be severe enough to result in major hypoxemia and hypercapnia. In these cases, knowledge of the underlying pathophysiology, combined with careful ventilator adjustments, may allow the selection of a specific I:E ratio, which results in better oxygenation and ventilation.

Traditional teaching to those managing ventilators dictates that the duration of inspiration should rarely exceed one-half the total ventilatory cycle. When reviewing the literature in an effort to discover the foundation for this gospel, it is quite confusing. Each study uses different animals, ventilators and modes, various flow patterns, and a variety of patient populations. The one consistent finding that emerged from studies done during the 1960s was that a short inspiratory time resulted in an increased deadspace ventilation (Vd/Vt) and decrease in dynamic compliance. This was thought to result from a worsening of ventilation/perfusion (V/Q) matching. Follow-up studies confirmed that prolongation of inspiration causes a decrease in Vd/Vt, which becomes more significant as lung disease progresses.

With this physiologic premise studied and confirmed, pediatricians were the first to question whether prolonging inspiration to the point of I:E ratio reversal might improve ventilation/perfusion. This seems only appropriate since pediatric ventilators were of the pressure limited, time cycled variety, having inspiratory and expiratory times as their major control variables.

In 1971, E.O.R. Reynolds looked at the effect of multiple alterations in mechanical ventilator settings on the pulmonary gas exchange of neonates with hyaline membrane disease. He concluded that the use of a very long inspiratory phase resulted in a large increase in PaO_2 and decrease in right to left shunt. In 1976, S.F. Fuleihan et al demonstrated that the addition of an end-inspiratory pause in adults with acute respiratory insufficiency, resulted in a decrease in Vd/Vt and improved efficiency of ventilation. This finding was further confirmed using an animal model 3 years later.

On the other hand, Connors et al (1981), showed that patients with severe chronic airway obstruction noted improvement in gas exchange and more even distribution of ventilation at short inspiratory times (higher flow). Although contrary to their expectations, and quite the opposite of what previous studies might have predicted, they conjectured that the increased time available for alveolar emptying allowed redistribution of ventilation to regions with longer time constants.

Can some sense be made from all of this? Is there a unifying model or concept which might provide guidelines for when I:E ratios should be longer or shorter?

Figure 1 demonstrates what happens when the time constant (Resistance × Compliance) is lengthened as it is in obstructive airway disease. Short inspiration with longer expiration (Fig. 1A) allows obstructed lung units to fully empty resulting in a more even distribution of ventilation with each new breath. As inspiration is prolonged (Fig. 1B), a relative shortening of expiratory time results in an increased Vd/Vt, functional residual capacity (FRC) and airtrapping, which are undesirable consequences of ventilating this type of patient. Figure 2 demonstrates what occurs when the time constant is shortened as it is in diseases such as acute respiratory distress syndrome (ARDS) (decreased compliance). A short inspiratory time (Fig. 2A) allows unstable lung units to collapse during the relatively longer expiratory phase. However, a prolonged inspiratory time (Fig. 2B) secondary to a pause, allows equilibration between lung units and a more even distribution of ventilation. If reinflation occurs rapidly after a short expiratory phase, less lung units will collapse if they can be reexpanded prior to attaining their closing volume.

Assuming this model is correct, then patients with obstructive diseases, such as asthma, emphysema, and bronchitis, should be ventilated with shorter inspiratory times. Patients with ARDS, having stiff lungs and shorter time constants (with minimal secretions to cause obstruction), should be considered for prolongation of the inspiratory time.

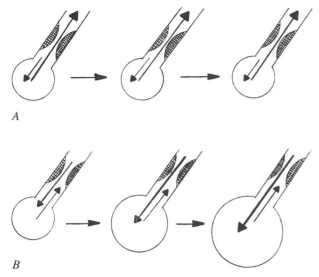

Figure 1 Consequences of increasing inspiratory time in regions of airflow obstruction (long time constant). *A,* short inspiratory times allow even severely obstructed lung units plenty of time to empty; *B,* at a constant respiratory rate, progressive lengthening of the inspiratory phase allows less time for complete exhalation to occur. This results in an increased FRC and Vd/Vt, air trapping, "auto PEEP" and possible barotrauma, none of which are desirable consequences when ventilating patients with airflow obstruction.

METHODS OF INCREASING THE I:E RATIO

How much to lengthen the inspiratory time and when to reverse the ratio are not yet known. Success depends on trial and error with close monitoring and observation until an optimum I:E ratio can be achieved. I increase the inspiratory time slowly in increments and watch for a desired effect. The least prolongation that provides a maximum therapeutic effect is "the best I:E ratio" as it maximizes oxygenation while minimizing hemodynamic compromise.

How the inspiratory time is prolonged when inverting the ratio appears to make a difference. Animal models have shown that inversed ratio ventilation (IRV) is more effective in a pressure-controlled mode rather than volume-controlled mode. The model shown in Figure 3 may help explain why.

Figures 3A and 3B show various ways by which the inspiratory time can be prolonged using a volume mode. By slowing the flow rate while maintaining a constant respiratory rate, the inspiratory time will encroach on the expiratory phase (see Fig. 3A). Inspiratory time can be prolonged by adding a pause after the tidal volume is delivered (see Fig. 3B). Pressure controlled inverse ratio ventilation allows a critical inspiratory pressure to be reached rapidly and maintained constant while the flow rate decelerates (Fig. 3C). This method of applying IRV may be more ef-

fective for the following reasons. In a volume modality, slowing the flow wastes the early portion of inspiration (dotted area) by allowing surfactant deficient lung units more time to collapse because early inspiratory pressures remain low. Adding a pause is helpful, but differences between peak and pause pressures may be significant, initially applying a pressure, which overventilates compliant units, then dropping to a pause pressure, which may be too low to maintain unstable lung units open.

Pressure controlled, time cycled ventilation allows flexibility and precision when prolonging inspiration to begin IRV (see Fig. 3C); however, it requires a shift from conventional thinking about the use of appropriate tidal volumes to the application of some critical and constant inspiratory pressure. This preset critical inspiratory pressure "splints" the lung, thereby allowing even inflation throughout inspiration while each new breath begins just prior to the end of terminal flow from the previous one. A "PEEP like effect" is thereby obtained as the lungs are immediately reinflated prior to the closing of unstable lung units. High peak airway pressures are avoided when

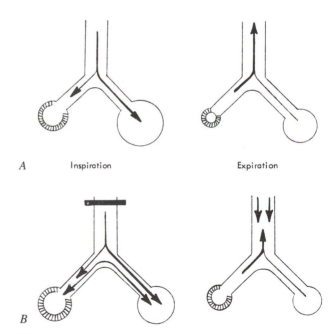

Figure 2 Consequences of increasing inspiratory time in lung units with decreased compliance (short time constant). *A,* short inspiration with longer expiration allows time for unstable lung units to collapse; *B,* stable, prolonged constant pressure occurs after a rapid insufflation with pressure controlled ventilation and similarly in volume control with pause. Equilibration occurs between lung units with differing time constants and results in a more even distribution of ventilation. If reinflation occurs rapidly after a shortened expiration, a PEEP like effect occurs, causing further recruitment of alveoli and less collapse of unstable lung units.

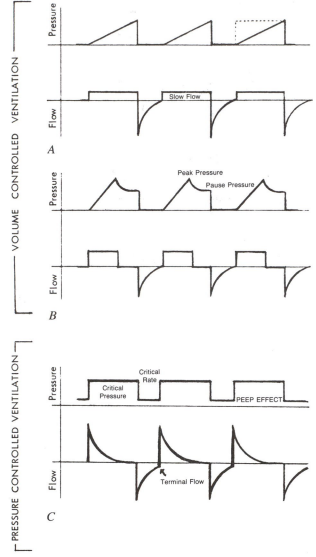

Figure 3 Methods of increasing the I:E ratio. *A,* slowing the flow while at a constant respiratory rate allows the inspiratory phase to encroach onto the expiratory period. This wastes the early portion of inspiration as many unstable lung units may still be continuing to empty despite being in the inspiratory portion of the cycle (dotted area). *B,* progressive prolongation of an end inspiratory pause results in eventual reversal of the I:E ratio. This results in peak pressures that can overinflate more compliant regions before dropping to a pause (static) pressure, which may be below the critical pressure necessary to maintain unstable lung units open. *C,* rapid insufflation with a decelerating flow maintains a preset pressure throughout inspiration. The critical rate is determined by setting each new breath to begin just prior to terminal flow returning to zero. Appropriate selection of an I:E ratio and respiratory rate will result in the desired PEEP effect.

a PEEP like effect is obtained in this manner providing the major impetus to consider this method.

As an example, let us consider a volume-ventilated patient who requires 50 cm H_2O pressure to move a 500 cc tidal volume. If a PEEP of 15 cm H_2O is added, the peak pressure will then rise to approximately 65 cm H_2O (50 cm H_2O for the tidal volume, on top of a PEEP baseline of 15 cm H_2O). Using IRV, a "PEEP-like" effect of 15 cm H_2O can be achieved in patients who are well ventilated with a peak pressure that may be no greater than 35 to 40 cm H_2O by selecting a special respiratory rate and I:E ratio that reinflates the lung prior to complete emptying. One of the major goals when utilizing this form of ventilation is to stop the lung damage that occurs as a result of shearing forces between adjacent hyperinflated and atelectatic regions. These forces ultimately result in further parenchymal damage and barotrauma as peak and PEEP pressures are increased. The alternative application of a lower constant pressure for a prolonged time period may prevent further lung damage while maintaining gas exchange.

HOW TO BEGIN

The Siemens 900C Servo Ventilator is currently the only ventilator that allows pressure controlled inverse ratio to be applied with full monitoring capabilities. A sample patient is one with severe ARDS, who has been hemodynamically stable (on no pressors), and begins failing traditional ventilatory measures. The PEEP is 15 cm H_2O, FIO_2 0.70, and peak pressure 65 to 70 cm H_2O despite full sedation. Radiographic infiltrates are progressing while compliance and PaO_2 are dropping. It is at this time that I would consider the application of IRV. Efforts to improve this patient must be started before there is further deterioration. "Onset hypoxemia," which frequently accompanies any modality change, can be noted when starting IRV and needs to be compensated for should it occur. In addition, it may take up to an hour before any improvement is noted if it is to occur with this modality, making it all the more difficult to begin implementation of IRV if the patient is already hypoxemic at an FIO_2 of 1.0.

Disposable ventilator circuits are replaced by stiff noncompliant-type tubing, and then a strip channel recorder, oscilloscope or computer module to monitor in line pressure and flow contours are added. If prior sedation has not been adequate to remove spontaneous respiratory efforts, additional sedation is tried and/or neuromuscular blockade added.

The ventilator is switched to its pressure control mode after an FIO_2 of 1.0 has been delivered for several minutes. Inspiratory time is increased to 67 percent (2:1) and the pressure control knob adjusted to between one-half to two-thirds of whatever peak cycling pressure had been in the previous mode. This should result in a tidal volume of approximately 400 to 600 cc. The respiratory rate is initially and arbitrarily set at 25 per minute and then adjusted up or down by watching the terminal flow curve as previously described. A rate is found that causes each new breath to be started just as end terminal flow approaches baseline (see Fig. 3C). The dialed-in PEEP level is reduced to no greater than 5 to 7 cm H_2O pressure and FIO_2 returned to its original setting. A complete line of data is then obtained from the ventilator, pulmonary artery catheter, and any noninvasive monitors available, i.e., oximeter or capnograph. The expiratory pause hold button is pressed momentarily to read the effective PEEP level and this is also recorded. An arterial blood gas is obtained 15 to 30 minutes later, after which time fine tuning is done by adjusting ventilating pressures, rate, and I:E ratios. Ventilating pressure and rate are adjusted to maintain a desirable $PaCO_2$, whereas the I:E ratio and rate are adjusted to obtain an "effective PEEP" level for adequate oxygenation. The total inspiratory time can be increased upward in increments of 5 percent by adding a pause, as total inspiratory time is equal to that dialed in plus the pause time selected.

PHYSIOLOGIC CONSEQUENCES

Certain physiologic principles must be understood when utilizing this mode of ventilation. Although patients are being ventilated at lower peak airway pressures, these pressures are being held for a longer time, and may result in mean airway pressures (MAP) that are actually higher than what had been noted prior to IRV. The higher MAP is felt by some to be the reason for improvement in oxygenation. Although correlation between increasing MAP and PaO_2 exists, MAP is not the major determinant of oxygenation. During ventilation at various combinations of inspiratory pressures and I:E ratios, significant changes in blood gases commonly occur, despite a constant MAP. It is of interest that changes in the respiratory rate do not change MAP, as in any given minute the same percent of time is spent in inspiration at the preset pressure. At I:E ratios around 2:1, MAPs are usually similar to those attained during conventional ventilation with PEEP, thereby allowing the benefits of IRV to be realized without hemodynamic compromise. At ratios approaching 4:1, however, the resultant drop in cardiac output may offset any improvement in PaO_2, thus emphasizing the importance of astute observation when applying IRV to this extreme. If cardiac output falls because of an increased MAP and decreased venous return, then intravenous fluids should be increased to maintain right ventricular preload much as one does when PEEP levels are increased. Because of this potential hemodynamic compromise, however, oxygen delivery (O_2 content × cardiac output) is the important parameter to follow.

Although tidal volume is not specifically set, it results as a consequence of the pressure change in going from an end-expiratory (PEEP) baseline to the preset inspiratory pressure (see Fig. 3C). The total PEEP is really a combination of the PEEP dialed into the ventilator plus the "PEEP effect," which occurs because of progressively shorter expiratory times. As the I:E ratio or respiratory rate increase, the PEEP baseline rises, causing a smaller pressure differential in going from a new higher baseline to the same preset pressure. The resulting decrease in tidal volume may cause $PaCO_2$ retention, which can be averted by decreasing the dialed-in ventilator PEEP. At a higher I:E ratio or respiratory rate the PEEP effect becomes significant without having to be superimposed on a dialed-in level, and often the dialed-in PEEP can be set to zero. As an alternative, preset inspiratory pressure can be raised to increase the pressure differential and thereby increase tidal volume, however, this also increases MAP—an increase which is usually undesirable.

As expertise is gained, one can frequently look at the expiratory flow tracing to determine whether the patient is a candidate for continued application of the inverse ratio mode. A prolonged expiratory flow suggests increased resistance and/or obstruction, and these patients have an increased $PaCO_2$. However, in appropriately selected patients, this mode decreases Vd/Vt and $PaCO_2$, thereby necessitating a lower minute ventilation than was used in conventional ventilatory modes. In these selected patients, it is hoped that there will be improved oxygenation and O_2 delivery at lower peak airway pressures.

Prolongation of the inspiratory time results in improved V/Q matching and decreased Vd/Vt in patients with normal or reduced lung compliance. Although prolongation of inspiration to the point of reversal of the I:E ratio has limited application, it may be effective in reducing peak airway pressure and improving oxygenation. A PEEP-like effect is created by setting a respiratory rate and I:E ratio that begin lung insufflation prior to complete exhalation from the previous breath. A critical inspiratory pressure is maintained throughout the remainder of each ventilatory cycle to provide alveolar stabilization and recruitment. Lower peak airway pressures sustained for a longer time period may prevent lung damage caused by excessive shearing forces that develop between inhomogenous lung units when they are ventilated at high peak and PEEP pressures.

Application of this modality should only be undertaken by those who are familiar with the equipment being employed and who are able to provide close observation and monitoring of these critically ill patients.

Suggested Reading

Boros, SJ. Variations in inspiratory:expiratory ratio and airway pressure wave form during mechanical ventilation: the significance of mean airway pressure. J Pediatr 1979; 94:114–117.

Bowe EA, Klein EF Jr, Buckwalter JA Jr. Mean airway pressure does not determine oxygenation [abstract]. Anesthesiology 1983; 59:106(A).

Cole AGH, Weller SF, Sykes MK. Inverse ratio ventilation compared with PEEP in adult respiratory failure. Intensive Care Med 1984; 10:227–232.

Connors AF Jr, McCaffree DR, Gray BA. Effect of inspiratory flow rate on gas exchange during mechanical ventilation. Am Rev Resp Dis 1981; 124:537–543.

Fairley HB, Blenkarn GD. Effect on pulmonary gas exchange of variations in inspiratory flow rate during intermittent positive pressure ventilation. Br J Anaesth 1966; 38:320–328.

Fuleihan SF, Wilson RS, Pontoppidan H. Effect of mechanical ventilation with end-inspiratory pause on blood gas exchange. Anesth Analg 1976; 55:122–130.

Gurevitch MJ. Observations on IRV [letter]. Chest 1986; 90:152.

Gurevitch MJ, Van Dyke J, Young E, Jackson K. Improved oxygenation and lower peak airway pressure in severe adult respiratory distress syndrome; treatment with inverse ratio ventilation. Chest 1986; 89:211–213.

Lachmann B, Danzmann E, Haendly B, Jonson B. Ventilator settings and gas exchange in respiratory distress syndrome. In: Prakash O, ed. Applied physiology in clinical respiratory care. Boston: Martinus Nijhoff, 1982:141.

Lindahl S. Influence of an end inspiratory pause on pulmonary ventilation, gas distribution and lung perfusion during artificial ventilation. Crit Care Med 1979; 7:540–546.

Reynolds EOR. Effect of alterations in mechanical ventilator settings on pulmonary gas exchange in hyaline membrane disease. Arch Dis Child 1971; 46:152–159.

Watson WE. Observations on physiological deadspace during intermittent positive pressure respiration. Br J Anaesth 1962; 34:502–508.

HIGH FREQUENCY JET VENTILATION

ISABELLE C. KOPEC, M.D.
ALAN L. VaNDERVORT, M.D.
GRAZIANO C. CARLON, M.D.

Conventional mechanical ventilators have evolved through progressively more sophisticated attempts to duplicate natural processes. The first devices used for long-term respiratory support ("iron lungs") expanded the chest wall, and consequently, the lungs, thereby generating a negative pressure. They were superceded in the late 1950s by ventilators, which expanded the lungs by increasing alveolar pressure, rather than by decreasing intrapleural pressure. Modern volume-cycled ventilators are substantially more efficient, versatile, and safer than their predecessors, but the basic principles of operation have not changed. A few major conceptual innovations have, however, been introduced; they include positive end-expiratory pressure (PEEP) and intermittent mandatory ventilation (IMV).

The development of PEEP illustrates what was probably the first attempt to treat acute respiratory failure according to its pathophysiology. The principal cause of hypoxemia was correctly identified in the presence of severe ventilation/perfusion (V/Q) inequality, rather than impaired diffusion process, as had previously been suggested. V/Q mismatch is caused by anatomic or functional collapse of alveoli and terminal respiratory units, precluding gas exchange within areas of the lungs which are still perfused. As a result, closing volume increases even while functional residual capacity (FRC) decreases. As long as perfusion through nonventilated areas occurs, these areas of anatomical or functional collapse contribute to increasing shunt fraction (Qs/Qt) and thus to hypoxemia. The conceptual basis of PEEP is thus remarkable for its simplicity; by raising the pressure within airways and alveoli to a value close to critical closing pressure, alveolar collapse at the end of each expiration should be prevented, maintaining adequate gas exchange throughout the entire respiratory cycle. PEEP not only increases the number of alveoli available for gas exchange, but also substantially expands the time during which alveoli are available for gas exchange. A major limitation of PEEP, especially when used at high levels, is that most patients with severe forms of respiratory failure have different degrees of involvement in various areas of the lung. Thus, application of a uniform mode of therapy may produce more injury in unaffected areas than benefit to the involved lung. Nonetheless, though PEEP therapy encountered a surprising amount of opposition for many years and controversy about its use still abounds, it is presently considered a standard component of conventional mechanical ventilatory support.

Despite an increased understanding of the pathophysiology of respiratory failure and technical advances in the design of mechanical ventilators, the mortality rate associated with acute respiratory failure remains high. Although statistics vary substantially in reports of different authors since the criteria used to define respiratory failure are different, mortality ranges from 30 to 60 percent in patients requiring mechanical support of ventilation for severe hypoxemia.

Though most patients improve, at least temporarily, when mechanical ventilation is instituted, in some cases therapeutic interventions aimed at increasing FRC may be accompanied by a deterioration of blood gases. In a few cases, the failure may be explained by substantial differences in the degree of involvement of the two lungs or by the presence of major airway disruption. However, in most instances obvious reasons may not be apparent. Use of conventional mechanical ventilation also carries the risk of serious complications. These include increased extravascular lung water, impaired surfactant function, and disruption of lung tissue.

The high mortality rate associated with acute respiratory failure and the existing therapeutic limitations have spurred the search for alternative modalities of mechanical support. High frequency ventilation (HFV)—the generic name applied to all ventilatory modes that use supraphysiologic breathing frequencies and small tidal volumes, at times less than anatomic dead space—is one such alternative modality.

Experimental demonstrations that life-sustaining gas exchange could be achieved with very small tidal volumes were available as early as 1915, but it was not until 1967 that a ventilator actually providing high frequency positive-pressure ventilation (HFPPV) was built. The purpose of this device was to support ventilation while minimizing interference with cardiac function (a complication frequently observed during mechanical support, especially when peak and mean airway pressures are greatly elevated). Several modifications of the prototype model were developed; in 1974, System H was built as the first commercially available system for HFPPV (Bronchovent, AGA

TABLE 1   Summary of Recommendations for the Use of High Frequency Jet Ventilators

HFJV should be connected to an adjustable pressure source that can operate up to 50 psi

Composition of gases delivered should be tested frequently

If a solenoid valve is used, it is advisable to change it every 2–3 months

Respiratory rates should be 100–200 bpm, with an I:E ratio of 1:2 to 1:3

Inspiratory line should be as short as possible, made of nondeformable material, such as Teflon or polyvinyl chloride

Injector cannula should have a diameter of 1.5–2.0 mm, inserted in the proximal end of the endotracheal tube and be centrally and coaxially oriented. Ratio between injector cannula and endotracheal tube cross-sectional area should be between 1:6 and 1:11

Reliable alarms and fail-safe mechanisms should be available

Adequate humidification of the gases should be assured

An initial tidal volume of 3.5–4.5 ml/kg should be used and then adjusted on the basis of $PaCO_2$ measurements

Driving pressure should be manipulated to adjust alveolar ventilation

Company, Sweden). That ventilator is still utilized for bronchoscopy as well as laryngoscopy and laryngeal surgery, including laser surgery of the larynx.

High frequency jet ventilation (HFJV) is another technique of ventilation at supraphysiologic frequencies, based on the principle of the jet injector. Although first described in 1956, it has been extensively studied only in the last 10 years. HFJV investigations have been directed toward three major areas: definition of the ideal technical characteristics of a jet ventilator; interactions between the ventilator and the patient; and identification of patients most likely to benefit from HFJV support.

COMPONENTS OF HIGH FREQUENCY JET VENTILATORS

In order to utilize HFJV optimally, a thorough understanding of the principles affecting gas delivery and of the operation of each component is necessary (Table 1). Several technical aspects of jet ventilation are different in function and design from those applicable to conventional ventilators. The most notable components include the pressure source, the gating mechanism, the inspiratory line, and the injector cannula.

For proper operation, gases must be delivered to the jet ventilator under pressures of 5 to 50 pounds per square inch (psi). The centralized oxygen and air supply of the hospital usually operates as the pressure source, although any other method of delivering compressed gases would be adequate. The minimum required pressure varies with the type of ventilator. Pneumatic and fluidic jet ventilators, which utilize part of the gas pressure to operate the controls, generally require higher operating pressures than electronic devices. The majority of commercially available devices are based on electronically operated solenoid valves.

Experimental and clinical evidence available with these systems suggest that gas pressures higher than 50 psi are rarely, if ever, necessary to maintain adequate ventilation. Thus, the centralized oxygen supply system of most hospitals, or the regulator of most compressed medical gas cylinders, could be used to operate HFJV with electronically-operated solenoid valves.

Gases delivered by the pressure source must pass through a gating mechanism before reaching the patient. This component of the jet ventilator determines the number of cycles (respiratory rate) and the percentage of time during which gas flow to the patient is allowed ("on time" or "duty cycle"). Ideally, opening and closing times of the gating mechanism should be instantaneous, and its function should be minimally affected by driving pressure and distal pneumatic impedance. Although electronic controllers generate remarkably precise time signals, the mechanical action does not have the same degree of accuracy. Accordingly, the response time of the gating mechanism can become a significant factor at high respiratory rates (several hundred breaths per minute). For instance, if opening and closing times are equal to 10 msec, an increase in respiratory rate or decrease in I:E ratio resulting in an inspiratory time of less than 100 msec would have a 20 percent error factor because of the time required for the valve to open and close.

The inspiratory line consists of the tubing between the gating mechanism and the injector cannula. This component of the jet ventilator must also conform to strict specifications to provide reliable gas delivery. In conventional ventilators, compressible volumes of 1.5 to 3.5 ml per cm H_2O are considered normal. This figure takes into account the effects of Boyle's law on the volume of gases present in the ventilator circuit, as well as the deformation of the conducting tubings. In HFJV, comparable compression values would result in very large gas losses, which might preclude effective gas delivery to the patient.

Just as significant as the actual reduction in tidal volume are the changes in pressure waveform, which are associated with anything but the most noncompliant tubing. The initial pressure rise after the opening of the solenoid valve is slow because part of the energy is dissipated to compress gases already present in the inspiratory line. After the solenoid valve closes, compressed gases in the inspiratory line expand, prolonging gas flow through the injector cannula. The magnitude of jet entrainment (discussed in detail later), is also dependent on gas flow and on the pressure gradient existing at the distal opening of the jet cannula (the "nozzle"). Tubing for the inspiratory line should be as short as practical, should be made of a virtually undeformable material, such as Teflon (compliance = 0.005 ml per cm H_2O), and should have a diameter three to four times that of the injector cannula.

Injector Cannulas

The inspiratory line of a jet ventilator terminates in an injector cannula through which gases enter into the patient's airway. Since the cannula has a small diameter, the gas pressure decreases as velocity increases to maintain a constant kinetic energy. Since jet entrainment depends primarily on volume and velocity of gases exiting from the nozzle, the characteristics of the injector cannula have a significant influence on the total tidal volume delivered. The principal variables controlling the ratio of directly delivered to entrained gas are (a) the diameter and length of the cannula; (b) the ratio of the surface areas of the injector cannula and endotracheal tube; (c) the axial orientation of the injector within the swivel connector and the endotracheal tube; and (d) the distance between cannula tip and entrainment source.

On the basis of available bench tests, animal experiments, and human studies, the following conclusions appear justified:

1. The diameter of the injector cannula should be 1.5 to 2.0 mm for application in adults. Cannulas with a smaller diameter cannot provide adequate gas flow, while those of larger size may cause dangerously high airway pressure. Smaller catheters (less than 1 mm diameter) may be sometimes used in pediatric patients.
2. The ideal ratio between the areas of the injector cannula and the endotracheal tube is 1:6 to 1:11. When the ratio exceeds 1:6, the cannula occupies an excessively large portion of the endotracheal catheter; as a consequence, excessive turbulence in the proximal part of the endotracheal tube may prevent forward gas motion and obstruct exhalation. At the other end of the spectrum, a ratio

at or greater than 1:11 will significantly reduce entrainment.
3. The optimal orientation of the cannula within the endotracheal tube is central and coaxial with its tip in close proximity to the source of entrainment.

SAFETY CONSIDERATIONS AND TECHNICAL PROBLEMS

Alarms

Reliable alarms are an indispensable component of every high frequency ventilator and should monitor the principal functions of the device.

Failure of the gating mechanism should be immediately identified and a fail-safe mechanism should guarantee that the valve remains open when inoperative.

An airway overpressure alarm is mandatory to prevent barotrauma and should be associated with a safety mechanism, which immediately discontinues ventilator operation while venting the airway to ambient pressure.

Humidification of Gases

Clinical and experimental evidence has convincingly proved that a minimum water content of 30 mg per liter of inspired gases, corresponding to 100 percent relative humidity at 30.1° C, is necessary for optimal airway function in intubated patients. On HFJV, it is usually difficult to humidify gases before they reach the solenoid valve because commercially available humidifiers are not designed to withstand pressures of 40 to 50 psi. Furthermore, water condensation may cause valve malfunction. On the other hand, placement of a humidifier in the inspiratory line distal to the gating mechanism adds a large compressible volume to the system, which limits effective ventilation.

An early solution, which had been considered, was restricting humidification to entrained gases only. However, the contribution of entrainment to the total delivered tidal volume is highly variable and depends on the type of HFJV application and on the characteristics of the system used. Also, radionuclide imaging has demonstrated considerable nonuniformity in the distribution of gas flow. Certain areas, such as the carina and medial aspects of the main bronchi, are in the path of a high-velocity gas stream, whereas the lateral aspects of the major airways are subjected to the low-velocity flow. If humidification were restricted to entrained gases only, severe regional drying of the areas exposed to the highest flow may occur with hemorrhagic mucosal necrosis, inspissation of secretions, and ultimately, airway occlusion. To obviate these problems, the jet flow itself can be used as a nebulizer by delivering 15 to 20 ml per hour of normal saline through a microdrip in the front of the nozzle with dispersion of saline by the respiratory gases. This method ensures adequate distribution of water particles to the level of the subsegmental bronchi.

Solenoid Valve

The solenoid valve has a life expectancy of over 100 million cycles. It is our policy to change the solenoid valve every 3 months after an average use of 10 million cycles. The cost is negligible and the increase in safety enormous.

Inadvertent PEEP

During mechanical ventilation, the inspiratory flow rate is higher than that of expiratory, since the mechanical device is more powerful than the alveolar elastic recoil. Accordingly, the expiratory time constant is longer than the inspiratory. When respiratory frequency increases or expiratory time decreases, alveoli fill with gas but cannot empty completely; thus, FRC continuously increases. Respiratory rates below 150 to 200 breaths per minute (bpm) with I:E ratios at or less than 1:2.5 are usually safe and have not been associated with clinically significant gas trapping.

Alveolar Ventilation on High Frequency Ventilation

Clinical studies indicate that tidal volumes of 3 to 4.5 ml per kilogram—approximately one-third of those required with conventional ventilators—maintain eucapnea on HFJV, even in patients with severe respiratory failure. Sound theoretical explanations of the observed CO_2 clearance at low tidal volumes exist. A markedly cone-shaped flow distribution allows a portion of any given tidal volume to move distally down the airways with each subsequent inspiration. Since the exhalation flow profile is also cone-shaped, a transitional volume of fresh gases, which were delivered but not exhaled, remain within the airways after each tidal exchange. With each new breath, these gases move further down the airway. After a finite period of time, a steady state is reached, masked by a continuous delivery of fresh gases at the alveolar level, though they may not derive from the tidal volume of the last breath delivered, but, rather, include gases inhaled over a number of preceding breaths. This theory has solid mathematical support and suggests that convective mechanisms alone can explain alveolar gas exchange during HFJV without the need to postulate enhanced diffusion, a mechanism that would operate poorly in adults at rates below the natural frequency of the lungs (8 to 10 Hz). Additional support

for the theory that diffusion is not the only, or even the primary, modality of gas exchange on HFJV comes from capnographic studies. Phasic changes of CO_2 concentration can be observed with each breath, indicating that CO_2 molecules are removed from the alveolar space with each breath.

CLINICAL APPLICATIONS OF HFJV

HFJV for Disrupted Airways

The ability of HFJV to maintain oxygenation and CO_2 clearance in the presence of large bronchopleural fistulas and other sources of pathologic gas leak has been thoroughly studied in animals and humans. In fact, long-term, successful ventilatory support has been achieved in patients with airway defects equal in cross-sectional area to the trachea. Patients can be supported for days or even weeks on HFJV, until the disrupted airway heals or the patient is able to breathe spontaneously. Some authors recommend instituting HFJV immediately for large air leaks if any difficulty is encountered in maintaining normal gas exchange during spontaneous ventilation or conventional mechanical support.

Airway disruption often begins as a slit or rent in the elastic tissue of the lungs. During positive pressure ventilation, airway pressure opens the hole, thus enlarging its cross-sectional area into an ellipse of area $A = d \times b$, where d is the long axis and b is the radius, or one-half the diameter of the short axis. If the radius of the slit doubles, the cross-sectional area also doubles. Since flow varies with the square of the area, the air leak will increase fourfold.

In addition to the higher peak pressure generated on conventional ventilation, time is also a factor in determining the amount of flow through the leak because the fraction of the respiratory cycle spent at the highest airway pressure is greater during conventional ventilation than during HFJV. Thus, both the period of time during which the area of disruption is enlarged and the pressure gradient across it are larger with conventional ventilation; a much larger portion of the tidal volume will be lost through the disrupted airway. In contrast, during HFJV, lower peak pressures are diffused for shorter periods of time, thus reducing the gas losses through pathologic disruptions.

Other Indications

Mechanical ventilators are used in operating rooms to manage anesthetized patients and in intensive care units (ICUs) to support patients with acute respiratory failure. Less commonly, mechanical ventilators may be employed for individuals with neuromuscular complications, which preclude spontaneous breathing, or with severe forms of chronic obstructive pulmonary disease.

HFJV has a potential role in the operating room for laryngeal and tracheal surgery, but HFPPV has been extensively and effectively used for many years, and the need for a substitute form of support is not apparent.

Some investigators have suggested that HFJV can be beneficial in thoracic surgery. Theoretical benefits include continuous lung expansion and a quiet surgical field. Evidence from clinical studies, however, is inconclusive from a practical point of view. It is difficult to propose radical changes in the ventilatory techniques used in anesthesia since the incidence of complications is currently nil with conventional approaches, and proof that HFJV is of added benefit would require a study involving a large number of patients.

HFJV is not indicated in patients who are unable to breathe as a result of neuromuscular dysfunction, since small portable volume-cycled units are effective. Also, HFJV has not been employed in patients with chronic obstructive pulmonary disease except during weaning, where HFJV has sometimes been beneficial. Some studies indicate that patients who have developed neuromuscular discoordination may have an easier transition to spontaneous breathing through a period of HFJV support. Theoretically, this may be a result of reduced fatigue of the diaphragm and respiratory muscles. Pulmonary stretch receptor stimulation suppresses the respiratory center during HFJV, even if the patient is awake and normocapnic. Other forms of weaning, such as IMV can overexercise the diaphragm and induce fatigue, thus precluding sustained respiratory efforts. These deleterious effects can be prevented by periodically resting the patient on HFJV; this also avoids the adverse consequences of conventional ventilation and the need for sedation or muscle paralysis.

Several psychological studies also suggest that most patients adapt easily to, and indeed often prefer HFJV, despite the unnatural respiratory frequency. This observation may be explained by several mechanisms. Suppression of the afferent stimulations from the J receptors of the lungs inhibits the respiratory center, thereby decreasing the subjective feeling of dyspnea. Cessation of spontaneous ventilation reduces fatigue of the diaphragm and inspiratory muscles, thus reducing oxygen demand and its appreciated discomfort. Finally, the added resistance to inspiratory flow imposed by IMV demand valves is removed.

HFJV has been successfully used to prevent aspiration in emergency surgical procedures. A cannula can be inserted transtracheally or transcricoidally in patients who have injuries involving the oral cavity and/or upper airways. Ventilatory support can be provided with reduced danger of aspiration of blood or other debris from the upper airway. This approach should be restricted to cases where tracheal intubation is difficult or contraindicated. There is always the risk of placing the injector cannula into the soft tissue of the neck, with consequent massive subcutaneous emphysema.

The most common reason for initiating mechanical respiratory support in the ICU is acute respiratory failure. Though mechanical ventilation is only a form of symptomatic support (not a therapy of acute respiratory failure), patients who fail to achieve adequate oxygenation invariably die. Several studies involving a few hundred patients have compared the efficacy of HFJV with conventional volume-controlled ventilation. All investigators confirm that survival rates are identical with the two types of ventilation, as are the total durations of ventilation in patients who survive and in those who die. Also, in the vast majority of cases, the immediate cause of death is not a failure of the mechanical ventilator to maintain life-supporting gas exchange, but rather a nonpulmonary event.

Thus, HFJV can successfully maintain arterial oxygenation and alveolar ventilation and appears to be as safe and effective as conventional ventilation.

Despite the lack of complications and the equivalent rates of survival, major airway disruption that is unmanageable by conventional ventilation remains the only current indication for HFJV. There is little justification to use a new device when older, more tested systems work as effectively.

HFJV shows great promise as an ancillary ventilatory technique, but physicians using HFJV should be aware of its experimental nature and of the availability of equivalent modalities of support for most patients requiring mechanical ventilation.

Suggested Reading

Carlon GC, Combs AH. Selection of mechanical ventilatory support based on respiratory pathophysiology. In: Hamilton LH, Neu J, Calkins JM, eds. High frequency jet ventilation. Boca Raton, FL: CRC Press, 1986.

Carlon GC, Combs AH, Groeger JS. Ventilation at supraphysiologic frequencies: theoretical, technical, experimental, and clinical basis. Acute Care 1983; 10(3–4):123–183.

Carlon GC, Howland WS, eds. High frequency ventilation in intensive care and during surgery. New York: Marcel Dekker, 1985.

Carlon GC, Howland WS, Ray C, Miodownik S, Griffin JP, Groeger JS. High frequency jet ventilation: a prospective randomized evaluation. Chest 1983; 84:551–559.

Turnbull AD, Carlon GC, Howland WS, Beattie BJ. High frequency jet ventilation in major airway or pulmonary disruptions. Ann Thor Surg 1981; 32:468–474.

HIGH FREQUENCY VENTILATION: CURRENT USE AND FUTURE PERSPECTIVES

ANIL S. MENON, Ph.D
ANTHONY S. REBUCK, M.B., B.S., M.D.
ARTHUR S. SLUTSKY, M.D.

Conventional mechanical ventilation attempts to reproduce the pattern observed during spontaneous breathing and is therefore characterized by tidal volumes that may exceed the anatomic dead space, cycled at rates of 10 to 20 breaths per minute. Although it is usually effective in achieving adequate gas exchange, the inevitable use of relatively large tidal volumes during conventional ventilation results in an increased risk of barotrauma and hemodynamic compromise. Recent additions to the techniques of respiratory support are those covered under the broad title of high frequency ventilation, in which frequencies of at least four times the normal resting breathing frequency are utilized. In addition, high frequency ventilation uses tidal volumes that are often less than the anatomic dead space. High frequency ventilation techniques can be categorized into three types: (1) high frequency positive-pressure ventilation, (2) high frequency jet ventilation also known as high frequency flow interruption, and (3) high frequency oscillation.

In this chapter we will confine our attention to HFPPV and high frequency oscillation since high frequency jet ventilation (HFJV) is discussed in detail elsewhere in this book (see the chapter on *High Frequency Jet Ventilation*). For each technique we will outline its basic principles, advantages, commercial availability, current clinical use, possible future applications, and present shortcomings.

HIGH FREQUENCY POSITIVE-PRESSURE VENTILATION (HFPPV)

This technique was developed in the late 1960s by Sjöstrand, whose original objective was not the design of a therapeutic modality but rather the design of an experimental tool. During studies of the carotid sinus baroreflex, Sjöstrand and colleagues wished to avoid respiratory synchronous variations in blood pressure that occurred with spontaneous breathing or conventional mechanical ventilation. They devised a method by which ventilation could be achieved using reduced tidal volumes, but with rapid respiratory rates. This technique, called high frequency positive-pressure ventilation (HFPPV), proved adequate in maintaining normoxia and normocapnia in animals and avoided large swings in intratracheal and intrapleural pressures. It also offered promise in reducing the complications of barotrauma and cardiac depression that accompany the use of conventional positive-pressure ventilation.

HFPPV employs stroke volumes usually approaching but greater than the anatomic dead space and frequencies of 1 to 2 Hz (1 Hz = 60 breaths per minute). The equipment includes a time-cycled, pressure-controlled ventilator that utilizes a pneumatic valve (Fig. 1). The valve consists of a small-bore (5 to 10 mm) side-arm tube that is attached to a main tube to form an acute angle. The main tube fits directly onto an endotracheal or tracheostomy tube. Conditioned, compressed gas is supplied intermittently to the side arm of the pneumatic valve, with most of the flow directed into the lung during inspiration. Some gas escapes to the atmosphere, thereby preventing entrainment. Since the main tube of the pneumatic valve is open, this arrangement has proved especially advantageous during bronchoscopic procedures. The inspiratory to expiratory time ratio is somewhat variable but is usually maintained at about 1:4. HFPPV requires a compressed gas source and a circuit in which the compressible volume and tubing compliance are very small. Exhalation is passive and is accomplished by the static recoil of the respiratory system (lungs and chest wall).

An HFPPV system (Bronchovent) was developed and marketed in Sweden by AGA Company and has found extensive clinical use. The ventilator operated at a fixed frequency of about 1 Hz and an inspiratory duration of 22 percent of total cycle time. A further modification, called "system H," incorporated a valve in the expiratory limb of the circuit. The rights for Bronchovent have been recently purchased by Siemen Elma of Sweden, and a new version incorporating adjustable frequencies and inspiration-expiration ratios and humidification is being developed.

HFPPV is now used in intraoperative, postoperative, long-term, and emergency treatments that require a low airway pressure with minimal interference with spontaneous breathing. It has become an established technique during laryngoscopy, bronchoscopy, and microlaryngeal surgery. The technique has also proved safe and satisfactory during esophagoscopy for laser treatment of diverticula. Since the extent of lung

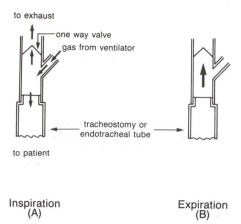

Figure 1 Schematic diagram of the pneumatic valve for HFPPV.

movement during HFPPV is small compared with that observed during conventional mechanical ventilation, HFPPV provides adequate ventilation without interfering with the operative field. Thus HFPPV is used in thoracic surgery for sleeve pneumonectomy, correction of tracheal stenosis, during open heart surgery, and in neonates and infants undergoing plastic surgery for repair of cleft lip or palate.

Conventional ventilators have also been used at high ventilatory frequencies to deliver HFPPV to ventilate neonates or adults with respiratory failure in whom serious complications have occurred. In general, however, it is disappointing to report that oxygenation, ventilation, cardiac performance, and oxygen transport during HFPPV are not significantly different from values observed using conventional ventilation. However, CO_2 elimination comparable to that produced by conventional ventilation is achieved with lower tidal volumes and lower mean airway pressures than with conventional methods. One potential advantage of HFPPV is that the need for sedatives to ensure patient-ventilator cooperation is reduced. Furthermore, the reduction in arterial oxygenation during tracheobronchial suctioning is comparatively less during HFPPV when compared with conventional ventilation.

HFPPV has also been used alone or in conjunction with conventional ventilation in the treatment of unilateral lung damage caused during surgery or by trauma or asymmetric pulmonary disease. Ventilating the injured lung with HFPPV and the normal one with conventional ventilation allows for better overall ventilation and oxygenation.

When should the use of HFPPV be considered as a substitute for conventional ventilation? Certainly when airway disruption has occurred through a bronchopleural fistula, HFPPV seems to be the best method available. The low intra-airway pressures markedly reduce the leaks from the existing bronchopleural fis-

tula. Theoretically, the low intrathoracic pressures make HFPPV attractive for patients who are hemodynamically unstable. The small HFPPV insufflation catheters offer a viable alternative for patients with large malignancies in the glottic area in whom intubation with an armored tube is not always possible or is contraindicated, as in the case of friable hemorrhagic tumors. HFPPV has potential use in neurosurgery, since experimental studies in animals have shown considerably reduced brain movements and decreased intracranial pressures with its use. It also offers promise for use in liver transplantation or resection or for procedures around the diaphragm.

HIGH FREQUENCY OSCILLATION

In 1973, Lunkenheimer and colleagues, while studying cardiac impedance in apneic dogs, fortuitously discovered that normocapnia could be maintained when they oscillated small volumes of air in the animals' airways at rates of 23 to 40 Hz. Subsequently, a large number of investigators have shown that adequate alveolar ventilation is possible with tidal volumes much less than the anatomic dead space. High frequency oscillation systems differ from those employed during HFPPV in that both inhalation and exhalation are active, i.e., by contrast with HFPPV (and HFJV), exhalation does not occur passively due to respiratory system recoil. A high frequency oscillation ventilator can consist of any device that can produce oscillatory flows at the required frequencies and tidal volumes. Systems that have been used include a piston pump, loudspeakers, or a servo-controlled linear magnetic motor, in line with the patient's airway. Since the ventilator does not provide "fresh gas" to the circuit, a bias flow of gas must be used between the ventilator and the patient to provide adequate oxygen and to remove carbon dioxide (Fig. 2).

The bias flow system consists of fresh gas, delivered at a rate of 5 to 60 L per minute across the tubing connecting the oscillator to the patient. Resistance of the line is controlled either by a spring valve or by adjusting the length of the tubing. The effluent gas is drained through a long tube placed in the line

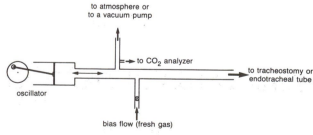

Figure 2 Schematic diagram of high frequency oscillation circuit.

connecting the patient to the oscillator. The drainage tube is sometimes connected to a vacuum source. Both tubes generally have a diameter less than that of the endotracheal tube. Depending on the geometry of the effluent line, bias flow systems have been categorized as either low or high impedance bias flow. The low impedance bias flow system presents a low impedance to the oscillations, is relatively simple to use, and allows for spontaneous ventilation by the patient. However, in this system the fraction of the stroke volume entering the lungs depends on the relative impedances of the circuit and the patient's respiratory system. By contrast, the high impedance circuit prevents loss of oscillatory volume to the bias flow. It is more difficult to use and has been employed largely under experimental conditions in which accurate determination of the tidal volume delivered to the subject is required, since it allows the installation of a flow measurement device (pneumotachygraph) between the patient and the bias flow without adding dead space to the circuit. Efficacy of gas transport can be affected by the bias flow configuration and flow rate. There is evidence that CO_2 elimination increases by placing the bias flow as far into the lung as possible, although this configuration may increase the risk of barotrauma.

Besides using oscillatory frequencies (2 to 30 Hz) that are higher than those used by either HFPPV or high frequency jet ventilation, high frequency oscillation utilizes tidal volumes that are much smaller than the anatomic dead space. The tidal volume delivered depends on the balance between the impedance of the patient's airway and that of the bias flow. Usually inspiration and expiration are of equal duration. Another important difference lies in the airway pressure profiles. In HFPPV and high frequency jet ventilation when the subject exhales passively, the airway pressure is near atmospheric. By contrast, during high frequency oscillation the return stroke of the ventilator may generate large subatmospheric pressures during exhalation. During HFPPV and high frequency jet ventilation, the mean airway pressure is adjusted by expiration retarding valves. For high frequency oscillation any desired tracheal pressure can be attained by adjusting the bias flow.

The use of high frequency oscillators offers another distinct advantage over both HFPPV and high frequency jet ventilation. It is possible to determine the efficacy of ventilation readily, by monitoring the CO_2 concentration in the effluent limb of the bias flow. Unlike high frequency jet ventilation systems in which humidification is difficult, humidification of inspired gas is relatively easy during high frequency oscillation with the low impedance circuit, since only the bias gas flow must pass through the humidifier. Consequently, the same humidification devices used for conventional ventilation can be used.

The current clinical literature contains a number of reports on the uses of HFPPV or high frequency jet ventilation or an assortment of combined modalities. Fewer clinical reports exist for high frequency oscillation, mainly because HFPPV and high frequency jet ventilators are easier to build, especially if the operating frequencies are limited to 1 to 4 Hz. Furthermore, the Food and Drug Administration (FDA) does not require a special investigative license for jet ventilators when they are operated at frequencies less than or equal to 2.5 Hz. Thus, a number of jet ventilators and HFPPV systems are available commercially, but there are few commercially available high frequency oscillators. An investigative license is required prior to clinical application, and hence the clinical data base is smaller than for HFPPV and high frequency jet ventilators. A recent study demonstrated that in infants with respiratory distress syndrome, high frequency oscillation reduced the inspired oxygen requirements from a mean of 0.66 to 0.41. The results from these short-term experiments in premature infants suggested that ventilation with high frequency oscillation gave better oxygenation at lower mean airway pressures than did conventional ventilation. Early publications theorized that the low mean airway pressures would result in reduced barotrauma, although there is little experimental evidence to support this conclusion. There is extensive clinical experience using HFJV in infants with pulmonary interstitial edema. Since high frequency oscillation uses much lower tidal volumes, this condition would appear to provide an ideal situation for such an approach. As in the case of HFPPV and high frequency jet ventilation, high frequency oscillation could find extensive use in the treatment of infants with pulmonary hypoplasia and in microsurgery when a stable operating field is required.

There is substantial evidence from animal studies that the use of large tidal volumes during conventional mechanical ventilation in the treatment of respiratory distress syndrome is associated with the formation of hyaline membrane. Mechanical ventilation in premature animals has been shown to induce epithelial injury, the foundation for protein leak, hyaline membrane formation, and sequestration and activation of granulocytes in the lung, which further enhance lung damage. High frequency oscillation techniques have been shown to reduce or even prevent hyaline membrane formation. However, the success of high frequency oscillation depends on its efficacy in resolving atelectasis by volume recruitment, i.e., the mean airway pressure should always be maintained above the airway opening pressure. The results obtained using high frequency oscillation are no better than those employing conventional mechanical ventilation, when the mean airway pressure is less than the airway opening pressure, but they are much better when ventilation is performed at airway pressures greater than the opening pressure. These encouraging results have formed the basis for the current National Institutes of Health's multi-centered trial on the use of high frequency oscillation in the treatment of infant respiratory distress syndrome.

Paradoxically, the greatest strength of high frequency oscillation, its ability to operate at low mean airway pressures, was perhaps its greatest adversary in terms of its overall success. Earlier investigators tried to maintain as low a lung volume as possible over extended periods of time, resulting in successive alveolar collapse, hypercapnia, and hypoxemia in both premature baboons and human neonates. The use of high frequency oscillation with intermittent sighs greatly improved the results. As an alternative to using a periodic sigh, high frequency oscillations have been imposed on conventional mechanical ventilation. While treating adults with ARDS using conventional mechanical ventilation, it was soon realized that a crucial factor that determined the success of the ventilatory therapy was the end-expiratory pressure. Although the maintenance of open alveoli is important, success depended on the ability to maintain their patency, thereby requiring the institution of high levels of positive end-expiratory pressure (PEEP). However, this inevitably resulted in a further increase in the peak airway pressures, a potent factor in the risk of developing barotrauma. High frequency oscillation can overcome this problem by using the traditional method of PEEP to maintain lung volume above closing volume without the necessity of imposing large excursions in lung volume. This method of instituting high frequency oscillation may result in improved performance and will help to determine whether it is superior to conventional modes of ventilation. The rationale for using the technique of alveolar recruitment is described below.

Maintenance of low lung volumes for extended periods of time results in alveolar collapse and concomitant hypoxemia. Furthermore, the relationship between mean airway pressure and lung volume is not a unique function because of pulmonary hysteresis, which is increased in diseased lungs. During conventional mechanical ventilation, the lung is inflated along the inflation limb, and most of the oxygenation occurs near peak inspiration when most of the alveolar units are open. The lungs then return to their original volume along the deflation limb. The end point depends on the extent of PEEP applied and the time available for expiration. Increasing PEEP can decrease the extent of "decruitment." However, increased peak airway pressure during conventional mechanical ventilation does increase the possibility of lung damage and also results in compromised cardiac performance. High frequency ventilation thus offers a distinctive advantage, since one could apply the PEEP necessary to

keep the alveoli open and yet the peak pressures are relatively low because of the small tidal volumes. It requires an element of skill to establish the minimal level of PEEP necessary to maintain adequate oxygenation by "safely" inflating the lungs to a given level, then allowing them to deflate to the desired end-expiratory position. If the arterial oxygenation falls progressively subsequent to inflation, the level of PEEP is increased. The procedure is repeated until a sustained high level of oxygenation is attained. This technique has proved to be both safe and efficacious in animal models of infant respiratory distress syndrome, although the clinical value of high frequency oscillation using this strategy remains controversial.

One potential advantage of high frequency oscillation compared with conventional mechanical ventilation arises from studies of gas transport mechanisms. At relatively low frequencies, distribution of ventilation is determined by the resistance (R) of the airways and the compliance (C) of the lung parenchyma. By contrast, at relatively high frequencies, the distribution of ventilation becomes less dependent on regional R-C constants but is dependent on regional resistance-inertance time constants of the airways. It has been found that at high frequencies and small tidal volumes (volumes still larger than anatomic dead space), the apices are better ventilated, but as the tidal volumes approach the dead space volume, the base of the lung is ventilated preferentially. It is therefore theoretically possible to direct ventilation to desired regions using high frequency oscillation, by choosing appropriate values of tidal volume and frequency. A clinical example of the use of this mechanism can be found in the treatment of bronchopleural fistula. A bronchopleural fistula can be viewed as a region of high compliance, and hence, during conventional mechanical ventilation the ventilation is directed to the high compliance region and results in a large percentage of ventilation being lost. Using high frequency oscillation, flow could be directed away from the high compliance region, since the airway rather than the parenchymal properties of the lung dominates the distribution of the flow.

SHORTCOMINGS AND COMPLICATIONS OF HIGH FREQUENCY VENTILATION

Although high frequency ventilation has potential beneficial effects, convincing data indicating that it is better than conventional mechanical ventilation in any specific clinical situation do not exist. Based on available information, compared with conventional mechanical ventilation high frequency ventilation has not been proved to offer sufficient benefits to warrant widespread clinical use. Although the reduction in peak airway pressure during high frequency ventilation is likely to reduce the incidence of barotrauma, this speculation remains unsupported by published data. Furthermore, high frequency ventilation has several problems that may be viewed as falling into two categories: (1) technical, and (2) physiologic.

Technical Problems. High frequency ventilation is potentially more dangerous than conventional mechanical ventilation because of the high flow rates and driving pressures used. The catheter through which the HFPPV or high frequency jet ventilation is delivered can kink and become obstructed. Care should be exercised in the clinical use of high frequency oscillation because the relatively high bias flow rates could result in rapid overdistention of the lungs and pneumothorax if the expiratory line becomes blocked. The tendency to use conventional ventilators with high internal and circuit compliances and valve systems not rated for the high frequency operation may result in loss of delivered tidal volume or ventilator failure. Pressure safeguard and alarm systems are generally not as effective as those for conventional mechanical ventilation. Furthermore, because of the high flow rates, adequate humidification can be difficult to attain, especially with the high impedance bias flow circuits. In terms of gas exchange, prediction of the effect of a given set of ventilator settings on gas exchange when compared with conventional mechanical ventilation is difficult; to a large extent, a trial and error approach is required.

Physiologic Problems. High frequency oscillation has been reported to cause dynamic hyperinflation of the lungs because of gas trapping; in such a situation, central airway pressure does not reflect alveolar pressure. One approach to check for this problem is to measure mean airway pressure under static conditions following airway occlusion (i.e., measure the airway pressure after occluding a valve between the airway and the oscillator). A mean airway pressure following occlusion that is significantly greater than the mean airway pressure during high frequency oscillation is indicative of gas trapping, which can lead to hemodynamic compromise. Another potential problem with high frequency oscillation is its effect on lung mucociliary transport. Animal experiments have indicated significant reduction in mucus transport during high frequency oscillation when compared with conventional mechanical ventilation or spontaneous breathing. Clinical experience with several high frequency ventilators indicates that problems with bronchial mucus plugging after long-term ventilator support can occur. This may result from inadequate humidification or disruption of mucociliary transport. Despite these limitations, there are reports in which intermittent high frequency positive-pressure ventilation has been associated with improvement in clinical, radiologic, and pulmonary function of adults with

chronic obstructive lung disease and in children with cystic fibrosis. It has been suggested that the high frequency device shakes free secretions from the mucosa, enabling major airways to be cleared more effectively by an improved cough mechanism or by mechanical means.

The ability to ventilate patients at a lower mean airway pressure during high frequency ventilation was the rationale for suggesting that it would reduce the incidence of barotrauma. However, the mechanisms responsible for barotrauma are incompletely understood. If shear forces rather than distending pressures are the major determinants of barotrauma, then high frequency ventilation could prove more detrimental than conventional mechanical ventilation in this regard. There have been recent reports in which necrotizing tracheobronchitis has been associated with various forms of high frequency ventilation. Animal studies and studies on neonates have shown that all forms of high frequency ventilation produced significant inflammation (erosion, necrosis, and polymorphonuclear leukocyte infiltration) in the trachea in the region of the endotracheal tube tip. The precise factors responsible for this complication are unknown, but they may be related to the ventilatory frequency; of note, necrotizing tracheobronchitis has also been reported during conventional mechanical ventilation.

In summary, although microscopic and ultrastructural examination of the lungs after several hours of high frequency ventilation has shown no evidence of structural damage, the problem of necrotizing tracheobronchitis needs to be addressed. A number of subtle changes induced by high frequency ventilation have been identified in animal models in the vascular response to hypoxia, fluid transport, mucociliary clearance, and the presence of hepatic lesions. Further controlled trials are needed to assess the risk:benefit ratio of high frequency ventilation in normal and diseased lungs.

FUTURE OF HIGH FREQUENCY VENTILATION

The initial optimism that high frequency ventilation might be clinically beneficial and cardiac-sparing has not been substantiated. The future of high frequency ventilation, although uncertain, is not bleak. Currently, research has been directed at addressing the following issues: (1) lung volume recruitment and oxygenation, (2) pattern of lung expansion and lung injury, (3) determination of operating tidal volumes and frequency, and (4) mechanisms of gas transport and distribution of ventilation.

The rationale and methods involved in alveolar recruitment during high frequency oscillation have already been discussed. The choice of ventilator frequency, especially during high frequency oscillation, has been rather arbitrary. Recent studies examining the pressure interrelationships in the lung during high frequency oscillation have suggested that the best frequency to operate at is the resonant frequency of the lung, since at this frequency pressure swings in the airways are at a minimum, resulting in minimum overall pressures and reducing the possibility of airway trauma. However, parenchymal damage is probably reduced by using the smallest tidal volume (i.e., usually using the highest frequency). Furthermore, since the compliance of the lung changes rapidly during recovery, selecting an optimal frequency based on the resonant frequency would require repeated assessments of pulmonary mechanics throughout the treatment and this, at present, is not practical.

Although high frequency ventilation offers potential solutions in the treatment of a number of clinical problems (bronchopleural fistula, pulmonary interstitial edema, and persistent pulmonary hypertension) and has the potential to reduce barotrauma, a number of important physiologic problems such as its effect on mucociliary clearance, lung lymph flow, pulmonary circulation, and tracheal damage remain to be resolved. In the final analysis, the clinical utility of high frequency ventilation will be determined by appropriate clinical trials, such as the current National Institutes of Health-sponsored multicentered trial on its use in infants with infant respiratory distress syndrome. We speculate that high frequency ventilation will prove to be useful in a limited number of clinical conditions but will not supplant conventional mechanical ventilation in the general treatment of respiratory failure.

Suggested Reading

Bryan AC, Froese AB. High frequency ventilation. Am Rev Respir Dis 135(6), Part 1:1363–1374.

Carlon GC, Howland WS. High frequency ventilation in intensive care and during surgery. In: Lung biology in health and disease. Vol. 26. New York: Marcel Dekker, 1985.

Drazen JM, Kamm RD, Slutsky AS. High frequency ventilation. Physiol Rev 1984; 64:505–543.

George RJD, Geddes DM. High frequency ventilation. Br J Hosp Med 1985; 33:344–349.

Kolton M. A review of high frequency oscillation. Can Anesth Soc J. 1984; 31:416–429.

Scheck PA, Sjöstrand UH, Smith RB. Perspectives in high frequency ventilation. Boston: Martinus Nijhoff, 1983.

Slutsky AS. Non-conventional methods of ventilation. Am Rev Respir Dis (In Press).

Smith RB, Sjostrand UH. High frequency ventilation. Int Anesthesiol Clin 1983; 21(3):1–208.

INDEPENDENT LUNG VENTILATION

COLE RAY JR., A.A.S., RRT

ASYMMETRIC LUNG DISEASE

Asymmetric lung disease (ALD) is a term used to describe the condition in which airspace loss and interstitial pathology is concentrated in one or more discrete areas rather than diffusely distributed through the pulmonary parenchyma. The therapeutic implications of this relatively uncommon state are profound, because in this setting such support modalities as high-volume positive pressure ventilation and positive end-expiratory pressure (PEEP) tend to produce a paradoxical deterioration in ventilation-perfusion matching and lung function. This is primarily due to compliance-mediated hyperinflation of the normal lung areas, resulting in redistribution of blood flow to shunt units, hypoxemia, and an increase in physiologic deadspace. The successful management of severe true ALD almost certainly requires endobronchial intubation and selective independent ventilation of each lung as the extreme compliance mismatch renders parallel ventilation ineffective or worse.

Diagnosis and Preendobronchial Intubation Management

Some of the diagnostic signs of this condition are radiographic evidence of asymmetric airway collapse and interstitial edema, intrapulmonary shunting and hypoxemia in the presence of normal to high compliance, and exaggerated gravitationally induced swings in oxygenation. Improvement of oxygenation with positional or gravitational maneuvers most frequently occurs with the nonaffected lung in the dependent position. In the setting of suspected ALD increasingly aggressive evaluations and interventions can and probably should be undertaken prior to the point of endobronchial intubation and institution of independent lung ventilation (ILV) if the patient's pulmonary status continues to worsen. These include (1) therapy for the primary disorder and (2) aggressive attempts to remedy reversible obstruction including high-output aerosol therapy, bronchodilator prescription, directionally guided suctioning, bronchoscopy (possibly with balloon occlusion), and insufflation reexpansion.

Failure of these measures to cause significant improvement may require a trial of standard endotracheal intubation and positive pressure ventilation with high volumes (12 to 15 ml per kilogram) and PEEP. Lack of improvement in oxygenation, particularly if the pulmonary compliance is normal to high or the shunt fraction rises with incremental increases in PEEP, is an indication that ILV may be needed. In this setting regional increases in pulmonary vascular resistance occur as ventilatory volume is distributed to compliant nonaffected lung areas causing hyperinflation and pulmonary capillary compression. Pulmonary blood flow so redirected finds its way to the relatively low-resistance shunt paths in the diseased portions of the lung. This causes hypoxemia as well as significant increase in physiologic deadspace and need for high minute ventilations.

Because high-frequency jet ventilation (HFJV) is a mode of support in which the distribution of gas within the lung is relatively compliance independent, it has been suggested that it might be a viable alternative to endobronchial intubation and ILV. My experience in a limited number of cases indicates that HFJV support through a standard endotracheal tube in patients suspected of having asymmetric lung disease has no advantage over conventional positive pressure ventilation.

Endobronchial Intubation

Endobronchial intubation is a technically demanding procedure, particularly in patients with severely compromised pulmonary function. Whenever possible it should be performed by staff with prior experience in the procedure. Although still not an ideal device, the Bronchocath endobronchial tube (Mallinckrodt Critical Care, Glens Falls, NY) is much better suited to the needs of the patients undergoing prolonged intubation than are the older Carlen, Robert-Shaw or Ravanian endobronchial tubes, which were designed primarily for short-term intraoperative use. Problems frequently encountered with prolonged endobronchial intubation include difficulty in suctioning and airway blockage due to retained secretions, loss of airway patency due to cuff prolapse or abutment of the distal lumen against the airway wall, kinking of the tube at the pharyngeal level, and mucosal erosion due to cuff pressure. These are common problems with a real likelihood of causing morbidity or mortality. Constant monitoring of airway pressures, cuff pressures, secretion volume and consistency, and humidifier function is extremely important.

Postendobronchial Intubation Evaluation

Following placement of the endobronchial tube, evaluation of the patient's individual lung compliance, airway resistance, and the partition of tidal volumes reveals whether the diagnosis of ALD is correct and whether a trial of ILV may be of benefit. Partition of tidal volume is determined by ventilating both lungs with a single ventilator. The circuit on this machine is configured so that the inspiratory line splits at a "Y" into an inspiratory line leading to a "Y" on each limb of the endobronchial tube. From the expiratory limb of the "Y" on each limb of the endobronchial tube, an expiratory line conducts exhaled gas through a standard mushroom exhalation valve to a PEEP valve and exhaled gas spirometer. The exhalation valve drive line from the ventilator is split at a Y-connector and attached to each of the mushroom exhalation valves. With this set-up, the tidal volume delivered by the ventilator is split between the two lungs in proportion to the difference in their impedances. (For our purposes the lung impedance may be considered to be the vector sum of the airway resistance and the compliance.) Compliance may be determined by introducing a volume into each lung in turn via a pulmonary function volume calibration syringe connected to the endobronchial tube and observing the associated back pressure on an attached manometer. A difference between lungs in compliance or tidal volume partition of more than 20 percent is considered indicative of a degree of ALD that may benefit from ILV.

Management of Independent Lung Ventilation

There are three general configurations for independent lung ventilation: one-ventilator ILV, two-ventilator synchronized ILV, and two-ventilator unsynchronized ILV.

Single-Ventilator Method

The single-ventilator method is set up in the same manner as the ventilator described above for the tidal volume partition determination. With this circuit PEEP can be independently applied to each lung but volume, flow, and FiO$_2$ cannot. A modification of this circuit, the installation of variable resistance in the inspiratory limb of the circuit supplying the healthy lung, can provide a measure of control over gas volume delivery to each lung. The variable resistance can be the type of large-bore stopcock used in pulmonary function equipment or found on the port of Douglas bags. Progressively closing the stopcock decreases the gas flow to the good lung, shunting a greater volume to the opposite side. This technique, however, has the drawback that it increases the time constant (ventilator compliance times ventilator flow resistance) to the point that only relative slow respiratory rates can be used to achieve the desired effect. Another problem is that the circuit in practice is bulky, confusing and a hindrance to nursing care. The large number of connections, adapters, pressure sampling ports, and so on make it prone to leaks and, worse, disconnections. For these reasons the single-ventilator setup is used at my institution only for determining the initial tidal volume distribution.

Synchronized Two-Ventilator Method

The synchronized two-ventilator setup has a number of advantages over the single-ventilator method. The first is that volume, flow, FiO$_2$, PEEP, and alarm limits are independently adjustable for each lung. In addition, the system is operationally simple, each lung has its own ventilator, and ventilatory parameters are controlled in the normal manner by using the ventilator's controls. This technique, however, requires that some method or device be available to synchronize the cycling of the two ventilators. To my knowledge, with the exception of the Siemens Servo 900C and 900D, none of the currently available adult ventilators has provision for synchronous cycling with another machine.

At my institution initial synchronized independent lung ventilation was achieved by the use of a digital timer and relay driver attached across the terminals of the manual breath switches of two Puritan Bennett MA1 ventilators. The device was designed so that device or power failure would leave the relays in the normal open position, allowing the ventilators to be cycled manually or operated asynchronously. In addition an audible alarm in the timer was present to alert staff to any fail to cycle condition. Because this device involved no modifications to the ventilator and was designed to avoid negative interactions with the ventilator even in a failure mode, it was a safe and simple solution. Synchronization for the next generation of ventilator, the Bear Medical Systems Bear I, required the creation of a circuit path including a cable to conduct a signal from the inspiration timer card of one ventilator to the manual breath-detect circuit on the second ventilator. The first machine was left in the control mode and the second or slave machine was set in the continuous positive airway pressure (CPAP) mode. The latest generation of ventilators typified by the Puritan Bennett 7200 and the Bear Medical Systems Bear 5 operate under the control of proprietary software and are exceedingly complex and thus cannot be safely user modified or operated outside of their designed operating modes. The current state of federal device regulation, the medicolegal climate, and the device complexity are such that life-support device modification of the current generation of devices is probably best left to the equipment manufacturer.

Unsynchronized Two-Ventilator Method

No long-term unsynchronized ILV has been carried out at my institution. However, during brief periods of asynchronous ILV occasioned by equipment switching or synchronizer cabling problems, no adverse blood gas or hemodynamic changes have been noted. The literature contains reports of successful management of ALD with ILV using two ventilators operating without any attempt at synchronization.

Monitoring

The management of patients undergoing ILV requires frequent monitoring because the time course of response to therapy varies greatly. Postoperative situations in which profound $\dot{V}/\dot{Q}$ mismatch follows sudden resolution of conditions causing vascular compression or sudden release of trapped lung may respond to ILV in a matter of minutes to hours, while the progression of the asymmetric distribution of acute pulmonary failure may be glacial. Frequent checking on the pressure-volume status of each lung is necessary in order to facilitate the adjustments in PEEP and volume to each lung necessary for the normalization of lung volumes. The compliance of each lung can be measured at one point or its pressure-volume loop can be measured by noting the recoil pressure for sequential volume increments and decrements. Another useful measure is to note the partition of tidal volume using a single ventilator setup with the split inspiratory or double expiratory circuit described above. Although it may seem cumbersome to involve three ventilators in the care of one patient, if the machines are available, the tidal volume partition determination is a quick method of evaluating the efficacy of the current independent tidal volume and PEEP settings. ALD is encountered occasionally at any institution doing a significant amount of mechanical ventilatory support. Because the prognosis for these patients is frequently poor when they are ventilated via a standard endotracheal tube, a case can be made for having available the equipment and trained staff to provide ILV when the need arises.

Suggested Reading

Carlon GC, Ray C Jr, Klein R, et al. Criteria for selective positive end-expiratory pressure and independent synchronized ventilation of each lung. Chest 1978; 74:501–507.

Hillman KM, Barber JD. Asynchronous independent lung ventilation. Crit Care Med 1980; 8:390–395.

Kvetan V, Carlon GC, Howland WS. Acute pulmonary failure in asymmetric lung disease. Crit Care Med 1982; 10:114–117.

DIAPHRAGM PACING

JACOB LOKE, M.D.

Diaphragm pacing by electrical stimulation of the phrenic nerve was first used in 1966 by Judson and Glenn to treat a patient with chronic ventilatory insufficiency. This form of artificial respiration allows patients to be free from dependence on mechanical ventilation, giving them greater mobility and independence. It has been successfully applied to many patients with intact phrenic nerves, lung, and diaphragm for the treatment of alveolar hypoventilation and respiratory failure. However, diaphragm pacing is not applicable in all forms of ventilatory insufficiency, and correct selection of patients for diaphragm pacing, together with an experienced surgical team, is a prerequisite for a successful outcome of this mode of therapy. Much of the pioneering work of diaphragm pacing and its subsequent refinement has to be credited to Dr. Glenn and his colleagues.

PHYSIOLOGY

The respiratory system consists of a gas-exchange organ, the lungs, and a pump that is controlled by the respiratory center that ventilates the respiratory system (which includes the thoracic cage and respiratory muscles with innervating nerves to the respiratory control centers). Respiratory insufficiency without parenchymal lung disease can occur from dysfunction of one or more components of the ventilatory pump leading to alveolar hypoventilation, hypoxemia, and hypercapnia. Abnormalities in the respiratory center, with or without central nervous system involvement, can cause alveolar hypoventilation. The cause of central alveolar hypoventilation is unknown and some cases are congenital in nature. Also, central alveolar hypoventilation may be present as a result of central nervous system involvement, of which the leading cause is cerebrovascular disease; other causes include encephalitis, medullary tumor and cyst, Shy-Drager syndrome, and Kleine-Levin syndrome. The hallmark of central alveolar hypoventilation is hypercapnia associated with hypoxemia and a normal alveolar-arterial oxygen difference. The alveolar hypoventilation is aggravated by sleep or narcotic and/ or sedative drugs. The consequences of the alveolar hypoventilation and hypoxemia are pulmonary hypertension and cor pulmonale. Ventilatory control studies during carbon dioxide inhalation and hypoxic stimulation show diminished to absent ventilatory responses in these patients. Voluntary hyperventilation leads to improvement in arterial oxygenation and a decrease in the carbon dioxide tension. Because the lungs and the components of the ventilatory pump are normal except for the dysfunction of the respiratory control centers that causes the alveolar hyperventilation, pacing of the diaphragm improves ventilation and arterial oxygenation.

Interruption of the innervating phrenic nerves to the diaphragm, which may be caused by organic lesions of the cervical cord or trauma, may be associated with complete paralysis of the diaphragm. The diaphragm is the principal muscle of respiration, and complete paralysis of both diaphragms leads to respiratory insufficiency, requiring ventilatory support with mechanical ventilation. Trauma to the cervical cord above the third cervical level (C3) results in respiratory paralysis, quadriplegia, and ventilator dependence. Because of the interruption of upper motor neurons of the phrenic nerve, respiratory paralysis and insufficiency are present. However, the lower motor neurons of both phrenic nerves are intact, so that by bypassing the interruption and electrically stimulating the phrenic nerve at the neck or upper thoracic area, adequate ventilation is restored.

Finally, the ventilatory pump can fail owing to mechanical defects in the thoracic cage (e.g., kyphoscoliosis) or inspiratory muscle fatigue in which the respiratory muscles are not functioning as effective force generators. Respiratory insufficiency due to abnormalities in thoracic cage or respiratory muscle function is not amenable to diaphragm pacing.

The intact phrenic nerve can be stimulated by placement of a monopolar electrode through a surgical incision in the cervical region of the neck or upper thorax. Earlier, the electrode was implanted in the cervical neck. However, in recent years, Dr. Glenn has performed a thoracotomy (second interspace anteriorly), and implanted the electrode in the upper thoracic region. The latter technique provides more effective diaphragm pacing, because it allows stimulation of the branches of the fifth cervical accessory nerve and below the segments of the cervical cord, which would be missed with an electrode in the cervical location. Pacing of the diaphragm can be performed unilaterally or bilaterally. In the early 1970s, diaphragm pacing for patients with central alveolar hypoventilation involved the near maximal stimulation of alternating hemidiaphragms for 12-hour periods, with equal periods of rest for each hemidiaphragm. This was needed to avoid diaphragm fatigue. For unilateral diaphragm pacing, the muscles were stimulated at higher frequencies, often leading to myopathic changes and diaphragmatic fatigue. Thus, diaphragm pacing was limited to a 12-hour period. Recently, continuous bilateral diaphragm pacing has produced effective ventilation similar to intermittent unilateral diaphragm pacing. In contrast to the high frequency used for stimulating the phrenic nerve in unilateral diaphragm pacing, low-frequency stimulation was used for bilateral diaphragm pacing, and with this mode of stimulation, histochemical studies of the muscle fibers showed increased oxidative metabolism without evidence of histologic or ultrastructural myopathic changes. Bilateral diaphragm pacing is definitely a more physiologic form of ventilation that more closely resembles the spontaneous respirations seen in normal individuals. In addition, both diaphragms can be paced continuously without evidence of diaphragm fatigue. A period of conditioning of the diaphragm is required for bilateral diaphragm pacing in patients with quadriplegia. During this phase, the time period for stimulating both hemidiaphragms is increased progressively over a several-month period to full-time ventilatory support. A progressive decrease in frequencies of phrenic stimulation is also performed. Periods of diaphragm rest without pacing are provided with mechanical ventilation. During bilateral diaphragm pacing, the tidal volume, minute ventilation, arterial blood gases, and transdiaphragmatic pressure are monitored.

SELECTION OF PATIENTS

The ideal patients for diaphragm pacing are those individuals with *chronic* ventilatory insufficiency who have no impairment of the phrenic nerves, lungs, or diaphragm. The ideal patient may have idiopathic central alveolar hypoventilation (Ondine's curse) or alveolar hypoventilation as a result of organic lesions of the brain stem or cervical cord. These patients may present with polycythemia, hypercapnia, hypoxia, somnolence, cor pulmonale, and congestive heart failure, or they may be ventilator dependent and unable to be discontinued or weaned from mechanical ventilation. Ventilatory control and sleep studies, together with tests of voluntary hyperventilation while monitoring arterial oxygenation, and a clinical history can identify the group of patients with idiopathic central alveolar hypoventilation. Patients with neck trauma and respiratory paralysis associated with quadriplegia usually have lesions of the cervical spinal cord involving the C1-C2 segments, although respiratory insufficiency can also occur with lesions involving the C3-C5 segments. There is edema and hemorrhage

around the cervical cord after trauma, and dysfunction of motor neurons to the phrenic nerve may be reversible with time. Those patients who are healthy before their spinal cord injury should not be referred for diaphragm pacing until there is no further improvement in the neuromuscular deficit (which can take 3 to 6 months). In patients with laboratory studies of alveolar hypoventilation, it is important to exclude systemic diseases, progressive neurologic or neuromuscular disorders, and other conditions that are potentially reversible with medical therapy. Phrenic nerve stimulation is ineffective in patients with myopathy associated with dermatomyositis and polymyositis, scleroderma, or systemic lupus erythematosus that affects diaphragmatic function. Hyperthyroidism and myxedema can produce respiratory muscle weakness. Neuromuscular diseases, including amyotrophic lateral sclerosis, myasthenia gravis, muscular dystrophies, and acid maltase deficiency have been reported to cause diaphragm weakness or paralysis. Cold cardioplegia during cardiac surgery can cause prolonged bilateral diaphragm paralysis that is potentially reversible.

In patients with severe parenchymal lung disease due to obstructive or restrictive ventilatory factors, there are abnormalities in the lung itself in addition to ventilatory pump failure. Periods of rest for the respiratory muscles are the goal of therapy for these patients in order to correct their short-term hypoventilation or respiratory failure by mechanical ventilation. When there is respiratory muscle fatigue or significant distortion of the chest cage owing to hyperinflation, pacing of the diaphragm is not effective. Furthermore, when the diaphragm is flattened (as in patients with emphysema), an effective contraction of the diaphragm is not produced with diaphragm pacing. Therefore, diaphragm pacing in patients with severe parenchymal lung disease is not indicated. However, in selected cases of chronic obstructive pulmonary disease, patients with severe hypoxia and hypercapnia, but with a normal dome-shaped configuration of the diaphragm and relatively mild impairment of respiratory muscle function, may be candidates for diaphragm pacing. In such patients, diaphragm pacing may be useful to permit administration of low-flow oxygen therapy without suppressing ventilation, a form of "pacing protected oxygenation."

DIAGNOSTIC EVALUATION OF PATIENTS

The clinical assessment in patients suspected to have alveolar hypoventilation should include clinical and laboratory examinations that exclude systemic metabolic disease, thyroid disorders, and neuromuscular disease. Pulmonary function tests are performed to exclude obstructive or restrictive pulmonary disease and any evidence of upper airway obstruction. Arterial blood gases or ear oximetry readings of oxygen saturation can be measured before and after voluntary hyperventilation to document alveolar hypoventilation, hypercapnia, hypoxia and the improvement in arterial oxygenation after hyperventilation. Hypercapnia and hypoxia may be present only during sleep study monitoring. The ability to decrease the carbon dioxide tension to normal with voluntary hyperventilation does not rule out the possibility of diaphragmatic weakness or paralysis. Therefore, more specific tests of diaphragm function, such as the measurement of transdiaphragmatic pressure, can be performed to exclude primary diseases of the diaphragm. Also, fluoroscopy of the diaphragm in the supine position is done to measure the descent of the diaphragm with maximal inspiration. The normal descent of the diaphragm is 5 to 10 cm with maximal inspiration. Bilateral elevations of both hemidiaphragms may indicate diaphragmatic paralysis on chest roentgenogram associated with respiratory insufficiency. Unilateral paralysis of one hemidiaphragm on chest roentgenogram is seldom associated with respiratory insufficiency in the presence of a normal lung.

The evaluation of the respiratory center requires ventilatory control studies using hypercapnic hyperoxia and normocapnic hypoxia inhalation challenges. In patients with central alveolar hypoventilation, diminished or absent ventilatory responses are noted to carbon dioxide and hypoxic studies. Sleep studies are required to evaluate patients for sleep apnea, evidence of upper airway obstruction in the form of obstructive apnea (be it central or peripheral in origin—the latter may require a tracheostomy), and oxygen desaturation, in addition to the breathing pattern during sleep. Exercise testing should be performed in patients with central alveolar hypoventilation to evaluate their ventilation and oxygenation during exercise, because their spontaneous ventilation during exercise may not be able to meet their metabolic oxygen demands.

Finally, in order to be able to perform diaphragm pacing, the phrenic nerve should be intact. The viability of the phrenic nerve can be tested by percutaneous stimulation in the neck, by transvenous stimulation in the thorax, or by direct stimulation at operation. Phrenic nerve conduction studies can also be used.

MANAGEMENT

Most of the patients who require diaphragm pacing have a tracheostomy performed and subsequently replaced with a tracheal button. Some patients with combined obstructive and central apnea experience worsening of their obstructive apnea with diaphragm pacing. Diaphragm pacing exaggerates upper airway obstruction secondary to facial and palatal deformities, macroglossia, or excessive obesity. A permanent tracheostomy is needed in these patients.

In order to have a successful outcome from diaphragm pacing, meticulous follow-up of these patients is needed by an experienced surgical and medical team, with full support by the family of the patient. The phrenic pacemaker should be checked periodically, and adequate ventilatory support with conventional mechanical ventilator should be available in the event of pacemaker failure.

Suggested Reading

Bradley TD, Day A, Hyland RH, Webster P, Rutherford R, McNicholas W, Phillipson EA. Chronic ventilatory failure caused by abnormal respiratory pattern generation during sleep. Am Rev Respir Dis 1984; 130:678–680.

Cohen CA, Zagelbaum G, Gross D, Roussos C, Macklem PT. Clinical manifestations of inspiratory muscle fatigue. Am J Med 1982; 73:308–316.

Glenn WWL, Gee JBL, Schachter EN. Diaphragm pacing. Application to a patient with chronic obstructive pulmonary disease. J Thorac Cardiovasc Surg 1978; 75:273–281.

Glenn WWL, Haak B, Sasaki C, Kirchner J. Characteristics and surgical management of respiratory complications accompanying pathologic lesions of the brain stem. Ann Surg 1980; 191:655–663.

Glenn WWL, Hogan JF, Loke JSO, Ciesielski TE, Phelps ML, Rowedder R. Ventilatory support by pacing of the conditioned diaphragm in quadriplegia. N Engl J Med 1984; 310:1150–1155.

Glenn WWL, Sairenji H. Diaphragm pacing in the treatment of chronic ventilatory insufficiency. In: Roussos C, Macklem PT, eds. The thorax, part B. Vol 29. New York: Marcel Dekker, 1985; 1407.

Laporta D, Grassino A. Assessment of transdiaphragmatic pressure in humans. J Appl Physiol 1985; 58:1469–1476.

Milic-Emili J. Recent advances in clinical assessment of control of breathing. Lung 1982; 160:1–17.

Roussos C, Macklem PT. The respiratory muscles. N Engl J Med 1982; 307:786–797.

Shaw RK, Glenn WWL, Hogan JF, Phelps ML. Electrophysiological evaluation of phrenic nerve function in candidates for diaphragm pacing. J Neurosurg 1980; 53:345–354.

INVASIVE MONITORING TECHNIQUES IN THE VENTILATED PATIENT

HERBERT P. WIEDEMANN, M.D.

This chapter focuses on two frequently utilized invasive monitoring techniques in the patient receiving mechanical ventilation: (1) peripheral artery cannulation, and (2) pulmonary artery catheterization. In each case, the goal is to provide practical advice to enable the skillful and timely application of these monitoring devices, avoidance of complications, and accurate physiologic interpretation of the resulting data.

PERIPHERAL ARTERY CATHETERIZATION

Cannulation of a peripheral artery is commonly performed in the intensive care unit and operating room, allowing (1) continuous monitoring and graphic display of the systemic arterial blood pressure, and (2) repeated analysis of the arterial blood gases.

Indications

Peripheral artery catheterization is warranted in all patients with hemodynamic instability. Not only is continuous monitoring of the arterial blood pressure essential in such patients, but frequent analysis of the arterial blood gases is also necessary.

In the hemodynamically stable patient receiving mechanical ventilation, the need for arterial cannulation must be more carefully considered. In such patients, the use of noninvasive monitoring techniques (such as transcutaneous monitoring of P_{O_2} and P_{CO_2} or oximeter monitoring of oxygen saturation) may suffice. These techniques can be supplemented by occasional "single stick" direct samples of arterial blood.

Methods of Insertion

The most common sites of insertion of a peripheral artery catheter are the radial, brachial, femoral, and dorsalis pedis arteries. The radial artery usually is chosen because of its accessibility and generally good collateral circulation via the ulnar artery. Prior to insertion, the status of this collateral circulation should be assessed with an Allen's test. In this test, both the ulnar and radial arteries are occluded by pressure at the wrist; after the hand becomes pale and cool, releasing only the ulnar circulation should rapidly restore adequate circulation. Preferably, palmar blush caused by filling via the ulnar artery should appear within 5 seconds. Longer refill times are associated with an increased incidence of ischemic complications.

Catheterization of a peripheral artery may be achieved via surgical cutdown or percutaneous insertion. Percutaneous insertion is generally performed by one of two techniques. In the transfixation technique, the entire catheter is advanced into the lumen of the artery and the posterior wall is then penetrated. The inner needle is then withdrawn and the outer plastic cannula is carefully and slowly withdrawn until blood flows freely from the end. The cannula can then be advanced farther up into the arterial lumen. Direct insertion is also possible, but the tip must be positioned so that the cannula is entirely within the arterial lumen before it is advanced over the needle. Either technique is acceptable, and there is no proven difference in the incidence of complications. Cannulation of a peripheral artery may be performed with an 18- or 20-gauge catheter.

Complications

The major complications of peripheral artery catheterization are infection and distal ischemia. Ischemia may be secondary to either thrombosis (local occlusion) or distal embolization.

Risk factors favoring the development of infection include (1) insertion by surgical cutdown rather than percutaneously, (2) duration of cannulation exceeding 4 days, and (3) inflammation of the catheterization site. Infection may often originate in the transducer or fluid delivery apparatus. This problem is reduced by the use of normal saline (rather than pathogen-supporting dextrose solution) and of disposable transducer domes. With careful adherence to the precautions outlined in Table 1, catheter-related septicemia can be reduced to less than 1 percent.

Clinically significant thrombosis or embolization is extremely rare. Necrosis of a finger or toe occurs in less than 0.2 percent of catheterizations. Clinical risk factors for acute distal ischemia include systemic hypotension, severe peripheral vascular disease, and the use of vasopressor drugs. Although clinically recognized ischemia is rare, angiographic studies have documented that reversible subclinical arterial occlusion or reduced flow is common. About one-quarter

TABLE 1   Recommendations for Inserting and Maintaining Systemic Artery Lines

Use sterile insertion technique (antiseptic preparation, gloves, drapes).
Perform Allen's test prior to radial artery cannulation. Ulnar refill time should
    be less than 5 seconds to minimize risk of ischemic complications.
Percutaneous insertion is preferred over surgical cutdown.
Use a 20-gauge catheter if wrist circumference is small.
The transducer should have a disposable dome.
Use continuous flush system with a nondextrose solution (e.g., normal saline)
    containing heparin.
Assess frequently
        Catheter site for evidence of inflammation,
        Distal extremity for evidence of ischemia.
Limit cannulation to 4–5 days at one site.
Remove catheter for
        Distal ischemia,
        Local infection,
        Persistently damped pressure tracing,
        Difficulty with blood withdrawal.

of arteries remain occluded 1 week following catheter removal. Risk factors for such occlusion include larger catheter size (18 gauge is worse than 20 gauge), smaller wrist size (as found in women and children), repeated attempts before successful cannulation, and duration of cannulation (risk increases after 3 to 4 days).

Once a catheter is in place, distal perfusion should be assessed frequently by noting skin color and temperature distal to the catheter. Catheters should be flushed with a continuous low flow (approximately 3 ml per hour) of normal saline solution containing heparin. This does not interfere with continuous pressure monitoring but reduces the incidence of thrombus formation on the catheter tip.

The overall safety of peripheral artery cannulation has been well established in several large studies. The incidence of complications can be maintained at a low rate by observing the few simple precautions listed in Table 1.

Future Directions

Arterial catheters with special probes capable of continuous on-line monitoring of arterial Po_2, Pco_2, and pH are becoming available commercially. With the use of such catheters, arterial blood gases can be monitored in a manner analogous to arterial blood pressure (e.g., continuous monitoring with preset alarm values). Since experience with this technology in routine clinical care is limited, it is too early to reach conclusions regarding risks, benefits, or ultimate clinical utility. However, the potential usefulness of this technology in monitoring of critically ill patients with cardiopulmonary instability is readily apparent.

PULMONARY ARTERY CATHETERIZATION

Bedside catheterization of the pulmonary artery became feasible with the introduction of the balloon-tipped catheter by Swan and colleagues in 1970. The inflatable balloon at the tip was an important adaptation that allowed the catheter to be directed by blood flow. Thus, fluoroscopy usually is not necessary for a proper placement, although patients with markedly reduced cardiac output or significant tricuspid regurgitation may still present difficulties. The so-called Swan-Ganz catheter is now utilized so frequently that there is concern about possible overuse. Although the pulmonary artery catheter often provides a more accurate hemodynamic evaluation than clinical assessment alone, it is important to distinguish the "need to know" from the "want to know." The pulmonary artery catheter should be reserved for instances when its use is likely to enhance patient management rather than used simply to provide a large collection of data. Appropriate utilization is impossible without an understanding of the physiologic information that can be obtained from the pulmonary artery catheter as well as an appreciation of the possible risks and pitfalls in the acquisition and interpretation of such data.

Indications

The pulmonary artery catheter provides important physiologic information regarding the assessment of intravascular volume status and cardiac performance. However, the wide potential of the Swan-Ganz catheter should not preclude a careful clinical and noninvasive (e.g., chest roentgenogram) assessment. In many patients, initial decisions and therapy can be based on such an assessment. Nevertheless, the pulmonary artery catheter is helpful and necessary in a wide variety of serious illnesses, including myocardial infarction complicated by shock or pulmonary edema, sepsis, and the adult respiratory distress syndrome (ARDS). In particular, patients receiving positive end-expiratory pressure (PEEP) at levels greater than 10 cm H_2O should be monitored with a pulmonary artery catheter. This is because higher levels of PEEP are often associated with a depression of cardiac output and oxygen transport.

Methods of Insertion

The pulmonary artery catheter can be inserted percutaneously through the subclavian, internal jugular, external jugular, femoral, or antecubital vein; cutdown may be necessary with the antecubital route. The physician's prior training and experience usually dictate the access route, but clinical considerations may favor a certain site. For instance, severe thrombocytopenia would be a relative contraindication to the subclavian approach, since it would be difficult or impossible to control bleeding complications. In such a case, the antecubital route would be favored. However, antecubital access is associated with difficulties, including phlebitis; also, movement of the arm may cause migration of catheter tip position. Pneumothorax is more commonly encountered with the subclavian than with the internal jugular route. In general, the internal jugular access seems to provide an appropriate balance between ease of catheterization and an acceptably low incidence of complications.

After achieving venous access, the catheter is advanced with continuous pressure monitoring from the distal tip and with continuous ECG monitoring of the cardiac rhythm. When the catheter tip reaches a central intrathoracic vein, a sudden increase in the respiratory fluctuation of the recorded pressures occurs. At this time, the balloon is inflated to the full recommended volume (1.5 ml for the typical No. 7 French catheter) for subsequent flow-directed passage through the right atrium and subsequently to the pulmonary artery. It is important to inflate the balloon fully to prevent the catheter tip from protruding. A protruding tip may cause endovascular damage and enhance the risk of ectopy during passage through the right ventricle. As the catheter is advanced from a central vein, the first waveform is the right atrial tracing, followed by the right ventricular, pulmonary artery, and pulmonary artery wedge tracings, in sequence.

The wedge tracing occurs when the balloon totally occludes the distal pulmonary artery segment; with absent flow, pressures rapidly equilibrate, and the pressure tracing from the distal orifice of the catheter now reflects left atrial pressure. Criteria that can be used to verify a true wedge position are listed in Table 2. Distal migration of the catheter tip frequently occurs after initial placement. Such peripheral migration is attributable in part to warming of the catheter, making it more compliant. This allows the loop taken by the catheter, especially through the right ventricle, to shorten. It is important to always note what balloon inflation volume is required to obtain a wedge pressure and to consider pulling back the catheter if less than 1.0 to 1.3 ml produces a wedge tracing. If less than this volume produces a wedge reading, the catheter tip is located too far distally in a small pulmonary artery. A proper proximal wedge position is important to reduce complications (such as pulmonary infarction) and ensure accuracy of thermodilution cardiac output and mixed venous oxygen saturation determinations.

Complications

The adverse effects of pulmonary artery catheterization are now well understood from over a decade of experience (Table 3).

Ventricular arrhythmias occur frequently during insertion of the catheter, but are usually self-limited. In critically ill patients, the incidence of ventricular tachycardia (three or more consecutive premature ventricular contractions) is reported to be 20 to 50 percent. However, sustained ventricular tachycardia requiring therapy occurs in only 1 to 2 percent of such patients. Risk factors for ventricular tachycardia include hypocalcemia, myocardial infarction or ischemia, hypotension, and hypokalemia. However, the

TABLE 2   Criteria for True Wedge Position

A waveform characteristic of left atrial pressure (e.g., including "a" and "v" waves) should be seen. A "damped" waveform, straight line, or waveform deflections solely related to ventilatory pressures are not acceptable. The "wedge" waveform should disappear promptly with balloon deflation (giving a pulmonary artery tracing) and return rapidly after balloon reinflation.

The mean pulmonary artery wedge pressure should be lower than or equal to the pulmonary artery diastolic pressure and lower than the mean pulmonary artery pressure. (In severe mitral regurgitation, the wedge pressure may transiently exceed the pulmonary artery diastolic pressure.)

Catheter obstruction is ruled out by the presence of a free-falling column of fluid or continuous flush.

Blood gas analysis of samples withdrawn from the distal tip with the balloon inflated should reflect alveolar capillary gas pressures rather than mixed venous gas pressures.

TABLE 3 Complications of Right-Sided Heart Catheterization

Complications at insertion site
  Pneumothorax
  Arterial puncture
  Venous thrombosis or phlebitis
  Air embolism
Arrhythmias
  Transient premature ventricular contractions
  Sustained ventricular tachycardia
  Ventricular fibrillation
  Atrial fibrillation
  Atrial flutter
Right bundle branch block
Pulmonary infarction
Pulmonary artery rupture
Catheter knotting
Catheter-related infections (e.g., endocarditis)
Endocardial damage
  Valve cusps
  Chordae tendineae
  Papillary muscles

two most significant risk factors are hypoxemia (Po_2 less than 60 mm Hg) and acidosis (pH less than 7.0). In such high-risk patients, the use of prophylactic lidocaine during catheter insertion should be considered.

During the initial years of Swan-Ganz catheter use, pulmonary infarction was one of the most common serious complications. The incidence of pulmonary infarction was found to be higher than 7 percent in the mid-1970s. However, more recent experience suggests that the incidence of pulmonary infarction is now at most 1 percent. The difference may be the result of better understanding of techniques that minimize this complication. For instance, the risk of a thrombus developing on the catheter tip is now reduced by the use of continuous flush with heparin solutions. Equally important is the avoidance of persistent wedging of the catheter tip. Distal migration of the catheter can be prevented by maintaining it in a position in which nearly the full recommended balloon inflation volume is required to produce a wedge tracing. Furthermore, the balloon should never be inflated for longer than is necessary to obtain a wedge pressure reading (15 to 20 seconds).

The incidence of pulmonary artery rupture is about 0.2 percent. This is a serious complication with an approximate 50 percent mortality rate. The major risk factor for pulmonary artery rupture is pulmonary artery hypertension. Proper technique can minimize the risk of this serious complication. The balloon should always be inflated slowly and with continuous pressure monitoring; inflation should cease as soon as a wedge tracing is obtained. Hand flushing of the catheter while it is in a wedge position should be avoided.

Septicemia related to the catheter (same pathogen growing from the blood and the catheter tip) complicates the use of the Swan-Ganz catheter in up to 2 percent of cases. Catheter-related infections are more common if the line is left in place for more than 3 to 4 days or if a known focus of infection existed prior to catheter insertion. The incidence of infection can be reduced by careful adherence to sterile technique during initial placement and subsequent repositioning of the catheter. Sheath systems are now available that simplify the task of maintaining a sterile portion of catheter for use in the event that catheter advancement should prove necessary later.

Physiologic Information Derived from the Right-Sided Heart Catheter

Pulmonary artery catheterization enables the direct measurement of three important physiologic variables (Table 4): cardiac output, mixed venous oxygenation, and intravascular pressures within the right side of the heart and pulmonary circulation. From these primary measurements, several important calculations can be performed to define further the cardiopulmonary status of the patient. These calculations are listed in Table 5, but a full discussion of such derived variables is beyond the scope of this chapter.

Cardiac Output

The thermodilution technique for measurement of cardiac output involves the bolus injection of a cold indicator solution of known volume (10 ml) into the proximal port of the right-sided heart catheter. The indicator solution exits the catheter in the right atrium; the thermistor bead located near the distal tip of the catheter detects the subsequent change in temperature that occurs in the pulmonary artery. A bedside microprocessor unit calculates and displays the numeric cardiac output. The procedure is safe and can be performed repeatedly.

The principle on which the thermodilution technique is based assumes a constant blood flow during the time the indicator solution travels the 10 cm from the right atrium to the thermistor. Obviously, the method is therefore inaccurate in the presence of intracardiac shunts or severe tricuspid valve incompet-

TABLE 4 Directly Measured Physiologic Information Obtained with Balloon Flotation Right-Sided Heart Catheterization

Cardiac output
Mixed venous oxygenation
Intravascular pressures
  Right atrial pressure
  Right ventricular pressure
  Pulmonary artery pressure
  Pulmonary artery "wedge" pressure

TABLE 5 Derived Calculations

Cardiac Index (L/min/m²)
$$CI = \frac{CO}{BSA}$$
Normal Range: 2.4–4.4

Systemic Vascular Resistance (dyne · sec · cm⁻⁵)
$$SVR = \frac{MAP - CVP}{CO} \times 79.9$$
Normal Range: 900–1,400

Pulmonary Vascular Resistance (dyne · sec · cm⁻⁵)
$$PVR = \frac{MPAP - PAOP}{CO} \times 79.9$$
Normal Range: 150–250

Stroke Volume (ml)
$$SV = \frac{CO}{HR}$$

Stroke Volume Index (ml/min/m²)
$$SVI = \frac{SV}{BSA} = \frac{CI}{HR}$$
Normal Range: 30–65

Left Ventricular Stroke Work (g · meters/m²)
$$LVSW = SVI \times (MAP - PAOP) \times 0.0136$$
Normal Range: 43–61

Right Ventricular Stroke Work (g · meters/m²)
$$RVSW = SVI \times (MPAP - CVP) \times 0.0136$$
Normal Range: 7–12

Oxygen Content (ml/dl blood)
$$CaO_2 = Hgb \times Arterial\ O_2\ Saturation \times 1.36 + (Po_2 \times 0.003)$$
Normal Range: ~19.5

Arteriovenous Oxygen Content Difference (ml/dl)
$$avDO_2 = CaO_2 - CvO_2$$
Normal Range: 3–5

Oxygen Delivery (ml/min)
$$O_2\ Delivery = CO \times CaO_2 \times 10$$
Normal Range: 800–1,200

Oxygen Consumption (ml/min)
$$VO_2 = CO \times (CaO_2 - CvO_2) \times 10$$
Normal Range: 180–280

Pulmonary Shunt (venoarterial admixture) (%)
$$\frac{Qs}{Qt} = \frac{CcO_2 - CaO_2}{CcO_2 - CvO_2}$$
Normal Range: <3–5%

BSA = body surface area; CaO_2 = arterial oxygen content; CcO_2 = Pulmonary capillary oxygen content (assume that capillary Po_2 is equal to alveolar Po_2); CI = cardiac index; CO = cardiac output; CvO_2 = mixed venous oxygen content; CVP = central venous pressure; Hgb = hemoglobin concentration; HR = heart rate; LVSW = left ventricular stroke work; MAP = mean arterial pressure; MPAP = mean pulmonary artery pressure; PAOP = pulmonary artery occlusion pressure (pulmonary artery wedge pressure); PVR = pulmonary vascular resistance; Qs/Qt = pulmonary shunt; RVSW = right ventricular stroke work; SV = stroke volume; SVI = stroke volume index; SVR = systemic vascular resistance.
Modified from Sprung CL, Rackow EC, Civetta JM. Direct measurements and derived calculations using the pulmonary artery catheter. In: Sprung CL, ed. The pulmonary artery catheter: methodology and clinical applications. Baltimore: University Park Press, 1983:105.

ence. However, the normal pulsatile nature of blood flow and respiratory variations in intrathoracic pressure also affect thermodilution measurements and explain why single measurements often exhibit poor reproducibility, especially during positive pressure ventilation and high levels of PEEP. Most of the variability can be overcome by averaging three separate measurements performed about a minute apart and timed to a particular phase of respiration (e.g., end expiration). When performed in this manner, the thermodilution determination of cardiac output has acceptable accuracy and reproducibility and correlates well with the Fick or dye dilution methods.

Controversy persists regarding the use of iced versus room temperature indicator solution. Ice temperature solution has the theoretic advantage of more contrast with body temperature (greater signal-to-noise ratio) but carries some practical disadvantages (e.g., maintaining sterility of ice-water emerged syringes). I feel that room temperature indicator solution is adequate for routine use, since studies show there is no significant loss of accuracy. However, for hypothermic patients (core temperature 10 to 20° F below normal), the use of ice temperature indicator solutions is mandatory.

Automated injection systems offer no significant advantage over manual injection by a well-trained operator.

Mixed Venous Oxygenation

Mixed venous blood is sampled by withdrawal of blood from the distal orifice of the pulmonary artery catheter with the balloon deflated. (The initial 2.5 ml, representing the dead-space volume of the No. 7 French catheter, should be discarded.) In patients receiving very high inspired oxygen fractions and mechanical ventilation, a fast rate of blood withdrawal may cause contamination of the specimen with oxygenated pulmonary capillary blood and lead to a false mixed venous sample with a measured Po_2 higher than that of true mixed venous blood. This problem is avoided by using a slow rate of blood withdrawal (<3 ml per minute).

Although severe mitral regurgitation can cause unreliable sampling because of retrograde pulmonary capillary flow, mild to moderate mitral insufficiency is probably not associated with significant errors. Left-to-right intracardiac shunts cause inaccurate mixed venous PO_2 and oxygen saturation determinations. This principle may be helpful in diagnosing atrial or ventricular septal defects (such as may occur during myocardial infarction); during passage of the catheter, blood samples may show an abnormal "step-up" in oxygen saturation as the catheter is passed through the right side of the heart.

The normal mixed venous oxygen tension is 36 to 42 mm Hg and the normal mixed venous oxygen saturation is about 75 percent. Mixed venous oxygenation is used to assess the adequacy of oxygen delivery to the tissues relative to the metabolic demand (oxygen consumption). In normal individuals and many patients with isolated cardiac dysfunction, oxygen consumption remains relatively unaffected by changes in oxygen delivery (until critically low values are reached). Thus, a decline in oxygen transport (cardiac output × oxygen content) will manifest as a drop in the mixed venous oxygenation.

However, such an interpretation often cannot be made in sepsis, since peripheral shunting of oxygenated blood past tissue beds may lead to maintenance of a high mixed venous oxygen level despite tissue oxygen deprivation indicated by elevated blood lactate levels. Furthermore, recent studies suggest an abnormal "supply dependency" of oxygen consumption in many patients with ARDS. In such patients, oxygen consumption appears to vary with the oxygen delivery, even at normal or high cardiac outputs. The reason for this phenomenon in ARDS is uncertain but may be related in part to abnormalities in the peripheral capillary circulation that prevent adequate capillary recruitment when increased oxygen extraction is required. Although the precise mechanism of the abnormal supply dependency is unknown, the result is that mixed venous oxygenation may remain relatively stable despite large and presumably important changes in tissue oxygen consumption, cardiac output, and oxygen delivery. The clinician therefore needs to monitor several parameters independently, including cardiac output and arterial oxygen saturation, in order to be informed regarding the hemodynamic status of patients with complex illnesses, including ARDS and sepsis.

Pulmonary artery catheters that provide a measurement of mixed venous oxygen saturation through use of fiberoptic reflectance oximetry are currently available. This technology provides no information that is otherwise unavailable through the direct intermittent sampling of mixed venous blood with standard catheters. However, the continuous and instantaneous monitoring of mixed venous oxygenation may provide a helpful early warning system for detecting adverse hemodynamic trends, especially in patients with cardiac dysfunction in the absence of sepsis or ARDS. The fiberoptic catheter may also be helpful in the rapid distinction between a true wedge tracing and a partially "damped" pulmonary artery pressure tracing, since oxygen saturation should rise when blood is withdrawn distally from a totally occluded pulmonary artery.

Finally, it is important to remember that the mixed venous oxygen saturation has an important influence on the arterial oxygen saturation when there is a high degree of shunt through the lungs, such as in ARDS. Although clinicians often automatically attribute a decrease in PaO_2 to a worsening of lung function, such as decrease may in fact be due to nonrespiratory factors that cause a reduction in mixed venous oxygen saturation (e.g., lowering of the cardiac output).

Pulmonary Artery Wedge Pressure

The measurement of the pulmonary artery wedge pressure (PAWP) is a major use of the Swan-Ganz catheter. The PAWP allows the clinician to make important assumptions regarding left ventricular preload and pulmonary capillary hydrostatic or filtration pressure. The normal PAWP is 2 to 12 mm Hg.

RELATIONSHIP OF PAWP TO LEFT VENTRICULAR PRELOAD

A major value of the PAWP is that it usually approximates the intracavitary left ventricular end-diastolic pressure or filling pressure. When this measure is taken in conjunction with assessment of left ventricular function (e.g., cardiac output), the clinician can reach important conclusions regarding left ventricular contractility according to the Frank-Starling principle. This principle states that the left ventricular preload determines the force of cardiac contraction for any given level of myocardial contractility. Thus, it is important to understand the relationship between PAWP and left ventricular preload, which are sometimes mistakenly assumed to be identical.

Preload refers to stretch of the myocardial fibers and therefore is best assessed by left ventricular end-diastolic volume. It is determined by the transmural ventricular distending pressure (intracavitary pressure, or PAWP, minus juxtacardiac pressure) and ventricular compliance (pressure-volume relationship). A given PAWP may be associated with different degrees of left ventricular filling in critically ill patients with altered juxtacardiac pressure (mechanical ventilation and PEEP) or ventricular compliance (myocardial ischemia, pericardial effusion).

Failure to understand the PAWP-left ventricular end-diastolic volume relationship may cause the clinician to misdiagnose underlying pathophysiology and institute inappropriate therapy. For instance, a hypotensive patient on high PEEP levels may have a measured PAWP that appears to reflect adequate left ventricular preload. Assuming that cardiac dysfunction exists, the physician may begin treatment with inotropic or vasopressor agents. However, it needs to be remembered that the PAWP (uncorrected for elevated pleural pressure) probably overestimates left ventricular transmural distending pressure in this patient; perhaps a volume infusion trial is the most appropriate initial therapy.

The influence of pleural pressure changes on PAWP is minimized through the practice of measuring vascular pressures at end expiration. Of course, this does not eliminate the problem, especially in patients receiving PEEP. Nevertheless, temporarily disconnecting PEEP in order to measure PAWP is discouraged. The resulting new measurements will be of questionable value, since hemodynamics will be altered (e.g., an acute increase in venous return). Furthermore, abrupt removal of PEEP may cause dangerous hypoxia, and this may not reverse rapidly with reinstitution of PEEP. Although a reasonably accurate estimation of juxtacardiac pressure can be achieved with an esophageal balloon, this is impractical for routine intensive care unit use. For most clinical purposes, it is sufficient to estimate the effect of PEEP; the change in pleural pressure at end expiration is usually less than one-half of PEEP in patients with poor lung compliance. Overall, it is most helpful to correlate changes in PAWP with other hemodynamic and clinical changes rather than attaching excessive significance to single measurements of PAWP.

RELATIONSHIP OF PAWP TO PULMONARY CAPILLARY HYDROSTATIC PRESSURE

A major clinical utility of the PAWP is that it provides a means of assessing the filtration pressure favoring the development of pulmonary edema. This information often allows for the distinction between cardiogenic and noncardiogenic origins of edema fluid. However, despite the tendency for people to refer to PAWP as "pulmonary capillary pressure," these two values are not equivalent. In fact, the PAWP usually underestimates true pulmonary capillary pressure. In some clinical settings, the discrepancy between these values may be large, perhaps accounting for the development of pulmonary edema when PAWP is relatively normal and there is no reason to suspect capillary injury.

Resistance in the pulmonary circulation is located on both sides of the capillary midpoint. Usually about 40 percent of the total pressure drop from the pulmonary artery to the left atrium occurs on the pulmonary venous side. Remembering that PAWP approximates left atrial pressure, pulmonary capillary pressure can be estimated as PAWP $+0.4$ (mean pulmonary artery pressure $-$ PAWP). However, many physiologic and pharmacologic agents (including hypoxia, sympathetic stimulation, histamine, serotonin, prostaglandins, and norepinephrine) are capable of altering the longitudinal distribution of pulmonary vascular resistance. It is therefore unrealistic to assume a fixed relationship between PAWP and pulmonary capillary pressure. Hydrostatic pulmonary edema may exist in the presence of a relatively normal PAWP if there is significant vascular resistance in the pulmonary venous system. This may partially explain the occasional observation of "normal wedge" pulmonary edema in myocardial infarction, neurogenic pulmonary edema, and other settings in which identifiable risk factors for ARDS are not found and there is no reason to assume capillary damage.

Suggested Reading

Boyd KD, Thomas SJ, Gold J, Boyd AD. A prospective study of complications of pulmonary artery catheterizations in 500 consecutive patients. Chest 1983; 84:245–249.

Connors AF Jr, McCaffree DR, Gray BA. Evaluation of right-heart catheterization in the critically ill patient without acute myocardial infarction. N Engl J Med 1983; 308:263–267.

Morris AH, Chapman RH, Gardner RM. Frequency of wedge pressure errors in the ICU. Crit Care Med 1985; 13:705–708.

O'Quin R, Marini JJ. Pulmonary artery occlusion pressure: clinical physiology, measurement, and interpretation. Am Rev Respir Dis 1983; 128:319–326.

Rowley KM, Clubb KS, Smith GJW, Cabin HS. Right-sided infective endocarditis as a consequence of flow-directed pulmonary-artery catheterization. N Engl J Med 1984; 311:1152–1156.

Sprung CL, ed. The pulmonary artery catheter: methodology and clinical applications. Baltimore: University Park Press, 1983.

Stetz CW, Miller RG, Kelly GE, Raffin TA. Reliability of the thermodilution method in the determination of cardiac output in clinical practice. Am Rev Respir Dis 1982; 126:1001–1004.

Wiedemann HP, Matthay MA, Matthay RA. Cardiovascular-pulmonary monitoring in the intensive care unit (Parts 1 and 2). Chest 1984; 85:537–549, 656–668.

MECHANICAL VENTILATION: FLUID AND PHARMACOLOGIC MANAGEMENT OF HYPOTENSION

BART CHERNOW, M.D., F.A.C.P.
DANIEL M. STEIGMAN, M.D.

Respiratory failure necessitating mechanical ventilatory support is a common problem, as is acute hypotension, in the critically ill patient. Hypotension may be a manifestation of respiratory failure, a consequence of positive pressure ventilation used to treat respiratory failure, or exist independent of the respiratory failure as a nonrelated variable complicating the patient's pulmonary problem. The hypotension observed following the initiation of mechanical ventilatory support is most frequently due to a decrease in cardiac preload. Positive pressure ventilation impairs venous return to the heart via its action to increase intrathoracic pressure. The addition of positive end-expiratory pressure may further reduce venous return and cardiac output. The hypovolemic patient is particularly predisposed to this adverse action of ventilatory support.

DIAGNOSING THE PROBLEM

As is emphasized throughout this text, monitoring the ventilated patient is essential. Not only should blood pressure be serially assessed but measurement of indices of tissue perfusion is the key to diagnosis. For example, hourly urine output is a useful determination that provides the clinician with a rough (but helpful) index of renal tissue perfusion. As a rule of thumb, the hourly urine output should equal or exceed 0.5 ml per kilogram per hour.

Oliguria (urine output <0.5 ml per kilogram per hour, or in most adults an output <30 ml per hour) is an important clue that renal tissue perfusion may be decreased. However, oliguria may also exist in patients with primary renal disease who may have normal renal perfusion. Microscopic urine analysis, measurement of the urine sodium concentration and urine osmolality (urine sodium concentration of <20 mEq per liter and urine osmolality >500 mOsm per liter

suggest a prerenal etiology), and review of the clinical situation (e.g., fluid intake versus output, physical examination, medication history) help the clinician to determine the etiology of oliguria.

If the patient has been administered diuretics (such as furosemide) as part of the therapy for a cardiopulmonary problem, the hourly urine output, urine sodium concentration, and urine osmolality may not reflect renal perfusion as accurately. Similarly, if the patient is hyperglycemic with glucosuria, the hourly urine output may reflect the impaired glucose homeostasis more than renal function or perfusion.

Other indices of tissue perfusion include the mental status examination (cerebral perfusion is likely to be adequate if mental status is normal), arterial pH (acidemia suggests the possibility of diminished oxygen delivery), and circulating lactate concentrations (increased levels indicate ongoing anaerobic metabolism).

Although some individuals may have adequate tissue perfusion and oxygen delivery with relatively low arterial blood pressures (e.g., 90/60 mm Hg), we believe that a mean arterial blood pressure of less than 60 mm Hg is highly suggestive of inadequate tissue perfusion, especially in a ventilated patient. Of course, when we treat "numbers," we are assuming the validity of the determined number. A sphygmomanometer that is not properly calibrated or an improperly functioning transducer may produce misleading results. In assessing results, intensive care practitioners have come to appreciate the importance of tube length between the catheter and the transducer, of bubbles in the system, and of the need for accurate standards of calibration.

Despite the availability of "high technology" in the intensive care unit, the clinician should not lose sight of the importance of the patient history and physical examination. The patient who indicates that he or she is thirsty, has a dry mouth, and feels dizzy when standing is probably intravascularly volume-depleted. A positive tilt test (a decrease in systolic blood pressure of more than 20 mm Hg and an increase in heart rate of more than 20 beats per minute) is an excellent sign of vascular volume depletion in patients who are free of autonomic diseases (e.g., Shy-Drager syndrome or idiopathic orthostatic hypotension).

CAUSES OF HYPOTENSION

The pulmonary artery flotation catheter may help the clinician to objectively determine if the hypotensive patient has diminished vascular volume, impaired cardiac pump function, or obstruction to blood flow. Diminished central venous, right atrial, and pulmonary artery occlusion pressures suggest hypovolemia, as does a decreased stroke volume (cardiac output/heart rate). High filling pressures and a low cardiac index (<2.2 L per minute per square meter) suggest a cardiogenic etiology for the hypotension. Equalization of pressures across the chest (such as central venous and mean pulmonary artery pressures) suggests obstruction to blood flow due to cardiac tamponade.

The causes of hypotension and circulatory shock (Table 1) alter either cardiac output or systemic vascular resistance. The mechanically ventilated patient may suffer from hypovolemia, cardiac problems, pneumothorax or pulmonary emboli (examples of processes that may cause hypotension via obstruction to blood flow), drug-induced hypotension (e.g., following barbiturate administration), or gram-negative septicemia.

The temporal relationship of the onset of hypotension to the timing of clinical events is often very revealing. Hypotension that immediately follows administration of a drug is likely to be drug-induced

TABLE 1 Etiologic Factors in Shock

Hypovolemia
  External fluid losses
    Hemorrhage
    Gastrointestinal
      Vomiting (pyloric stenosis, intestinal obstruction)
      Diarrhea
    Renal
      Diabetes mellitus
      Diabetes insipidus
      Excessive use of diuretics
    Cutaneous
      Burns
      Exudative lesions
      Perspiration and insensible water loss without replacement
  Internal sequestration
    Fractures
    Ascites (peritonitis, pancreatitis, cirrhosis)
    Intestinal obstruction
    Hemothorax
    Hemoperitoneum
Cardiogenic
  Myocardial infarction
  Arrhythmia (paroxysmal tachycardia or fibrillation, severe bradycardia)
  Severe congestive heart failure with low cardiac output
  Cardiac mechanical factors
    Acute mitral or aortic regurgitation
    Rupture of interventricular septum
Obstruction to blood flow
  Pulmonary embolus
  Tension pneumothorax
  Cardiac tamponade
  Dissecting aortic aneurysm
  Intracardiac (ball valve thrombus, atrial myxoma)
Neuropathic
  Drug-induced
    Anesthesia
    Ganglion-blocking or other antihypertensive drugs
    "Ingestion" (barbiturates, glutethimide, phenothiazines)
  Spinal cord injury
  Orthostatic hypotension (primary autonomic insufficiency, peripheral neuropathies)
Other
  Infection
    Gram-negative septicemia (endotoxin)
    Other septicemias
  Anaphylaxis
  Endocrine failure (Addison's disease, myxedema)
  Anoxia

Reproduced with permission from Braunwald E, et al, eds. Harrison's principals of internal medicine. 11th ed. New York: McGraw-Hill, 1987:154.

or perhaps is caused by anaphylaxis. Hypotension that develops upon initiation of positive pressure ventilation or PEEP or both is probably mechanical (ventilator- or PEEP-induced) in origin.

External fluid losses (that result in hypovolemia) are usually obvious; however, internal sequestration of fluid may be occult. The other causes of hypotension have varying degrees of diagnostic difficulty. It is the responsibility of the physician, nurse, and respiratory therapist to be constantly attentive to possible causes of hypotension.

TREATMENT OF HYPOTENSION

Once hypotension occurs, the clinician must rapidly restore blood pressure and tissue perfusion to normal or be faced with organ failure. Multiple organ system failure is a major cause of death in critically ill, mechanically ventilated patients. The choice of treatment of hypotension depends on the cause.

Hypovolemia. The first step in managing any hypotensive patient is to assume concomitant hypovolemia until proven otherwise. For that reason, patients are immediately placed in the Trendelenburg position (so as to increase preload to the heart). A fluid bolus (500 ml of crystalloid normal saline or lactated Ringer's solution) is rapidly administered over 10 minutes. If the patient's blood pressure rapidly responds to this vascular volume repletion, then the diagnosis of hypovolemia is strongly supported. To confirm the diagnosis and to define the cause of hypovolemia, a rapid physical examination, review of laboratory data (e.g., hemogram, blood and urine glucose levels, chest roentgenogram, serum sodium concentration), and analysis of hemodynamic data are performed. During this period of rapid evaluation, the diagnosis may become clear and may turn out not to be hypovolemia. For example, the patient may be recognized to have a pneumothorax, in which case insertion of a chest tube may rapidly result in blood pressure normalization.

If hypovolemia is confirmed, the cause and degree must be determined. If the ventilated patient is having an upper gastrointestinal hemorrhage, the clinician must replete intravascular volume, determine the coagulation status of the patient, ensure adequate availability of blood products (and venous access for fluid administration), consult a general surgeon, consider diagnostic procedures (e.g., endoscopy), and initiate therapy to stop the bleeding (e.g., iced water lavage of the stomach, intravenous vasopressin, intravenous histamine-2 receptor antagonists, or fresh frozen plasma, or platelets—the choice of therapy dependent on the pathogenesis of the hemorrhage).

The choice of resuscitation fluid in the treatment of many forms of hypovolemia remains controversial. However, certain guidelines may be useful. If the hypovolemia is due to diabetes insipidus and if the serum sodium concentration is less than 155 mEq per liter, replacement therapy should be with hypotonic crystalloid fluid such as 5 percent dextrose in water or one-quarter or one-half normal saline. In this condition, it is a water deficit that is being replaced. (Sixty percent of the body weight is water; therefore, a 70-kg person has 42 L of water. Water deficit can be calculated by first multiplying the observed sodium over predicted sodium times the normal water content. In this case, $155/140 \times 42 = 46.5$ L. The difference between this number and the normal water content equals the water deficit, that is, $46.5 - 42 = 4.5$ L = water deficit). If the hypovolemia is caused by excessive use of diuretics or diabetes mellitus, isotonic saline (with appropriate electrolytes as additives) is the fluid of choice, since both electrolytes and volume are needed. Similarly, many cases of hypovolemia resulting from diarrhea or emesis or both may be appropriately treated in this fashion.

Colloids Versus Crystalloids. The controversy as to colloids versus crystalloids enters when we discuss volume repletion required because of hemorrhage, sepsis, pancreatitis, or peritonitis. The pros and cons of the two therapies relate to variables such as cost, rapidity of resuscitation, and time within the vascular compartment. Numerous experimental and clinical studies support the arguments of advocates for each type of fluid. Several authorities suggest (and we agree) that for mild to moderate hypovolemia (up to 25 percent loss of acute blood volume), the less expensive isotonic crystalloid is appropriate. For volume loss greater than this amount, blood products (if indicated) plus colloid are thought to be preferable because they will maintain vascular volume and tissue perfusion without overexpanding the volume of the interstitium.

The choice of colloid varies among clinicians. Most scholars in the field agree that fresh frozen plasma should be reserved for those with deficiencies in clotting factors that have resulted in prolongation of the activated partial thromboplastin time. This point has been underscored by the conclusions of a National Institutes of Health Consensus Conference.

Critically ill patients may become deficient in fibronectin, which is important for normal opsonic activity of macrophages and cells of the reticuloendothelial system. Increasing experimental and scientific evidence supports the concept that fibronectin replacement may increase survival after critical illness, trauma, or burns. Since cryoprecipitate is rich in fibronectin, some clinicians have been infusing cryoprecipitate as a type of resuscitation fluid. In the near future, pure fibronectin itself will be available for infusion.

Packed red cells are an excellent replacement product in the hypovolemic patient, especially if oxygen-carrying capacity is reduced by anemia. However, since blood products are a scarce resource and because of the advent of the AIDS epidemic, our use of red cells has been reduced. Arbitrary hematocrit levels (such as 30 percent) at which red cell transfusion therapy used to be instituted have been reduced. In our practice, we consider the patient's oxygen delivery, and if it is reduced and the patient is anemic (hemoglobin, for example, less than 8 g per deciliter), we administer packed red blood cells. However, a chronically anemic patient with renal failure may have adequate oxygen delivery with a hemoglobin of 8 g per deciliter and, thus, may not require transfusion therapy. Therefore, as with our previous comments, the clinical decision concerning the type of volume replacement therapy must be individualized based on the patient's condition.

Albumin, dextran, hydroxyethyl starch, hypertonic saline, and other fluids are discussed in other texts. (The reader is directed to the Suggested Reading section.) Regardless of the type of resuscitation fluid chosen, the clinician should monitor the physiologic and biochemical responses to this form of therapy. Volume replacement should be titrated so as to normalize tissue perfusion, acidemia (if present and if the acidemia is due to hypovolemia–induced volume depletion), and cardiac performance, without causing pulmonary edema.

If filling of the vascular "tank" fails to normalize tissue perfusion and oxygen delivery, other approaches must be taken. If this failure is drug-induced, the offending drug should be removed. If the failure is mechanical in origin, the problem is corrected (e.g., by draining pericardial fluid if cardiac tamponade is present, or by placing a chest tube if pneumothorax exists). Beyond these therapeutic moves, a pharmacologic approach becomes requisite.

PHARMACOLOGIC THERAPY OF HYPOTENSION AND SHOCK

A first-line medication in the treatment of hypotension is the sympathomimetic phenylephrine hydrochloride (Neo-Synephrine). This alpha$_1$-adrenergic receptor stimulant is a well-tolerated vasoconstrictor and vasopressor. Administered at an initial intravenous infusion rate of 100 to 200 μg per minute, it usually results in prompt reversal of hypotension. Once the blood pressure normalizes, the phenylephrine infusion rate should be decreased to 40 to 60 μg per minute or it should be discontinued if a vasopressor is no longer needed. Phenylephrine may be problematic in patients receiving halothane anesthesia, monoamine oxidase inhibitors, or oxytocic drugs. As mentioned above, intravascular volume must be normalized and the *cause* of the patient's hypotension diagnosed and treated (if possible). Although blood pressure may

be normalized by phenylephrine administration, an assessment of tissue perfusion is needed, since this is the variable of greatest importance.

In patients with profound hypotension that responds poorly to fluid administration or phenylephrine or both, norepinephrine bitartrate (Levophed) should be considered. This catecholamine is a potent alpha$_1$-adrenergic receptor agonist that causes vasoconstriction. It is, therefore, particularly useful in vasodilated hypotensive patients. It is such a potent vasoconstrictor that it may cause tissue hypoxia in the volume-depleted patient. Therefore, assessment of the patient's vascular volume is essential. Norepinephrine should be infused into a large vein via a centrally placed catheter, since extravasation may cause tissue necrosis. Like phenylephrine, norepinephrine should be used with extreme caution in patients receiving monoamine oxidase inhibitors or certain other antidepressants. We begin norepinephrine therapy at an infusion rate of 4 μg per minute and adjust the rate based on the response of the patient.

Epinephrine (1 : 1,000 for injection) is rarely used to reverse hypotension except in the setting of anaphylaxis or anaphylactoid reactions (0.01 mg per kilogram subcutaneously) or cardiac arrest (0.5 mg IV or intracardiac in adults). It has other uses, such as for hemostasis and for relief of hypersensitivity reactions to drugs and allergens, bronchospasm, serum sickness, urticaria, or angioneurotic edema. It is also used to prolong the action of local anesthetics. Some experienced critical care physicians infuse epinephrine in cases of hypotension that are refractory to other therapies.

Dopamine hydrochloride is a unique catecholamine in that its physiologic actions are mediated by three types of adrenergic receptors (alpha, beta, and dopamine). Dopamine's actions vary in a dose-dependent manner. At low infusion rates (0.5 to 3.0 μg per kilogram per minute), dopamine causes renal artery vasodilation (leading to a diuresis), and it inhibits aldosterone release (leading to a natriuresis). At higher infusion rates (5 to 10 μg per kilogram per minute), it acts as a potent inotropic agent. At the highest infusion rates (>20 μg per kilogram per minute), dopamine causes vasoconstriction. Although this dose response information is fairly true in normal subjects, it often fails to be accurate in the critically ill patient. The variability in the response to dopamine probably has several mechanisms. One putative mechanism is that dopamine, as the precursor of norepinephrine (in the endogenous biosynthetic pathway of catecholamines), may trigger the synthesis and release of norepinephrine. Regardless of mechanisms, clinicians should be aware of this variability. We prefer to use dopamine at low infusion rates (1 to 2 μg per kilogram per minute) in an attempt to benefit from its ability to maintain urine output and a natriuresis. Experimental data suggest that low-dose dopamine may prevent norepinephrine-induced renal artery vasoconstriction. Therefore, in the vasodilated hypotensive patient, we prefer to simultaneously administer both norepinephrine and low-dose dopamine. Clinicians should be mindful of the fact that some authors report that catecholamines like dopamine may worsen hypoxemia in ventilated patients (possibly because of drug-induced increases in shunt).

Isoproterenol hydrochloride (Isuprel) is rarely used to reverse hypotension unless it is accompanied by bradycardia or in some cases bronchospasm or both. If used, an infusion rate of 0.5 to 5.0 μg per minute is appropriate.

Like isoproterenol, dobutamine is a beta>alpha adrenergic receptor agonist catecholamine. Dobutamine (infused at 5 to 15 μg per kilogram per minute) is an effective inotropic agent that is particularly useful in the patient with low cardiac output and high ventricular filling pressures. We find that it has minimal effect on arterial blood pressure; however, cardiac output increases while pulmonary artery occlusion pressure and systemic vascular resistance decrease. Therefore, dobutamine is usually used in patients with diminished cardiac output, despite normal or high ventricular filling pressures.

EXPERIMENTAL THERAPEUTIC APPROACHES

As our knowledge of the biochemical basis of hypotension has improved, new potential therapies have emerged. Among those medications with a firm experimental basis for reversal of hypotension are naloxone hydrochloride (Narcan, an opiate receptor antagonist), thyrotropin-releasing hormone (a "physiologic" opiate-leukotriene antagonist), ATP magnesium chloride, glucagon, BAY k 8644 (a calcium-channel agonist), and antagonists to platelet-activating factor. In addition, monoclonal antibodies are being developed for use against mediators of hypotension—especially as they relate to the sepsis syndrome. Controlled clinical trials of these medicines are needed before they can be recommended in the treatment of hypotension.

This chapter was written during Dr. Steigman's tenure as a fellow under NIH research training grant No. HL 07354.

Suggested Reading

Chernow B, ed. The pharmacologic approach to the critically ill patient. 2nd edition. Baltimore: Williams & Wilkins, 1988.

Chernow B, Roth BL. Pharmacologic manipulation of the peripheral vasculature in shock—clinical and experimental approaches. Circ Shock 1986; 18:141–155.

Chernow B, Soldano S, Cook D, et al. Positive end-expiratory pressure increases plasma catecholamine levels in non-volume loaded dogs. Anaesth Intensive Care 1986; 14:421–425.

Demling RH. Shock and fluids. In: Chernow B, Shoemaker WC, eds. Critical care state of the art. Vol 7. Fullerton, CA: Society of Critical Care Medicine, 1986:301–351.

Houston MC, Thompson WL, Robertson D. Shock—diagnosis and management. Arch Intern Med 1984; 144:1433–1439.

National Institutes of Health Consensus Development Conference. Fresh frozen plasma—indications and risks. Vol 5-5. Washington, DC: NIH Publication, 1984.

Saba TM, Blumenstock FA, Shah DM, et al. Reversal of opsonic deficiency in surgical, trauma and burn patients by infusion of purified human plasma fibronectin—correlation with experimental observations. Am J Med 1986; 80:229–240.

NONINVASIVE MONITORING TECHNIQUES IN THE VENTILATED PATIENT

ROBERT M. KACMAREK, Ph.D., RRT

Invasive approaches to the monitoring of gas exchange have seemed to dominate the management of the mechanically ventilated patient. However, recent technologic developments, along with continued interest in evaluating pulmonary mechanics as well as ventilatory reserves, have expanded noninvasive approaches to monitoring the mechanically ventilated patient. Specifically, four areas are addressed in this chapter: (1) determination of pulmonary mechanics (compliance and resistance); (2) evaluation of ventilatory reserve (vital capacity, inspiratory force, tidal volume, respiratory rate, and minute volume); (3) oximetry and transcutaneous P_{O_2} monitoring; and (4) end-tidal CO_2 and transcutaneous P_{CO_2} monitoring.

PULMONARY MECHANICS

The term *pulmonary mechanics* in relation to mechanically ventilated patients refers to the evaluation of compliance and airways resistance. Reference is made to three distinct measurements: effective static compliance (Ces), dynamic compliance (Cdyn), and airways resistance (Raw). The term Ces implies that the determined value corresponds to laboratory determinations of total lung compliance, while Cdyn is a value that reflects total respiratory system impedance. In the determination of Ces, an inspiratory equilibration pressure (plateau pressure, Pplat) is used, and with Cdyn determinations the peak airway pressure (PIP) is employed. The Raw determination provides a gross estimate of the total gas flow resistance of the patient, artificial airway, and ventilatory circuitry.

Determination of Ces and Cdyn

Since compliance (C) is a measure of distensibility, it can be defined as:

$$C = \Delta V / \Delta P$$

where ΔV is change in volume, and ΔP is change in pressure. In mechanically ventilated patients, the ΔV used is the exhaled tidal volume (Vet) measured ideally at the patient's airway. Vet is used in preference to inspired tidal volume (VT) to ensure that gas having leaked out of the system during the generation of positive pressure is not included in the calculation. Change in pressure used is either the PIP or Pplat. Figure 1 depicts an inspiratory pressure-time curve during normal delivery of a positive pressure breath. Point A represents the PIP, while point B is the Pplat. In establishing the Pplat, a 1.5 to 2.0 second inflation hold is performed to ensure complete equilibration of pressure.

Thus, Ces is determined as follows:

$$Ces = \frac{Vet}{Pplat}$$

Cdyn is calculated as shown below:

$$Cdyn = \frac{Vet}{PIP}$$

Effect of Applied and Intrinsic Positive End-Expiratory Pressure (PEEP)

The pressure used to calculate both Ces and Cdyn should reflect only pressure required to distend the lung from its end expiratory position, or, more simply stated, the pressure needed to deliver the Vet. Applied PEEP (PEEPa) and intrinsic (auto) PEEP (PEEPi) elevate both peak and plateau pressure and result in diminished compliance calculations if the pressure recorded is not corrected.

The magnitude of PEEPa is obvious and easily noted, while the presence of PEEPi is more difficult to establish. PEEPi can be determined by occluding the expiratory port just prior to a mechanical positive pressure breath. If PEEPi is present, system pressure immediately increases to the PEEPi level. Remember, PEEPi may be present even if PEEPa is present. The effects of PEEPa and PEEPi on the determination of Ces are depicted in Figure 2.

The following formulas for determination of Ces and Cdyn should be employed if PEEPa is employed or if PEEPi is noted.

$$Ces = \frac{Vet}{Pplat - PEEPa - PEEPi}$$

$$Cdyn = \frac{Vet}{PIP - PEEPa - PEEPi}$$

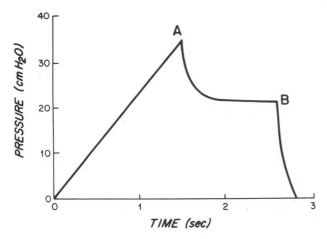

Figure 1 Inspiratory pressure curve with pressure plateau, constant square wave inspiratory flow pattern. A = PIP, B = Pplat, $A-B$ = pressure change reflective of Raw.

Compressible Gas Volume

Correction of Vet for ventilator system compressible volume loss is recommended by some. Since ventilator circuits are expandable and circuits with humidifiers contain large gas volumes, a gas compression factor (CF) exists for all systems. In most adult circuits, 3 to 5 ml per centimeter H_2O PIP is lost as compressed volume. Failure to account for compressible gas volume in calculating Ces results in an erroneously high compliance determination, since the volume delivered to the lung would be overestimated. On the other hand, if the same type of ventilator circuitry is used and serial measurements are

performed consistently, the error included in each calculation is constant. Thus, the percent error in serial determinations is the same and values determined can be used to trend change over time. Concern over the effect of CF can be eliminated if measurements of Vet are performed at the airways, not at the system exhalation valve. The following formulas should be used if Vet is to be corrected for compressible volume:

$$Ces = \frac{Vet - (Pplat - PEEPa - PEEPi)(CF)}{Pplat - PEEPa - PEEPi}$$

$$Cdyn = \frac{Vet - (PIP - PEEPa - PEEPi)(CF)}{PIP - PEEPa - PEEPi}$$

Determination of Raw

The calculation of Raw is used to reflect the total system resistance to gas flow. Resistance (R) in a dynamic gas flow system is determined by the following formula:

$$R = \frac{\Delta P}{Flow}$$

For the determination of R to be accurate, flow must be constant. In ventilated patients, the ΔP used is that pressure required to maintain gas flow or PIP − Pplat, while flow is the peak flow setting on the ventilator. For the most accurate determinations of Raw, as well as Cdyn, the ventilator must deliver a constant square wave flow. Other inspiratory flow patterns result in inaccurately low calculations of Raw and Cdyn. The following formula is used to calculate Raw:

$$Raw = \frac{PIP - Pplat}{Peak Flow}$$

Sources of Error

As already mentioned, PEEPa, PEEPi, and CF can affect Cdyn and Ces determinations, while a nonconstant square wave flow pattern affects Cdyn and Raw. Additionally, all of these determinations are affected by patients' spontaneous breathing capabilities. The greater the patient's involvement in the process of ventilation, the less likely will any of the measured values reflect actual pulmonary mechanics. Ideally, a completely cooperative or apneic patient is necessary for the most accurate results.

I also do not recommend basing the above determinations on programs incorporated into the new generation of mechanical ventilators unless provisions to maintain a 1.5 to 2.0 second inflation hold are included to establish a true plateau pressure. Some of these programs hold pressure for much less than 0.5 seconds. In the presence of alterations in distribution

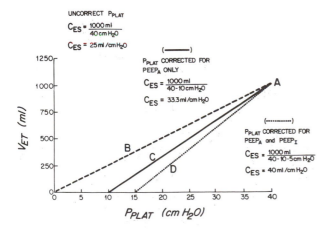

Figure 2 Effects of PEEPa and PEEPi on determination of Ces. A = Pplat, B = Atm pressure, C = PEEPa level, and D = PEEPi level. BA represents Ces curve, without correction for PEEPa or PEEPi. CA represents Ces curve, with correction for PEEPa only. DA represents Ces curve, with corrections for PEEPa and PEEPi. See text for details.

of ventilation, these programs result in erroneously high estimates of plateau pressure.

Utilization of Results

Data obtained from the serial determination of pulmonary mechanics can be used to (1) select appropriate Vets, (2) determine optimal PEEP levels, (3) evaluate the effectiveness of pharmacologic bronchodilatation, and (4) monitor the progression of pulmonary disease.

Most assume that a tidal volume of 12 to 15 ml per kilogram of ideal body weight is appropriate for the majority of patients. However, a more accurate determination of the ideal maximum tidal volume for a given patient can be determined by plotting a patient's Ces curve. This technique is depicted in Figure 3, where the Pplat is plotted against progressive 200 ml increases in Vet. The ideal maximum Vet is that volume at the top of the steep portion of the compliance curve.

As we are all aware, no single factor can be used to determine the optimal PEEP level on a given patient. However, Ces does provide data that assist in this determination. As alveoli are recruited, Ces normally improves and, in turn, decreases with overdistention. Thus, monitoring Ces with increases in PEEPa assists in determining optimal PEEPa settings.

Bronchospasm, mucosal edema, and secretions all contribute to increased airways resistance and this results in a decrease in Cdyn and an increase in Raw. Monitoring of these values is helpful in determining the efficacy and the necessity of systemic or aerosolized bronchodilatation, as well as the effects of chest physical therapy.

The progression and resolution of pulmonary pathology demonstrates alterations in both elastic and nonelastic resistance to ventilation. The monitoring of Ces and Cdyn compliance curves provides quantitative data on changes in pulmonary pathology. Figure 4 illustrates Ces and Cdyn curves, representative of various pathophysiologic conditions.

The evaluation of pulmonary mechanics on a routine basis is not required in all mechanically ventilated patients. However, in those patients presenting with long-term ventilatory courses that are directly a result of pulmonary pathology, the daily monitoring of Ces and Cdyn curves does provide valuable information on the progression of pathology and the efficiency and appropriateness of therapy. Actual calculations of Raw, in my opinion, do not add significantly to the information provided by Ces and Cdyn, because measurements of Cdyn, when compared with Ces measurements, reflect actual changes in Raw. Additionally, few mechanical ventilators are truly capable of delivering the square wave inspiratory flow pattern required for accurate Raw determinations.

VENTILATORY RESERVE

Shortly after instituting mechanical ventilation, most of us begin to contemplate discontinuing ventilatory support. Along with the evaluation of data indicating resolution of the pathophysiologic condition requiring ventilatory support and a review of blood gas results is normally an assessment of the patient's ability to breathe spontaneously. I have found the frequent evaluation of vital capacity and inspiratory force as well as spontaneous respiratory rate, tidal volume,

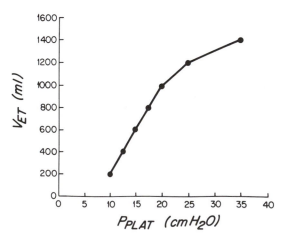

Figure 3 Ces curve developed by increasing Vet in 200-ml increments. The ideal maximum Vet in this example remaining on the steep aspect of the compliance curve is about 1,000 ml. Vet over this level markedly increases static and dynamic pressures. See text for details.

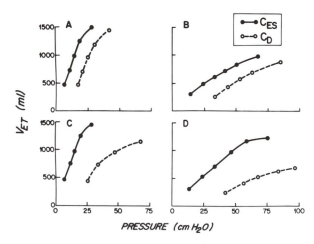

Figure 4 Ces and Cdyn curves under various pathophysiologic conditions. *A*, Normal pulmonary mechanics. *B*, Decrease in lung-thorax compliance, Raw normal. *C*, Normal lung-thorax compliance with increased Raw. *D*, Decrease in lung-thorax compliance, Raw increased. See text for details.

and minute volume invaluable in evaluating patients' readiness for sustained spontaneous ventilation.

Vital Capacity

The ability to sustain spontaneous ventilation appears to be well correlated to the vital capacity (VC), particularly in patients without chronic pulmonary disease. In the chronic disease group, VC is frequently diminished markedly before the acute insult and is less prognostic of spontaneous breathing capability and ventilatory muscle strength. Generally, a VC of greater than 10 to 15 ml per kilogram of ideal body weight supports decisions for ventilator discontinuance or weaning trials.

The major drawback in monitoring VC is the requirement of patient cooperation. Many patients do not provide maximum effort in performing the VC maneuver. This difficulty is also compounded by central nervous system pathology and language impairments.

Inspiratory Force

In my opinion, the best indication of ventilatory reserve and ventilatory muscle strength is the inspiratory force (IF) measurement. This is primarily because patient cooperation is unnecessary. IF of −25 to −30 cm H_2O correlate well with VCs of 10 to 15 ml per kilogram and are predictive of spontaneous ventilatory ability.

Appropriate technique must be assured when evaluating IF. Occlusion of the airway should occur at end exhalation. This is to ensure that the diaphragm has returned to its resting position and has the maximum mechanical advantage when contracting. Ideally, a one-way valve is attached to the IF meter (Fig. 5) to allow exhalation to occur, so that with each subsequent inspiration the mechanical advantage of the diaphragm is improved. Finally, the IF should be determined over a 20-second period. Measurement during the 20-second period should be discontinued only if (1) cardiovascular stress is noted (arrhythmias, tachycardia, bradycardia, or hypo- or hypertension); (2) arterial desaturation (pulse oximetry) occurs; or (3) the maximum level achieved begins to deteriorate (i.e., at 10 seconds a force of −15 cm H_2O is noted, but on subsequent breaths −12 and −10 cm H_2O is seen). If performed properly, this simple measurement provides valuable and useful information.

Spontaneous Rate, Tidal Volume, and Minute Volume

In addition to the frequent evaluation of VC and IF, the monitoring of spontaneous rate, tidal volume

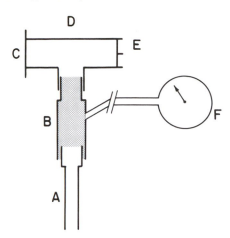

Figure 5 Set-up for determination of inspiratory force. *A*, Endotracheal tube. *B*, Adapter for attachment of pressure manometer. *C*, Point of occlusion by thumb. *D*, Briggs T-piece. *E*, One-way valve. *F*, Pressure manometer. During inspiration, occlusion at *C* prevents inspiration. During expiration, gas exits at point *E*. See text for details.

(VT), and minute volume provides data on patients' ability to sustain spontaneous ventilation. Generally, VTs of 2 to 3 ml per kilogram, rates of less than 25 per minute, and minute volume less than 10 L are consistent with prolonged spontaneous ventilation. I have found spontaneous ventilatory rates to be most useful in predicting prolonged spontaneous ventilatory capabilities.

When to Monitor

I monitor spontaneous respiratory rate, tidal volume, and minute volume each time the ventilator-patient system is checked if the patient is in the intermittent mandatory ventilation (IMV) and synchronized IMV (SIMV) mode. In patients being ventilated in the assist-control mode, or solely maintained on pressure support, rate, VT, and minute volume are evaluated every 8 hours.

In patients not actively weaning, VC and IF are evaluated each morning. During IMV or pressure support weans, VC and IF are evaluated each shift. In patients on T-piece or continuous positive airway pressure (CPAP) weans, I evaluate VC, IF, rate, VT, and minute volume at the start and completion of each weaning period. These serial measurements provide quantitative data for the ongoing assessment of ventilatory reserve.

OXIMETRY AND TRANSCUTANEOUS P_{O_2}

Continuous monitoring of oxygenation status has become the standard in neonatal and pediatric ICUs as well as operating suites because of the frequency and severity with which oxygenation status may change in these arenas. In the adult ICUs noninvasive monitoring of oxygenation status has also become more common. Practitioners presently have a choice between two technologies: transcutaneous Po_2 and pulse oximetry.

Transcutaneous Po_2

Transcutaneous monitoring of Po_2 requires the placement of a heated miniaturized Clark electrode on the skin. If peripheral perfusion is good and sensor temperature is maintained, good correlation between transcutaneous Po_2 ($PtcO_2$) and PaO_2 is maintained. However, $PtcO_2$ monitoring systems require about a 20-minute warm-up period before functioning accurately, provide inaccurately low results in decreased perfusion states, require electrode relocation every 4 hours, may cause skin burns, are technically elaborate, require calibration, and lag behind the actual PaO_2 change. For these reasons I prefer to use pulse oximetry.

Pulse Oximetry

Oximeters employ the principle of spectrophotometric analysis of the light absorption by blood perfusing peripheral vascular beds. They have demonstrated excellent correlation with actual saturations measured with co-oximeters. In addition, their response to actual changes in arterial oxygen saturation is almost instantaneous.

Pulse oximetry provides rapid, real-time monitoring of a change in oxygenation status. Ideally, these devices should be employed on all acutely ill, mechanically ventilated patients and those spontaneously breathing patients at risk of developing ventilatory failure. Since sufficient numbers of oximeters are rarely available, I employ this monitor on all acutely unstable, mechanically ventilated patients, patients in ICUs at risk of developing ventilatory failure, and long-term ventilator-dependent patients during weaning trials.

END-TIDAL CO_2 AND TRANSCUTANEOUS Pco_2

Improvement in the technology of noninvasive monitoring of CO_2 has led to the development of two different approaches: transcutaneous CO_2 ($PtcCO_2$) and end-tidal CO_2 ($etCO_2$) monitoring.

Transcutaneous Pco_2

As with the monitoring of $PtcO_2$, the $PtcCO_2$ electrode is a miniaturized blood gas electrode, spe-

cifically, a Severinghaus CO_2 electrode. In order for proper function it must be heated to 44–45°C. As a result, the same problems occur as with $PtcO_2$ (i.e., movement every 4 hours and surface burns). In addition, warm-up time is required, performance in low flow states is limited, and response to changes in $PaCO_2$ is slow. As a result of the limitations in this technology I have not employed $PtcCO_2$ monitoring in the adult population.

End-Tidal CO_2

Spectrophotometric analysis of exhaled gas is used to determine the end-tidal CO_2. Actual sampling is performed by two different methods: mainstream and sidestream. With mainstream analyzers, actual analysis is performed at the airway and there is no delay between sample and presentation of data. With sidestream analyzers, a capillary tube extracts a small sample of exhaled gas, and actual analysis is performed away from the airway. A delay between actual sampling and presentation of the data occurs, and water may accumulate in the capillary tube. Mainstream analyzers are frequently bulky and difficult to maintain at the airway without increasing torque on the artificial airway.

One of the major nontechnical problems with on-line monitoring of $etCO_2$ is interpreting the capnograph produced, as well as the $etCO_2$ level, with changes in clinical status. Significant continuing in-service and clinical use are necessary if maximum use is to be made of the data provided.

I find $etCO_2$ monitoring most useful in two settings: the management of the unstable, acutely-ill patient, wherein multiple alterations in ventilatory and cardiovascular management are required, and during weaning trials of the long-term ventilator-dependent patient who must be closely monitored.

Suggested Reading

Bone RC. Compliance and dynamic characteristic curves in acute respiratory failure. Crit Care Med 1976; 4:173–179.

Boysen PG. Respiratory muscle function and weaning from mechanical ventilation. Respir Care 1987; 32:572–583.

Harris K. Non-invasive monitoring of gas exchange. Respir Care 1987; 32:544–557.

Hubmayer RD, Gay PC, Tayyab M. Respiratory system mechanics in ventilated patients: techniques and indications. Mayo Clin Proc 1987; 62:358–368.

Milic-Emili J, Gottfried SB, Rossi A. Non-invasive measurements of respiratory mechanics in ICU patients. Int J Clin Monit Comput 1987; 4:11–20.

Pierson DJ. Weaning from mechanical ventilation in acute respiratory failure: concepts, indications, and techniques. Respir Care 1983; 28:646–662.

Rossi A, Gottfried SB, Higgs L, et al. Respiratory mechanics in mechanically ventilated patients with respiratory failure. J Appl Physiol 1985; 58:1849–1858.

Rossi A, Gottfried SB, Zocchi L, et al. Measurement of static compliance of the total respiratory system in patients with acute respiratory failure during mechanical ventilation: the effect of intrinsic positive end-expiratory pressure. Am Rev Respir Dis 1985; 131:672–677.

Sahn SA, Laksminarayan S, Petty TL. Weaning from mechanical ventilation. JAMA 1976; 235:2208–2212.

WORK OF BREATHING

JOHN J. MARINI, M.D.

QUANTIFYING THE WORK OF BREATHING

Indices of Muscle Metabolism

Oxygen Consumption

The attempt to quantify breathing effort can be approached in three quite different but related ways. The first is to measure the O_2 consumed by the ventilatory muscles during the application or removal of a breathing stress, attributing the difference in total oxygen consumption ($\Delta \dot{V}_{O_2}$) to the activity of the respiratory pump. In theory, this method has the advantage of quantifying effort at its most basic level, i.e., at the level of cellular metabolism. Because the breathing effort involves muscular activity that is not strictly associated with useful chest movement, the $\Delta \dot{V}_{O_2}$ technique takes into account the grossly inefficient nature of the ventilatory musculature that often characterizes critical illness, as well as the energy expended by nonrespiratory muscle groups. Expiratory as well as inspiratory muscle activity influences the measurement. Although theoretically attractive, this methodology has several major drawbacks for the clinical setting. First, the energy cost of breathing is normally a small portion of the total body O_2 requirement, so that precise measurement may not be easy when breathing efforts are small. This inherent problem of signal detection is multiplied in the clinical setting by a second factor. High inspired fractions of O_2 and elevated minute ventilations may be needed to adequately support the patient suffering a crisis of oxygenation. As a result, large volumes of O_2 are inspired and expired with every breath. By comparison, total body O_2 consumption is small, and the O_2 consumed in the breathing effort much smaller still. Consequently, the instrument used to detect O_2 in the inspired and expired gas must be very accurate to prevent large percentage errors from occurring. The recent introduction of equipment that bases the O_2 consumption estimate on volumetric measurements may circumvent some of these problems, but has not yet been thoroughly evaluated.

Stability, both of the patient (regarding total body O_2 consumption) and of the inspiratory gas composition (regarding F_{IO_2}) must be excellent, or large errors will also be introduced on this account. Computation of $\dot{V}_{O_2}$ from the product of cardiac output and the O_2 content difference between arterial and mixed venous blood is easily accomplished. However, although theoretically attractive, this invasive technique is subject to multiplicative arithmetic errors of inherently imprecise measurements (cardiac output, CaO_2, CvO_2), in addition to transient imbalances between arterial and venous blood at the time of sampling. Perhaps the most serious indictment of either technique for estimating respiratory O_2 consumption is that repeated measurements are time consuming and require an active intervention in the patient's ventilatory status.

Electromyography

Respiratory muscle activity can also be monitored electromyographically. The integrated electromyogram (EMG) provides an indirect indication of the tension and metabolic activity of the muscle it monitors. Indeed, for any given patient, there appears to be a close relationship between the magnitude of the integrated electromyogram and oxygen uptake by the muscle. Unfortunately, the EMG cannot be compared across patients, because its amplitude varies widely from person to person, so there is no absolute standard for intensity. Furthermore, tracking the activity of any single muscle group may not faithfully reflect the global activity of all respiratory muscles. Finally, the electromyogram of the diaphragm is difficult to record in many patients without semi-invasive techniques. I consider electromyography to be a valuable tool for research, but not for clinical application to the respiratory problems of ventilated patients.

Measures of External Mechanical Work

Estimating the Work of a Spontaneous Cycle

From a practical standpoint, ventilatory effort is more conveniently indexed from measurements of the pressures and flows generated by the respiratory musculature, as reflected by the external mechanical work of breathing $W_B = \int P V dt$. Energy is consumed and work is done when a passive structure (e.g., the lung) is moved by a pressure gradient (the transstructural pressure, P_{TS}) through a volume change (the time integral of air flow $\int V dt$). For example, when the passive thorax is expanded by positive pressure, as during controlled mechanical ventilation, the airway is pressurized, a volume change occurs, and the machine performs work. Note that exhalation normally occurs passively, so that the mechanical work of breathing is most often calculated only over the inspiratory half cycle. The P_{TS} applied across the entire thorax during inspiration is the airway pressure minus atmospheric pressure. If we are interested only in the work done across the lung, the relevant P_{TS} is airway pressure minus intrapleural pressure, whereas, for the passive chest wall the relevant pressure difference is pleural pressure minus atmospheric pressure. These pressure-volume (work) integrals can be computed electronically by integrating the product of P_{TS} and flow, or graphically by plotting cumulated inspired volume versus pressure, thereby quantifying the area enclosed by the relevant portion of the resulting figure (Fig. 1).

The lung is an inherently passive structure that moves equally well, whether inflated by negative intrathoracic pressure or by positive pressure applied at the airway opening. If an estimate of pleural pressure is available (for example, as monitored by an esophageal catheter), the work done across the lung can be easily measured in either case. However, the work done in moving the chest wall cannot be quantified during active breathing by such an analysis. The pressure that moves the chest wall is generated deep within the muscles themselves and is not directly accessible to a measuring instrument. The negative intrapleural pressure opposes chest expansion. Therefore, although intrapleural pressure (P_{pl}) may be thought of as an index of the afterload to muscular contraction, it does not act to *displace* the chest wall. For this reason, indirect methods must be used to quantify the work done in inflating the thoracic cage. The most common of these techniques, undoubtedly imprecise, is to measure the work of inflating the passive chest wall during voluntary relaxation, sedation, or neuromuscular paralysis, assuming that a similar value applies during active contraction. This value is then added to the measured value for work done across the lungs to estimate the work of moving the entire system.

When a passive patient is ventilated with positive pressure delivered at a constant flow rate, the geometric figure described by the airway pressure volume curve closely resembles a trapezoid (Fig. 2). Under these specific conditions, time is a linear analogue of volume, so that the airway pressure measured at mid cycle ($\bar{P}$), multiplied by the tidal volume, yields work. $\bar{P}$ estimates work performed per liter of ventilation at the selected values of tidal volume and inspiratory flow. For example, if the pressure at mid cycle were 25 cm H_2O, the work per liter of ventilation would be 2.5 joules per liter. Incidentally, the airway pressure tracing can be easily recorded at the bedside using the standard transducer and strip-chart recording apparatus normally employed for pulmonary arterial pressure measurement. (To avoid the potential for infection or gas embolism, the transducer used must be dedicated exclusively to this purpose.) An even simpler method is to estimate the airway pressure at mid cycle from the difference in peak dynamic (P_D) and peak static (P_s) pressures under passive constant flow conditions. The expression ($P_D - \frac{1}{2}P_s$) yields a rough estimate of $\bar{P}$. Such estimates of W_B would be reasonably accurate for the values of tidal volume and flow delivered by the mechanical ventilator, but are not valid indicators for the tidal volumes and flows of the spontaneously breathing patient with greatly different parameters. For accuracy, the patient must be inflated passively by the mechanical ventilator at a tidal volume and flow rate that reflect the average spontaneous values. This matching of V_T and $\dot{V}$ is often difficult to accomplish at the bedside without deep sedation or neuromuscular paralysis.

The mean inflation pressure, $\bar{P}$, can also be expressed in terms of measured resistance, compliance, tidal volume, and mean inspiratory time (T_i) accord-

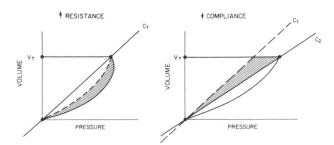

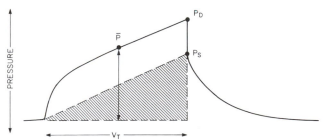

Figure 1 Measuring the inspiratory work of breathing from a plot of distending pressure (horizontal axis) against inspired volume. C_1 and C_2 refer to conditions of normal and reduced compliance, respectively. In the lefthand figure, the unshaded area enclosed by the three heavy dots and dashed line quantifies the workload under basal conditions. The shaded areas indicate the increments of work needed under conditions of high resistance (left panel) or decreased compliance (right panel) conditions.

Figure 2 Tracing of airway pressure against inspired volume during controlled inflation of a passive subject under constant flow conditions. Designated points refer to the pressures that correspond to peak dynamic (P_D), peak static (P_s), and mean ($\bar{P}$) values. $\bar{P}$ reflects the work done per liter of ventilation. The shaded area corresponds to inspiratory work done against elastic impedance of the lung and chest wall, whereas the unshaded area reflects work done against frictional impedance.

ing to a simplified modification of the "equation of motion" formulated by Otis: $\bar{P} = R(V_T/T_i) + V_T/2C$. Once resistance, compliance, and tidal volume have been estimated or measured, T_i can be determined directly from a strip tracing of airway pressure. This expression is valid both for passive inflation and for active breathing. However, when it is used to estimate the work of spontaneous breathing, care must be taken that R, C, and V_T, as well as T_i refer to the spontaneous values (Table 1).

Thus, we have several means for estimating the mechanical work of spontaneous breathing in the clinical setting. The work of lung inflation can be measured directly from a plot of esophageal pressure and inspired volume during unassisted breathing, with the work of chest wall inflation estimated from published literature values. During passive inflation, the mechanical work required to expand the entire thorax can also be measured—without the need for an esophageal catheter—from a plot of airway pressure and volume. Finally, when inspiratory flow is constant, the work per liter of ventilation, $\bar{P}$, can be estimated from mid-cycle airway pressure. $\bar{P}$ can be directly measured from a strip chart record of airway pressure. It can also be estimated from peak dynamic and static pressure values or from the measured components of the modified equation of motion. Any method of estimating spontaneous work from airway pressure data is only valid if flows and tidal volumes mimic spontaneous values and if inflation proceeds passively. Furthermore, it must be kept in mind constantly that these mechanical measures are very indirect indicators of underlying metabolic activity of the muscle itself and may bear no relation whatever to the sense of dyspnea.

Estimating the Work of a Triggered Machine Cycle

Although mechanical support for ventilation is intended to reduce or eliminate the work of breathing, this is not always the case. Typical volume-preset machine cycles differ markedly from spontaneous tidal breaths. Ventilators are commonly set to deliver flows

TABLE 1   Measures of Inspiratory Effort During the Breathing Cycle

---
Metabolism-Based Measures
  O$_2$ Consumption
  Electromyography

Measures of External Work Output
  Spontaneous Breathing
    Equation of Motion: $\bar{P} = R(V_T/T_i) + V_T/2C$
    Pressure-Volume area (Lung only)
  Mechanical Ventilation
    Passive: $\bar{P}$ during constant flow
    Active: P − V area difference for passive and
          machine assisted cycles
---

and tidal volumes that exceed their natural values. Furthermore, the flow contour of the delivered breath varies markedly from the natural pattern, in that its waveform follows a stereotypic pattern and remains invariant from cycle to cycle. It may not be surprising, therefore, that the patient (especially when dyspneic) often fails to quickly terminate the inspiratory effort that initiates a machine cycle.

During ventilator-aided cycles, the patient's inspiratory work of breathing can be estimated by comparing the machine work done during active and passive cycles. Provided that inspiratory flow rate and tidal volume are held constant, the difference in machine work between assisted and controlled cycles estimates the patient's contribution to chest inflation during the active effort.

DETERMINANTS OF THE WORK OF BREATHING

Spontaneous Cycles

As suggested by the equation of motion already discussed, the key determinants of the work of breathing *per liter* of ventilation (W$_B$) are: tidal volume, mean inspiratory flow rate (V$_T$/T$_i$), and the impedance characteristics of the chest—R and C. The total work *per breath* is influenced by the quotient of W$_B$ and by the size of the breath, whereas the total work *per unit time* is determined by the product of W$_B$ and minute ventilation.

The clinical circumstances that influence the primary components of the work equation are those that determine the impedance characteristics of the chest, the rate of inspiratory airflow, and the depth of each tidal breath. Thus, unless counterbalanced by another component of the equation, pathologic conditions that increase resistance (bronchospasm, retained secretions, external loads), elastance (lung edema, pleural effusion, lung or chest wall restrictive disease), inspiratory flow rate or V$_T$ (high V̇$_E$ requirement) will increase the ventilatory workload. Note that V̇$_E$ is doubly important to patient effort, by influencing both work per liter of ventilation and the minute ventilation itself.

Ventilator-Assisted Cycles

The determinants of patient work for assisted cycles are in many ways similar to those of spontaneous cycles, but there are important differences. Apart from muscle strength, the key determinant of how much work is done during an assisted cycle is the patient's ventilatory drive. Drive is of central importance because the machine is sufficiently powerful to perform the entire work of chest inflation—were the patient able to relax immediately after triggering the cycle. Minute ventilation requirement ($\dot{V}_E$) and breathing discomfort are both important indirect determinants of W_B, because they influence drive. It is interesting to note that the impedance to inflation (chest compliance and airway resistance) does not influence the amount of work performed, so long as the inspiratory flow delivered from the machine exceeds the patient's spontaneous inspiratory demand. When delivered flows are sufficient, resistance changes within the patient's airway or the machine circuitry are met by increased pressure output from the ventilator, not by patient effort.

Having emphasized that ventilatory drive is the single most important determinant of the work performed by the patient during a machine-aided cycle, it follows that manipulation of certain machine settings can impressively influence W_B. The trigger sensitivity setting is one of these. The less sensitive the machine's activation threshold, the more work will be done per liter of ventilation during the inspiratory cycle. (In terms of percent, the effect of trigger threshold is most evident at lower levels of stress.) As already noted, the inspiratory flow setting of the ventilator can also make an important difference when it is set lower than the patient's spontaneous need for inspiratory flow. Under these circumstances the resistance of the patient and the machine circuit, as well as the compliance of the thorax, reemerge as important determinants of how much work is performed.

To my knowledge, no ventilator settings other than trigger sensitivity and flow have been systematically investigated in the clinical setting. However, on theoretic grounds, any factor that augments output of the ventilatory center may influence the work of breathing. Variations in V_T, flow profile, and positive end-expiratory pressure (PEEP) level may be important to the extent that they influence ventilatory drive. PEEP may also influence W_B when associated chest distention weakens the ability of the inspiratory muscles to perform external work, despite unchanging or increased oxygen consumption. Note that in this instance, metabolic and external mechanical measures of effort could lead to opposite conclusions regarding the impact of PEEP on patient effort. Conversely, if expiratory muscle activity prevents PEEP from recruiting lung volume, PEEP or continuous positive airway pressure (CPAP) may help to ventilate the lungs during the inspiratory cycle.

POTENTIAL IMPORTANCE OF THE WORK OF BREATHING DURING MECHANICAL VENTILATION

During spontaneous ventilation, the oxygen cost of breathing appears to be quite high in patients who require mechanical support. One study of patients with acute respiratory failure indicated that the oxygen cost of spontaneous breathing averaged approximately 25 percent of total body oxygen consumption, with occasional patients expending several times this amount. Such requirements represent at least a tenfold increase over the normal resting value. Consequently, if the ventilatory burden were alleviated, additional oxygen might be freed for delivery to other vital organ systems, provided that overall oxygen delivery remained unchanged. Experimental studies of animals placed into circulatory shock by pericardial tamponade seem to confirm this, thereby indicating a survival advantage for those receiving mechanical ventilation. Thus, it appears that when tissue oxygenation is compromised, mechanical ventilatory support may improve the overall matchup of oxygen delivery and demand.

A second major reason to be concerned about the work of breathing experienced by patients during mechanical ventilation is that it could impose a burden sufficient to prevent recovery from muscle fatigue. In such instances, reducing the inspiratory work of breathing during mechanical ventilation would become a central therapeutic focus necessary for expedient removal of machine support. At the present time, it is unclear to what extent the work of initiating the ventilator cycle contributes to ventilator dependence. However, from recent studies of active breathing effort during mechanical ventilation it seems likely that the level of muscle activity is at least sufficient to prevent disuse atrophy of ventilatory musculature.

Although the mechanical work of breathing is easily measured, it must be borne in mind that W_B correlates imprecisely with ventilation-associated oxygen consumption ($\dot{V}_{O_2}r$). These two values are interrelated via the expression: $W_B = \dot{V}_{O_2}r \times \epsilon$, where ϵ is the efficiency of converting consumed oxygen to useful mechanical work. External work may not reflect the tension developed by the muscle fibers in a straightforward way, particularly when loading conditions vary (as during synchronized intermittent mandatory ventilation [SIMV]). At the bedside, the product of the pressure developed by the muscles and the time over which it is generated (the pressure time product), may be a preferable index of effort under conditions of changing afterload.

MEASURES TO REDUCE THE WORK OF BREATHING DURING MECHANICAL VENTILATION

Breathing cycles during mechanical ventilation are of two essential types: spontaneous and machine-aided. The inspiratory work required for a spontaneous breath is influenced by the impedance for chest inflation and by the breathing pattern, as reflected in the depth, rate, and configuration of the pressure waveform. The potential for additional work imposed by the external apparatus to which the patient is connected has received (deservedly) a great deal of recent attention. An endotracheal tube presents resistance to gas flow in direct proportion to its length, and in inverse proportion to the fourth power of its radius when flow is laminar. Even when measured in a constant-flow experimental system the resistance of standard endotracheal tubes may exceed the total resistance of the normal respiratory system. Resistance increases dramatically when rapid flows move through tubes of narrow diameter. Thus, a first approach to minimizing the work of breathing is to ensure that the endotracheal tube is of adequate diameter and free of intraluminal kinks, constrictions, and adherent secretions. Nasotracheal tubes present greater resistance than do orotracheal tubes or tracheostomy tubes and are therefore less desirable when the goal is to minimize patient work of breathing. The use of pressure support and/or PEEP can help to offset the effort needed to overcome tube resistance.

Although it is common knowledge that endotracheal tubes present an important source of flow resistance, many practitioners remain unaware that the valving systems of the machinery they employ also affect the ease with which spontaneous breaths can be drawn through the circuit. Some demand-valve systems for delivering CPAP are slowly responsive and/or impose considerable resistance to ventilation once flow is established. On the inspiratory side, demand-valve resistance impacts the work of breathing during spontaneous cycles and during assisted machine cycles when the inspiratory flow demanded exceeds the set rate of flow delivery. As a general rule, continuous-flow systems seem less resistive than demand-flow systems, but there is some controversy on this point. Undoubtedly, there is considerable variance from manufacturer to manufacturer of ventilator equipment. Similar problems impact the expiratory work of breathing. The mushroom and scissor valves that gate exhalation offer considerable flow resistance, especially when PEEP is applied, thus adding to the total respiratory burden. For all of these reasons, many patients tolerate extubation more easily than low-level intermittent mandatory ventilation.

The mode chosen for ventilation support greatly influences the work of breathing. When all patient effort is silenced during controlled mechanical ventilation, no respiratory work is performed by the patient. Conversely, during CPAP breathing, each cycle is powered by spontaneous effort. Assisted mechanical ventilation (AMV) is the least energy consumptive of the modes that allow the patient to control the onset of the breathing cycle. Under normal circumstances, AMV appears to be about 25 to 50 percent as energy costly as fully spontaneous breathing, but the percentage can increase greatly during vigorous breath-

ing. During SIMV, the lowest levels of machine support are associated with the greatest breathing efforts.

Assuming that the machine, mode, endotracheal tube, flow and sensitivity settings are chosen appropriately, what specific measures should be taken to minimize WB during mechanical ventilation? (Table 2). For a start, the airway should be kept free of secretions. Secretions both obstruct the bronchial lumen and cause increased turbulence, thereby raising the pressure differential needed to drive flow. Such factors are almost inconsequential when the airway lumen is of normal size, but cause a marked increase in airway resistance in patients with endogenous airflow obstruction or those breathing through a narrow tube lumen. The patient should be positioned in such a way that elastance of the chest wall is minimized, i.e., sitting upright rather than supine, so that the hydrostatic forces of abdominal weight do not press on the underside of the diaphragm, thereby loading inspiration. If there is a component of reactive airways disease, bronchodilators should be used liberally, and modest doses of glucocorticoids may be helpful. Diuretics can be used to minimize the amount of lung water and improve lung compliance, especially in the setting of cardiogenic pulmonary edema. Large air pockets and fluid collections should be drained from the pleural space. If the goal is to minimize the respiratory workload, while allowing patient control of $\dot{V}E$, then AMV is most often the appropriate ventilatory mode. Trigger sensitivity should be minimized and inspiratory flow rate should be set at a level that exceeds the peak inspiratory flow demand of the patient—generally in the range of 60 to 80 L per minute. Above all, the patient should be made comfortable. For some patients this may mean adjusting the VT and peak inspiratory flow rate so that the inspiratory cycle lengths of patient and machine are synchronized. Such matching minimizes dyspnea and the attendant work. For this reason, pressure support ventilation may be preferrable to an equivalent level of SIMV in some patients.

In many patients, the single most important factor determining the patient's workload is the $\dot{V}E$ re-

TABLE 2 Reducing WB During Mechanical Ventilation

↓ $\dot{V}E$	Correct acidosis, fever, agitation, excessive deadspace
↓ Impedance	R: Address bronchospasm, secretions, endotracheal tube
	C: Administer diuretics, drain pleural space, position optimally
↓ Dyspnea	Improve patient-ventilator interactions
	Change to different ventilator mode
	Match inspiratory cycle length and rate of delivered flow to inspiratory flow demand
	Improve trigger sensitivity

quirement. Therefore, whatever steps can be taken to reduce $\dot{V}E$ (reduction in CO_2 output or physiologic deadspace) have a clear and immediate impact on total work. Any metabolic influence that increases CO_2 production is to be avoided. Specifically, the patient should be kept from becoming agitated or febrile; shivering, seizures, and myoclonus must be prevented. Analgesics, antipyretics, or sedatives may be needed to reduce agitation, drive, and workload. Although adequate nutrition is essential, patients must not be overfed or supported on a diet that has a high percentage of carbohydrate; (CO_2 production may increase in both of these circumstances). Deadspace can be minimized by shortening the length of tubing between the ventilator Y-piece and the endotracheal tube, by avoiding hypotension, overdiuresis, pulmonary embolism, and excessive PEEP.

In my own practice, I have often encouraged compensatory bicarbonate retention to allow $PaCO_2$ to increase without incurring acidemia. In this way, $\dot{V}E$ can be reduced, as each tidal exhalation vents a greater volume of the generated CO_2. Currently however, I am more cautious about adopting this strategy, since elevating $PaCO_2$ may simultaneously impair muscle function—at least when hypercarbia develops acutely. When judiciously applied, PEEP may improve lung compliance and dilate airways as lung volume is recruited, thereby reducing WB. Yet, hyperinflation must be avoided because it places the inspiratory musculature at a mechanical disadvantage, thus reducing the efficiency of the muscular pump in accomplishing external work. (PEEP may also increase deadspace and $\dot{V}E$). Therefore, there should be special awareness of the potential problems of the patient with decompensated airflow obstruction (CAO).

In the setting of CAO, reducing the $\dot{V}E$ requirement as well as the severity of airflow obstruction must be key goals. Many such patients have positive pressure continuously at the alveolar level, even when it is not applied intentionally. Not only does the resulting hyperinflation mechanically disadvantage the respiratory muscles, but also the associated "autoPEEP" (AP) effect increases the work of breathing and blunts the effective trigger sensitivity of the machine. To initiate inspiratory flow in the presence of AP, expiratory flow must first be stopped by counterbalancing the alveolar recoil pressure. This not only adds to the inspiratory work during spontaneous cycles, but also increases the pressure deflection needed to activate a machine-assisted cycle. The effective trigger sensitivity becomes the set value plus the level of autoPEEP. The AP level may be minimized by reducing $\dot{V}E$ requirement and by improving airflow obstruction. Some recent experimental data indicate that low levels of PEEP purposely added to the machine circuit may help to offset the inspiratory work requirement of autoPEEP, without markedly increasing end-inspiratory

pressures. This technique, although rational from a physiologic viewpoint, is still undergoing evaluation. PEEP should not be considered appropriate therapy for such patients until outcome data from a prospective trial become available.

COMPENSATING FOR AN INCREASED WORKLOAD

Because the ability to wean a patient from a mechanical ventilator depends upon restoration of balance between ventilatory demand and capability, it is important to attack both problems simultaneously. Although it is not the purpose of this chapter to discuss respiratory muscle function, a few points deserve emphasis. Muscle bulk should be improved by a nutritional program geared to maintain positive nitrogen balance. Whenever possible, the patient should be placed in a supported upright posture. Muscle strength and endurance are optimized by achieving the levels of hemoglobin, arterial oxygen tension, cardiac output, and electrolytes (Ca^{+2}, K^+, Mg^{+2}, PO_4^{-3}) vital to neuromuscular performance. Other measures are more controversial. Experimentally, theophylline and beta-adrenergic agents appear to marginally increase diaphragmatic contractility, whereas acute CO_2 retention has the opposite effect.

Few would argue with attempting to minimize respiratory effort during the initial phase of machine support for ventilatory failure. However, soon thereafter many physicians use IMV to withdraw support to the point of tolerance, hoping to keep the respiratory system exercising and strong. Yet, it has been cogently argued that patients who fail to wean from mechanical ventilation may be chronically on the verge of respiratory muscle fatigue. If so, adequate rest may be essential to their treatment. The correct approach has not been determined and may well vary from patient to patient. However, in the difficult-to-wean subject, alternating periods of nearly complete muscle rest (achieved by using AMV) with incremental periods of ventilatory stress (to exercise the system) would seem to be a strategy with a good rationale for allowing fatigued muscle to recover.

Suggested Reading

Field S, Kelly SM, Macklem PT. The oxygen cost of breathing in patients with cardiorespiratory disease. Am Rev Respir Dis 1982; 126:9–13.

Gibney RTN, Wilson RS, Pontoppidan H. Comparison of work of breathing on high gas flow and demand valve continuous positive airway pressure systems. Chest 1982; 82:692–694.

Katz JA, Kraemer RW, Gjerde GE. Inspiratory work and airway

Supported in part by Grant No. HL-19153 from the National Institutes of Health.

pressure with continuous positive airway pressure delivery systems. Chest 1985; 88:519–526.

Marini JJ, Capps JS, Culver BH. The inspiratory work of breathing during assisted mechanical ventilation. Chest 1985; 87:612–618.

Marini JJ, Rodriguez RM, Lamb VJ. Bedside estimation of the inspiratory work of breathing during mechanical ventilation. Chest 1986; 89:56–63.

Marini JJ, Rodriguez RM, Lamb VJ. The inspiratory workload of patient-initiated mechanical ventilation. Am Rev Respir Dis 1986; 134:902–909.

Marini JJ, Smith TC, Lamb VJ. Rapid estimation of the inspiratory work of breathing in ventilated patients. Am Rev Respir Dis 1986; 133:120(A).

Otis AM, Fenn WO, Rahn H. Mechanics of breathing in man. J Appl Physiol 1950; 2:592–607.

Pepe PE, Marini JJ. Occult positive end-expiratory pressure in mechanically ventilated patients with airflow obstruction. The auto-PEEP effect. Am Rev Respir Dis 1982; 126:166–170.

Peters RM. The energy cost (work) of breathing. Ann Thorac Surg 1969; 7:51–67.

Smith TC, Marini JJ, Lamb VJ. The effect of PEEP on auto-PEEP. Chest 1986; 89 (Suppl 22):443.

Viale JP, Annat G, Bertrand O, Ing D, Godard J, Motin J. Additional inspiratory work in intubated patients breathing with continuous positive airway pressure systems. Anesthesiology 1985; 63:536–539.

WEANING TECHNIQUES

LEONARD D. HUDSON, M.D.

The official definition of *wean* is "to accustom (a child or young animal) to food other than its mother's milk." The Random House Dictionary offers an additional meaning that is perhaps more apropos to mechanical ventilation: "to withdraw from some object, habit or form of enjoyment or the like." Weaning, whether from a mechanical or biological support system implies a gradual—not sudden—withdrawal. Most patients receiving mechanical ventilation do not require weaning, but rather can be removed abruptly once the reason for mechanical ventilatory support has abated.

No one method for the gradual weaning of a patient from mechanical ventilatory support in order to achieve total spontaneous ventilation is favored currently by experimental evidence (i.e., support of an appropriately controlled clinical study). The clinician must choose a method based on individual preference, experience, logic, and bias. The choice is further complicated by our limited understanding of the physiology of respiratory muscles and their training. Because respiratory muscle physiology is currently an area of great research interest, studies may soon provide us with new information that will more strongly support one method of weaning over another. Until then I recommend an empirical approach to weaning from mechanical ventilation.

The first consideration concerns the appropriateness of weaning: Is the patient ready, and is weaning necessary? If so, the weaning method must be determined and implemented and the process closely evaluated to ensure steady progress toward resumption of completely spontaneous breathing. If this goal is not accomplished within a reasonable period of time, then another method should be tried.

WHO NEEDS TO BE WEANED?

It is important to determine whether weaning as defined above is necessary. Most patients receiving mechanical ventilation do not require weaning. Once the reason for mechanical ventilation is resolved, the patient can be removed from mechanical ventilatory support in one step. Determining the proper timing for this sudden cessation of mechanical ventilatory support is particularly important. There are two aspects to this determination: (1) deciding whether the underlying disease processes have resolved or are improving and (2) obtaining evidence that the patient has enough respiratory muscle strength and reserve to maintain spontaneous ventilation.

Clinical evaluation of the underlying disease should include a review of the patient's symptoms and physical examination, arterial blood gases, and review of the chest roentgenograph. A history of the presence and degree of chronic respiratory disease is important. Patients with severe underlying chronic airflow obstruction or severe neuromuscular disease are most likely to require gradual weaning from mechanical ventilation. Other candidates for weaning include patients with acute lung injury that is healing with considerable destruction or scarring. Acute lung injury patients with a complicating nosocomial necrotizing pneumonia often fall into this category. Acute diffuse lung injury superimposed on chronic lung disease, especially chronic airflow obstruction, is another clinical circumstance in which weaning may be required.

Patients with respiratory muscle fatigue are often difficult to remove from mechanical ventilation. Respiratory muscle fatigue is manifested by three findings: (1) Rapid shallow respiration is the most common but is not specific for muscle fatigue. More specific but less sensitive are (2) paradoxical abdominal breathing and (3) respiratory alternans. During normal breathing the abdomen moves outward as the chest wall moves outward during inhalation. Paradoxical abdominal breathing is present if the abdominal wall moves inward on inhalation. Respiratory alternans consists of periods of almost total use of the diaphragm and abdominal muscles for breathing interspersed with periods of almost total use of the chest wall muscles for breathing. If these findings are present it is less likely that weaning from mechanical ventilation can be achieved. However, it should be kept in mind that one study has demonstrated paradoxical abdominal breathing in outpatients with severe chronic obstructive pulmonary disease (COPD) who are able to breathe spontaneously. Therefore, although these findings imply a poor prognosis for successful weaning, especially if they were not present prior to initiation of mechanical ventilation, they do not totally preclude a weaning attempt. However, they do indicate the need for careful clinical evaluation and judgement. Also, a period of total respiratory muscle rest should be considered.

Other aspects of the patient's clinical status should

be considered in addition to evaluation of the respiratory status. It is unlikely that the patient will be able to be successfully weaned from mechanical ventilation if he remains clinically septic or is hemodynamically unstable, even with improvement in the respiratory status.

Evidence of sufficient respiratory muscle strength and reserve to maintain spontaneous ventilation can be obtained by simple bedside measurements of pulmonary function and respiratory muscle function, commonly referred to as *ventilatory parameters*. These measurements commonly consist of the patient's spontaneous tidal volume (V_T), spontaneous vital capacity, and inspiratory effort as indicated by the negative airway pressure achieved with an inspiratory attempt during occlusion of the airway. The minute ventilation ($\dot{V}_E$) required during mechanical ventilatory support and the $\dot{V}_E$ during a brief period of spontaneous breathing are also important variables in making an appropriate clinical decision.

Measurement of $\dot{V}_E$ on mechanical ventilatory support with relation to this finding to the arterial P_{CO_2} gives an indication of the amount of ventilation required to maintain adequate CO_2 removal and avoid respiratory acidosis. If the $\dot{V}_E$ is greater than 20 L per minute it is unlikely that any but the strongest patient will be able to maintain this level of ventilation. On the other hand, if the minute ventilation is less than 10 L per minute and the negative inspiratory pressure is less than -25 cm H_2O, then it is very likely that the patient will be able to achieve this amount of ventilation indefinitely. Another important measurement during mechanical ventilation is that of arterial P_{O_2}, making sure that the arterial oxygen tension is adequate on a fraction of inspired oxygen (F_{IO_2}) that can be achieved easily during spontaneous ventilation by nasal prongs or face mask. If the patient is stable clinically with improvement in the underlying pulmonary disease and the tidal volume is greater than 5 ml per kilogram of body weight, vital capacity is greater than 10 ml per kilogram and negative inspiratory pressure is less than -25 cm H_2O, then the patient can nearly always maintain adequate spontaneous ventilation.

If these respiratory function variables are borderline, then measurement of maximal voluntary ventilation (MVV) may be helpful. A study by Sahn and Lakshminarayanan, one of the few to evaluate systematically the usefulness of spontaneous ventilatory parameters, tested whether adequate spontaneous ventilation could be predicted from the patient's resting minute ventilation and the ability to double this on an MVV maneuver in patients who met the other clinical criteria reviewed above. In this study, all patients who had a resting minute ventilation of less than 10 L per minute and were able to double their resting minute ventilation by an MVV maneuver, were able

to be successfully removed from mechanical ventilation. Some patients who did not meet these criteria were also able to be successfully removed from mechanical ventilation. Usually these patients had a minute ventilation that was only slightly greater than 10 L per minute or were not quite able to double their minute ventilation with an MVV effort. Also, all of these patients had a negative inspiratory pressure of greater than -20 cm H_2O. Sahn and Lakshminarayanan showed that often the patient with borderline values for these tests could more than double the resting minute ventilation during MVV once the endotracheal tube was removed, reflecting the increased airway resistance resulting from some artificial airways. Patients who did not achieve a negative inspiratory pressure of less than -20 cm H_2O were unsuccessful in breathing spontaneously when removed from mechanical ventilation.

If these simple bedside measurements demonstrate that the patient is extremely likely to be able to breathe spontaneously, then any method that results in a gradual reduction of ventilatory support is inappropriate. For example, the use of intermittent mandatory ventilation (IMV) rather than going directly to a T-piece trial could result only in the addition of unnecessary arterial blood gases. More importantly, it could prolong the period of mechanical ventilation by delaying the onset of spontaneous ventilation and thus continue to expose the patient to the risks of an artificial airway and mechanical ventilation.

Some have argued that sudden removal from mechanical ventilation represents an unnecessary "sink or swim" test for the patient and that gradual reduction of the mandatory rate on IMV is indicated in all patients. This does not seem logical, however, if it can be predicted by simple bedside tests that virtually all patients who pass such a test are able to "swim." In fact, it seems reasonable that there should be an occasional failure of direct removal from mechanical ventilation as judged by clinical evaluation and measurement of ventilatory parameters. A reasonable surgical analogy is evaluation of appendectomies. Unless an occasional negative appendix is found by the pathologist following appendectomy there will be some patients who actually have appendicitis but are not operated on. In this case, if everyone who is removed from mechanical ventilation succeeds then it suggests we may be keeping many patients on mechanical ventilation for an excessively long period, well past the time when they would be able to breathe spontaneously. Therefore, it is acceptable to try a patient with borderline measurements on spontaneous breathing by T-piece as long as the patient is carefully and appropriately evaluated. This practice should not result in an untoward clinical result, because any patient in this condition should be in an intensive care unit where close monitoring by respiratory therapy and nursing staff can be accomplished.

AVAILABLE METHODS FOR WEANING FROM MECHANICAL VENTILATION

Three ventilatory methods are commonly used for weaning from mechanical ventilation: (1) IMV with a gradual reduction in the rate of mandatory breaths; (2) pressure-support ventilation (PSV) with a gradual reduction in the amount of pressure used to augment spontaneous ventilation; and (3) intermittent T-piece trials (spontaneous breathing) with ventilatory muscle rest between the periods of spontaneous ventilation.

Intermittent Mandatory Ventilation

IMV was first described as a method of weaning from mechanical ventilation. For this use the mandatory breathing rate should be gradually decreased with clinical evaluation carried out with each rate reduction as well as periodic arterial blood gas measurements. The mandatory rate should be reduced as rapidly as the patient can clinically tolerate. In the patient who truly requires a weaning method, this reduction rate is usually relatively slow, being one to four breaths per day depending on the clinical situation and the initial mandatory rate.

Pressure-Support Ventilation

PSV is a relatively new method of ventilation in terms of widespread availability and practical use. PSV allows the ability to augment spontaneous breaths with a variable amount of inspiratory positive pressure. The level of positive pressure is preset. When the patient begins a spontaneous breath, the inspiratory pressure rapidly rises to the preset level (as opposed to the relatively slow rise with intermittent positive pressure ventilation delivered by older pressure-cycled ventilators, a form of ventilation with which PSV is often confused). The inspiratory flow rate capabilities are very high. The signal that terminates the positive inspiratory pressure varies from machine to machine but often is a fall in inspiratory flow to 25 percent of the peak value. The patient has control of the ventilatory rate and the inspiratory assist time and can interact with the set inspiratory pressure to determine the inspiratory flow and the delivered tidal volume. One of the main advantages appears to be an improvement in patient comfort, perhaps related to the degree of patient control and the high inspiratory flow capabilities.

PSV allows control of the amount of work of breathing done by the patient versus that done by the ventilator. The inspiratory pressure assist level can be set such that nearly all of the inspiratory work is done by the machine. If the pressure level is gradually lowered, the amount of work done by the patient will progressively increase.

Intermittent Spontaneous Breathing (T-piece Trials)

In intermittent spontaneous breathing the patient is removed from mechanical ventilation for short periods while breathing through a T-piece with a high flow of oxygen mixture. This is followed by a longer period of nearly total respiratory muscle rest by mechanical ventilatory support, usually in the assist-control mode. The time period of spontaneous breathing necessary to result in training and the length of rest necessary to recover from muscle fatigue are unknown. The patient usually breathes spontaneously for approximately 15 minutes initially and this is repeated two to four times per day. The spontaneous breathing periods are then gradually lengthened as tolerated by the patient.

RESPIRATORY MUSCLE TRAINING

Whether one of the above methods is more appropriate than the others depends on the type of training regimen to which respiratory muscles best respond. Some respiratory muscle physiologists argue that it is necessary to work the respiratory muscles to the point of fatigue and then allow recovery from fatigue in order to achieve a training effect. This would best be accomplished by intermittent T-piece trials with rest between the periods of spontaneous ventilation. These investigators argue that IMV (1) does not cause muscle fatigue and so training is not achieved (or, if it does, it is not being appropriately used) but (2) also never allows complete rest of the respiratory muscles with a chance for total recovery.

Other workers in this area believe that respiratory muscles are endurance muscles and so need to be trained more as a distance runner than a sprinter. This approach consists of lower-level exercise over much longer periods to achieve improvement in endurance as a goal of training. Under this philosophy, partial assumption of the work load makes most sense. This reasoning favors use of the PSV or IMV method of weaning. More information is needed to distinguish which of these practice philosophies actually carries more physiologic benefit to the patient. Other important questions deal with disuse atrophy and its prevention: Does a prolonged period of complete rest result in atrophy of the respiratory muscles, and if so, do IMV or PSV methods of ventilatory support prevent such muscle atrophy? Also, if disuse atrophy does occur, what period of complete muscle rest is required before it becomes clinically important? Obviously, the answers to these questions will have an important effect on clinical practice.

FACTORS OTHER THAN THE STATE OF RESPIRATORY MUSCLES

Several factors besides the state of the respiratory muscles are of prime importance in choosing an optimal time for attempted weaning. The underlying pulmonary disease state is of special concern. Improvement in the underlying condition for which the patient was ventilated should be apparent before weaning is attempted. An optimal bronchodilator regimen should be in place for the patient with airflow obstruction.

Nonpulmonary clinical factors are also important. Continuing sepsis and hemodynamic instability have already been discussed. The nutritional state of the patient and the nutritional support being given can influence weaning. Chronic malnutrition can lead to muscle weakness. Excessive calorie intake, on the other hand, results in increased CO_2 production ($\dot{V}CO_2$) and increased ventilatory requirements. This is especially true if the nutritional intake is heavy in carbohydrates. An increase in carbohydrates relative to fats and proteins results in an increased respiratory quotient (ratio of $\dot{V}CO_2$ to oxygen consumption) and thus a higher $\dot{V}CO_2$ for a given amount of calories. If $\dot{V}CO_2$ increases, a greater $\dot{V}E$ is required to maintain the same arterial PCO_2. Failure to wean could result from an increase in $\dot{V}E$ in a patient with limited pulmonary function, and several clinical papers have strongly suggested that respiratory failure can either result from or be increased in degree by this mechanism. Although nutrition can contribute to respiratory failure, it is my belief that this problem has been overemphasized. The decision for the level of nutritional support and the nutritional constituents should be based on other factors until this has been demonstrated to be a problem in the weaning process. Nutritional support should not be changed on this basis until the patient is actually ready to be weaned and then only after failure of progressive weaning has been demonstrated. Once weaning has started, if it does not progress in a satisfactory fashion, the level and type of nutrition should be evaluated. This problem usually can be handled simply by decreasing the total caloric intake, although the composition of the nutrition may also have to be changed.

The psychological state of the patient is critical to successful weaning. The patient must be properly prepared for weaning attempts. A positive approach with realistic goals for the patient is important and a consistent approach to the patient must be assured. The entire team involved in the weaning effort, including physicians, respiratory therapists, and nurses as well as family members and social workers who are involved in the patient's care, need to be aware of the goals and methods of weaning. For example, in the patient receiving intermittent T-piece trials it should be recognized that there may be times when the T-piece trial has to be aborted because of patient discomfort or for other reasons. An occasional problem such as this should be anticipated and should not be viewed as a significant setback in the patient's weaning process. Rather the goal should be viewed over the long term as steady progress toward complete weaning from the ventilator.

HOW TO CARRY OUT WEANING: THE PROCESS

The first step in the weaning process is deciding whether weaning is appropriate and timely. A current history and physical examination and laboratory records should be reviewed to evaluate the need for ventilation. This evaluation should include a review of the minute ventilation on and, for a brief period, off of the ventilator and the accompanying blood gases; discussion of any intermittent changes in the patient's respiratory status and respiratory needs with the respiratory therapists and nurses; review of nutritional status and current nutritional support; and measurement of ventilatory parameters. This evaluation should allow a decision on whether the patient is a candidate for sudden removal from mechanical ventilation. If it is thought that this is likely to be successful (or if the patient is borderline in this regard), then a T-piece trial should be attempted. If the patient remains comfortable for 15 to 30 minutes breathing an air-oxygen mixture that can be achieved by nasal or face mask oxygen administration and the arterial blood gases remain acceptable, then the patient should be removed from mechanical ventilation and the endotracheal tube removed. Longer T-piece trials in this clinical situation are not warranted because they place the patient at a disadvantage owing to the added airway resistance from the endotracheal tube. If a tracheostomy tube is in place, oxygen supplementation by tracheostomy mask should be initiated.

The weaning plan should be developed if it is decided that the patient is not likely to be successful in abrupt withdrawal from mechanical ventilatory support. A sample plan for weaning is discussed below. Once a plan has been established it should be explained to everyone involved in the weaning process. The patient should be strongly encouraged in the plan, and all team members should be supportive. It should be emphasized to the patient that the initial method of weaning is not the only available option. If the possibility of other methods has been appropriately discussed, the patient may not be as discouraged if the first weaning method is not immediately successful.

What is a reasonable plan for weaning? In the past several years I have often used IMV with a progressive reduction in the mandatory rate as the initial weaning attempt, mainly because of the ease of applying this method. If no progress in weaning was achieved over a relatively short period of time such as 2 to 3 days, then the weaning method was changed to that of intermittent T-piece trials. I have since modified this weaning approach because of increasing experience with the PSV method. The advantages of PSV are that (1) it allows regulation of the amount of work of breathing by the patient and (2) it offers improvement in patient comfort. The enhanced comfort seems to be particularly significant.

Because of this advantage in patient comfort, I currently start with PSV in a patient who is thought to be difficult to wean. I start with a level of inspiratory PSV adequate to supply essentially all of the ventilatory demands of the patient. This level is progressively decreased relatively rapidly so that the patient takes on more and more of the active work of breathing. It is important to evaluate continually whether the patient is clinically tolerating the level of spontaneous breathing work.

If there is no improvement after a few days of PSV or if it appears that progress has stalled, I proceed to intermittent T-piece trials. The short periods of spontaneous breathing often result in fatigue and are followed by longer periods of rest in which recovery from muscle fatigue occurs. These rest periods may be very important in the weaning process. We previously thought that the assist-control mode of mechanical ventilation in which the patient consistently triggers the ventilator breaths resulted in almost total rest of the respiratory muscles, because apparently the only work required was that to create a small negative inspiratory pressure, which would then trigger active delivery of a ventilator breath. It has recently been shown, however, that some patients continue to inhale actively using their respiratory muscles during assist-control breathing, even when the ventilator is delivering the breath. The inspiratory flow rate is an important variable in this regard in that patients receiving a slow inspiratory flow rate have a greater tendency to inhale actively throughout inspiration. Careful observation of the patient during mechanical ventilation usually discloses whether this active inspiratory work is occurring with the assist-control mode. Studies I have carried out measuring CO_2 production as an indication of work suggest that on the average assist-control still results in less work by the patient than IMV with a mandatory rate half that of the assist-control mode.

This weaning plan occasionally fails and complete spontaneous ventilation is not achieved, despite the best efforts of the respiratory management team. If this occurs, then a thorough reevaluation should be carried out to see if anything can be changed that will increase the patient's advantage. Possible measures that may ultimately result in successful weaning include increasing muscle strength by better nutritional support while total mechanical ventilatory support is being carried out or reducing the CO_2 production by nutritional management changes during weaning attempts. Hypophosphatemia as a cause of muscle weakness should be considered. Inadequate nutrition (semistarvation) can be a cause of reduced drive to ventilation. The patient's underlying disease status, both pulmonary and nonpulmonary, should be carefully reviewed to see if any pharmacologic changes will result in patient improvement. If none of the patient's problems is subject to remedial therapy, then a plan should be developed for continued ventilatory support at home or in an extended care facility. It is important periodically to reevaluate the patient who is discharged from the hospital on continuous mechanical support. Occasionally patients, including those with severe neuromuscular problems that are thought to be stable, have enough improvement that they can eventually be removed from mechanical ventilation. Another option is available for the patient who is able to stay off the ventilator for an extended period of time during the day but who then tires and requires mechanical ventilation overnight. The so-called wrap ventilator, a new portable version of a negative pressure ventilator using the principle of the old cuirass ventilator, has been developed and appears to be ideal for overnight ventilation.

PERSPECTUS

Information about training respiratory muscles currently is in a state of flux. This type of information is critical for making decisions about the optimal methods of weaning patients from mechanical ventilation. At the present time, the selection of weaning method and its application is largely empirical. However, there is no substitute for careful clinical evaluation and monitoring. It first should be determined whether the patient actually needs to be gradually weaned from mechanical ventilation or whether abrupt removal is appropriate. Adequate ventilatory parameter measurements usually allow prediction of successful removal from mechanical ventilation with a high degree of certainty, after the underlying pulmonary and cardiovascular states that led to the need for mechanical ventilation have stabilized. A weaning method should be chosen empirically if it is determined that initiation of the weaning process is appropriate. Available methods include PSV, IMV, and intermittent T-piece trials interspersed with rest periods. A recommended plan is to begin with PSV with progressive reduction in the amount of pressure used or IMV with progressive steady reduction in the mandatory rate. If these methods do not result in progressive weaning over a 2- to 3-day period, then intermittent T-piece trials should be substituted as the weaning method. Important factors in weaning success include optimal therapy of the underlying disease states, appropriate decisions regarding nutritional support, careful psychological preparation of the patient for the weaning process, a consistent and optimistic approach to weaning by all members of the team, and continuing evaluation of weaning progress and any confounding factors or complications. A plan for home ventilation should be developed for the occasional patient who cannot be weaned from mechanical ventilation, with periodic reevalution of the need for ventilatory support.

Suggested Reading

Aubier M, Murciano D, Lecocguic Y, et al. Effect of hypophosphatemia on diaphragmatic contractility in patients with acute respiratory failure. N Engl J Med 1985; 313:420–424.

Cohen CA, Zagelbaum G, Gross D, Roussos C, Macklem PT. Clinical manifestations of inspiratory muscle fatigue. Am J Med 1982; 73:308–316.

Gilbert R, Auchincloss JH Jr, Peppi D, Ashutosh K. The first few hours off a respirator. Chest 1974; 65:152–157.

Jung RC. Weaning criteria for patients on mechanical respiratory assistance. West J Med 1979; 131:49–55.

Klein EF Jr. Weaning from mechanical breathing with intermittent mandatory ventilation. Arch Surg 1975; 110:345–347.

Morganroth ML, Morganroth JL, Nett LM, Petty TL. Criteria for weaning from prolonged mechanical ventilation. Arch Intern Med 1984; 144:1012–1016.

Pierson DJ. Weaning from mechanical ventilation. Respir Care 1983; 28:646–662.

Sahn SA, Lakshminarayan S. Bedside criteria for discontinuation of mechanical ventilation. Chest 1973; 63:1002–1005.

Sahn SA, Lakshminarayan S, Petty TL. Weaning from mechanical ventilation. JAMA 1976; 235:2208–2212.

Williams MH Jr. IMV and weaning. Chest 1980; 78:804–810.

NUTRITIONAL CONSIDERATIONS IN RESPIRATORY FAILURE

MARCIA S. KEMPER, B.A., CRTT
JEFFREY ASKANAZI, M.D.

The relationship between nutrition and respiratory failure is well established. As has frequently been stated in the literature, starvation is often respiratory in origin.

MALNUTRITION DEVELOPMENT IN PATIENTS WITH RESPIRATORY DISEASE

Malnutrition and semistarvation occur in many disease states, including some respiratory diseases. The patient diagnosed with chronic obstructive pulmonary disease (COPD) frequently suffers from accompanying malnutrition. One mechanism by which malnutrition may develop is an increased metabolic rate resulting from the disease process. An increased resistance to airway gas flow and a reduced respiratory muscle efficiency cause work of breathing to increase in COPD patients. This increased work of breathing leads to an increased caloric demand. Failure to meet the increased caloric needs by altering an established eating pattern results in chronic nutritional depletion. Any disease state that can cause an increase in metabolic rate that is not met with increased caloric intake can ultimately cause malnutrition and accompanying respiratory failure.

MALNUTRITION AND PREDISPOSITION TO RESPIRATORY FAILURE

The mechanism by which malnutrition may predispose to respiratory failure is only partially understood. When caloric needs are not met, the body catabolizes tissue to provide protein, which in turn is converted to glucose, an obligatory fuel for the central nervous system. Adipose tissue is mobilized for free fatty acids to be used as fuel for the peripheral tissues. Earlier literature reported that vital organs that sustain life, such as the heart and diaphragm, were spared from the catabolic process during starvation. Recent studies have shown that this is not true. The muscles of respiration and the heart are subject to the same catabolic process, to the same degree, as are skeletal muscles. This chronic catabolic process results in weakened respiratory musculature that may rapidly fatigue and deteriorate to respiratory failure, particularly if an acute process intervenes.

MALNUTRITION AND PROLONGATION OF RESPIRATORY FAILURE

When respiratory failure presents as a consequence of malnutrition, recovery can be protracted. The repletion of weak and fatigued muscles is a slow process. Furthermore, body systems depleted of protein stores are unable adequately to incorporate large infusions of nutrients. Massive repletion efforts have been associated with cardiopulmonary dysfunction and death and hence must be avoided. Cardiac muscle compromised by malnutrition is unable to increase cardiac output to the level necessary to handle any larger increase in volume load. When the heart is forced to pump a volume load that is beyond its capabilities, failure may result. Refeeding the severely depleted patient requires a nutrient intake that exceeds resting energy expenditure only by moderate amounts. More concentrated solutions can supply the required calories and reduce the volume of infusion; hence, nutrients such as a 20 percent dextrose solution and a 20 percent solution of lipid instead of 10 percent solutions are useful.

EVALUATION OF THE NUTRITIONAL STATE

The initial clinical observation of the patient's physical appearance should contribute to any tests or measurements in assessing the nutritional status. The loss of subcutaneous fat with bony protrusion represents malnutrition. An early manifestation of nutritional depletion is an expansion of the extracellular fluid compartment (ECF). Because of this third space expansion, nutritional assessment is separated into an assessment prior to nutritional support and an assessment during administration of adequate nutritional support.

The intensive care unit (ICU) patient who is not receiving adequate nutrition remains particularly difficult to evaluate, because disease states and therapies alter normal physiologic events. A 15 percent loss of body weight is an accepted guideline for nutritional depletion. Knowing body weight and comparing it against predictive tables is a commonly accepted form of evaluating weight loss. However, in the ICU, patients present with a range of problems from severe dehydration to excessive fluid overload. Altered fluid volumes make actual current body weight difficult to assess. A reliable pre-illness body weight may also be difficult to obtain from the relatives. Predictive table weights from measured heights actually vary 20 percent from the mean. All this makes a 15 percent loss of body weight a difficult assessment in the ICU. By the same token, skin fold thickness is not a useful measurement.

Plasma protein measurement, a primary means of assessing nutritional status in normal patients, may have low values owing to an expansion of the ECF space that may be due to either malnutrition or an underlying disease process. The creatinine–height index is useful only in patients with properly functioning kidneys, without sepsis or trauma, and who are not receiving steroids. The maximal inspiratory pressure measurement (PImax) is useful to determine respiratory muscle strength but may be affected by chronic lung disease. A PImax of at least -20 cm H_2O should be generated to demonstrate adequate inspiratory strength.

As the above problems indicate, the means available for determining malnutrition in the normal individual are not applicable to the critically ill patient. It is unwise to let the clinical observation of obvious wasting occur before initiating nutrition, because repletion is a very slow process. Thus, we are left with the clinical judgment of whether the patient will be able to eat within the week or whether there are clear indications of wasting that justify initiating nutrition in the critically ill. When it is clear that a patient will not be able to eat, nutritional support as early as possible is of benefit.

The nutritional state of a patient receiving full nutritional support can be judged by assessing the ECF. When, during the course of nutrition, the ECF compartment contracts and a weight loss due to diuresis is experienced, a normal nutritional status has been achieved. Until the loss of third space fluid is observed in the depleted patient, normal nutritional status has not been achieved. It is the diuresis, with its accompanying weight loss, that is the indication of a successful nutritional support regime. The contraction of the ECF compartment can take weeks of adequate nutritional coverage to achieve in the depleted patient.

INITIATION OF NUTRITIONAL SUPPORT

Nutritional support of the depleted patient must be instituted as early in the disease process as possible. For ICU patients, nutritional support should be started as soon as it is clear that they will not be able to eat within a week. Nutritional support in any form becomes progressively less effective as the severity of the stress response increases. If supportive therapy is to benefit the patient maximally, it must be started as early as possible. Knowledge of the proper number of calories to administer is critically important. Semistarvation or gross overfeeding are stresses in themselves. The resting energy expenditure (REE) equation can provide the number of calories an individual will burn in 24 hours if he or she remains completely at rest. Because patients do not remain at rest but are subjected to therapies, additional calories must be added to the REE to cover the caloric needs of patient activity. ICU studies have shown that the mean total energy expenditure in the critically ill for a 24-hour period is 5 percent above the REE, and that the day-to-day variability of the REE is 15 percent. Thus, the surgical ICU patient requires an additional 20 percent calories above the REE per day to meet nutritional needs.

Predictive equations for determining the REE are available but are unreliable in the critically ill. Fluid overload and severe nutritional depletion are some of the problems that can deviate predictive values from 70 percent to 140 percent of the true value. Actual bedside measurement of the critically ill patient's metabolic rate is the best way of determining the individual patient's REE. The accuracy of equipment must be validated for use in the ICU and properly calibrated. The patient should be awake, motionless, and undisturbed for 20 minutes before the REE is determined.

ROUTE OF NUTRITIONAL SUPPORT ADMINISTRATION

The most appropriate route of delivery for nutritional support in an individual patient is based on clinical assessment (Table 1). Routes available include enteral, central vein, peripheral vein, and a combination of enteral and central vein or enteral and peripheral vein. Enteral nutrition is preferable to the use of central or peripheral vein catheters whenever possible because it uses the gut, is the cheapest form of nutrition, and is the least invasive. If the patient's gut is working, enteral solutions can be used. The primary problems with enteral solutions are that most contain over 50 percent carbohydrates and they create a full stomach. Also, rapidly delivered enteral solutions in nutritionally depleted patients can cause diarrhea owing to atrophy of the gut and reduced enzyme activity. In malnourished patients, enteral solutions are often initiated at slow infusion rates and at less than full strength. If diarrhea presents, the enteral solutions should be stopped until the diarrhea subsides and then restarted at a lower rate. Use of less than full-strength solutions, slow start-up rates, and frequent stopping and starting because of diarrhea prevent immediate, full nutritional coverage. Only as patients tolerate gradually increasing rates of administration at more concentrated levels, without diar-

TABLE 1   Routes of Administration for Nutritional Support

	Indications	Advantages	Disadvantages	Limits	Hazards
Enteral	A working gastrointestinal tract	Line placement is easier than a central venous catheter placement	Full nutritional coverage may take up to 2 weeks to achieve	Full absorption of nutrients not assured	Increased risk of aspiration because the stomach always has solution in it
		Many types of solutions to choose from	Poor absorption of nutrients when sepsis present		Feeding lines can end up in the trachea
		Uses the gastrointestinal tract	Must be stopped for various diagnostic tests		Errors in types of solution to give certain patients
			The feeding lines kink and clot off		Diarrhea
			Can cause diarrhea		
Central venous	A nonworking gastrointestinal tract	Full nutritional support can be achieved on day of catheter insertion	Infusion line placement is highly invasive	Nutrient solution supports sepsis	Line or solution sepsis
	A need for full nutritional support immediately	The nutritional components solution can be manipulated without trauma to vessels	Lines can become septic		
	A need to minimize stool	Adjustment of solution components is easy	Blood sugar can rise requiring insulin therapy		
Peripheral venous	A nonworking gastrointestinal tract	Less invasive than the central catheter, therefore easier to start nutrition	Nutritional solution is caustic to peripheral veins	The patient must tolerate large volume loads	Insertion site or solution sepsis, fluid volume overload
	A supplement to enteral		Very large volumes are needed for full nutritional support		
	An alternative to central line placement		The intravenous site must be changed every 4 days		

rhea, can the strength of the solution be increased and the number of calories provided be brought up to 1.20 × REE. Full caloric coverage with enteral solutions in the ICU may take up to 2 weeks, or longer if diarrhea persists. Patients with pressing nutritional needs should not be started on enteral feeding if the goal is that the nutritional needs be met soon. Also, with enteral solutions, the amount of carbohydrate included may be over 50 percent of the solution. As many reports have shown, giving patients nutritional support high in carbohydrates produces large increases in CO_2 production. Critically ill, nonmechanically ventilated patients should not be subjected to the increased ventilatory requirements caused by higher CO_2 loads.

Unless patients are ventilator dependent and an increase in minute ventilation ($\dot{V}E$) can be effected mechanically, these increased ventilatory loads should not be added. Patients being weaned from mechanical ventilation who are subjected to large additional CO_2 loads frequently fail to wean. Finally, enteral solutions are usually administered directly into the stomach, although sometimes they are dripped into the duodenum. Patients with aspiration syndromes can be at risk with a full stomach. Patients with continuous infusions of foodstuffs must have the endotracheal tube cuff inflated at all times, the head of the bed elevated 30 degrees, and their sputum observed for color and consistency similar to those of the enteral solutions.

Central venous catheters provide an excellent route for total parenteral nutrition (TPN), but certain factors must be considered. For patients who already have had a number of invasive procedures, adding one more may be met with resistance. Sepsis from the peri-infusion site may occur and must be closely monitored. Also, TPN is more costly than enteral solutions. Pending those problems, central venous catheterization is an excellent way to begin immediate coverage of $1.20 \times$ REE to the ICU patient.

In patients who can tolerate enteral nutrition but need full caloric coverage immediately, a combination of central venous catheter and the enteral route may be effected. The enteral route can then be initiated very slowly so as not to cause problems with diarrhea. The central route can be adjusted to supply the remaining calories to achieve $1.20 \times$ REE. The parenteral route is then tapered as enteral administration is increased. The central line can be discontinued as soon as enteral feeding reaches the desired caloric level and there are no problems with diarrhea. With this method, full nutrition is achieved early and the gut is used to its maximum capabilities.

Peripheral parenteral nutrition (PPN) is infused via a peripheral vein. This route is generally not used in the ICU, because PPN solutions are very dilute and thus require large volumes to achieve REE. The solution is necessarily dilute so as to be tolerated by peripheral vessels.

Traditionally, TPN and PPN were administered with the carbohydrates and amino acids in one container and the lipid in a second container. The lipid was then piggybacked into the carbohydrate-amino acid solution. The hypertonicity of the carbohydrate and amino acid solution was thus reduced to near isotonic by the addition of the lipid solution and well tolerated by the vein. However, lipids were generally administered over a 12-hour period, while carbohydrates-amino acids were administered over 24 hours. Recently, all three nutritional components—carbohydrates, amino acids, and lipids—have been mixed together in one bag. This is called the three-in-one system of administering nutrients and is much better

tolerated by the vein than the two-container system. With the three-in-one infusion system, inflammation may be a result of the venous cannulation or the solution itself. The PPN infusion site must be changed every 4 days as a matter of protocol to prevent gross irritation or breakdown of the peri-infusion site. PPN solutions are generally used for short-term nutritional supplementation of 3 weeks or less. If fluid volume is not a problem and the patient's gastrointestinal tract can be used, PPN can be used to supplement enteral feedings until the enteral nutritional support is at full strength and full nutritional coverage.

DETERMINATION OF THE COMPOSITION OF HYPERALIMENTATION FLUIDS FOR PATIENTS WITH RESPIRATORY FAILURE

The composition of TPN for patients with respiratory failure has been specifically defined (Table 2). All three nutritional components are included in specific amounts. Because amino acids drive the respiratory system, the amino acid component is kept at 20 percent of the TPN solution. The provision of 1.0 to 1.5 g per kilogram body weight per day of a balanced amino acid mixture is normally used. Of the remaining 80 percent of the caloric intake, approximately 40 percent should be given as fat and 40 percent as carbohydrates. Supplying one-half the nonprotein calories as fat keeps the metabolized carbohydrate (CO_2) load as low as possible but still provides adequate carbohydrate volume (Fig. 1). Fats are an excellent source of calories for the patient with respiratory compromise, because they provide fuel for the body but do not produce increased CO_2 loads or drive the respiratory system. However, fats should not exceed 3 g per kilogram because alveolar-capillary diffusion problems have been noted above this level.

ALIMENTATION OF THE DIFFICULT-TO-WEAN PATIENT

Alimenting the difficult-to-wean ICU patient can be done successfully if close attention is paid to metabolic and respiratory parameters. Nutritional support must begin as early as possible. It is best actually to measure the REE, because narcotics, beta-blockers, inotropic drugs, and other factors may affect the metabolic rate, rendering predictive equations of limited value. Third space volume does not affect metabolic rate but does contribute to body weight, also affecting predictive tables. Because it is possible to overfeed and stress the system or underfeed and semistarve the patient, a measured value is the best way to determine how many calories to give an ICU patient. Also, because the measured metabolic rate includes increases or decreases in the metabolic rate, correction factors do not have to be considered.

TABLE 2   Recommended Amounts and Effects of the Administration of Amino Acids, Carbohydrates, and Lipids

Nutrient	Hazards	Recommended Amount
Amino acids	Increase respiratory drive	1.0–1.5 g/kg/day equalling 20% of TPN solution
Carbohydrates	Produce high resting levels of carbon dioxide, which manifests in increased $\dot{V}E$	4–5 mg/kg, not exceeding 6 mg/kg/min
Lipids	May enhance $\dot{V}O_2$ in hypermetabolism	Should account for 40% of a TPN solution
	May cause temporary hyperlipidemia	1–2 g/kg/day, equalling 40% of the TPN solution
	May cause O_2 diffusion problems	

One-half of the nonprotein calories must be given as fat in the diet of the difficult-to-wean patient. Any diet high in carbohydrates produces excessive CO_2 and compromises weaning. It is very useful to know resting $\dot{V}E$ before and one day after instituting nutri-

EFFECT OF GLUCOSE INTAKE ON THE $\dot{V}E$ – $\dot{V}CO_2$ RELATIONSHIP

(Mean ± SEM)

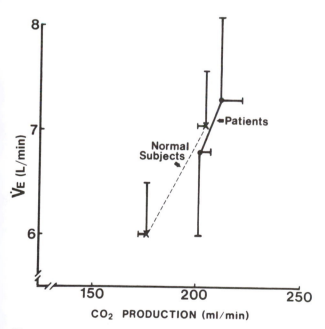

Figure 1 Relationship of minute ventilation to endogenous CO_2 production. With increasing glucose intake, the rise in CO_2 production is accompanied by a parallel increase in $\dot{V}E$. (From Rodriguez JL, Askanazi J, Weissman C, et al. Ventilatory and metabolic effects of glucose infusions. Chest 1985; 88:512–518.)

tional support. If a resting $\dot{V}E$ can be obtained before alimenting and compared to the resting $\dot{V}E$ during full $1.20 \times$ REE, the clinician will know the amount of $\dot{V}E$ caused by the feeding program. It is not unusual to find the $\dot{V}E$ doubled on many forms of enteral nutrition, most of which are 55 percent carbohydrate, and on TPN solutions in which more than 50 percent of the nonprotein calories are carbohydrates. Switching the patient to a diet in which 40 percent of the nonprotein calories are fat can significantly reduce required $\dot{V}E$. There are commercially available enteral solutions high in fat for use in the difficult-to-wean patient whose gut can be used.

The PaO_2, $PaCO_2$, and respiratory rate (RR) are also important parameters to follow before and during nutritional support. The PaO_2 should not fall with the onset of nutrition. The $PaCO_2$ and RR should not rise significantly with the onset of nutritional support. If the $PaCO_2$ rises with no increase in respiratory rate, the patient has a poor response to CO_2 and will be unable to handle the additional CO_2 load the nutrition demands. If the patient is on a ventilator the $\dot{V}E$ will have to be increased to keep the $PaCO_2$ within normal limits. If the $PaCO_2$ is unchanged but the RR rises, the patient is coping with the additional CO_2 load. If the $PaCO_2$ rises with a commensurate rise in the respiratory rate, the patient is trying but unable to cope with the additional CO_2 demands and is likely to develop respiratory failure. If neither the $PaCO_2$ nor RR rises, the nutrition has not added significant amounts of CO_2 to the system and there need be no worry about coping. These patients should be reassessed if their nutritional coverage is increased.

RESPIRATORY HAZARDS OF HYPERALIMENTATION

The respiratory hazards of TPN should be well known by clinicians caring for patients in respiratory failure. These hazards should be remembered and watched for when initiating nutrition. Proteins drive the ventilatory system and should be provided at 1.0 to 1.5 g per kilogram per day balanced amino acids, and not used as a caloric source. Carbohydrates increase V_{CO_2} and drive the metabolic system; consequently, no more than one-half of the nonprotein calories should be carbohydrate. Fats are an excellent source of calories that have minimal impact on the respiratory system; however, excesses should be avoided. TPN solutions should be concentrated from 10 percent to 20 percent dextrose and lipid concentration when fluid volume overload is a danger.

Suggested Reading

Arora NS, Rochester DF. Effects of general nutritional muscular states on the human diaphragm. Am Rev Respir Dis 1977; 115:84–89.

Askanazi J. Principles of nutritional support. Am Soc Anesthesiologists. Philadelphia: JB Lippincott, 1986:14.

Askanazi J, Rosenbaum SM, Hyman AI, et al. Respiratory changes induced by the large glucose loads of total parenteral nutrition. JAMA 1980; 243:1444–1447.

Askanazi J, Weissman C, LaSala PA, Charlesworth P. Nutrients and ventilation. Adv Shock Res 1983; 9:69–79.

Baker JP, Lemoyne M. Crit Care Clin 1987; 3(1).

Dmochowski JR, Moore FD. Choroba glodowa. N Engl J Med 1975; 293:356–357.

Keys AB, Brozck J, Henschel A, et al. Biology of human starvation. Minneapolis: University of Minnesota Press, 1950.

Rodriguez JL, Askanazi J, Weissman C, et al. Ventilatory and metabolic effects of glucose infusions. Chest 1985; 88:512–518.

Starker PM, LaSala PA, Askanazi J, et al. The response to TPN: a form of nutritional assessment. Ann Surg 1983; 198:720–724.

Vandenberg E, Van de Woestijne KP, Gyselen A. Weight changes in the terminal stages of chronic obstructive pulmonary disease; relation to respiratory function and prognosis. Am Rev Respir Dis 1978; 95:556–566.

Weissman C, Kemper M, Askanazi J, Hyman AI, Kinnery JM. Resting metabolic rate of the critically ill patient: measured vs. predicted. Anesthesiology 1986; 64:673–679.

ANESTHETIC AND PARALYTIC TECHNIQUES IN THE INTENSIVE CARE UNIT

THOMAS L. HIGGINS, M.D., F.A.C.P.

The mechanically ventilated patient presents many challenges to the intensive care clinician. The patient must be made comfortable and relaxed in a confining, sometimes painful, and anxiety-inducing environment. In addition, clinical goals include reduction of ventilator-induced barotrauma, facilitation of varying modes of ventilation, abolition of energy-wasting agitation or shivering, and preservation of the patient's cooperation for ease of examination and eventual weaning from the ventilator. This chapter gives a broad overview of the sedative, anesthetic, and paralytic techniques that I find useful in the intensive care setting and addresses the questions of when to sedate and induce neuromuscular blockade in ventilated patients, when to perform epidural and intercostal nerve blocks, the role of neuroleptic agents and deliberate hypothermia, and monitoring of these interventions and their potential complications.

SEDATION AND PAIN RELIEF IN THE INTENSIVE CARE UNIT

For the patient, the intensive care unit (ICU) is an unfamiliar, stressful, and often chaotic place. The ventilated patient lacks control over his or her environment, down to such basic bodily functions as feeding, elimination, and the ability to take a deep breath. Normal circadian rhythm may be disturbed by noise, the effects of medication, and lack of environmental cues such as daylight and regular meals. Loss of sleep tires the patient, inhibits cooperation with therapy, and may result in a situational psychosis. Add to this picture the uncertainties of outcome from a serious medical illness, and it is not hard to understand why patients in the intensive care unit become anxious, agitated—or even psychotic. The sequelae of anxiety and agitation include tachycardia, hypertension, and difficulty in medical and nursing management. Most critically ill patients who are still aware of their surroundings benefit from judicious sedation, and this becomes mandatory when the patient endangers his or her own care with nonpurposeful movement and agitation to the point of pulling out monitoring lines, chest tubes, or in-dwelling catheters. Provision of a good night's sleep each evening facilitates restoration of a normal sleep-wake cycle, leaving the patient awake and better able to cooperate with physical and respiratory care during the day.

Disadvantages of sedating patients include respiratory depression and alterations of mental function. Patients who are fully ventilated do not need a respiratory drive, but the process of weaning is facilitated when a hypercapnic drive is present. Preservation of mental status becomes important in evaluating head trauma or neurosurgical patients, in serving as a monitor for intracranial events in the patient on heparin or thrombolytic therapy, or when weaning from long-term ventilation. Pain relief in the acute setting is unlikely to cause drug addiction, but long-term use of sedatives and narcotics can induce tolerance and require gradual withdrawal of these agents.

Four broad classes of drugs are useful in the ventilated ICU patient. Choosing between a narcotic, benzodiazepine, barbiturate, or butyrophenone involves considering the problem to be treated, coexisting problems that may limit therapy, side effects to be employed or avoided, and interactions with other drugs. Frequently, two or more agents can be combined in a synergistic manner. On the other hand, use of multiple agents, particularly in elderly patients, may result in profound confusion, complicate evaluation, and lead to addition of yet another agent to an already muddy therapeutic situation.

Narcotics

Narcotic analgesics are natural or synthetic derivatives of opium, derived from the poppy plant. Narcotics act at receptors within the central nervous system and gut to produce analgesia, respiratory depression, drowsiness, changes in mood, and decreased bowel motility. Endogenous morphine-like substances, termed endorphins, are released by the anterior hypothalamus in response to stress, and some of the variability in patient response to pain can be explained by the presence of this system. Dozens of narcotic compounds exist, differing in activity at various opioid receptors, duration of action, and side effects. Specific narcotic antagonists, such as naloxone, can be used to reverse inadvertent overdosage. Compounds such as nalbuphine and butorphanol have both agonist and antagonist effects. Although each of the various agents has therapeutic potential, morphine, fentanyl, and naloxone are the opioids I find most useful.

Morphine is an ideal sedative whenever there is a concurrent need for pain relief, peripheral vasodilation, suppression of airway reflexes, or reduction of dyspnea due to acute left ventricular failure or pulmonary edema. Depression of respiratory drive and airway reflexes occurs within 7 minutes of intravenous administration and lasts for up to 5 hours, facilitating mechanical ventilation. In the spontaneously ventilating patient, hypercarbia and resultant increased intracranial pressure may be produced, making morphine relatively contraindicated for head trauma or neurosurgical patients. Morphine is commonly used intravenously at doses of 2 to 10 mg every 1 to 4 hours to provide postoperative pain relief. Hypotension due to histamine release is common with bolus administration and more likely to develop with postural changes or in the presence of volume depletion. Other cardiovascular effects include systemic venodilation and reduction in pulmonary vascular resistance.

For the chronically ventilated patient, continuous intravenous morphine infusion at rates of about 10 (range 2 to 30) mg per hour provides a constant level of pain relief and sedation. In patients with renal failure, morphine metabolites begin to accumulate after 24 hours; these metabolites add to the depressant effects and may cause further clouding of consciousness. Morphine dosage must also be reduced in elderly or debilitated patients, during induced hypothermia, and with severe metabolic derangements. Continuous morphine infusion decreases bowel motility and may interfere with provision of enteral nutrition.

Meperidine (Demerol) is a commonly used postoperative analgesic, which at doses of 80 to 100 mg provides analgesia, sedation, and respiratory depression equivalent to 10 mg of morphine. Meperidine is useful in treating shivering in patients emerging from anesthesia. I avoid the use of meperidine in the ICU, since its duration of action is shorter than that of morphine, and with repeated doses, there is accumulation of the excitatory metabolite normeperidine, which may cause seizures.

The fentanils (fentanyl, sufentanil, alfentanil, and others) are synthetic opioids related to meperidine. Fentanyl (Sublimaze) is approximately 80 times as potent as morphine. Unlike morphine and meperidine, which can cause histamine release and hypotension, clinically relevant doses of fentanyl rarely result in hemodynamic instability. Fentanyl can be given in doses of 25 to 200 μg (0.5 to 4.0 ml) to relieve pain and blunt the sympathetic response to intubation, dressing changes, and diagnostic procedures. Respiratory muscle rigidity is seen after rapid intravenous injection of fentanil-class drugs, and although it is rare in the above dosage, it is prudent to give these drugs slowly and in a setting in which mask ventilation and neuromuscular relaxation can be rapidly provided if necessary. Since the fentanils are more expensive than morphine, and tolerance to their anesthetic effects develops rapidly, I reserve their use for situations in which morphine is contraindicated by allergy or hemodynamic instability.

Naloxone (Narcan) is a narcotic antagonist that acts competitively at opiate receptor sites to reverse the effects of both endogenously and exogenously administered opioids. Animal laboratory evidence and anecdotal clinical reports suggest that naloxone, when given in very high doses, has an antihypotensive effect in patients with hemorrhagic or septic shock. It should probably not be used as a pressor agent for the chronically narcotized patient, since it will produce a very dramatic and disturbing reversal of analgesia. Intractible ventricular fibrillation has been reported following reversal of general anesthesia with as little as 0.8 mg of intravenous naloxone. Thus, if naloxone is deemed necessary in the narcotized ICU patient (for neurologic evaluation or reversal of inadvertent overdose, for example), it should be given cautiously in increments of 0.08 mg (0.2 ml) until the desired effect is achieved.

Tolerance to narcotics develops rapidly, and escalating dosages may be needed to adequately sedate patients. When narcotics alone are insufficient, or it is important for the patient to be asleep, I add a benzodiazepine or barbiturate, keeping in mind that depressant effects are potentiated with combination therapy.

Benzodiazepines

The benzodiazepines are useful for induction of anesthesia, for reducing anxiety, and for providing amnesia. The important differences among the benzodiazepines are in their duration of action, not in the action itself. Although a large number of oral or intravenous preparations are available, I rely on diazepam (Valium) as an all-purpose agent when long-term sedation is needed. For suppressing anxiety, 2 to 5 mg of diazepam intravenously, repeated every 6 to 8 hours as needed, is usually sufficient. To induce sleep, to provide anesthesia for cardioversion, or to control agitation or seizures, I give intravenous diazepam in increments of 5 mg to a total of 20 mg over the course of 10 to 20 minutes. At times, patients require 30 mg or more of diazepam; although the benzodiazepines as a class of drugs have a high margin of safety, prolonged sedation is common with increasingly high doses.

Midazolam (Versed), a newer, shorter acting, and more expensive agent, is particularly useful for short-term sedation, in doses of 1 to 5 mg intravenously.

Midazolam may also be given by continuous intravenous infusion, starting with a dose of 2.5 µg per kilogram per minute and titrating back to 0.4 µg per kilogram per minute once the desired effect is seen. Lorazepam (Ativan; 1 to 2 mg intravenously) may offer a slight advantage when amnesia is desirable, as, for example, during painful dressing changes or line placement. Finally, chlordiazepoxide (Librium; 50 to 100 mg intramuscularly or intravenously initially, repeated in 2 to 4 hours if needed) is the classic agent for the treatment of alcohol withdrawal syndromes. Although benzodiazepines alone are less likely than barbiturates or narcotics to suppress respiratory drive or affect the circulation, combinations of these central depressants must be used cautiously.

Barbiturates

Barbiturates cause dose-related central nervous system depression ranging from mild sedation to coma. Short-acting agents such as thiopental sodium (Pentothal; 3 to 5 mg per kilogram intravenously) or methohexital (Brevital; 1 mg per kilogram intravenously) are primarily used as anesthetic induction agents for dressing changes or cardioversion. Medium-acting agents such as pentobarbital (Nembutal) or phenobarbital may be used in an initial adult dose of 30 mg for sedation or 100 mg for sleep. The longer-acting agents, such as phenobarbital, 150 to 300 mg, are preferred as anticonvulsants or for inducing barbiturate coma. In the ICU, barbiturates are best given as an adjunct to narcotics, since when given alone in low doses they have a hyperalgesic effect and may cause excitement, restlessness, or delirium. Respiratory depression is produced by loss of central nervous system, hypercapnic, and eventually hypoxic respiratory drives. Cardiovascular effects at low doses are minimal, but hypotension may be seen in hypertensive patients and rarely with histamine release. Higher doses of barbiturates diminish cardiac output and provoke hemodynamic instability.

Butyrophenones

Haloperidol (Haldol) and droperidol are related compounds. Droperidol is a neuroleptic agent normally used in combination with fentanyl for anesthesia. Droperidol (0.6 to 5.0 mg intravenously) has antiemetic effects and causes a state of indifference to environmental stimuli. When given alone, droperidol often produces dysphoria and a sensation of restlessness; thus it is often given in combination with a narcotic or benzodiazepine. Respiratory depression is minimal, and cardiovascular effects of droperidol include a moderate decrease in systolic and diastolic blood pressure without significant changes in heart rate.

Haloperidol is an effective antipsychotic agent. Its calming and sleep-inducing effects are useful in the critically ill patient suffering from agitation after other causes (hypoxia, hypercarbia, hypoglycemia) have been ruled out. Haloperidol alone has minimal effects on blood pressure, pulmonary artery pressure, heart rate, or respiration, but it does potentiate the effects of other drugs. For acute agitation or confusion, haloperidol can be given in geometrically increasing increments starting with 2 mg intramuscularly or intravenously and doubling the dose until adequate sedation is achieved, or a total dose of 64 mg is given. One-half the effective dose is then given at bedtime, or when agitation reoccurs. A third dose, one-quarter of the original dose, may be needed 12 hours later. Control can then be achieved with as little as 1 to 3 mg at bedtime. I prefer this regimen to the more common method of giving a fixed dose every 6 hours, which may result in oversedation by the third or fourth day of therapy.

Extrapyramidal reactions (Parkinson's syndrome, akathisia, acute dystonic reactions, and tardive dyskinesias) may occur during or following the use of antipsychotic drugs, including haloperidol. Acute dystonic reactions respond to administration of diphenhydramine (Benadryl), but tardive dyskinesia has no effective treatment. Side effects are more common in older patients, females, and patients with prior brain damage but may occur in otherwise healthy patients. Therefore, haloperidol should be used with due consideration, in its minimally effective dosage, and for the shortest time possible. The neuroleptic malignant syndrome, a rare, potentially fatal idiosyncratic reaction to antipsychotic medication, is characterized by fever, muscle rigidity, autonomic dysfunction, and altered consciousness. It is occasionally misdiagnosed as sepsis and is often complicated by rhabdomyolysis. If this syndrome is properly recognized, treatment includes cessation of the offending agent, hydration, supportive care, and probably administration of dantrolene sodium.

Neuromuscular Blockade

In some cases, narcotics alone or in combination with other central nervous system active agents may not sedate the patient adequately to allow for mechanical ventilation. Indications for induction of neuromuscular blockade include stiff (low-compliance) lungs, the presence of seizure activity, and spontaneous ventilatory efforts that are dysynchronous with the ventilator and produce unacceptably high peak pressures. When using deliberate hypothermia, neuromuscular blockade is essential to prevent energy-wasting shivering. The inability to make respiratory efforts or to move one's limbs is a particularly stressful condition; thus I believe neuromuscular blockade *should never be induced unless adequate sedation is provided*. Patients on neuromuscular blockade cannot move but may signal their distress with mydriasis, diaphoresis, hypertension, and tachycardia. Neuromuscular blockade plus narcotic sedation is, in essence, a form of general anesthesia and carries with it attendant risks and monitoring responsibilities.

Several nondepolarizing neuromuscular blocking drugs are available for use, and decisions on the ideal agent involve duration of action, mode of termination, side effects, and cost. The prototypic and least expensive agent is *d*-tubocurarine (Curare, dTc). Neuromuscular blockade can be induced with an initial dose of 0.6 mg per kilogram and maintained with an intravenous infusion of 0.3 mg per kilogram per hour. *d*-Tubocurarine causes histamine release and may provoke hypotension when given as a rapid bolus, but it has minimal cardiovascular effects when given as an infusion. Normally, *d*-tubocurarine is cleared primarily by the kidneys, but in the presence of renal failure an alternate hepatobiliary mechanism becomes more important. Metocurine (Metubine) is approximately 1.5 times as potent as *d*-tubocurarine and less likely to release histamine but has essentially only renal excretion. Pancuronium (Pavulon) is the most commonly used agent for paralysis in the ICU. The dose of pancuronium is 0.05 to 0.1 mg per kilogram initially, repeated as required. Pancuronium has a vagolytic effect and often produces an undesirable tachycardia; it is eliminated mainly by the kidneys but also via biliary excretion. Atracurium (Tracrium) and vecuronium (Norcuron) are newer, shorter-acting neuromuscular blocking agents. Vecuronium offers the advantages of hepatic elimination, minimal hemodynamic pertubation, and less than 1 hour of blockade at a dose of 0.1 mg per kilogram. The effects of atracurium (0.05 to 0.5 mg per kilogram) are also dissipated in under an hour, partly by Hoffman elimination (spontaneous degradation at body temperature and pH), which makes it useful in patients with combined hepatic and renal failure. In the intensive care setting, vecuronium and atracurium are costly to use for intravenous infusion, but they do offer an advantage over succinylcholine (Anectine) as short-acting agents for intubation, particularly in burn, renal failure, or paraplegic patients who have a tendency to hyperkalemia. Gallamine (Flaxedil; 2 to 3 mg per kilogram), a nondepolarizing neuromuscular blocking drug with near-total renal elimination, tends to cause tachycardia and is rarely used in the intensive care setting.

The major hazard of neuromuscular blockade is abolition of all respiratory function. Thus, it is essential that paralyzed patients be closely monitored and ventilators equipped with disconnect alarms. The paralyzed patient cannot move, and special nursing attention is necessary to prevent pressure necrosis at bony prominences. Unit personnel should be cautioned that although the paralyzed, sedated patient is immobile, he or she may hear and remember bedside conversations. To avoid corneal drying, the eyes must be filled with a lubricating gel and taped closed. I monitor the level of neuromuscular blockade, periodically back off on the infusion rate, and watch for diaphragmatic motion or other signs of muscular activity.

Neuromuscular blockade is generally allowed to dissipate by discontinuing the drug and maintaining full ventilation until the return of muscle activity is apparent. More rapid reversal is seldom needed but can be accomplished by administering an anticholinesterase drug, such as neostigmine (Prostigmine), pyridostigmine (Mestinon), or edrophonium (Tensilon), along with an anticholinergic agent such as atropine or glycopyrrolate (Robinul) to prevent anticholinesterase-induced bradycardia. Consultation with an anesthesiologist familiar with the use of these drugs is well advised. Monitoring of neuromuscular blockade prior to weaning of the patient from mechanical ventilation can be accomplished with a train-of-four nerve stimulator looking for return of four equal muscle contractions, or clinically by sustained grip, head lift, or vital capacity measurements. Neuromuscular blockade may be prolonged with aminoglycosides, hypermagnesemia, hypothermia, and hepatic or renal dysfunction. Patients with myasthenia gravis will be exquisitely sensitive to the effects of the neuromuscular blocking agents and may have prolonged blockade following their use.

Continuation of Anesthesia Postoperatively

Indications for the induction or maintenance of anesthesia in the ICU continue to grow with advances in surgical technique and anesthetic management. The balanced narcotic–muscle relaxant anesthetic technique, first used for cardiac surgery, combines a high initial dose of narcotic with neuromuscular blockade and provides a high degree of cardiovascular stability intraoperatively. Since abrupt antagonism of narcotics with naloxone or reversal of neuromuscular blockade may precipitate hypertension or tachycardia or both, patients are often ventilated postoperatively until the agents have been eliminated or metabolized. The advantages of this technique were soon extended from the cardiac unit to the care of other patients with coronary artery disease, particularly those undergoing vascular surgery procedures, and it is now common for patients to arrive from the operating room fully ventilated. Fluid balance, temperature, and hemodynamic control can gradually be achieved as the patient is allowed to awaken and ventilate spontaneously.

Epidural Anesthesia and Analgesia

Systemic narcotics rarely produce complete relief of pain, and their use is complicated by respiratory depression and other side effects. Systemic narcotics also fail to prevent reflex muscle spasm or vasospasm or the development of a stress hormone response to surgery. In contrast, properly conducted regional anesthesia interrupts the transmission not only of pain but also of reflex responses, without effects on ventilation. Epidural anesthesia via in-dwelling catheter is a preferred method for major vascular surgery and can be used for other abdominal and lower extremity procedures. Epidural anesthesia results in less hemodynamic perturbation and better abolition of the stress response than general anesthesia. Once a continuous epidural catheter is in place, the anesthetic can potentially be continued for 1 to 3 days into the postoperative period. Advantages of postoperative epidural anesthesia include improved nitrogen balance and decreased risk of lung morbidity compared with conventional pain relief. Problems with this approach include orthostatic hypotension, toxicity of local anesthetics, urinary retention, inability to ambulate, and lack of skilled personnel to properly monitor the anesthetic.

Narcotics can also be administered via the epidural route and are highly effective in alleviating pain and improving respiratory function in post-thoracotomy patients. Although epidural local anesthetics may result in seizures, hypotension, or even cardiovascular collapse, the selective blockade of pain by epidural narcotics is less likely to cause serious side effects. Early and late respiratory depression are the major concerns. The other side effects of epidural narcotics (pruritus, nausea and vomiting, urinary retention) can usually be reversed with small systemic doses of naloxone without affecting pain relief.

The technique of epidural insertion is beyond the scope of this chapter and best left to experienced personnel. Pain relief is most effective if the first dose of narcotics is given in the operating room or before the epidural local anesthesia has worn off. The catheter may migrate into an epidural vein or, less commonly, into the subarachnoid space. Before the first dose of epidural narcotics, I inspect the placement of the catheter and give a test dose of 3 ml of 2 percent lidocaine mixed with epinephrine, 1:100,000. If the catheter is subarachnoid, a moderate spinal level will result; and if the catheter is intravascular, tachycardia will be noted from the epinephrine. If both tests are negative, I then give 5 mg of preservative-free morphine (5 ml volume) mixed with 5 ml of preservative-free saline for a total volume of 10 ml. Careful attention should be paid to keeping the catheter end sterile, a bacterial filter should be utilized, and an attempt should be made to aspirate blood before each epidural injection. If there is any doubt about the proper placement of the catheter, the lidocaine-epinephrine test is repeated, or the catheter is removed and replaced. I generally limit use of the catheter to 72 hours and remove it earlier if there is evidence of skin inflammation or suspicion of sepsis.

At present, only preservative-free morphine (Duramorph) is approved for epidural use. Fentanyl, 50 to 100 μg, is also commonly used, and some clinicians feel that as a highly lipid-soluble drug, fentanyl offers more rapid onset and less late respiratory depression than morphine. A single dose of epidural morphine can be expected to have an effect 45 minutes after injection and to last for 15 to 20 hours, but there is considerable individual variation. I have given repeated doses as often as every 3 hours in patients with severe pain from terminal cancer. Respiratory depression may rarely occur as late as 12 hours after administration, and I keep patients in a monitored setting for at least that long after their last dose.

Intercostal Nerve Blocks

Post-thoracotomy pain can be effectively relieved and respiratory function improved by placing local anesthetic along the neurovascular bundle at the lower rib margin of the incision level and two interspaces above and below that level. This technique is best suited for patients with lateral chest wall incisions and chest tubes after lobectomy, since effective pain relief will result in better expansion of the remaining lung segments. Intercostal nerve blocks may also be used after pneumonectomy, but the benefit of pain relief must be balanced against the potential of introducing infection in a closed space. Cutaneous infection at the site of entry is the only absolute contraindication to intercostal nerve block.

Either 1 percent lidocaine or 0.5 percent bupivacaine may be used; if the patient is free of significant heart disease, an epinephrine-containing solution can be given to limit systemic absorption and perhaps extend the duration of action. The patient can be positioned prone with a pillow under the midabdomen, laterally, or leaning over the bedside table; in all cases attempt to increase the size of the intercostal spaces and to widen the distance between the scapula and the midline. To include the lateral cutaneous division of the intercostal nerve, the block must be performed at or posterior to the midaxillary line; I find that about four finger breadths from the spine gives good results. Under sterile conditions, I draw up 30 ml of local anesthetic in three 10-ml syringes. The patient's back is prepped with a sterile iodine-containing solution, and a 1.5 inch 23-gauge needle is gently walked off the lower rib border and inserted another one-eighth inch. After aspirating for blood, 3 to 5 ml of local anesthetic are deposited at each of five ribs, and the remaining anesthetic is used at the point of entry for the chest tubes. Duration of pain relief is variable, and while one treatment is adequate for a minority of patients, most require retreatment at 8 to 12 hours. Potential adverse effects include local anesthetic toxicity, inadvertent intravascular injection, injection directly into the nerve, and pneumothorax, but the most common problem encountered in inexperienced hands is incomplete block due to misplacement of the anesthetic.

Rectal Indomethacin

If epidural or intercostal nerve blocks are not feasible and systemic narcotics are insufficient in safe doses, rectal indomethacin (Indocin) provides an adjunct to pain relief. One hundred mg of indomethacin can be given per rectum every 8 hours for control of early post-thoracotomy pain. In one study, indomethacin was helpful in reducing pain on movement, and patients receiving the drug required less opiate analgesia and showed improved respiratory peak flow values.

Induced Hypothermia

Patients with severe respiratory failure may reach a point in their illness where, despite toxic levels of oxygen, high levels of positive end-expiratory pressure, and various adjustments in ventilatory pattern, adequate tissue oxygenation cannot be sustained. Evidence of this state would include an A-aDO$_2$ (alveolar-arterial oxygen difference) of 500 mm Hg or more, or shunt greater than 40 percent on 100 percent oxygen. Initial efforts should include reduction of fever, avoidance of overfeeding, and appropriate sedation. Further decreases in metabolism can be achieved by deliberate cooling to temperatures of about 32° C. This mode of therapy is controversial and perhaps even heroic and is justified primarily as a means of buying time by reducing oxygen consumption and carbon dioxide production while any reversible processes are treated and/or spontaneous improvement in lung function occurs. Cooling may also be employed in the treatment of massive bronchopleural fistulas to reduce the inspired oxygen concentration to less than 60 percent in order to delay oxygen toxicity, and to decrease intracranial pressure. Induced hypothermia is of unproven efficacy with regard to outcome and introduces many potential complications, including a rise in systemic vascular resistance, hyperglycemia, increased blood viscosity, left-sided shift of the oxygen-hemoglobin dissociation curve, acid-base abnormalities, masking of febrile response to infection, decreased gastric motility, and inability to assess mental status.

Hypothermia is accomplished in a patient on full ventilatory support by first inducing sleep with narcotics and barbiturates or benzodiazepines and then inducing neuromuscular blockade to prevent shivering. With the patient placed on a cooling blanket, the temperature is gradually lowered to approximately 32° C. At this temperature, oxygen consumption and carbon dioxide production decrease by 40 to 50 percent, with minimal hemodynamic instability. Lower temperatures offer little additional benefit but increase the risk of ventricular irritability. Monitoring of temperature is essential. I use core temperature measured from the thermistor tip of the pulmonary artery catheter when available; alternatives include posterior nasopharyngeal, esophageal, rectal, or thermocouple-containing Foley catheter temperature probes. Interpretation of arterial blood gases is more difficult, since the patient is at 32° C and the laboratory typically measures the samples on a machine calibrated for 37° C. Although nomograms exist to correct back to the patient's temperature, I find it easiest to interpret pH and Pco$_2$ as reported (*uncorrected*) to adjust ventilation, since the error will result only in moderate hyperventilation and hypocarbia. On the other hand, interpretation of Po$_2$ is safest if the corrected values are used, since the value as read off the blood gas machine will be artificially elevated. I believe the corrected Po$_2$ value more accurately represents the actual pressure gradient within the patient, and thus the oxygen delivery at the cellular level, but the point is controversial. More research needs to be done in this area.

While in a hypothermic state, the patient needs appropriate protection against pressure sores, nerve injury, stress ulceration, and eye trauma. All signs of intracranial, intra-abdominal, or intrathoracic catastrophe may be masked, so special vigilance is needed, particularly in looking for pneumothorax. I draw daily blood for cultures for early identification of sepsis. Rewarming is attempted as soon as clinical conditions permit and is best achieved by passive rewarming while maintaining sedation.

Suggested Reading

Calabreze JR, et al. Incidence of postoperative delirium following myocardial revascularization. Cleve Clin J Med 1987; 54:29.

Cousins MJ, Mather LE. Intrathecal and epidural administration of opioids. Anesthesiology 1984; 61:276–310.

de la Rocha AG, Chambers K. Pain amelioration after thoracotomy: a prospective, randomized study. Ann Thor Surg 1984; 37:239–242.

Greenblatt DJ, Shader RI, Abernethy DR. Current status of benzodiazepines. N Engl J Med 1983; 309:358, 410–416.

Keats AS. The effect of drugs on respiration in man. Annu Rev Pharmacol Toxicol 1985; 25:41.

Keenan DJM, Cave K, Langdon L, Lea RE. Comparative trial of rectal indomethacin and cryoanalgesia for control of early post-thoracotomy pain. Br Med J 1983; 287:1335–1337.

Merriman HM. The techniques used to sedate ventilated patients: a survey of methods used in 34 ICUs in Great Britain. Intensive Care Med 1981; 7:217–224.

Nathanson C, Shelhamer JH, Parrillo JE. Intubation of the trachea in the critical care setting. JAMA 1985; 253:1160–1165.

Pflug AE, Bonica JJ. Physiopathology and control of postoperative pain. Arch Surg 1977; 112:773–781.

EXTRACORPOREAL MEMBRANE OXYGENATION

THOMAS W. RICE, B.A.Sc., M.D.

Extracorporeal membrane oxygenation (ECMO) is a technique of temporarily replacing or augmenting the gas exchange function of the lungs. Life is supported by preventing hypoxia and hypercarbia, allowing time for the acute lung injury to resolve. Although ECMO has no pulmonary reparative properties, its use may avoid the complications of aggressive ventilation, i.e., oxygen toxicity and barotrauma.

HISTORY

In the early 1950s total cardiopulmonary bypass was introduced to support cardiac and pulmonary functions during the repair of intracardiac defects. These early uses of extracorporeal circulation were limited to short periods of support. The oxygenator was the weak element in these circuits. The discovery of the excellent gas transfer properties of silicone rubber allowed for the development of the membrane oxygenator. These oxygenators, which were highly efficient gas transfer units, were much less damaging to blood elements and allowed for the long-term support of patients with acute respiratory failure.

ECMO was first used in 1966 to support a patient whose respiratory failure did not respond to conventional mechanical ventilation therapy. This was followed by a flurry of activity in multiple centers. Various causes of acute respiratory failure were treated using many different ECMO circuits and oxygenators. In the ensuing 10 years, over 200 patients were placed on ECMO support, and an overall survival rate of 10 to 15 percent was realized. During this period, it became evident that early use of ECMO in patients with reversible lung injury was necessary for survival.

These discoveries prompted a multicenter randomized prospective study of partial venoarterial ECMO in acute respiratory failure. The study had rigid entry and exclusion criteria. The majority of people who were treated for acute respiratory failure suffered from pneumonia. This study showed that ECMO could support respiratory gas exchange for prolonged periods, but there was no survival advantage of ECMO over conventional mechanical ventilation. Contrary to the results of previous studies, none of the patients with pulmonary embolism or post-traumatic acute respiratory failure survived. Those patients who died showed progression of their pulmonary disease, with extensive fibrosis and necrosis. This study was the death knell for ECMO support of adult patients with acute respiratory failure in the United States.

This failure of conventional venoarterial ECMO to improve survival of patients suffering from acute respiratory failure led some researchers in Europe to consider another means of ECMO support. This system was called LFPPV-ECCO$_2$R. Low frequency positive pressure ventilation (LFPPV) at 3 breaths per minute was used as a means of oxygenation by diffusion. Extracorporeal removal of CO_2 (ECCO$_2$R) was done by the venovenous route. The early report was promising, with two of three treated patients surviving. Since this study, little else has been reported. In the 1980s the use of ECMO in the support of adult respiratory failure has been a stagnant research topic.

In the neonatal population, ECMO has been used successfully to support infants with reversible causes of acute respiratory failure that have failed to respond to conventional management. The most commonly seen successfully treated causes of respiratory failure were meconium aspiration, persistent fetal circulation, hyaline membrane disease, congenital diaphragmatic hernia, and total anomalous pulmonary venous drainage. Spectacular results have been reported, with 55 to 85 percent of infants being weaned from ECMO and ventilatory support. In a randomized prospective study using the "randomized play the winner" statistical method, the survival of ECMO-treated infants directed all 11 survivors to the ECMO arm of the study.

ECMO CIRCUITS

Although four modes of extracorporeal circulation have been described (arteriovenous, venovenous, venoarterial, and mixed [venovenous, venoarterial]), only two are now clinically used. The most common mode, venoarterial, removes blood from the systemic venous system, oxygenates it, and returns it to the systemic arterial system. A drawback of this circuit is that there may be maldistribution of the oxygenated blood. If femoral cannulation is used, cerebral hypoxia is possible. For this reason special cannulas have been developed for venoarterial perfusion in which the arterial return line is introduced into the common femoral artery and advanced into the aortic arch to assure adequate oxygenation of all vital organs. The effects on the pulmonary circulation of venoarterial bypass are also in question. It has been shown that in bypassing the lungs, pulmonary injury may result. There is increased sludging and thrombosis in the pulmonary vasculature with venoarterial bypass. This may aggravate and accelerate pulmonary injury. Venoarterial bypass, however, does provide right-sided heart support by unloading the right ventricle and returning a portion of the right-sided heart return to the systemic arterial system. This appears to be beneficial in the pediatric population.

The other circuit used in ECMO support is venovenous. Blood is drawn from the systemic venous system, and after oxygenation, it is returned to that system. Difficulties with this circuit arise from the return of blood to the venous system. The right heart is not supported, and the pulmonary arterial pressure is not reduced, since all the cardiac output returns to the right heart, and it must be pumped through the lungs. Inadequate systemic oxygenation may result from short circuiting. Here a portion of the returned oxygenated blood is picked up by the drainage cannula before adequate mixing can occur. This parallel path through the ECMO circuit decreases oxygenated return to the patient. Venovenous ECMO does assure full pulsatile pulmonary flow and reduces the risk of systemic emboli.

Since 1979, there has been little impetus to improve ECMO technology. Most new equipment development has resulted from work with cardiac support. The choice of cannulas for both venous withdrawal and oxygenated blood return is variable. In neonates nasogastric feeding tubes and chest tubes are commonly used. Venous drainage is usually provided by a 14 to 16 F catheter; arterial return is generally adequate with a 8 to 10 F catheter. For adults, modified chest tubes or specially constructed catheters are used. These catheters should assure flow rates of 40 to 100 ml per kilogram per minute. For partial bypass, catheters of 12 F have been successfully used; however, catheter sizes larger than 20 F are best suited for large adults who require higher flow rates. A sterile surgical approach is required for both insertion and removal of cannulas. Recently a successful percutaneous system of cannulization has been reported. This system speeds insertion and eliminates surgery for cannulation or decannulation. In the past, the roller pump has been used for ECMO support; however, recently the centrifugal pump (Bio-Medicus) has been used. The pump head must be changed to avoid thrombosis and embolization. However, single pump heads have been used for periods of 1 week. Multiple membrane oxygenators have been used in the past for ECMO support. Only one oxygenator is available commercially at present for long-term support (Sci-med).

INDICATIONS

In an appropriate critical care setting, ECMO is an accepted means of supporting neonates with acute respiratory failure due to reversible causes. At present in the adult population there is no indication for the generalized use of ECMO support of patients with acute respiratory failure. ECMO may be indicated in certain experimental settings. It has been used to successfully support lung transplant patients who have developed acute respiratory failure in the early post-transplantation period.

THE FUTURE

There is no question that ECMO can support gas exchange in patients with acute respiratory failure. However, most commonly, the acute respiratory failure is not reversible and progresses in spite of this support. ECMO is a useful technique but its widespread use awaits our increased knowledge of acute lung injury. Not until effective therapies that halt the progression of acute lung injury and speed the reparative process are developed will ECMO be a useful clinical tool.

Suggested Reading

Bartlett RH, Andrews AF, Toomasian JM, et al. Extracorporeal membrane oxygenation for newborn respiratory failure: forty-five cases. Surgery 1982; 92:425–433.

Bartlett RH, Gazzaniga AB, Wilson AF, et al. Mortality prediction in adult respiratory insufficiency. Chest 1975; 67:680–684.

Bartlett RH, Roloff DW, et al. Extracorporeal circulation in neonatal respiratory failure: a prospective randomized study. Pediatrics 1985; 76:479–487.

Gattinoni L, Pesenti A, Rossi GP, et al. Treatment of acute respiratory failure with low-frequency positive-pressure ventilation and extracorporeal removal of CO_2. Lancet 1980; 2:292–294.

Gille JP, Bagniewski AM. Ten years of use of extracorporeal membrane oxygenation (ECMO) in the treatment of acute respiratory insufficiency (ARI). Trans Am Soc Artif Intern Organs 1976; 22:102–108.

Hill JD, O'Brien TG, Murray JJ, et al. Prolonged extracorporeal oxygenation for acute post-traumatic respiratory failure (shock-lung syndrome). N Engl J Med 1972; 286:629–634.

Krummel TM, Greenfield LJ, Kirkpatrick BV, et al. Clinical use of an extracorporeal membrane oxygenator in neonatal pulmonary failure. J Pediatr Surg 1982; 17:525–531.

Loe WA Jr, Graves ED III, Ochsner JL, et al. Extracorporeal membrane oxygenation for newborn respiratory failure. J Pediatr Surg 1985; 20:684–688.

Pratt PC, Vollmer RT, Shelburne JD, et al. Pulmonary morphology in a multihospital collaborative extracorporeal membrane oxygenation project. Am J Pathol 1979; 95:191–205.

Zapol WM, Snider MT, Hill JD, et al. Extracorporeal membrane oxygenation in severe acute respiratory failure. A randomized prospective study. JAMA 1979; 242:2193–2196.

HOME CARE AND PULMONARY REHABILITATION

PULMONARY REHABILITATION

JOHN E. HODGKIN, M.D.

In 1942, the Council on Rehabilitation defined rehabilitation as "the restoration of the individual to the fullest medical, mental, emotional, social, and vocational potential of which he or she is capable." Traditionally, the process of rehabilitation has been applied to patients with neuromuscular and musculoskeletal disorders. More recently, rehabilitation programs for patients with cardiovascular and pulmonary disease have become more common.

In 1974, an Ad Hoc Committee of the American College of Chest Physicians developed the following definition: "Pulmonary rehabilitation may be defined as an art of medical practice wherein an individually-tailored, multidisciplinary program is formulated which through accurate diagnosis, therapy, emotional support, and education stabilizes or reverses both the physio- and psychopathology of pulmonary diseases and attempts to return the patient to the highest possible functional capacity allowed by his pulmonary handicap and overall life situation." Subsequently, an Ad Hoc Committee of the American Thoracic Society Scientific Assembly on Clinical Problems developed an official position statement on pulmonary rehabilitation, which was published in 1981. This statement listed the recommended sequence for a pulmonary rehabilitation program and summarized the services that should be available if a facility is to offer such a program.

STRUCTURE OF THE PULMONARY REHABILITATION PROGRAM

One of the crucial members of a pulmonary rehabilitation team is a physician who is knowledgeable about respiratory disease. A careful history and physical examination of the patient to identify specific medical problems is vital to the team in developing an appropriate treatment program for the individual. A multidisciplinary team that includes a respiratory nurse, respiratory therapist, occupational therapist, physical therapist, dietitian, social worker, chaplain, and psychologist or psychiatrist is particularly useful for programs to which large numbers of patients are referred and for teaching or research purposes. It is possible to perform a thorough assessment and deliver similar services with fewer allied health professionals if the individuals on the team are specifically trained in the evaluation and management of patients with respiratory disorders. The specific provider of essential services varies from program to program depending on the size of the facility and the availability of allied health professionals who are trained to assess patients with pulmonary disease.

Pulmonary rehabilitation is currently accomplished in the outpatient setting because third-party payers are reluctant to pay for inpatient care for those who are not acutely ill. However, it is very useful for members of the pulmonary rehabilitation team to perform an initial assessment and outline an appropriate treatment program when a patient is hospitalized for an acute exacerbation in order to help ensure a smooth transition from hospital to outpatient setting.

SEQUENCE OF PULMONARY REHABILITATION

Table 1 presents the recommended sequence for an individual participating in a pulmonary rehabilitation program. Any individual with respiratory symptoms should be considered for pulmonary rehabilitation. Most patients participating in a pulmonary rehabilitation program have chronic obstructive pulmonary disease (COPD), e.g., emphysema or chronic bronchitis. Many patients with bronchial asthma can also benefit by participating in a structured pulmonary rehabilitation program. Patients with very mild or very severe disease are not usually placed on as intensive and comprehensive a rehabilitation program as are those with moderate to moderately severe disease.

**TABLE 1 Sequence of Pulmonary
Rehabilitation**

Select patient
Evaluate patient to determine needs
Determine goals
Outline components of care
Assess progress
Arrange for long-term care

**TABLE 2 Components of Pulmonary
Rehabilitation**

General
  Patient and family education
  Proper nutrition including weight control
  Avoidance of smoking and other inhaled irritants
  Avoidance of infection (immunization, etc.)
  Proper environment
  Adequate hydration
Medications
  Bronchodilators
  Expectorants
  Antimicrobials
  Corticosteroids
  Cromolyn sodium
  Digitalis
  Diuretics
  Psychopharmacologic agents
Respiratory Therapy Techniques
  Aerosol therapy
  Oxygen therapy
  Home use of ventilators
Physical Therapy Modalities
  Relaxation training
  Breathing retraining
  Chest percussion and postural drainage
  Deliberate coughing and expectoration
Exercise Conditioning
Occupational Therapy
  Evaluate activities of daily living
  Outline energy-conserving maneuvers
Psychosocial Rehabilitation
Vocational Rehabilitation

A proper identification of the patient's specific respiratory problem is useful in order to outline a treatment program that is best designed to meet the patient's needs. Essential diagnostic information generally includes pulmonary function studies, a chest radiograph, an electrocardiogram, an arterial blood gas measurement, and often sputum analysis and blood theophylline measurements. Some type of emotional screening is important because many of these individuals have anxiety or depression, which may significantly affect performance in the program and compliance in the future. It is important to determine what personal and environmental assets are available to help the individual, including family and social support, employment possibilities, and community resources, because the mobilization of these resources may be crucial to improving the patient's overall ability to function.

Often physicians fail to develop or discuss with the patient and family short- and long-term goals. If such goals are not developed or discussed with the patient and family, hostility often develops between the patient and the care provider. Patient and family members must be realistic with regard to achievable goals.

Table 2 lists the various components of pulmonary rehabilitation. These are discussed briefly in this chapter. All of these components of care are not essential for every individual; however, some member of the team must be qualified to describe each of these components of care for those individuals needing it.

The patient's progress should be monitored throughout the pulmonary rehabilitation program and appropriate changes made based on the patient's response to the various components of care being used. It is important to outline a long-term program for the patient at the time of completion of the pulmonary rehabilitation program, and a summary of the patient's assessment and recommendations should be sent to the individual's primary care physician to help assure high-quality care in the future. Periodic reassessment should be offered to the individual as a way of objectively evaluating progress so that any appropriate changes can be made and educational reinforcement can be achieved.

COMPONENTS OF PULMONARY REHABILITATION

General Considerations

Encouraging the patient to quit smoking is one of the most important components of care if one hopes to slow down the disease process. The most successful technique is for a physician to discuss personally with the patient the adverse effects of smoking and the importance of stopping. Many other techniques have been used with some individuals responding better to one technique than another. Nicotine chewing gum may be a useful adjunct in helping some patients who are truly addicted to nicotine to withdraw from cigarettes. Most pulmonologists recommend that patients with chronic respiratory disease have an influenza vaccine yearly and a pneumococcal vaccine one time. In an effort to try to liquefy airway secretions, adequate fluid intake (e.g., eight to ten glasses per day) should be recommended. Teaching the patient and family that the therapeutic program should be intensified at the first sign of an exacerbation can help reduce the need for hospitalization and probably lessen morbidity and mortality.

Medications

Bronchodilators are the mainstay of pharmacologic therapy for patients with obstructive airway disease. The fact that some individuals with chronic obstructive pulmonary disease (COPD) who do not show dramatic response to bronchodilator inhalation on spirometric testing still seem to benefit from bronchodilator therapy suggests that bronchodilator medications may, in fact, have actions other than relief of bronchospasm. Indeed, theophylline preparations have been reported to increase diaphragmatic contractility, and beta-adrenergic agents have been reported to improve mucociliary function. Antimicrobials should be used at the first sign of a respiratory infection to help reduce airway damage resulting from infection. Corticosteroids can decrease inflammation of the airways in patients with reactive airway disease and also have been reported to enhance bronchodilator action.

Other medications that are occasionally useful include digitalis for patients with left ventricular failure, diuretics to reduce excess fluid retention in those with either left ventricular or right ventricular decompensation, and cromolyn sodium in patients with asthma. Psychopharmacologic agents can enhance the COPD patient's functional ability by reducing anxiety, agitation, and depression. Almitrine holds promise as a way to improve arterial oxygen levels and reduce carbon dioxide blood levels, and may allow some COPD patients to avoid oxygen therapy, at least for a period of time.

Respiratory Therapy Techniques

Aerosolization of many medications, including bronchodilators, corticosteroids, mucolytic agents, bland mist, and antimicrobials has been used in COPD patients. Although there is little evidence to support aerosolization of the latter three agents, clearly bronchodilator and corticosteroid inhalation are useful. Sympathomimetics inhaled by aerosol work more quickly and have fewer side effects than when the same agent is administered orally or parenterally. Ipratropium bromide (Atrovent) is another type of bronchodilator that has recently become available in the United States as a metered-dose inhaler. Certain inhaled corticosteroids, i.e., beclomethasone, dipropionate (Vanceril, Beclovent) triamcinolone acetonide (Azmacort) and flunisolide (AeroBid) have the major advantage of providing corticosteroid benefit to the airway while avoiding the systemic side effects seen with administration of oral corticosteroids. Holding chambers (spacers) may enhance proper use of metered-dose inhalers and minimize topical and systemic side effects, i.e., sore throat, hoarseness, and palpitations, which occur in some patients.

Oxygen has been reported to reverse pulmonary hypertension and polycythemia and improve neuropsychologic dysfunction in hypoxemic patients with COPD. The National Heart, Lung and Blood Institute (NIH) Nocturnal Oxygen Therapy trial and the British Medical Research Council (MRC) multicenter trial have both clearly shown that oxygen improves survival in COPD patients with significant hypoxemia. In the NIH study, patients with an arterial Po_2 of 55 mm Hg or less when stable and those with an arterial Po_2 up to 59 mm Hg with evidence of pulmonary hypertension or polycythemia were randomized between nocturnal oxygen therapy and continuous oxygen therapy. The nocturnal oxygen therapy group ended up using oxygen approximately 12 hours per day, and the continuous oxygen therapy group used oxygen approximately 18 hours a day. In the British MRC study, COPD patients with significant hypoxemia were randomized between room air and oxygen for 15 hours a day. The results indicate that oxygen for 12 to 15 hours a day was preferable to room air only, and the best survival was achieved in patients who were advised to use oxygen continuously. On the basis of these studies, continuous oxygen therapy is recommended for individuals who, when stable, have a PaO_2 on room air of 55 mm Hg or less or a PaO_2 of 56 to 59 mm Hg with evidence of right heart failure or polycythemia. If a patient's Po_2 drops to 55 mm Hg or less (equivalent to an O_2 saturation of 88 percent or less) during the level of exercise prescribed in an exercise prescription, supplemental oxygen during exercise training is advised. Nocturnal oxygen can be beneficial for patients with significant hypoxemia occurring during sleep.

Intermittent positive pressure breathing (IPPB) has no proven advantages in outpatients with COPD over less expensive and simpler methods of aerosol therapy, i.e., cartridge inhalers and compressor nebulizers. In the National Heart, Lung and Blood Institute study comparing IPPB with compressor nebulizer therapy in stable outpatients with COPD, there was no significant difference in any of the variables monitored, including survival between the two groups. Home use of mechanical ventilation in patients who need ventilatory support for part or all of the day has allowed many of these individuals to return home rather than remain hospitalized. Preparing the ventilator-assisted patient to make the transition from hospital to home is a prime example of a situation in which a pulmonary rehabilitation team is crucial.

Chest Physiotherapy

Patients with COPD should be taught to slow their respiratory rate with a prolonged exhalation phase as a way of improving alveolar ventilation, reducing shortness of breath and decreasing the alveolar-arterial oxygen difference. Using pursed lip breathing is a common way to achieve this slowing of the respiratory rate. In patients with a large amount of secretions, i.e., greater than 30 ml per day, clapping, vibration, and postural drainage may be a helpful adjunct to a proper cough in clearing secretions from the airways. Most COPD patients do not need clapping and postural drainage. These techniques are particularly likely to be of benefit in those with a large amount of thick secretions, i.e., those with bronchiectasis or cystic fibrosis.

Exercise Conditioning

Exercise training should be a routine component of any pulmonary rehabilitation program. An enhanced ability to function is the end result of improving exercise capability. Although a walking program is usually prescribed, swimming or bicycle riding can also achieve similar benefits. The mode of exercise to be recommended should be readily accessible and something the patient is willing to do. Although respiratory muscle training has been shown to improve exercise ability in some COPD patients, I prefer to have the patient pursue an aerobic-type exercise program, e.g., walking for 20 to 30 minutes at least three to four times per week. Respiratory muscle training has not yet been shown to add anything of clinical significance to a rehabilitation program that incorporates aerobic-type exercise conditioning.

Activities of Daily Living

An evaluation of activities of daily living can identify problem areas in which appropriate changes can reduce energy expenditure, allowing people to perform activities more efficiently. Occupational therapists and physical therapists can teach individuals to modify their activities so as to consume less oxygen. Teaching these patients to relax, particularly during periods of panic or dyspnea, can decrease the respiratory rate, heart rate, and oxygen consumption.

Psychosocial Rehabilitation

Depression, fear, anxiety, hostility, and denial are common among COPD patients. Although various members of the pulmonary rehabilitation team can usually assist in reversing these problems, individualized treatment with a psychologist or psychiatrist is sometimes necessary. Psychotherapy and psychopharmacologic agents may help patients with more severe disorders to cope with their disease more effectively. Sexual dysfunction is another area that unfortunately is commonly avoided by many physicians. This area should routinely be addressed by pulmonary rehabilitation team members, because it is so common.

Vocational Rehabilitation

Some patients with COPD may be able to return to productive occupations. It is important to evaluate the job for any adverse effect on the respiratory system, i.e., exposure to pollutants in the air, and to ensure that the energy requirements for the job do not exceed the patient's work capacity. Unfortunately, many patients do not come in for pulmonary rehabilitation until they are severely disabled and thus unable to return to useful employment. For patients with more mild to moderate impairment of function, vocational rehabilitation should routinely be considered.

Nutrition

A dietitian or nutritionist is an essential member of the pulmonary rehabilitation team because so many of these patients have nutritional problems. Certain medications, ulcers, smoking, and increased work of breathing can all lead to impaired appetite and poor nutrition in patients with COPD. Assuring adequate protein is important for the individual who is losing weight excessively. Using nutritional supplements between meals and multiple feedings per day can improve the caloric intake in those with anorexia. In obese patients, a weight reduction program including regular exercise should be prescribed to help lessen the work of breathing. It is important to measure the patient's potassium, magnesium, and phosphorus levels because deficiency of any of these can result in muscle weakness, respiratory failure, and cardiac arrhythmias.

BENEFITS OF PULMONARY REHABILITATION

A summary of the benefits that have been reported through the use of the components of care considered to be part of pulmonary rehabilitation are listed in Table 3. A reduction in respiratory symptoms, reversal of anxiety and depression, and an improvement in ego strength have been reported commonly. Also, all programs have described an improved ability for patients to carry out activities of daily living, enhanced exercise capacity, and achievement of a better

TABLE 3 Demonstrated Benefits of Pulmonary Rehabilitation

Reduction in respiratory symptoms
Reversal of anxiety and depression and improved ego strength
Enhanced ability to carry out activities of daily living
Increased exercise ability
Better quality of life
Reduction in hospital days required
Prolongation of life in selected patients, i.e., use of continuous oxygen in patients with severe hypoxemia

quality of life. Patients with mild to moderate disease are often able to continue or return to gainful employment.

A reduction in hospitalization in patients with COPD following pulmonary rehabilitation has been reported by several groups. In a study of 80 patients at Loma Linda University Medical Center (LLUMC), patients achieved an average reduction from approximately 19 days of hospitalization in the year prior to the program to approximately 6 days of hospitalization during the first year following completion of the program. This trend has continued for the 8 years for which follow-up data have been analyzed. As can be seen from evaluating Figure 1, the reduction in hospital days was not simply due to the death of the sickest patients during the initial years of follow-up because the curve for only those patients surviving during the 8 years of follow-up was similar to the curve for all patients. A reduction in hospital days needed can result in a significant decrease in costs.

No pulmonary rehabilitation study to date has shown a significant alteration in the mean rate of decrease in pulmonary function measurements such as the forced expiratory volume in 1 second (FEV_1). The decrement in FEV_1 for patients with COPD ranges from 40 to 80 ml per year, rather than the 20 to 30 ml per year decrease reported for normal individuals. The fact that pulmonary function may improve significantly or even return to normal in patients with early obstructive airway disease who stop smoking provides hope that by applying the principles of pulmonary rehabil-

itation to patients earlier in the course of disease it will be possible to alter the ultimate course of the disease, i.e., slow down the progression of, or even improve, the obstructive airway defect.

There is a variation in survival curves that has been reported by pulmonary rehabilitation programs (Fig. 2). Table 4 compares information relating to the patients in the four pulmonary rehabilitation study groups depicted in Figure 2. A possible reason for the improved survival curve in the study by Hodgkin and associates is that patients entered into that pulmonary rehabilitation program with milder disease (see Fig. 2). The Hodgkin study did, however, compare the cumulative survival rate for only those patients with an initial FEV_1 above 1.24 L with patients with a similar degree of airway obstruction from the Burrows study (Fig. 3). The survival rate for the patients in the Hodgkin study was significantly better (P value <0.05) for years 2 to 7. This could be related to the fact that the patients in the study reported by Hodgkin and associates participated in a comprehensive pulmonary rehabilitation program and had continuing follow-up by team members, including home visits. It has been suggested that the improved survival in the Postma study, as compared with the Petty and Burrows studies, might be related to the fact that the patients were younger, very responsive to bronchodilator, and probably included asthmatic patients who were excluded from the other studies depicted in Table 4 and Figure 2.

The possibility that a comprehensive pulmonary

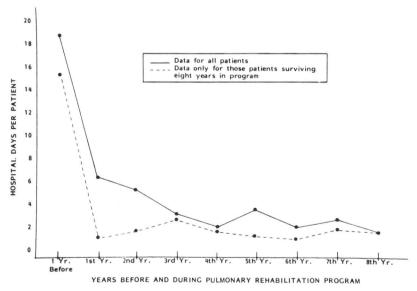

Figure 1 Analysis of hospital days before and during pulmonary rehabilitation program at the Loma Linda University Medical Center. (Reproduced from Hodgkin JE, Branscomb BV, Anholm JD, et al. Benefits, limitations, and the future of pulmonary rehabilitation. In: Hodgkin JE, Zorn EG, Connors GL, eds. Pulmonary rehabilitation: guidelines to success. Boston: Butterworths, 1984; 405.)

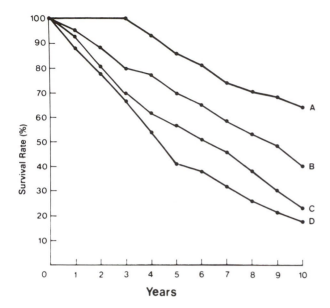

Figure 2 Cumulative survival rates of COPD patients. *A*, Hodgkin and associates. *B*, Postma and associates. *C*, Burrows and associates. *D*, Petty and associates. (Reprinted from Bebout DE, Hodgkin JE, Zorn EG, et al. Clinical and physiological outcomes of a university-hospital pulmonary rehabilitation program. Respir Care 1983; 28:1472.)

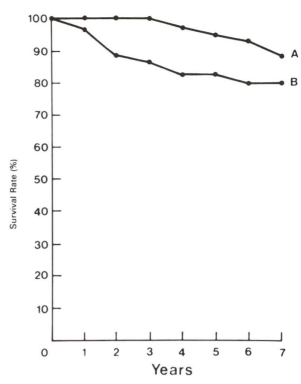

Figure 3 Cumulative survival rates of COPD patients with $FEV_1 > 1.24$ L. *A*, Hodgkin and associates ($N = 46$). *B*, Burrows and associates ($N = 52$). (Reprinted from Bebout DE, Hodgkin JE, Zorn EG, et al. Clinical and physiological outcomes of a university-hospital pulmonary rehabilitation program. Respir Care 1983; 28:1472.)

rehabilitation program, including close follow-up, may improve survival was also suggested by cumulative survival curves for patients in the NIH IPPB Study. The patients in this study had moderate to severe COPD (mean FEV_1 was 1.03 L and was 36 percent of predicted).

Mortality in the IPPB study patients with a baseline postbronchodilator FEV_1 of at least 50 percent of predicted was only slightly worse than in a group of healthy smokers. The baseline FEV_1 was clearly a predictor of survival.

Prolongation of life has also been reported in those

COPD patients with severe hypoxemia who use supplemental oxygen continuously. If significant hypoxemia is corrected with continuous supplemental oxygen, patient survival appears to be no different from that in those with similar obstruction to airflow but without baseline hypoxemia.

In order to achieve a significant reduction in the

TABLE 4 Comparison of Pulmonary Rehabilitation Study Groups

	Hodgkin*	Postma†	Burrows‡	Petty§
Number	75	129	200	182
Mean age (years)	60	54	59	61
Mean FEV_1 (L)	1.55	0.61	1.04	0.94
Mean PaO_2 (mm Hg)	68	—	—	—
Mean $PaCO_2$ (mm Hg)	42	44	44	—
Nonsmokers (%)	23	36	38	—

* Bebout DE, Hodgkin JE, Zorn EG, et al. Clinical and physiological outcomes of a university-hospital pulmonary rehabilitation program. Respir Care 1983; 28:1468–1473.

† Postma DS, Burema J, Gimeno F, et al. Prognosis in severe chronic obstructive pulmonary disease. Am Rev Respir Dis 1979; 119:357–367.

‡ Diener CF, Burrows B. Further observations on the course and prognosis of chronic obstructive lung disease. Am Rev Respir Dis 1975; 111:719–724.

§ Sahn SA, Nett LM, Petty TL. Ten year follow-up of a comprehensive rehabilitation program for severe COPD. Chest 1980; 77(suppl):311–314.

rate of respiratory function deterioration and a definite prolongation of life, it would seem reasonable that the components of care outlined in Table 2 must be instituted earlier in the course of the disease rather than waiting until severe irreversible impairment of function has occurred.

The National Heart, Lung and Blood Institute is currently sponsoring a multicenter study in patients with mild obstructive airway disease to determine whether interventions such as smoking cessation and inhalation of bronchodilator early in the course of the disease may significantly alter the course of the disease and survival.

COST EFFECTIVENESS OF PULMONARY REHABILITATION PROGRAMS

Cost studies have been performed in an attempt to evaluate in economic terms the benefits of pulmonary rehabilitation. If a program is to be cost effective, increased tangible benefits when compared with traditional treatment programs must be identified in terms of the program's monetary worth and its health-related benefits. It is estimated that there are at least 7.9 million Americans with chronic bronchitis, 6.8 million with asthma, and 2.5 million with emphysema. The total cost of health care related to diseases of the respiratory system was estimated in 1975 to be $19.7 billion, and of course is much higher now. It has also been estimated that the cost of health care, lost wages, and time away from work for people with asthma, chronic bronchitis, and emphysema exceeds $15 billion. Pulmonary rehabilitation programs would seem justifiable if they result in less suffering and an improved quality of life. However, if such programs can also result in a reduction in the cost of medical care, this is an added economic bonus.

For those individuals who, because of the process of pulmonary rehabilitation, are able to maintain or return to gainful employment, there is a cost benefit to society. In addition, by helping patients to achieve independence in their activities of daily living, there is an economic savings by reducing the individual's dependence on health care providers. Indicators of this kind of improvement include a reduction in the need for hospitalization, emergency room visits, doctor's office visits, extended care facility placements, and home care visits.

A reduction in hospital need achieved by those COPD patients depicted in Figure 1 resulted in an estimated savings in hospitalization costs during the first year following the pulmonary rehabilitation program of approximately $1,935 per patient and more than

TABLE 5 Cost of the Loma Linda University Medical Center Respiratory Rehabilitation Program from July 1981 to June 1982

Total direct labor	$354,785
Indirect labor	92,244
Space	52,343
Supplies	6,591
Travel	11,452
Miscellaneous	2,527
Total	$519,942

$150,000 for the 80-patient group. The cost of the pulmonary rehabilitation program at LLUMC from July 1981 to June 1982 amounted to $519,942 (Table 5). In 1982, the LLUMC Pulmonary Rehabilitation Team was following approximately 1,150 COPD patients; consequently, the cost per patient was about $452 per year. For an 80-patient group, this would amount to a cost of $36,160 per year. Clearly, the cost of rehabilitation when one takes into account the savings achieved by the reduction in hospital days required alone makes the program seem justifiable.

PERSPECTUS

Any patient with respiratory symptoms is a candidate for pulmonary rehabilitation. By following a proper sequence, the pulmonary rehabilitation team can outline a program that should allow the individual to achieve the established goals. An increase in the availability of pulmonary rehabilitation programs will allow more patients with respiratory disease to enhance their ability to carry out daily activities, resulting in an improved quality of life and reduction in the cost of medical care. It seems logical that the course of the disease is more likely to be altered favorably by instituting the principles of pulmonary rehabilitation earlier than has traditionally been done.

Suggested Reading

Anthonisen NR, Wright EC, Hodgkin JE, et al. Prognosis in chronic obstructive pulmonary disease. Am Rev Respir Dis 1986; 133:14–20.

Hodgkin JE, Petty TL, eds. Chronic obstructive pulmonary disease: current concepts. Philadelphia: WB Saunders, 1987.

Hodgkin JE, Zorn EG, Connors GL, eds. Pulmonary rehabilitation: guidelines to success. Stoneham, MA: Butterworth, 1984.

Nocturnal Oxygen Therapy Trial Group. Continuous or nocturnal oxygen therapy in hypoxemic chronic obstructive lung disease. Ann Intern Med 1980; 93:391–398.

Pulmonary rehabilitation: official American Thoracic Society statement. Am Rev Respir Dis 1981; 124:663–666.

The Intermittent Positive Pressure Breathing Trial Group. Intermittent positive pressure breathing therapy of chronic obstructive pulmonary disease. Ann Intern Med 1983; 99:612–620.

VENTILATORY MUSCLE TRAINING

MICHAEL J. BELMAN, M.D.

Already a decade has passed since the publication of the first study to show that specific training of the ventilatory muscles improves their endurance capacity. This study was performed in young healthy subjects. Because patients with chronic obstructive pulmonary disease (COPD) suffer from impaired ventilatory mechanics and the potential for diaphragmatic fatigue, it was predictable that the idea of ventilatory muscle training would be extended to these patients. Several studies concerning the value of ventilatory muscle training in patients with COPD have already been published. A great deal of experience in ventilatory muscle training (VMT) has been accumulated and several different methods of training have been advocated. Training has been used mostly in patients with obstructive airways disease, such as COPD and cystic fibrosis, but neuromuscular diseases, such as quadriplegia, have also been investigated. Despite the relatively long period of time since the first description of ventilatory muscle training, there is still no unanimity of opinion regarding its efficacy.

RATIONALE

The response to endurance training depends upon several factors including intensity, duration, and frequency of exercise. The appropriate components of training have been the subject of intense study, and recently, the American College of Sports Medicine made recommendations concerning the appropriate mixture of intensity duration and frequency required to improve overall aerobic capacity. These conclusions for overall aerobic capacity were reached after an extended period of investigation; it is therefore not surprising that final recommendations for ventilatory muscle training cannot be made as yet. Ventilatory muscle training is still in its infancy.

In normal subjects, oxygen delivery via the cardiovascular system appears to be the major limiting factor during high intensity exercise. At these levels, normal subjects are operating at submaximal ventilatory levels. In contrast, the patient with COPD achieves peak exercise levels at submaximal cardiac frequencies, but at ventilatory levels that are close to or even exceed the maximum voluntary ventilation (MVV). Because of the probable ventilatory limitation to exercise in COPD patients, there is strong support for the view that training directed specifically at ventilatory muscles would not only improve ventilatory muscle function, but also increase overall exercise capacity. The factors that contribute to impairment of ventilatory muscle function in obstructive airways disease include not only the increased airways resistance, but also the fact that the diaphragm is operating at a disadvantage because of the hyperinflation associated with pulmonary emphysema. This hyperinflation shortens the muscle so that it operates at a suboptimal point on its length-tension curve. Malnutrition, which coexists with pulmonary emphysema in many cases, aggravates the situation because it adversely affects diaphragm muscle structure and function.

METHODS OF TRAINING

Three main methods of ventilatory muscle training have emerged. These are (1) resistive training, (2) hyperpneic training, and (3) threshold load training.

Resistive Method

The resistive method utilizes inspiratory devices with small orifices through which the patients breathe, thereby loading the ventilatory muscles (Fig. 1). During this form of training, expiration is unimpeded.

Hyperpneic Method

In the hyperpneic method, the patient performs voluntary hyperpnea in a rebreathing circuit so constructed as to maintain the inspired oxygen and carbon dioxide concentrations within physiologic limits. In addition, this system provides a target ventilatory level so as to stimulate the patient to maximum performance. Sustained ventilatory levels are usually between 70 percent and 90 percent of the MVV, and the breathing frequency is usually between 40 and 60 breaths per minute (bpm).

Threshold Load Method

The threshold load method uses an inspiratory valve, which is weighted so that it only opens when a predetermined threshold inspiratory pressure is attained. Inspiration can only proceed as long as this threshold pressure is exceeded. Mechanical devices

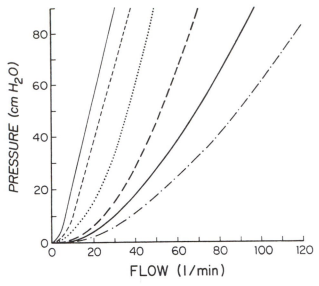

Figure 1 The relationship between flow rate and pressure developed across the orifices of an RTD. Each line represents the values obtained for one orifice. Regression lines from left to right represent orifices 6 through 1. (Reproduced with permission from Belman MJ, Thomas SG, Lewis MI. Resistive breathing training and ventilatory muscle training in patients with COPD. Chest 1986; 90:662–669).

for all three methods of ventilatory muscle training are available.

CLINICAL STUDIES OF VENTILATORY MUSCLE TRAINING

Resistive Training

Because of the simplicity of resistive training, it has been utilized by most published studies to date. A simple plastic resistive training device (RTD) is now marketed (Pflex) and, in principle, is similar to the other RTDs described. Resistive training is performed by breathing through an orifice while expiration is unloaded. Patients are instructed to start resistive breathing through the largest orifice. If they can tolerate this for a pre-determined time (usually 15 minutes), they then proceed to consecutively smaller orifices as tolerated. The results of these studies are summarized in Table 1. In general, the duration of the training was from 4 weeeks to 2 months and included patients with COPD and cystic fibrosis. In a few of the studies, normal subjects were also evaluated. In general, these studies showed that at the completion of the training, the patients were able to breathe through smaller orifices. Investigators concluded that findings implied improved ventilatory muscle function. It should be noted, however, that in the study by Bjerre-Jepsen in 1981, both patient and control group improved to the same degree.

However, in all of the initial studies, breathing strategy (including respiratory rate), inspiratory flow rate, inspiratory time, and tidal volume were not controlled. It is now clear that this is a major drawback since alterations in breathing strategy dramatically alter the inspiratory resistance and, consequently, the load applied to the respiratory muscles. As the orifices of inspiratory devices function as alinear resistances, increases in inspiratory flow rate increase the inspiratory resistance. Even in the presence of constant flow rates, an increase in breathing frequency increases the total load applied to the muscles. Because data on breathing strategy are not available in these studies, it is conceivable that the improved performance might just reflect alteration in breathing strategy (rather than a real improvement in ventilatory muscle performance). In fact, it has recently been demonstrated that a breathing pattern that utilizes slow, deep breaths improves resistive breathing performance. The reason for this is that the decreased flow rates and breathing frequency reduce the work rate and oxygen consumption of the respiratory muscles. Furthermore, as perception of effort during resistive breathing is closely related to peak mouth pressure, a reduction in this index results in a reduced sense of discomfort.

Preliminary data are now available from studies in which a feedback signal of the breathing strategy was shown to the patient so that breathing pattern could be regulated during the training and testing of the ventilatory muscles. In the study by Clanton and co-workers, the subjects followed a preset pattern of breathing by watching a record of their breathing pattern on an oscilloscopic screen. More recently, a portable feedback devise has been developed, which helps patients regulate breathing frequency and inspiratory mouth pressure. By this means, it is possible to control inspiratory time, expiratory time, mean inspiratory flow rate, and peak mouth pressure. Early data from these studies indicate that this "targeted" form of resistive breathing is efficacious.

As noted above, the load on the respiratory muscles with RTDs varies with the breathing pattern. With the RTDs patients are instructed to increase the load by breathing through a smaller orifice. However, if the breathing pattern is altered as the patient changes to a smaller orifice, it is possible to decrease the load on the respiratory mucles such that it may be the same or even less than that experienced while breathing through a large orifice. In our experience, the use of small orifices (hole #3 and smaller of the Pflex) may be associated with hypercapnia, whereas if large orifices are used (hole #1 of the Pflex) hypocapnea may result. Empirically we have found that COPD patients generally maintain normocapnia when breathing through an orifice of 0.46-cm diameter (hole #2 of the Pflex device) and that this orifice provides a wide

TABLE 1   Effect of Ventilatory Muscle Training on Ventilatory Muscle Endurance and Exercise Capacity

Author	Subjects	Type and Duration of Training	Effects on Ventilatory Muscle Endurance	Exercise Capacity
Anderson, 1979	COPD (28) & normal	Resistive 2 mo	Increased	
Pardy, 1979	COPD (12)	Resistive 2 mo	Increased	6/12 Increased walking performance
Bjerre-Jepsen, 1981	COPD (18) & control	Resistive 6 wk	Both groups improved	
Sonne, 1982	COPD (6)	Resistive 6 wk	Increased	Increased
Asher, 1982	CF (11)	Resistive 4 wk	Increased	Not increased
Chen, 1985	COPD (12) & control	Resistive 4 wk	Increased	Not increased
Leith, 1976	Normal (4)	Hyperpneic 5 wk	14% increase in MSVC	
Keens, 1977	CF & Normal	Hyperpneic 6 wk	55% increase in MSVC	
Belman, 1980	COPD (10)	Hyperpneic 6 wk	33% increase in MSVC	Increased walking performance
Levine, 1986	COPD, (15-VMT), (17-IPPB)	Hyperpneic 6 wk		ADLs and exercise improved in both groups
Larson, 1986	COPD	Threshold load 2 mo Low and high intensity groups	Increase Pimax Increase in SIP	Increase walking (high intensity group)

Pimax = maximal mouth inspiratory pressure
SIP = sustained inspiratory pressure

range of work rates when a constant breathing strategy is used. It is our impression, therefore, that resistive trainers in the future should employ a feedback device to control breathing strategy. Furthermore, a single orifice rather than multiple orifices is adequate. This system should make resistive training easier to accomplish and make the results more predictable.

Several of the studies of resistive breathing have evaluated overall exercise capacity, in addition to assessment of ventilatory muscle function. This has been done by means of tests of walking endurances such as the 12-minute walk or by endurance tests of cycling. However, it is only in the minority of patients that improvements in exercise capacity are found. There are many reasons to account for the lack of increase in walking performance. These include the fact that the ventilatory muscles may not play a limiting role in COPD and that there may have been a lack of real improvement in ventilatory muscle endurance after the resistive training. It has also been postulated that the pattern of breathing in resistive training with the low frequency of breathing and inspiratory flow rates is not appropriate to improve ventilatory muscle function during exercise when there is a high breathing frequency and rapid inspiratory flow rates.

Hyperpneic Training

The hyperpneic method was used in the original study by Leith and Bradley in 1976, but because of the complexity of the rebreathing system required for this form of training, it has been used in only a few subsequent studies. This training is also performed for approximately 30 minutes daily and in the published studies it has been done for approximately 6 consecutive weeks. The main index of measurement has been the maximal sustained ventilatory capacity (MSVC), which is defined as the maximal ventilation that can be sustained under isocapnic conditions for 15 minutes. In most subjects this ranges from about 60 to 80 percent of the MVV. Table 1 summarizes the studies performed using hyperpneic training. In these studies normal subjects, patients with COPD, and children with cystic fibrosis have been evaluated. All studies show a consistent increase in the MSVC, which ranged from 14 percent in normals to as high as 55 percent in patients with cystic fibrosis.

In two of the studies, exercise performance was evaluated in addition to the ventilatory muscle function. One study showed a 12-percent increase in the walking performance and similar increases in arm and leg cycle ergometry. A more recent study examined COPD patients and compared their results to a control group treated with intermittent positive pressure breathing (IPPB). Only the group that underwent the ventilatory muscle training showed a significant increase in the MSVC, but both treated and control groups showed an improvement in exercise capacity and in performance of activities of daily living (ADL). The investigators ascribed the improved exercise tolerance in the control group to a desensitization to dyspnea, which they felt occurred as a result of the multiple exercise tests that the patients underwent as part of the study protocol. Nevertheless, the fact that the control group showed an improvement in exercise capacity, does cast doubt on the limiting role of the ventilatory muscles in exercise capacity in patients with COPD. Clearly, other factors must be important. Despite this, there were impressive improvements in ventilatory function per se in all of the studies that used the hyperpneic breathing method. It remains to be seen whether improved ventilatory muscle endurance per se is an adequate measure of the efficacy of VMT or whether there should also be an improvement in overall exercise capacity.

Threshold Load Method

The original threshold device was relatively complex in its construction, but recently a more simple device has been developed.

This device overcomes the problem of varying inspiratory flow rates that occur with the RTD. Irrespective of the inspiratory flow rate, the valve opens when the threshold pressure is reached, after which inspiration proceeds as long as the inspiratory pressure is higher than the threshold. However, it should be pointed out that breathing frequency and inspiratory time need to be regulated so as to maintain work loads at a constant level. A patient who breathes at a high breathing frequency with a long inspiratory time performs more inspiratory work than a subject who breathes slowly with a short inspiratory time even though the threshold pressure is identical.

Weaning and Ventilatory Muscle Training

Some authors have suggested that intermittent mandatory ventilation (IMV) is potentially detrimental to the weaning process. This hypothesis is based on the supposition that fatigued ventilatory muscles should be rested completely in order to facilitate recovery. This school of thought has suggested that intermittent periods of spontaneous breathing (as in T tube trials), interspersed with periods of controlled ventilation, is a superior method of weaning than IMV.

We and others have tried either hyperpneic or resistive training in patients being weaned from mechanical ventilation as a means of accelerating improvement in ventilatory muscle function. These data are preliminary, but indicate that improvements in ventilatory function can be accelerated by means of specific training. However, in view of the preliminary nature of the data, it is not possible at present to endorse either resistive or hyperpneic training during weaning. Further studies are necessary before firm recommendations can be made.

Suggested Reading

Aldrich T. Inspiratory muscle resistive training in respiratory failure. Am Rev Respir Dis 1985; 131:461–462.

Anderson JB, Dragsted L, Kann T, et al. Resistive breathing training in severe chronic obstructive pulmonary disease. Scand J Resp Dis 1979; 60:151–156.

Asher MI, Pardy R, Coats AL, et al. The effect of inspiratory muscle training in patients with cystic fibrosis. Am Rev Respir Dis 1982; 126:855–859.

Belman MJ, Sieck GC. The ventilatory muscles: fatigue endurance and training. Chest 1982; 82:761–766.

Belman MJ, Thomas SG, Lewis MI. Resistive breathing training and ventilatory muscle endurance in patients with COPD. Chest 1986; 90:662–669.

Belman MJ, Mitman C. Ventilatory muscle training improves exercise capacity in chronic obstructive pulmonary disease patients. Am Rev Respir Dis 1980; 121:273–280.

Bjerre-Jensen K, Scher NH, Koh-Jensen A. Inspiratory resistance training in severe chronic obstructive pulmonary disease. Eur J Resp Dis 1981; 62:405–411.

Braun NMT, Faulkner J, Hughes RL, et al. When should respiratory muscles be exercised. Chest 1983; 84:76–84.

Chen H, Dukes R, Martin BJ. Inspiratory muscle training in patients with chronic obstructive pulmonary disease. Am Rev Respir Dis 1985; 131:251–255.

Clanton TL, Dixon G, Drake J, et al. Inspiratory muscle conditioning using a threshold device. Chest 1985; 87:62–65.

Flenley DC. Short review: inspiratory muscle training. Euro J Respir Dis 1985; 67:153–158.

Keens TG, Krastins IRB, Wannamaker EM, et al. Ventilatory muscle endurance training in normal subjects and patients with cystic fibrosis. Am Rev Resp Dis 1977; 116:853–860.

Larson JL, Kim MJ, Sharp JT. Inspiratory muscle training with a threshold resistive breathing device in patients with COPD. Am Rev Respir Dis 1986; 133:100A.

Leith ED, Bradley M. Ventilatory muscle strength and endurance training. J Appl Physio 1976; 41:508–516.

Levine S, Weiser P, Gillen J. Evaluation of a ventilatory muscle endurance training program in the rehabilitation of patients with chronic obstructive pulmonary disease. Am Rev Respir Dis 1986; 133:400–406.

Pardy RL, Rivington RN, Despas PJ, et al. The effect of inspiratory muscle training on exercise performance in chronic air flow limitation. Am Rev Resp Dis 1981; 123:426–434.

Sonne LJ, Davis JA, Increased exercise performance in patients with severe COPD following inspiratory resistive training. Chest 1982; 81:436–439.

EXERCISE TECHNIQUES DURING PULMONARY REHABILITATION

CYNTHIA COFFIN ZADAI, P.T., M.S.

Exercise conditioning is currently perceived as a relative newcomer among the therapeutic modalities available to treat the functionally limited pulmonary patient. The most likely cause of this perception is the long held, reasonable assumption that exercise would be counterproductive by exacerbating the symptoms of a patient population that is frequently dyspneic at rest. The historical physical therapy literature actually emphasizes the positive effect of corrective breathing patterns and walking exercise or stair climbing for the victims of pulmonary injury or disease. Today, the techniques of breathing retraining and exercise conditioning have been investigated in greater depth and specificity and applied across a broader range of patients to include individuals with cystic fibrosis, reactive airways disease, and restrictive disease of both neuromuscular and pulmonary origin. The common denominator among these individuals is dyspnea, the primary symptom that limits their functional performance.

Dyspnea, regardless of its origin, stimulates and produces the vicious cycle of self-imposed functional limitation leading to deconditioning and more pronounced limitation. Exercise conditioning for individuals with pulmonary impairment differs significantly from its use in either the normal or the predominantly cardiac-impaired population. The predicted response to exercise and the standardized exercise response values are not valid in the pulmonary-impaired population. The complexity of dyspnea as a symptom and the multiple components of the response to exercise combine to present a significant challenge to the clinician evaluating an individual whose primary complaint is dyspnea on exertion.

EVALUATION AND PATIENT ASSESSMENT

Exercise that involves repeated isotonic, skeletal muscle contraction for any length of time demands an increase in oxygen delivery to the exercising muscle. Oxygen delivery is dependent upon:

1. effective ventilatory muscle contraction,
2. compliant, patent airways,
3. adequate surface area and pressure gradient for gas exchange,
4. sufficient blood supply and oxygen-carrying capacity,
5. efficient and effective cardiac pumping,
6. successful O_2 kinetics, and
7. effective gas transport into and out of the cell.

Impairment of any of these components can limit exercise performance and produce symptoms. The clinical challenge is to determine the limiting factor(s) by means of evaluating the patient and exercise testing (Table 1). The goal of treatment is to minimize functional limitation secondary to the patient's lung disease and to use exercise conditioning to maximize pulmonary and cardiovascular performance.

Exercise testing and functional assessment prior to training are components of the comprehensive evaluation process. The goals of this assessment include:

1. evaluating the efficacy of the current therapeutic program during activities of daily living (ADL),
2. eliciting and documenting the factors that limit functional activity, and
3. assessing the medical safety of exercise through monitoring during several activity levels, and serving as a baseline for exercise prescription.

Individuals referred for evaluation and treatment with functional/exercise testing and training are diverse in their diagnoses and level of disease (Table 2). Patient evaluation begins with summarizing all available clinical data related to the patient's historically documented or currently described functional baseline. This summary indicates the patient's current functional level and estimates the optimum baseline that can be achieved. Short-term and long-term goals are planned based on objective and subjective findings and the individual patient's desires.

Interview and Examination

Patient interview questions focus on the patient's or family's perception of the individual's current functional level. Symptoms of pulmonary disease, such as cough and dyspnea, are related to both ADL and environment, e.g., sleep habits and occupational tasks or changes in season, temperature, and humidity. The patient is observed throughout the interview for breathing rate, rhythm, pattern, posture, and use of musculature as well as frequency and efficacy of cough. A standard thoracic physical examination is performed, including a comprehensive posture evalua-

TABLE 1   Exercise Limits: Interpretation Considerations

Ventilatory pump:	Low maximal inspiratory pressure, achievement of predicted maximal voluntary ventilation, respiratory rate 50–60, development or worsening of discoordinated breathing pattern
Airway reactivity:	Bronchospasm, wheezing, decreased FEV_1, change in ventilatory muscle use and breathing pattern
Cardiac dysfunction:	ECG abnormality, dyspnea, rapid inappropriate increase in heart rate, falling blood pressure, angina, hypertension
Gas-exchanging organ:	Decreasing O_2 saturation, increasing $PaCO_2$, dizziness, nausea, ECG abnormalities
Deconditioning:	Appropriate cardiopulmonary physiologic response to exercise that quickly reaches predicted maximal heart rate or is symptom-limited by noncardiopulmonary conditions (e.g., fear, weak extremities, lack of coordination)

tion to observe functional versus structural abnormalities and breathing patterns in various positions. Simple spirometry, oxygen saturation at rest, vital signs, and resting electrocardiogram are recorded and matched to baseline values available from either the referring source, an old chart, the patients themselves, or used to serve as a baseline if no other information is available. This initial examination identifies patients who require additional medical or therapeutic management prior to exercise testing or training. Examples include:

1. patients with acute reactive airways at rest who require bronchodilators;
2. individuals with cardiac conditions, e.g., congestive heart failure, angina, arrhythmia;
3. patients with resting oxygen saturation below 85 percent;
4. patients with adventitious breath sounds and productive cough requiring bronchopulmonary hygiene; and
5. patients with asynchronous or discoordinated breathing patterns regardless of position.

Patients evaluated for functional activity and exercise conditioning are assessed in this manner to determine which components of their oxygen delivery system may be limited prior to testing. Those underlying abnor-malities are treated when possible to minimize limitations.

Exercise Testing and Functional Evaluation

When the patient's pulmonary status is optimized, he or she can be exercised. Each patient's age, prior and present activity level, and degree of disease impairment determine the exercise modality, test protocol, and prescription. Integration of the physical examination findings and patient goals directs the clinician's choice in selecting the safest, most appropriate mode for exercise testing, the parameters to be monitored, and the eventual exercise prescription (Table 3).

Exercise Mode

The exercise test assesses the patient's physiologic response during performance of the activity that will be prescribed for training.

The terms training or exercise conditioning are not synonymous with aerobic conditioning when used in reference to a pulmonary-impaired population. Exercise conditioning in this population has not consistently demonstrated the central and peripheral adaptations commonly seen with normals and cardiac-

TABLE 2   Potential Population for Exercise Conditioning

Mechanically ventilated patients: deconditioned/unable to wean
COPD patients: frequent exacerbations that limit function requiring hospital admission
Cystic fibrosis patients: potential to increase exercise and decrease frequency of bronchopulmonary hygiene
Patients with multiple system disease (primarily of cardiopulmonary origin) that results in deconditioning
Patients with exercise-induced bronchospasm
Patients with neuromuscular or musculoskeletal disease limiting cardiopulmonary function

TABLE 3 Physiologic Parameters: Exercise Testing

Predicted Maximum Heart Rate (HR$_{max}$)
  220-Age for individuals 60 or younger
  60 and older; males plateau around 170, females plateau
  around 160
	Ability to reach 85% maximum or greater without
	  cardiopulmonary symptoms or limitation; good indicator
	  that patient is capable of exercise conditioning

Clinical Predictor for Maximum Ventilatory Capacity (MVV)
  35 × FEV$_1$ (actual)
	Individuals who reach this level of ventilation with minimum
	  intensity exercise may have difficulty with or be unable to
	  benefit from exercise conditioning

Oxygenation: resting PaO$_2$: 104 − (.42 × age)
    exercise O$_2$ sat: should be 85% or above
	Resting levels should be above 60 mm Hg and 85%
	  saturation. Levels below this at rest or with activity
	  require supplemental O$_2$

Carbon Dioxide: remains within 10 torr of resting level	Individuals who are unable to maintain this level of gas exchange will be unable to condition with exercise

Maximum Inspiratory Pressure (mouth): critical level 40–60
  cm H$_2$O
	Below this level ventilatory muscle strength training will
	  precede or accompany exercise conditioning

impaired patients. Consistent benefits do include an increased ability to perform functional activities that require walking and an increased endurance level during performance of the activity the patient is trained for. Since the most common functional limitation in pulmonary disease is inability to perform walking for ADL, the training modality most frequently prescribed is walking.

In some situations walking programs are not desirable or possible. Patients who are limited by lack of available space, attachment to a ventilator, environmental exposure (heat, cold, humidity, or allergens), lack of access to safe walking conditions, physical disabilities such as paraplegia, amputation, or musculoskeletal impairment, or preference for a more easily accessible modality (stationary bicycle) require testing on and prescription using a different exercise mode. Other options include stationary arm and leg ergometers or rowing ergometers.

Aerobic activities such as organized sports, dance clubs, and circuit training are generally not useful for this population. Pulmonary patients frequently require low-level, controlled intensity activities with easy access for daily programming. Activities that require transportation and specific timed participation without intensity control can be more problematic than helpful. The patient must be reasonably familiar with the activity and have control and access to increase comfort and security, promoting motivation to comply. The testing mode should be the training mode so the patient can easily document and see improvement from testing and goal setting through training and retest.

Protocol

The test protocol specifics for each patient may differ, but the following components are common among all tests. The stress test utilizes the exercise mode on which the patient will be training. It objectively provides a record of the patient's physiologic response to the activity, and it elicits the symptoms or physiologic responses that limit exercise. The two protocols that provide the greatest amount of useful information with the least patient discomfort are described in Table 4.

The two-stage intermittent test is administered to patients who will be exercising on either ergometers or treadmills during their exercise program. This test is administered only after the patient's ability to ride or walk on the equipment has been confirmed. Patients unfamiliar with the exercise and monitoring equipment require practice trials prior to choosing a mode or protocol. Stage I is performed at a low level for 6 minutes. This stage assesses the patient's level of dyspnea and symptoms elicited with minimal functional activity. A 6-minute time period allows the patient to reach a steady state if that is physiologically possible. Values obtained during the first stage provide objective data and direct the selection of the exercise level chosen for stage II. If the patient is unable to complete stage I, that is considered a maximum, symptom-limited test, and the values and symptoms elicited are recorded. If the patient experiences arterial desaturation below 85 percent during stage I, a second stage is performed with oxygen (O$_2$) to determine the patient's symptomatic and objective response to exercise with O$_2$. Patients who reach steady state, are not symptom-limited, and are physiologically capable of greater exercise intensity proceed to stage II after their vital signs have returned to baseline. The intensity of exercise selected for stage II patients is based on the minute ventilation, percentage of maximal heart rate achieved, and perceived exertion recorded during stage I. Most commonly either the treadmill grade or the pedal resistance is increased rather than the speed. This adjustment is more likely to produce the necessary heart rate and ventilatory responses to exercise. Increased speed generally produces fear, inability to coordinate the activity, or patient refusal. Stage II attempts to elicit a symptom-limited maximum or to determine the limits of safety and function for each patient. Patients who complete 6 minutes of stage II and approach 85 percent of

TABLE 4   Exercise Test Protocols

Two-Stage Intermittent Test
Stage I: *Dyspnea Index, Baseline Function*
      Treadmill/1–2 mph, 0% grade
      Ergometer/0.5 kpm @ 60 rpm
  Patient walks, rides, or cranks for 6 minutes steadily if possible. Collect expired gases during final 2 minutes if possible.
  Monitor and calculate: blood pressure, heart rate, respiratory rate, ventilatory muscle use, maximum inspiratory pressure at
     initiation and completion, ECG, $\dot{V}E$, $\dot{V}O_2$.
  Patient rests and returns to baseline.

Stage II: *Maximum Function*
    Treadmill: Increase grade to elicit 85% of predicted maximal heart rate based on response to stage I. If patient was
            well below predicted maximums and without symptoms during stage I, increase both speed and grade.
            These patients will use two stages to elicit their maximum. An increase to 2.5 mph and 5% grade equates
            to approximately 4 times resting metabolic level.
    Ergometer: Increase resistance to elicit 85% of predicted maximal heart rate without producing extremity fatigue based
            on response to stage I. If patient is coordinated enough to pedal or crank faster and has already
            complained of cramping, increase intensity by increasing speed.

Timed Walk Test
  Measure walkway in 10-foot increments/Time distance walked for either 6 or 12 minutes.
  Instruct patient to walk as far as possible as fast as possible for the timed segment. Record distance walked.
  Monitor: Blood pressure while walking (rolling sphygmomanometer), heart rate, ECG, respiratory rate, ventilatory muscle
      use, O_2 saturation.

maximal heart rate are not put through a third stage. Stage III is used when the patient does not reach his or her physiologic limitation and does not develop severe symptoms of dyspnea or fatigue in stage II.

Patients either below or above the level of function necessary for a two-stage intermittent test require a different protocol. Patients who only experience dyspnea with a high level of exercise require a continuous protocol such as the Bruce protocol, or a bronchial challenge. Patients who are unable to walk on a treadmill or ride an ergometer can be tested with a time-distance protocol (see Table 4). Objective information can also be collected with this protocol; it simply requires additional personnel to watch the patient and to monitor and record vital signs while the patient walks. This protocol is also extremely useful in situations in which little or no equipment is available.

Monitoring and Test Interpretation

Common monitoring parameters for all patients include measuring maximum inspiratory mouth pressure (MIP) prior to exercise, vital signs at rest and every 2 minutes throughout the test, continuous single-lead ECG for arrhythmia detection, continuous oxygen saturation (O_2 sat), and observation of breathing patterns. For patients who can progress to higher or to maximal levels of exercise and breathe through a mouthpiece, expired gas collection provides minute ventilation ($\dot{V}E$), oxygen consumption ($\dot{V}O_2$), expired oxygen (F_EO_2), and carbon dioxide (F_ECO_2). Analysis of the patient's documented response to exercise provides the objective information necessary to set realistic goals and make an exercise prescription.

EXERCISE PRESCRIPTION

Design of an exercise prescription or functional activity program is completely individualized and must be prescribed within both useful and achievable levels for each patient. Pulmonary patients who exhibit ventilatory pump limitations are questionable candidates for exercise conditioning programs. Comprehensive care for these patients is aimed at maximizing airway function through bronchodilation and airway clearance; supplementing O_2 as necessary; maintaining strength and endurance of the ventilatory muscles; providing psychosocial and nutritional support when necessary; and maintaining exercise function and endurance by means of performing ADL that routinely stress their ventilatory system to maximum. If all components of their system are performing at a maximal level with this management, they may not benefit from additional exercise training. Goal setting for these individuals, then, may be maintenance of present function and prevention of deterioration or frequent exacerbation.

Patients who do not reach a ventilatory maximum with exercise do appear to benefit from functional exercise training. Training for these individuals has consistently demonstrated improvements in exercise performance and functional ability, fewer hospitalizations, and an improved sense of well-being. Exercise sessions, however, must be performed regularly and continuously to achieve and maintain benefits.

Warm Up

Pulmonary patients who achieve high workload levels during testing can safely and effectively warm up at low levels of exercise on the modality with which they will be training. Individuals whose maximum exercise level was limited, for example, to 4 minutes of walking at 1.5 mph, 0 percent grade, cannot use walking to warm up. Rhythmic posture exercises with coordinated breathing patterns and simple passive or progressive stretch maneuvers serve to minimally increase the metabolic rate and make the patient aware of his or her breathing pattern. These exercises also mobilize the musculoskeletal system in preparation for exercise. Patients who require bronchopulmonary hygiene for airway clearance prior to exercise can consider that treatment a warm up. Many patients who need bronchopulmonary hygiene to maintain patent airways find exercise a suitable alternative and may alternate exercise and bronchopulmonary hygiene daily. Patients who require inhaled bronchodilators for exercise should administer them 15 to 30 minutes prior to warm-up exercise.

Intensity, Duration, and Frequency

The parameters of an exercise prescription designed to increase and maintain conditioning have been defined for normals and patients with cardiovascular impairment. Experience and research indicate that prescriptions should be individualized to achieve an intensity of at least 60 percent of maximal heart rate, a duration of 20 to 30 minutes, and a minimum frequency of three times per week. These minimums have been established to ensure achievement of the physiologic adaptations to training. Pulmonary patients, however, have not demonstrated either peripheral or central training effects with exercise. Despite an elevated heart rate and ventilatory response to exercise, pulmonary patients are either symptom-limited with exercise initiation or limited prior to achievement of anaerobic threshold and actual Vo_2 maximum. This limitation may be cardiopulmonary (as described in Table 1) or due to patient uncoordination, fear, or peripheral muscle limitation. Consequently, it seems that the use of heart rate as a correlate to oxygen consumption or exercise intensity is inappropriate, and physiologic training levels are not achieved. Initially, patients often cannot maintain any level of exercise for 20 to 30 minutes. Exercise prescription for pulmonary patients is based on the individual patient's actual achievement during his or her exercise test and functional assessment. Those achieved values are turned into an exercise prescription. For example, a patient who can walk for 6 minutes at 2 mph, 0 percent grade but for only 4 minutes at a 3 percent grade will be returned to the initial setting and exercised at that level (2 mph, 0 percent grade). An intermittent walk-rest program is used until the patient can accomplish a minimum of 20 minutes of continuous walking at that level. The program continues with an intermittent prescription, gradually increasing the walk time and decreasing the rest time until 20 to 30 minutes of continuous walking, biking, or arm cranking has been achieved. Once the duration of exercise time has reached 20 to 30 minutes, the intensity can be increased. Duration is the most significant element in the exercise prescription for pulmonary patients, since we are attempting to increase their functional endurance. Frequency is prescribed as daily until the patient achieves the 20-minute continuous minimum.

Similar principles apply to patients who require a time-distance test and stop frequently during the test period. These individuals are given a prescription that calls for gradually extending the duration of walking and shortening the rest period until they can walk for 20 continuous minutes. Patients who can walk initially for 20 minutes are progressed to 30 minutes before increasing intensity. Frequency of exercise also depends on the individual. Patients capable of high-level exercise who complete 30 minutes of continuous exercise receive prescriptions for three to four exercise sessions per week. Low-level or symptomatic patients who can only walk intermittently require daily sessions (i.e., two 10-minute walks per day). Often environment or symptoms prevent compliance with a daily regimen. New patients are given an exercise prescription card that lists either the distance to be covered in a given time or the workload and revolution rate to be ridden or cranked for specific time segments rather than a target heart rate. Frequency of exercise is also described.

Cool Down

Relaxed walking and rhythmic upper extremity exercise with controlled pursed/lip pattern breathing is excellent for cool down. This refocuses the patient's attention on breathing pattern, relaxes accessory muscles, and slows and controls the patient.

SUPPLEMENTAL OXYGEN

Our present method of oxygen use is based on current recommendations and clinical experience. Patients who record values below 85 percent saturation at rest are given oxygen prior to exercise testing and set up for continual home use. Oxygen is also used with individuals who desaturate below 85 percent when exercise is performed. Nasal oxygen is delivered throughout the test in amounts necessary to maintain O_2 saturation above 85 percent during exercise, and the appropriate liter flow is noted and indicated on the prescription card. There are some patients who demonstrate oxygen saturation levels in the low 90s at rest and then desaturate to borderline levels with exercise. These patients are also retested with a trial of oxygen. If their exercise performance changes (i.e., increased time at the previous maximal load, normalization of ECG, heart rate or blood pressure response, and decrease in symptoms), these patients are initially exercised while on oxygen. We have found that individuals with a marginal oxygen requirement often need less oxygen or no oxygen at all as they progress through the program.

EXERCISE PROGRESSION AND PROPHYLACTIC CARE

It is quite common in this patient population to initially document rapid although small gains on a daily or weekly basis. This is particularly true in patients who maintained an active lifestyle or who participated in an exercise program prior to their functional limitation. A 4- to 6-week program generally produces significant measurable results in patients who do not suffer an exacerbation of their underlying disease. Patients who achieve higher levels of work are also able to maintain and/or recover more quickly during exacerbations when managed aggressively medically. Frequent, regular contact every 2 to 3 months follow-ing the initial program provides patients with feedback on their achievements and allows for alteration in the exercise prescription. This contact also provides a means of communication if the patient begins to deteriorate. Aggressive management and quick return to the program interrupt the vicious cycle that precipitates physiologic decline. The program must be sustained to maintain benefits. The greatest benefit of long-term exercise conditioning may be the decreased frequency or severity of acute respiratory illnesses in addition to improved function. Retesting on a biannual basis provides an objective basis for patients to observe the continuation of their functional achievement.

Suggested Reading

Astrand P. Textbook of work physiology: physical basis of exercise. 3rd ed. New York: McGraw-Hill, 1986.
Loke J, guest ed. Symposium on exercise: physiology and clinical applications. Clin Chest Med 1984; 5(1).
Make BJ, guest ed. Pulmonary rehabilitation. Clin Chest Med 1986; 7(4).
Cardiopulmonary aspects of aging. Top Geriatr Rehabil 1986; 2(1):

CHOOSING A HOME CARE MECHANICAL VENTILATOR

JOHN E. THOMPSON, RRT
P. PEARL O'ROURKE, M.D.

The increasing popularity and the safety of home mechanical ventilation readily show that the need for chronic ventilation is no longer a deterrent for home care. Although home mechanical ventilation has become relatively easy, the decision to place a ventilator in the home is a multifactorial one that must include an analysis of the patient, of the patient's disease, of the family structure, and of medical and community supports. Once these issues are addressed and home mechanical ventilation is deemed appropriate and possible, the next step is to carefully evaluate the interface between the patient, the home, and the ventilator. This chapter discusses some of the issues that should be considered when selecting a positive pressure ventilator for home use.

There are a number of companies that supply positive pressure ventilators and service contracts, but the advantages and disadvantages vary. Because the physician and the hospital are responsible for the selection of the ventilator system, it behooves these providers to be able to critically evaluate the machine and the accompanying service contract.

Although the optimal home positive pressure ventilator should be tailored for each patient, such customization is impractical. However, there are a number of basic features that should be carefully considered when choosing a ventilator (Table 1). These features include appropriate ventilation capabilities, user-friendly simplicity, reliability, and, if possible, a compact size that is easily portable. The "best" specific ventilator varies for different patients, depending on their disease, the need for constant versus intermittent ventilation, and the issue of whether home ventilation is custodial or if the patient has potential for rehabilitation or for growth and hence the possibility of changing ventilator needs.

All home ventilators are ideally small and easily portable. However, the importance of portability varies in practice. If the patient requires constant ventilation and/or if patient mobility is a priority, then a small compact machine should be considered (Table 2). In contrast, if patient mobility is limited because of other medical problems, or if the patient needs only intermittent ventilation, then a larger less portable ventilator (i.e., Emerson, MA-I) can be just as easily used. When a portable machine is selected, the machine should have safe mounting to a cart or a wheelchair and any attachments, such as humidifiers or monitors, must be firmly attached.

The type of lung disease and the patient's ventilatory requirements determine the needed ventilator capabilities. Patients who are appropriate for home ventilation can be divided into two basic groups (Table 3). Group I is composed of patients with reasonably normal lungs who suffer neuromuscular disease with secondary respiratory weakness or abnormal control of breathing. Group II patients have abnormal lungs. These two groups of patients have different needs. The patients in Group I (neuromuscular or control of breathing disease) need a ventilator that delivers a reliable tidal volume, but these patients do not usually need high inflating pressures or positive end-expiratory pressure (PEEP) and rarely need oxygen. Generally, these patients need a less sophisticated machine than patients in Group II with abnormal lungs who need higher inflating pressures, who may need PEEP, and who usually do need a higher FIO_2. For these people, the ventilator must deliver a reliable tidal volume (V_T) in order to avoid hypoventilation and/or hyperventilation. Unfortunately, the delivered tidal volume in both home care and hospital ventilators is variable because it is affected by changes in the patient's lung or in the ventilator circuit. In a patient with normal lung compliance and airway resistance, routine changes in tidal volume are not extremely significant. In the patient with abnormal lungs who requires high inflating pressures, any changes in the delivered tidal volume may have profound effects on minute ventilation. Although no ventilator is perfect, generally speaking, hospital ventilators have the most reliable tidal volume delivery and, hence, are most frequently used for those patients with primary lung disease.

Spontaneous ventilation must be able to be done with ease because most home ventilated patients do have a spontaneous respiratory rate. This is particularly important in the patient with neuromuscular weakness. The ventilator should have a low resistance demand system or a continuous flow in order to minimize the work of breathing. Unfortunately, most home ventilators have neither of these options. Therefore the resistance of the existing exhalation valve and the humidifier must be carefully assessed to guarantee that the system is low resistance so that the patient does not have to significantly increase his or her work of

TABLE 1 Basic Ventilator Requirements

Reliable V$_T$
Low work of breathing
PEEP-compensated sensitivity
Apnea-rate back-up
Circuit breakers
Automatic change from AC to DC power
Alarms
   Power loss
   Low pressure (disconnect)
   High pressure
Stable settings with varying line voltage
Protection from inadvertent parameter changes
Safe and easy mounting of accessory equipment
Quiet
Hour meter
Accessible inlet filter

breathing to execute spontaneous breaths. The continued ease of spontaneous ventilation should be critically assessed whenever a new exhalation valve or a humidifier is designed or applied to the ventilator. In addition, if the patient requires positive end-expiratory pressure and assisted ventilation, the ventilator's sensitivity should be PEEP-compensated to minimize the work of breathing during spontaneously generated breaths. PEEP compensation allows the patient to initiate a mechanical breath by creating a negative pressure equal to the sensitivity setting. An uncompensated ventilator would require the patient to create a negative pressure equal to the PEEP setting plus the sensitivity setting.

A back-up system for apnea is needed if the patient has abnormal control of breathing. An audible alarm and a predetermined mechanical rate should be activated during any preset period of apnea. The activation of this system should be a minimum of 20 seconds.

The concerns of delivered tidal volumes and of increased work of breathing are more critical in the child than in the adult on home ventilation. Because the child has a smaller tidal volume than the adult, even small changes in the delivered tidal volume can have a large impact. In addition, the child's spontaneous ventilation may be more difficult with a greater increase in the work of breathing because not only must the child generate enough pressure for each spontaneous breath, but the mechanical deadspace encountered in the exhalation system is often large. This deadspace may be 40 to 100 ml, a volume that is not significant when compared to an adult tidal volume, but a volume that is unquestioningly large when compared to the tidal volume of a child.

The home ventilator must be able to deliver the required mode of support, and must not make the patient's own respiratory effort less effective. In addition, all of the parameter settings should be simple with no extraneous modes or knobs that might confuse the operator and increase the chance of error. The parameter knobs should be difficult to turn and protected from accidental changes—a plexiglas cover over the "control panel" may be useful.

With infants, the question of time-cycled pressure-limited ventilators versus volume-cycled ventilators must be considered. In the hospital, pressure-limited ventilators are generally used for children under 10 kg; these ventilators have a continuous flow of gas that facilitates spontaneous ventilation. There are a number of children less than 1 year of age and less than 10 kg who are candidates for home ventilation. For the aforementioned reason, the time-cycled pressure-limited ventilators are perfect, but there are a few problems. These ventilators require a 50 PSI gas source for operation; the required air compressor or tanks limit portability. In addition, the tidal volume can change as a function of water levels in the humidifier, of water accumulation in the inspiratory line of the circuit, and of changes in the patient's lung compliance. Pressure-limited ventilators are not usually used for patients who are larger than 10 kg. Hence, as a patient grows, if home ventilation is still required, a new ventilator must be purchased and mastered by care givers. Because of these limitations, at The Children's Hospital, Boston, we usually use volume-cycled ventilators for home ventilation of all patients, regardless of size. We feel that these are easier, more reliable, and eliminate the need to introduce a new ventilator as the patient grows. The only pa-

TABLE 2 Modern Home

	Tidal Volume Range	Respiratory Rate	Variable Inhalation: Exhalation	Apnea Back-Up	PEEP Compensation	Circuit Breaker
Puritan Bennett 2800	50–2,800 ml	1–69 breaths/min	Yes	12 breaths/min after 45 sec	Yes	Yes
Life Products LP-6	100–2,200 ml	1–38 breaths/min	Yes	10 breaths/min after 20 sec	Yes	Yes
Life Care PLV-100	50–3,000 ml	2–30 breaths/min	Yes	No	No	Yes
Bear 33	100–2,200 ml	2–40 breaths/min	Yes	No	Yes	Yes

tients that we send home on a pressure-limited ventilator are children less than 10 kg who require a low ventilator rate and who will most likely be weaned from all ventilator support within the foreseeable future.

ELECTRICAL CONSIDERATIONS

Home ventilators are usually electrically, rather than pneumatically, driven. The reason for this lies in the fact that storing enough gas supply to operate a pneumatic device is cumbersome and expensive. Hence, a discussion of pneumatic valves is not necessary. However, a sound understanding of the electrical system in the home is mandatory. There are a number of electrical considerations that, although not important for the in-hospital ventilator, become extremely important for the home ventilator.

Most homes are exposed to varying line voltage ranging between 95 to 135 volts. The ventilator should accommodate to these changes in voltage with no effect on the accuracy of the ventilator settings and on performance.

Preferably the home and ventilator are fitted with circuit breakers, rather than fuses. Circuit breakers simplify the situation because fuses can be difficult to replace, especially at inopportune times.

A continual power source for the ventilator must be available. The ventilator itself should have both an internal and an external battery. The internal battery should have a long battery life (approximately 1 hour) in order for emergent problems to be corrected or to connect to the external battery. The external battery should have a life of at least 4 hours. The switch-over from AC to DC should be completed automatically, and the ventilator should alert the operator whenever the mode is switched. The internal and external battery should automatically recharge whenever the ventilator is attached to an electrical outlet.

Patients who are totally ventilator-dependent may require a gas-powered generator in the event of a prolonged electrical failure. The gas-powered generator can supply power for days and can save the patient a possible hospital admission until power is restored.

Often, community fire stations can be helpful in securing and maintaining portable generators.

Internal specifics of the ventilator should be understood and discussed. Brushless motors may be safer in the home setting. Although brushless motors do not have a track record in mechanical ventilators, they have an excellent record of reliability and of low maintenance in the business world.

MECHANICAL CONSIDERATION

Quiet operation is mandatory for the home ventilator. The noise level should not exceed 70 dB, above which normal conversation is difficult.

Ventilator cleaning must also be planned. The auxiliary equipment, i.e., tubing, exhalation valves, and humidifier, should be easy to disassemble and to reassemble with the fewest parts necessary. A minimum of three sets of all equipment is needed for proper cleaning: one set on the ventilator, another being cleaned, the other ready for use. Disinfecting the equipment can be done in different ways. The easiest and the simplest is to place the equipment in a dishwasher. In our experience, this method has the best patient compliance.

There are also a number of seemingly minor features that could simplify home ventilators. The inlet filter should be accessible and easily changed without tools. An operational hour meter would be helpful for scheduling preventive maintenance programs. In addition, ventilator controls should require a two step procedure to alter their settings.

There are a number of alarms required for a safe home ventilator. There should be loud audible and/or visual alarms, and one alarm should be easy to distinguish from another. The basic alarms should be for true or impending power loss, patient disconnect, and excessive pressure. Remote alarms can also be installed as an accessory. In addition to alarms, another safety feature is an antisuffocation valve or system to allow the patient to breathe through the circuit if the ventilator fails.

Care Ventilators

| | Alarms | | | | | | |
Low Voltage	Low Pressure	High Pressure	Sigh	Weight	O₂ Accum	Flow Rate
Yes	Yes	Yes	Yes	31 lb	Yes	40–125 L/min
Yes	Yes	Yes	No	32 lb	Yes	No flow adjustment (inspiratory time)
Yes	Yes	Yes	No	28 lb	No	20–120 L/min
Yes	Yes	Yes	Yes	29 lb	Yes	20–120 L/min

TABLE 3   Indications for Home Ventilation

Group 1
  Abnormal control of breathing
    Primary central hypoventilation
    Central hypoventilation secondary to tumor, trauma, or postoperative
      complication
  Neuromuscular diseases
    Neurologic lesions
      Cord transection
      Phrenic nerve palsies
      Anterior horn cell disease
        Werdnig-Hoffmann disease
        Poliomyelitis
        Other viral infections
      Postinfectious polyneuritis: Guillain-Barré syndrome
      Neuromuscular junction disease: myasthenia gravis
    Muscle disease
      Muscular dystrophies
      Myopathies
      Congenital muscle defects
        Abdominal wall defects
        Chest wall defects
        Diaphragm abnormalities
Group II
  Pulmonary disease
    Lung hypoplasia, i.e., congenital diaphragmatic hernia
    Bronchopulmonary dysplasia
    Chronic obstructive pulmonary disease
    Pulmonary fibrosis

If a patient is totally dependent on mechanical ventilation, then a back-up ventilator must be in the home. Ideally, the back-up machine should be the same as the primary machine to guarantee that the family and patient are comfortable with the back-up. This extra machine should be used periodically to assure proper operation in an emergency.

If the patient needs mechanical ventilation only at night or intermittently for rest, a back-up ventilator may not be necessary. However, emergency plans for repair or for replacement should be discussed and planned ahead. A back-up ventilator should be available if the response time for repair or for delivery is too lengthy.

OXYGEN

A number of additional concerns arise when oxygen is required for home ventilation. First, an adequate oxygen supply must be carefully planned and monitored. The basic supply should be adequate for a minimum of 3 days, preferably for a week. The types of oxygen sources include cylinders, concentrators, and liquid oxygen (see *At-Home Administration of Oxygen*). The practicality of supplying oxygen in the home severely limits the mobility of the patient on home ventilation. There is also a limit to a reasonable FIO_2 that can be safely and consistently delivered in the home; because of this limit, patients who need an FIO_2 greater than 0.40 usually require in-hospital care.

When oxygen is required, the oxygen delivery system should preferentially be connected to the inlet of the mechanical system (i.e., at the piston or the bellows). Attempts to "bleed" oxygen into the inspiratory limb of the patient tubing have proved unsatisfactory. When the patient spontaneously breathes with this type of oxygen delivery, the FIO_2 of each spontaneous breath varies. In addition, the bled-in oxygen changes the delivered tidal volume of the set ventilator breaths. Compensating by adjusting the set tidal volume leads to discrepancies, depending on the patient's own minute ventilation.

DURABLE MEDICAL EQUIPMENT (DME) SUPPLIER

The choice between leasing or purchasing a ventilator is dictated by the patient's long-term prognosis, as well as more and more by the specifics of the insurance company. Regardless of whether the ventilator is owned or leased, some basic company policies and servicing should be considered. A service and preventive maintenance contract with a factory authorized service center should be included with the sale or the lease. In addition to maintenance, this service contract should provide a back-up ventilator in the event one is needed. The DME supplier should provide 24-hour availability with a 1- to 2-hour response time.

Comprehensive manuals should be supplied by the manufacturer. There should be three different manuals. One should be written in lay terms containing a simple explanation of the mechanical aspect of the ventilator and a comprehensive explanation of terms, such as tidal volume and FiO_2. The second should be for the hospital clinician with more technical aspects of the ventilator discussed, i.e., intermittent manditory ventilation and PEEP. The third manual, for the service personnel, should contain detailed descriptions of the electrical circuits and the preventive maintenance program.

Most patients with home ventilators need a respiratory therapist for help with the initial set-up and then intermittently for home supervision and monitoring. This therapist should be an employee of the DME supplier, thereby guaranteeing that the therapist has ongoing inservice education and is up to date with the policies and the procedures that relate to the specific ventilator.

Finally, the home care company (DME) should accept appropriate insurance or third party payers and should provide liability insurance for all equipment failures, as well as for any procedural errors made by the therapist or the service department that result in injury to the patient.

Suggested Reading

Dull WL, Sadoul P. Home ventilators in patients with severe lung disease. Am Rev Respir Dis 1981; 123:74.

Dunkin LJ. Home ventilatory assistance. Anaesthesia 1983; 38:644–649.

Gilmartin M, Make B. Home care of ventilator-dependent persons. Respir Care 1983; 28:1490–1497.

Kacmarek RM, Spearmen C. Equipment used for ventilatory support in the home. Respir Care 1986; 31:311–328.

Kacmarek RM, Thompson JE. Respiratory care of the ventilator-assisted infant in the home. Respir Care 1985; 31:7.

Long term mechanical ventilation guidelines for management in the home and at alternate community sites. Chest (Suppl.) 1986; 90:1.

Pediatric home mechanical ventilation. Pediatr Clin North Am 1987; 34:47–60.

Sivak ED, Cordasco EM, Gipson WT, Stelmach K. Clinical considerations in the implementation of home care ventilation. Cleve Clin Q 1983; 50:219–225.

Snider GL. Thirty years of mechanical ventilation: changing implications. Arch Intern Med 1983; 143:745–749.

Splaingard ML, Frates RC Jr, Harrison GM, et al. Home positive-pressure ventilation: twenty years' experience. Chest 1983; 84:376–382.

POSITIVE PRESSURE MECHANICAL VENTILATION: ALTERNATIVE APPROACHES

NORMA M. T. BRAUN, M.D.

In 1832 Dr. John Dalziel of Scotland developed the first negative pressure respirator generated by a manual bellows. In 1864 A. F. Jones of Kentucky patented a manually powered iron lung that he claimed "cured paralysis, neuralgia, rheumatism, seminal weakness, asthma, and dyspepsia." In 1876, Dr. Woillez of Paris built the first workable iron lung, called a spirophore. Since that time several designs of negative pressure devices to support respiration were made on both continents. Spurred by the poliomyelitis epidemics, a reliable iron lung was developed at Harvard Medical School by Drinker and Shaw in 1928. The efficacy of ventilatory support by iron lungs was shown by the reduction of mortality from respiratory muscle paralysis to 50 percent. Following widespread polio vaccination these respirators were used only by a handful of post-polio patients with residual respiratory muscle weakness. Since the mid-1960s, however, better ventilators and improved clinical skills in the management of acute and chronic respiratory failure resulted in patients who survived their acute decompensation episodes but could not sustain independent ventilation for 24 hours a day despite all efforts. This has been paralleled by the increased knowledge of the pathophysiology of respiratory muscle dysfunction and the awareness of sleep-associated gas exchange deterioration in many diseases. Better methods of clinical evaluation, earlier diagnosis, and a wider range of management options for respiratory muscle dysfunction evolved. Since positive pressure ventilation via chronic tracheostomy stomas has inherent problems of infection, speech impairment, discomfort, and increased nursing needs, negative pressure respiratory support became a considered alternative. This is particularly applicable to home management of patients with chronic or sleep-associated respiratory failure. Other therapies not requiring an artificial airway include a rocking bed, a pneumobelt with pressure applied to the abdomen, and a positive pressure system using a lip seal or face or nasal continuous positive airway pressure (CPAP) mask. The focus of this chapter is the application of these devices for the home ventilation of patients.

The hallmarks of patients who might benefit from chronic ventilatory support are hypercapnia and progressive decline of intellectual and daily functional capacity due to severe ventilatory impairment. Patients disabled by severe intractable dyspnea, repeated ("revolving-door") hospitalizations, and otherwise irreversible deterioration after successful weaning are candidates. They should have stable ventilatory demands, minimal secretions, no upper airway obstruction or esophageal reflux during use, and periods of time when independent ventilation can be sustained.

Physiologic criteria include reductions of pulmonary function capacity to 25 percent predicted of the vital capacity (VC), or forced expiratory volume in the first second (FEV_1), or the maximum voluntary ventilation (MVV). Maximal inspiratory muscle pressure generation capacity below -50 cm H_2O in patients with chronic obstructive pulmonary disease (COPD) and below -25 cm H_2O for patients with neuromuscular diseases are levels more likely to be associated with chronic hypercapnia. When the maximal expiratory pressure is less than 40 cm H_2O, cough capacity is reduced. The expiratory muscles also augment inspiratory muscles and can effectively move a paralyzed diaphragm when the subject is upright. When oxygen therapy is associated with a rising $PaCO_2$ a patient may suffer worsening gas exchange, especially during sleep. Because both hypercapnia and hypoxemia further impair ventilatory muscle performance, a vicious cycle is established.

There are numerous diseases that may render patients ventilator dependent for either part or all of each day. Although the list is not complete it includes patients with central and peripheral nervous system and muscle disorders. Patients who usually require continuous ventilatory support are those with failure of central drive after cortical vascular accidents or encephalitis. Loss of brain stem respiratory automatic drive, as in Ondine's curse or Arnold-Chiari malformation, brain stem syringobulbia, brain stem hemorrhage from AV malformations or localized infarcts, or localized degenerative disorders as in multiple sclerosis or Leigh's encephalomyelopathy or after head trauma may need only nocturnal ventilation. Spinal cord injuries and cervical syringomyelia may render patients ventilator dependent during sleep. Disorders of the anterior horn cells include spinal muscular atrophies, amyotrophic lateral sclerosis and post-poliomyelitis. Phrenic neuropathies are usually idiopathic but also include chronic Guillain-Barré syndrome, systemic lupus erythematosus, and diabetes. Sleep-associated hypoventilation is common in phrenic neuropathies. Primary muscle diseases, such as Duchenne muscular dystrophy, and the metabolic myopathies, especially acid maltase-deficient glycogen storage disease, are the most common.

Patients with irreversible thoracic wall dysfunction such as kyphoscoliosis, fibrothorax, or post-thoracoplasty processes are potential candidates for nocturnal ventilatory support. Several patients with chronic lung diseases, especially COPD, who having survived acute respiratory failure revolve back into repeated episodes, are candidates for nocturnal support. These patients may develop respiratory muscle fatigue when the work of breathing cannot increase to meet their ventilatory requirements. Their muscles are further compromised by worsening blood gases during sleep. Other lung diseases include severe bronchiectasis, bronchiolitis obliterans, and cystic fibrosis.

Patients with advanced interstitial fibrosis and hypercapnia can also benefit, as do children with bronchopulmonary dysplasia. While obesity hypoventilation-sleep apnea syndrome and diseases of the heart may result in hypercapnic respiratory failure and require ventilatory support, home ventilation is not recommended by the devices discussed at this time.

NEGATIVE PRESSURE VENTILATION

Decision for home ventilation depends on the nature and the severity of the disease process and the capacity of the patient and the health care team to learn and assume responsibility for the care program.

The major advantage of negative pressure respiration is that it is a means of providing ventilatory support without an artificial airway. The success of a system depends on matching the patient to the equipment for his ventilatory needs. Patient acceptability, availability of home help, and the type of disease affect the choice of equipment. The patient and family's lifestyle demands, the portability of a unit, the financial resources, and the geographic location influence the device chosen. Generally speaking, patients with COPD need faster inspiratory flow rates and slower expiratory times. Patients with neuromuscular diseases or chest wall diseases usually need slower inspiratory flow rates. Neuromuscular diseases require lower negative pressure settings than do chest wall diseases. In chest wall deformities the pressure required to deform the noncompliant chest cage could exceed the capacity of the negative pressure pump device.

Iron Lung

Negative pressure ventilators apply intermittent subatmospheric pressure around the thorax and the abdomen, producing a physiologic method of respiration akin to normal. The resultant pressure gradient expands the chest wall and inflation of the lungs proceeds. Expiration occurs passively from a recoil of the chest wall and lungs. A reasonably compliant chest wall is necessary for successful application, and a patient's pulmonary reserve should be sufficient to allow safe periods without support because it takes time to seal the patient into the device. The main disadvantages include lack of airway protection, uncertain tidal volumes, and potential pain from pressure points. Because the iron lung applies negative pressure to the entire body, it is the most efficient negative pressure ventilator. However, such pressure development causes blood to pool in the lower extremities and abdomen, resulting in a reduction of venous return. This unit is rate adjustable between 16 and 32 breaths per minute (bpm) and negative pressure can be generated up to -30 cm H_2O of pressure. Inspiratory flow rate is set by the pressure and the rate. The I:E ratio is fixed. Adjustments are made until the patient and the machine are synchronized and the desired minute ventilation is achieved as measured by arterial blood gases obtained several hours after the ventilator has been in operation. Positive pressure at end exhalation can be applied to assist cough, although it is usually not needed. The major disadvantages of the tank are its size (90 × 60 × 32 inches), bulkiness (650 lb), and nonportability. Restriction of position to one posture can result in back discomfort.

A modified version of an iron lung is a fiberglass model weighing 100 lb (Porta Lung) designed by a post-polio patient. It is powered by a separate negative pressure pump and remains cumbersome. For comfort and portability, body wraps of a suit or poncho design (pneumosuit or pulmowrap) connected to a negative pressure pump are available. There are several pumps suitable for use with these garments.

Negative Pressure Pumps

The Emerson pump has a variable I:E ratio, rates up to 45 bpm that are set by the inspiratory and expiratory time, and a pressure range up to -60 cm H_2O. It can develop high flow rates. Its major disadvantages include noise and the insecurity of not having specific numbers for rate and pressure settings. The brushes in the system need regular maintenance and replacement.

The Thompson-Maxivent is quiet, has a rate range of 8 to 24 bpm, and can generate pressures to -80 cm H_2O with a good seal. It has a fixed I:E ratio and is more costly.

The Monaghan 107C negative pressure pump develops maximum negative pressure slowly and no more than -40 cm H_2O. It has a fixed I:E ratio and has a rate range from 10 to 40 bpm.

The Emerson unit is best for patients with COPD and chest wall disorders. The Maxivent can be used for all disorders but may be inadequate for some patients with COPD. The 107C unit is best reserved for patients with neuromuscular disorders.

Suit or Poncho

The suit or poncho is worn over a rigid plastic or metal chest grid, which is usually applied onto a rigid back plate on which the patient lies. Only the metal grid can be individually tailored. Because the lower abdomen and legs are excluded from negative pressure, a positive transextremity pressure is developed and results in increased venous return during the inspiratory cycle. It is not necessary to lie supine in this unit. The patient can turn to his side or have the head raised up to 30 degrees, the limit being determined by the pressure exerted by the grid on the thighs. Omitting the back plate might result in greater back comfort but can cause the patient to be pulled upward and forward, resulting in discomfort to the shoulders and back and less transthoracic pressure change. Back discomfort can be overcome by adequate padding of the back plate with $1^1/_2$ to 2 inches of foam rubber. Air circulation, particularly through the neck area, may cause patients to be cold. However, applying a neck scarf or placing a heater nearby can increase the comfort. The pneumosuit has been successfully used in patients with COPD, cystic fibrosis, Duchenne dystrophy, kyphoscoliosis, thoracoplasty, fibrothorax, and interstitial lung disease. The poncho is most effective when pressures less than -40 cm H_2O are required because the suit tends to be sucked over the abdomen, paradoxically compressing it during inspiration.

Chest Cuirass

The chest cuirass or shell has been available in several models and sizes since the polio epidemic and is made of fiberglass. It consists of a rigid shell that fits firmly over the anterior portion of the chest with a port for connection to a negative pressure generator. This applies negative pressure over a much smaller surface area than either the iron lung or the pneumosuit and therefore is the least efficient of the negative pressure ventilators. It allows movement of only the anterior chest wall. Some models (Huxley) extend to the upper pelvis, which includes the upper abdomen. This improves efficiency because of greater diaphragmatic excursions from added abdominal expansion. Patients with deformities of the chest cage may require custom-made units in order to achieve adequate ventilation and comfort. The points of contact along the upper and lateral chest wall may chafe or blister. This can be reduced by careful fitting and use of talcum powder. The pressures achieved rarely exceed -30 cm H_2O regardless of the pump. Patients with neuromuscular disorders have low muscle mass and often have normal lungs and airways. Thus ventilatory requirements are quite low and the lesser level of ventilation needed to maintain such patients may be adequately provided by the cuirass respirator. Occasionally some patients prefer to couple a positive pressure system via a mouthpiece to the negative pressure cuirass to provide adequate ventilation, forestalling the need for a tracheostomy. These patients tend to have stable, or very slowly progressive disease such as the post-polio syndrome. When ventilatory requirements are great, (severe lung disease or rigid chest cages) and a large pressure differential for ventilation is needed, then the shell system is inadequate.

Application

The iron lung and Porta lung are easy to apply. The patient is placed in the unit, sliding the head through the neck portal. The unit is closed and turned on, and then the neck is closed in as snugly as the patient will allow with the least air leak so that adequate pressure is generated. Dyspnea may increase in the supine posture and reassurance needs to be given that this sensation is temporary. The patient can speak and move inside the unit more easily when instructed to do so during the exhalation phase.

The pneumosuit or poncho wrap takes longer to apply, but with practice, it can be accomplished within 10 minutes. Current pneumosuit models have a Velcro attachment for the back plate, (assuring its position and nonmobility), to which additional foam padding is added. An extra-long zipper facilitates its rapid application with the least patient effort. The grid can be tailored to accommodate the individual's chin and arms for comfort. The grid should extend from chin to the umbilicus for the greatest chest cage and abdominal expansion. The Velcro closures at the wrists and ankles, or a belt at the hips on the poncho, are snugly closed. The pump is turned on before the neck closure is secured and closed last. The rate and pressure is adjusted to achieve the desired tidal volume and minute ventilation. If the patient receives instruction to speak or move during the exhalation phase, it reduces anxiety and facilitates synchronization. The head can be elevated or a decubitus position assumed when minor adjustments may be needed for comfort. Allowing the patient to set the rate for increasing time of use facilitates adaptation. For example, a patient with COPD demanded -80 cm H_2O because she was exquisitely sensitive to a Pco_2 level greater than 45 mm Hg, which caused headaches. She would not accept a lower level of ventilation at less pressure.

ROCKING BEDS

There are several other systems that can support ventilatory function by displacing the abdominal contents. A rocking bed uses gravity to move the abdominal contents passively to displace the diaphragm.

The bed tilts the head downward 15 degrees, causing a cephalad movement of the diaphragm when exhalation occurs. Its rostral rock at 30 degrees moves the diaphragm downward when inspiration occurs. Larger rocking arcs can increase ventilation but are usually not tolerable. The patient can ventilate even more in the lateral decubitus position because the chest cage is in the more inspiratory position. The advantages of the rocking bed are that there is freedom from restriction of appliances and that no special size is required. However, sliding can occur when the lower extremities are flaccid or the patient weighs less than 70 lb. Use of pillows for head positioning and support of the knees can be tried to offset this. A foot board and side rails also help. The rate ranges between 15 and 26 bpm. A rocking bed is especially useful for patients with primary diaphragmatic paralysis. The accessory muscles reduce their effective contraction when supine because gravity puts them in the expiratory position. They cease to contract during rapid eye movement (REM) sleep. The most recent application of a rocking bed has been to patients who have suffered diaphragmatic dysfunction following phrenic nerve injury during coronary artery bypass surgery. The chest cage has been rendered less functional by the median sternotomy as well. It may require 6 to 8 months for the phrenic nerve to recover. The rocking bed has provided sufficient ventilation to allow extubation when copious secretions, severely impaired cough, or extensive pneumonia is not present. The major impediment to its use is lack of portability and relative bulkiness. A sense of motion sickness rapidly fades with use. The major advantages include the ease of use and the security provided by a patient-activated, hand-held switch to control the bed. Rocking beds have been used for over 20 years usually when the disease process does not progress and the lungs are normal.

PNEUMOBELT

A pneumobelt also displaces the abdominal contents to effect ventilation. This consists of a cloth corset, containing stays in the back and an inflatable rubber bladder in the front. The bladder portion is fitted over the abdomen and inflated intermittently by a positive pressure pump. During inflation the abdominal contents are pushed inward, displacing the diaphragm cephalad and causing active expiration. Bladder deflation allows passive downward movement of the diaphragm when inspiration occurs. This belt functions only when the patient is upright. It is best used in wheelchairs or on patients who can sleep sitting upright. The pressures generated are between 15 and 45 cm H_2O pressure. Cough can be assisted for secretion clearance with transient higher pressures. If the patient is too thin there will be insufficient abdominal contents to move. In severe scoliosis the distortion can preclude adequate displacement to effect ventilation. If the patient is too obese, the pressures required to move the abdominal contents may exceed the capacity of the positive pressure pump, and the diaphragm has already been displaced upwards. The simplicity of the belt and its portability allows for wheelchair use and daytime ventilatory assist, freeing the patient's arms for other activities. It is most useful in patients with low ventilatory requirements. Other devices will be needed for nocturnal ventilatory support.

GLOSSOPHARYNGEAL BREATHING

Another alternative method of ventilation not using body ventilators or airway intubation consists of glossopharyngeal or "frog" breathing. An intact upper airway is mandatory. The technique is usually learned by patients with neuromuscular diseases that have spared the upper airway. It consists of gulping motions of the tongue and submandibular and oropharyngeal muscles to force small boluses (50 to 60 ml) of air into the lungs. Rapidly repeated efforts allow tidal volumes up to 600 to 800 ml and minute ventilations of 6 to 8 L per minute. The sitting position is required, and with practice patients can perform this breathing for hours and can use this technique to sustain normal speech and ventilation to work 8 hours per day. This technique can also augment a cough effort. Many patients learn this spontaneously. Some patients can use this breathing for only short periods of time to allow application of another respiratory assist device. This allows for greater independence for movement.

Another form of alternate ventilatory assist device is the phrenic nerve pacemaker.

POSITIVE PRESSURE DEVICES

Although positive pressure devices are beyond the scope of this chapter, the application of positive pressure with either a mouthpiece, a lip seal system, a face mask, or CPAP mask using a positive pressure pump is an effective alternative modality to support nocturnal ventilation. A lip seal mouthpiece system has been in use for over 20 years. More recently it has acquired wider attention because better-fitting masks are now available. A portable positive pressure pump is attached to the selected system and set for rate and volume or pressure. The weakest patients with low ventilatory requirements tend to adapt most rapidly. Some may require gradually increasing time of use in order to trust the system enough to sleep with it. Facial or lip discomfort may limit use. The most troublesome problem with a mouthpiece system is the difficulty of handling increased salivary secretions. Drying agents and adaptation usually resolve this. The potential for air loss through the alternate orifice is usually compensated for quickly. Aerophagia can result in belching or reflux. The latter can be reduced with metoclopramide before bedtime and no food ingestion for 3 hours before sleep. The portability of these systems is the major advantage. The mouthpieces can be attached to support devices so that the patient need only turn his head toward the device and initiate its use. Sleeping with a CPAP mask may be the most effective alternative for patients who do not want airway intervention or negative pressure systems and who do not have secretions as a major component of their illness. Thus patients with kyphoscoliosis and neuromuscular diseases with nocturnal sleep disturbance are the best candidates.

Institution of ventilatory assist devices should be carefully considered. Reconstruction of a hospital setting at home is not the goal. Rather, facilitation of enhanced life quality, improved physical and physiologic function, and a reduction of morbidity are the goals. Life extension alone is not sufficient to initiate a system. Assist devices are generally best applied in the hospital first, where efficacy can be assessed and appropriate individual adjustments can be made before the final prescription is written for home use.

APPLICATION AND ACCLIMATION

Patients must be given the option to try different units to fit their needs, lifestyle, and the other requirements including financial resources. Determined and motivated patients adapt successfully to almost any system, especially when they have family support. Patients who are severely depressed and continually focus on losses or unrealistically focus on a "cure" almost never succeed. Make comfort and setting adjustments for acceptance prior to measuring the ventilatory and gas exchange effects. Once the best setting is achieved, arterial blood gas measurements can be made to assure the adequacy of gas exchange prior to discharge. Usually improvement continues at home with regular ventilatory support. Whether the improvement is due to a resetting of central respiratory drive or improved ventilatory capacity from resting over burdened muscles or to restoration of sleep is uncertain. If nocturnal use is not sufficient to reduce daytime CO_2 levels below 55 mm Hg then either additional time or additional or alternative devices may be needed. A change in body weight greater than 10 percent may require setting readjustment. Respiratory tract infection, or fatigue after increased physical exertion from rehabilitation training or shopping, may require a short period (1 to 3 hours) of use to relieve dyspnea and allow rest. The use of negative pressure supported ventilation during exercise reconditioning is now undergoing trials.

Attention to function of other organ systems and appropriate nutrition should parallel the focus on assisted ventilation. Continued education of the patient and family, coordination of the care team, adjustment of a system when it does not suffice, and careful monitoring by the primary physician may effect long-term stabilization of patients.

OUTCOME

To date, I have successfully applied the various systems described to over 100 patients in the home. Approximately 50 percent are those with thoracic disorders including COPD, bronchiectasis, cystic fibrosis, fibrothorax, interstitial lung disease, post-thoracoplasty, and kyphoscoliosis, and the remaining 50 percent have various neuromuscular diseases including myopathies, anterior horn cell diseases, phrenic neuropathies, and central drive dysfunction lasting for periods greater than 15 years.

In the group with thoracic diseases, mortality has occurred because of neoplasia, either in the lung or elsewhere, sudden death from a myocardial event or antibiotic-resistant gram-negative pneumonia rather than progressive hypercapnia and cor pulmonale. Neuromuscular patients have poorer cough and lower pulmonary reserve and tend to expire more quickly from pulmonary infections or alcohol- or drug-related CNS depression at home, especially when a minimal delay in instituting airways clearance and positive pressure ventilation is apt to result in more rapid deterioration of organ function.

Thus, expanding knowledge of the pathophysiology of respiratory muscle function and control and their physiologic interaction with sleep in thoracopulmonary and neuromuscular disorders has allowed the application of several types of ventilatory support or assist devices to improve the life of many patients. Although these alternative approaches have limitations, their advantages occasion consideration of their use in selected patients. Only from continual reassessment of supported patients can we finally learn how best to use them.

Suggested Reading

Braun NMT. Respiratory muscle dysfunction. Heart Lung 1984; 13:327–332.

Braun NMT, Marino WD. Effect of daily intermittent rest of respiratory muscles in patients with severe chronic airflow obstruction COPD. Chest 1984; 85:595–596.

Hill S. Clinical applications of body ventilators. Chest 1986; 90:897–905.

Johnson DL, Giovonni RM, Driscoll S, ed. Ventilator assisted patient care. Planning for hospital discharge and home care. Rockville, MD: Aspen Publishers, 1986.

O'Donohue WJ, et al. Long term mechanical ventilation guidelines for management in the home and at alternate community sites. Report of Ad Hoc Committee, Respiratory Care Section, ACCP. Chest 1986; 90:1S–37S.

Roussos C, Macklem PT. The thorax, part B, part V. Therapeutic approaches. New York: Marcel Dekker, 1985.

HOME DISCHARGE OF THE VENTILATOR-ASSISTED PATIENT

JANETTE JONES WALSH, R.N., RRT
PETER A. KIRKPATRICK, M.D.

In the last decade, changing health care economics have combined with improvements in respiratory care technology to provide increased impetus toward home care of chronically ventilator-assisted patients and improved capability to provide such care. Obstacles to home ventilator care are no longer technological or organizational, but instead are social, perceptual, and emotional. Most ventilator care has been provided in acute care hospitals, in a smaller number of chronic care hospitals, and in hospital-based ventilator rehabilitation units. Recently, a few nursing homes have begun to accept ventilator patients, but for most patients the only alternative to hospital care is home care. It has become increasingly clear that home ventilator assistance is not as difficult as we, in the medical community, had believed and that, although very few families or patients believe at first that they can cope with home ventilation, an intact family with average intelligence can sustain an alert patient at home on a ventilator when properly trained, supported, and motivated. No study has found, and our experience does not suggest, increased morbidity or mortality when home care of ventilator-assisted patients is provided by appropriately trained family members or by personal care attendants.

Ventilator-assisted patients have much more rehabilitation potential than previously believed, but their medical complexity has prevented the realization of this potential in the acute care setting. The traditional association of ventilator therapy with critical care perpetuates an emphasis on the treatment of disease. This inhibits effective rehabilitation, which seeks to improve the quality of life within the patient's limitations and often places less importance on weaning than is usual in critical care settings. A change in emphasis to rehabilitation to maximize function in areas of "ability" permits staff and patient to adopt achievable goals, thus preventing both the frustration associated with repeated failure to wean and the boredom associated with maintenance care. Effective rehabilitation is impractical in an intensive care unit and is best done outside the critical care areas or in a specialized ventilator rehabilitation unit, if one is available. The more common terminology for a chronically ventilated patient is "ventilator-dependent," but we prefer "ventilator-assisted." The label, "ventilator-dependent," is psychologically crippling to the patient and counterproductive to the rehabilitation philosophy, which we believe, is the best approach to discharging these patients to as fulfilling and independent a lifestyle as their limitations permit.

Most ventilator-assisted patients have multisystem impairment and require interdisciplinary cooperation for effective rehabilitation. As soon as the patient is stable, the physician should consult occupational, physical, and speech therapists to address systematically such quality of life issues as communication, mobility, eating (distinct from nutrition), dressing, and self-care. Communication with these disciplines should be frequent throughout the hospital course.

We believe that successful home discharge flows from a well-organized team approach to the rehabilitation of the ventilator-assisted patient in the hospital. We suggest the use of an interdisciplinary discharge team in order to allow the team- and goal-oriented rehabilitation approach to be applied in the acute care setting. Such a team regularly brings together all the disciplines involved in the patient's care and systematizes and organizes the discharge process.

THE DISCHARGE TEAM

At the initial meeting the patient's status is reviewed by each discipline, and any possible obstacles to home discharge are identified and discussed. If the decision to attempt home discharge is reaffirmed, each discipline develops a plan, establishes goals to be accomplished, and sets a target date for discharge. Thereafter, the team meets weekly to review progress and to reassess goals.

The discharge team should include the patient's attending physician (and a pulmonary specialist if the attending physician is not one); a respiratory therapist; the patient's primary nurse or the nearest analogue in the institution's nursing structure; a physical therapist; a social worker; a continuing care nurse; and the home care case manager or the home care therapist from the company chosen to provide the patient's home respiratory care equipment. A dietician is a valuable addition to the team for patients with specialized dietary requirements.

243

The Physician

Physician input must be frequent both to the staff and to the patient. Although the individual members of the discharge team function autonomously within their disciplines and collaboratively in the team setting, most families and patients do not understand this and need periodic explanations and reassurance from the physician personally. Likewise, the team members need the medical expertise, the emotional support, and the leadership of the physician in dealing with these complex patients.

Medical follow-up of home ventilator patients requires subspecialty-level expertise. If medical follow-up cannot be provided by the pulmonologist caring for the patient in the hospital, a pulmonary physician in the patient's community should be contacted to provide follow-up medical care. This action is particularly important in referral centers whose patients may live far from the hospital and have primary physicians who are either not involved in the care of the patient in the hospital or are not expert in respiratory care.

Resuscitation status must be clearly established and communicated to all concerned before discharge. Implementation of do not resuscitate (DNR) orders for patients on home ventilation may present special problems not encountered with hospitalized patients, and legal advice may be needed. Some home health care agencies involve their legal counsel if DNR status is decided upon, and their advice may be useful.

The Primary Nurse

The primary nurse is the central figure in the day to day management of the patient's rehabilitation and bedside care. To this end, the nurse develops a care plan that coordinates the patient's many therapies and activities and that teaches the patient to manage his or her own activity schedule within his or her capabilities.

The nurse plays a central role in dealing with the many psychosocial issues that arise daily in the care of ventilator-assisted patients and in planning for home discharge. Although the plan for dealing with such issues is usually developed by the entire team, the nurse bears the responsibility for carrying out the plan in innumerable daily interactions with patient and family. The nurse and the social worker can be of great help to each other in dealing with these problems, and they need to communicate frequently.

The primary nurse must constantly foster patient independence. Often this is an unusual experience for the patient, who may have recently come from an intensive care unit where he or she is used to receiving total care. Most patients in this situation have become dependent on their nurses and become angry when asked to do things for themselves. The primary nurse must not only insist on maximum independence by the patient, but must ensure that all other members of the care team do likewise. Consistency is vital.

Some patient teaching is appropriate once it is clear that long-term ventilator assistance is necessary, even before the patient is considered for home discharge. We have found that teaching the patient to "bag" himself during suctioning is particularly helpful; this gives the patient a sense of control over his breathing and is a step toward learning tracheostomy care and self-suctioning. As discharge approaches, the primary nurse also teaches the patient and the family problem-solving and troubleshooting algorithms for common respiratory problems and teaches the Visiting Nurses Association (VNA) or other home care nurses the care plan of the patient.

The Respiratory Therapist

Respiratory therapists are expert resources for patient, staff, and family with respect to respiratory therapy techniques and equipment. The therapist must convey to the patient a sense of familiarity with and confidence in the equipment being used. In many cases, this requires special training or preparation, since many of the devices used in the home setting are not commonly used in the hospital (e.g., the PLV-100) or are used only occasionally in any setting (the pneumobelt or the rocking bed). Unconventional devices, like the rocking bed, may not receive a fair trial without significant staff support and encouragement; therefore, patience and a positive attitude are vital when trying these devices. Patients are often tried on several different types of ventilatory support before a final choice is made of the best device or devices for long-term home use.

When a decision is reached on the device to be used, the therapist needs to make the use of the device as simple as possible for the patient and the family. We recommend the assist-control mode, rather than intermittent mandatory ventilation (IMV), for home positive pressure ventilation both for simplicity and to provide better rest for the respiratory muscles.

Other tasks appropriate for the respiratory therapist include

1. Titrating FIO_2 to the lowest level compatible with adequate oxygenation, both on and off the ventilator and during rest and exercise.
2. In some institutions, teaching the patient and the family the operation and care of the ventilator; in others the home care therapist may do this teaching. The best approach is probably for this teaching to be the responsibility of the hospital therapist in collaboration with the home care therapist.
3. Providing the home care therapist with a detailed list of all respiratory equipment and supplies needed

and informing the therapist of the respiratory plan of care and of any special needs or problems.

The Social Worker

The social worker plays a vital role in the home discharge process for several reasons. Severe chronic illness places great stress on the family unit and often changes roles within the family. Because the family must play an important part in patient care after discharge, awareness of the previous family structure and the changes in that structure caused by the patient's illness must be appreciated by the discharge team if the family's cooperation is to be obtained and preserved. Awareness of the family's motives for accepting the responsibility for home care may forestall problems in cases where guilt is a motivating force. High quality social work input is essential in obtaining this information and in helping the family cope with the stresses of the patient's illness and impending discharge.

Social supports in the community should be contacted by the social worker before discharge. Church groups and medically oriented groups, such as "breathing clubs," may be useful. The International Ventilator User's Network (St. Louis, MO) publishes a newsletter with practical tips, many written by patients and families, on home ventilator living.

The Rehabilitation Therapies (Occupational, Physical, and Speech Therapies)

These disciplines measure the patient's level of function in activities of daily living, mobility, swallowing, and speech and recommend programs to increase function. Therapy should be started as soon as the patient is medically stable. The goal of these therapies is not just to maintain function with passive range-of-motion exercises, but to maximize function within the limits of the patient's capabilities, thereby focusing on techniques for strengthening, endurance, and energy conservation. By participating in family team meetings and by home visits they define the relationship between the patient's physical capabilities and his home environment and make recommendations for environmental modifications, adaptive equipment, or further therapy to maximize the patient's function after discharge. These recommendations must be communicated to hospital nursing staff and to family so that techniques that are taught are reinforced in the hospital and not lost after discharge.

Most ventilator-assisted patients benefit more from exercise that is performed while on the ventilator because longer exercise sessions are tolerated. Most outpatient therapists are unaccustomed to exercising patients with this technique. Therefore, if therapy is to be continued after discharge the outpatient therapist

may need an inservice on the patient's program and equipment before discharge.

The Continuing Care Nurse

In collaboration with the primary nurse and the physician, the continuing care nurse determines the level and the amount of nursing care the patient needs after discharge and works with community health care agencies to provide and to fund the necessary care. Agency nurses are unlikely to be familiar with home ventilator care and should be familiarized with the family and the specifics of the patient's care in the hospital setting. If professional nursing care is necessary, this care can often be decreased or eliminated after discharge on a planned schedule as the family becomes more comfortable with home ventilation. Failure to establish such a schedule may result in excessive family dependence on agency personnel. In our experience, most adult patients on home ventilator assistance have not needed credentialed nursing care, other than skilled nursing visits.

In most acute care facilities the continuing care nurse is the one designated to deal with more traditional discharge planning matters, such as obtaining nursing services at home, arranging transportation, obtaining new or handicapped housing, and researching and applying for the available community services and financial sources appropriate for the patient. In some institutions the social worker may perform these functions.

The Case Manager and the Home Care Therapist

More expert and comprehensive home care management is needed as home care becomes more sophisticated. The position of the home care case manager developed in response to this need. The case manager should be expert in the respiratory care of home ventilator-assisted patients and knowledgeable in the rehabilitation process. Ideally, the case manager participates in the entire discharge process, beginning with patient selection and continuing after discharge, to bridge the gap that has existed in the past between hospital care and home care.

The responsibilities and the capabilities of the case manager exceed those of the traditional home care therapist. In addition to the usual durable medical equipment (DME) provider functions, such as providing trial equipment, training, and predischarge home assessment, the case manager collaborates with the hospital staff to make the patient's care plan and respiratory program more suitable for the home environment. After discharge, the case manager is responsible for coordinating home care services and for maintaining communication with the referring physician or facility. Although not all companies presently use case managers as we have described them, we believe that this model of home care management is a good one for ventilator-assisted patients, and we expect and hope that case managers will be more widely used.

The case manager works with a home care therapist in organizations that have both positions; companies that do not use the case manager model always provide a home care therapist, and we recommend that this person be included in team meetings, especially as discharge nears. Responsibilities of the home care therapist include instructing the patient and the family on the oxygen system they will use at home; assessing the home for a respiratory equipment setup and cleaning area; ensuring that the electrical system is satisfactory; labeling the circuits to be used for respiratory equipment; and completely setting up the equipment in the home 1 to 2 days before discharge. On the day of discharge the therapist meets the family at home to assist in "settling in." For the first week the therapist visits daily to review the equipment and to teach cleaning procedures. The goal of the first week is to increase the patient's confidence and independence, thus minimizing the need for daily therapist visits beyond the first week.

CHOOSING A HOME CARE VENDOR

The home care company should be viewed as an extension of the hospital and evaluated critically for high quality and for comprehensive services. Not all respiratory DME vendors are capable of providing the close supervision and the attention to detail necessary in a ventilator discharge. Vendor choice should be individualized and based on the following considerations.

Program

The company should have an organized, documented home ventilator program that includes predischarge training of care providers, postdischarge clinical assessment and monitoring of equipment and of patient compliance, ongoing care provider instruction, and contact with utility companies for priority listing. They should provide coverage 24 hours a day, 7 days a week, by credentialed respiratory therapy staff who are experienced in home ventilation. This respiratory staff should have a high ratio of full-time to part-time staff.

Personnel

Home care vendors vary in the amount of patient assessment (as opposed to equipment monitoring and maintenance) they provide. If a hospital based clinician is not available for home follow-up, an experienced home care therapist with good assessment skills is particularly important. Case managers are provided by some home care companies, in addition to the home care therapist.

Geography

The company should have an office within 40 miles of the patient's home. This is particularly important when the patient requires 24 hour ventilation. For these patients, a response time of 1 hour or less from the time of the patient's call to the therapist's arrival in the home is desirable. Most of the larger companies have branches throughout the region or the country, thereby making travel more feasible for those patients who wish to undertake it.

Equipment

The company should be able to provide a wide variety of equipment and should make the equipment available before discharge for in-hospital trial and training. The company should have monitoring equipment, such as oximetry and capnography (which is helpful in some cases). Most home care companies do not provide arterial blood gas measurements, but monthly oximetry is inexpensive, noninvasive, and informative. Replacement equipment should be locally and promptly available. Provision of a backup ventilator and a second suction machine is not always reimbursed by third party carriers, but nevertheless, some companies provide these units in the home for added safety or convenience.

Reimbursement Services and Policies

Some companies have formally organized reimbursement teams that have longstanding relationships with a network of third party payers and that negotiate actively with third party payers on the patient's behalf.

Insurance coverage, no matter how extensive, may be limited in time or in amount, and the company's commitment to continue services to the patient if insurance limits are reached should be established at the beginning.

PATIENT AND FAMILY

Ideal candidates for home ventilation are ventilated part time; are alert and able to participate, at least verbally, in their own respiratory care; are on stable, low FiO_2 and no PEEP; and have intact and supportive families with at least two caregivers willing to learn the patient's care. Unfortunately, ideal candidates are rare, and many patients who do not meet all of these criteria can be ventilated at home. Most home ventilator patients have either COPD or neuromuscular disease. Pulmonary fibrosis patients are more difficult technically and rarely become chronic ventilator patients.

Certain obstacles to family and patient acceptance of home ventilation occur repeatedly and need to be overcome to allow the patient and the family to consider home ventilation as an option.

One common obstacle is the belief that ventilator operation and tracheostomy care are too technically difficult for "lay people" to learn. This belief is not surprising, since most patients have ventilator therapy begun in an intensive care unit and carried out by highly trained personnel in a "life or death" atmosphere, with frequent measurements of arterial blood gases and with frequent changes in the ventilator settings. The patient and the family (and often the physician and the staff, as well) need to "demystify" the ventilator and stop associating ventilator therapy with critical care and critical illness. One of the major goals of ventilator rehabilitation is to stabilize the patient's ventilator program so that few changes need to be made and frequent monitoring of blood gases is not necessary.

A second common obstacle to home discharge on a ventilator is excessive emphasis, by patient, by physician, or by both, on weaning at the expense of function. The patient must cease to see himself as *debilitated,* or sick, and therefore able to get better to the point of not needing "the machine." The patient must come to view himself as *handicapped,* so that he can adopt the goal of maximizing his function within his capabilities by the use of whatever aids are available, including the ventilator. The ventilator patient needs to accept the ventilator as an assistive device to enhance function, just as a paraplegic accepts a wheelchair. We do not use the term "ventilator-dependent" in our practice. Patients who can be fully weaned to a stable and a functional state should certainly be weaned. However, once it becomes clear that complete weaning is impossible, the goal should become one of weaning for defined periods and of maximizing function, both on and off the ventilator.

Some patients continue to believe they can wean completely from the ventilator, even after the medical team has concluded that long-term weaning is impossible. Chronically ventilator-assisted patients usually have experienced numerous weaning attempts that end in failure and that occur at longer and longer intervals. Often, no specific decision is made to abandon weaning as a goal; rather, the medical team "burns out" and stops trying. A conscious decision to accept the impossibility of fully weaning such patients is preferable to a passive abandonment of weaning attempts because this decision permits the setting of new goals: the optimization of function and of quality of life on the ventilator and, possibly, home discharge.

Even when a conscious decision is made by the medical team to accept some amount of daily ventilator assistance for the foreseeable future, the patient may not accept the idea that he is "unweanable" and may interpret such a decision as a failure on his part or a "giving up" by the care team. Often, these patients insist on further weaning attempts and do not accept a stable weaning schedule, such as nocturnal ventilation. We have found that, for such patients to accept home ventilation, they must often try things "their way" and must be allowed to fail under close observation to ensure safety. If this process is not understood by the physician and by other caregivers, conflict can arise between the patient and the medical staff, and the patient may never reach his full potential.

The Family-Team Meeting

The suggestion to attempt home ventilation may arise from the patient, the family, or the staff. Once the idea is broached, the physician should discuss the suggestion with the family and the patient to establish its safety and its technical practicality and to allow them to ask the many medical questions that inevitably arise. If the family wants to proceed after this discussion, they should meet with the social worker so that detailed information about the family's resources, relationships, and structure can be obtained to guide the planning. This meeting also provides an opportunity for the social worker to assess the family's motives, problems, reservations, and strengths. Often, the family will more freely express their true feelings in a private meeting with the social worker than with the physician or in a formal family-team meeting.

A formal family-team meeting is scheduled if after reviewing all the available information, the discharge team still feels home discharge is a realistic goal. When the family-team meeting is held, the social worker's skills may make him or her the best choice to lead the meeting. At this meeting, all the members of the discharge team explain their role in the discharge process to the family and discuss the team's plans and goals. Frank discussion between the family and the team members often brings to light previously unappreciated problems and allows the discharge plan to be personalized and to be made more realistic. We recommend that the patient participate in the family-team meeting, despite the initial discomfort the family may feel with this idea. After the initial family-team meeting, at which goals and target dates are set, meetings are held (1) after milestones, such as a "transition room" experience or a leave of absence, (2) whenever the patient's condition changes significantly, and (3) immediately before discharge.

Patient and Family Education

Specific care skills must be detailed by team members, must be taught to the patient and the family

TABLE 1 Comparative Costs of Patient Care

	Home Care	Home Care with RN (24 hr/day)	Chronic Hospital	Acute Hospital non-ICU	ICU
Respiratory Care	2,000	2,000	7,500	7,700	7,700
Room & Board			7,500	10,600	27,000
Nursing Care		14,000			
Total per Month	2,000	16,000	15,000	18,300	34,700

in the hospital setting, and then must be systematically transferred to progressively less supervised settings. We recommend the use of education checklists to organize the many details that must be taught. Such checklists may be developed by the institution or be obtained from the home care company or the literature.

As discharge approaches and as the teaching is finalized, the patient and the caretakers are "put to the test" in a familiar, but less directly supervised, environment. We have used a "transition room" in the hospital to allow the family to stay overnight near the patient. This simulates the home care situation. Distant supervision is provided by hospital staff.

The final stage in the learning process consists of one or more unaccompanied home visits during which the family and the patient perform all the necessary care, independent of hospital staff. These visits have proven to be invaluable in building confidence in both the patient and the caregivers and in identifying unanticipated problems.

FINANCIAL CONSIDERATIONS

Costs

Although home care is usually assumed to be cheaper than institutional care, the cost of full-time RN care at home, plus the cost of equipment, can exceed the cost of care in the hospital, especially in chronic care facilities. Table 1 gives representative costs for ventilator care at institutions with which we are familiar. Obviously, the more independent the patient and the more participatory in his or her own care, the fewer highly trained home care personnel are needed.

Home care respiratory therapy procedures may differ from those used in the hospital with resultant cost reductions. For example, "clean," rather than sterile, technique for suctioning reduces costs for supplies by more than 80 percent and has not been shown to be associated with increased infection in the home setting. Most of the variable costs of home ventilation are oxygen costs and, therefore, reduction in oxygen utilization provides the greatest opportunity for overall cost reduction. Some patients who need supplemental oxygen when off the ventilator require only room air when on the ventilator, and oxygen requirements should be established separately for each situation in patients not on continuous ventilation.

Reimbursement

Securing adequate reimbursement for home ventilation may be difficult; the quest for coverage should start early in the patient's course. Reimbursement practices vary from state to state for private insurances and for programs such as Medicare and Medicaid.

The insurance industry has not yet fully adapted to the reality of home ventilator assistance. Each case is individually assessed by the insurer for both cost effectiveness and safety. Active negotiation with the insurer is often necessary, and even then, many private insurers prefer to pay 100 percent of hospital charges versus only 80 percent of a defined range of home services. Detailed knowledge of home care costs for each case is essential for effective negotiation with insurance carriers; diplomacy and appeals to the standards of fairness and the quality of life often make negotiation more successful than more assertive approaches.

More than one source of funding may be necessary to cover home ventilator care adequately. If the patient's primary insurance is not adequate, other sources should be sought; philanthropic organizations, community groups, and organizations such as the Muscular Dystrophy Association may help by funding specific pieces of equipment. Often a diligent effort enables an adequate program to be pieced together. Many home care companies are skilled and experienced in these matters and can provide helpful advice, as may home health care agencies and the American Lung Association. Physical modifications of the patient's home are generally not covered by insurance; some nonprofit community agencies may provide funding.

Written confirmation for the funding of DME and the salaries of allied health care providers should be obtained from private insurers or from state agencies before discharge.

Suggested Reading

Fischer DA, Prentice WS. Feasibility of home care for certain respiratory-dependent restrictive or obstructive lung disease patients. Chest 1982; 82:739–743.
Gilmartin M, Make BM. Home care of the ventilator-dependent person. Respir Care 1983; 28:1490–1497.

Johnson DL, Giovannoni RM, Driscoll SA, eds. Ventilator-Assisted patient care. Rockville, MD: Aspen Publishers, 1986.

Kopacz MA, Moriarty-Wright R. Multidisciplinary approach for the patient on a home ventilator. Heart Lung 1984; 13:255–262.

Make BM, Brody JS, Snider GL. Rehabilitation of ventilator-dependent subjects with lung diseases. The concept and initial experience. Chest 1984; 86:358–365.

O'Donohue WJ. Long term mechanical ventilation. Chest 1986; 90 (Suppl):1–37.

Sivak ED, Cordasco EM, Gipson WT, Stelmch K. Clinical considerations in the implementation of home care ventilation: observations in 24 patients. Cleve Clin Q 1983; 50:219–225.

Sivak ED. Long-term management of the ventilator-dependent patient. Preparation for home care. Cleve Clin Q 1985; 52:307–311.

HOME CARE PATIENT: VENTILATORY MANAGEMENT

EDWARD D. SIVAK, M.D.
JAN A. STEINEL, R.N., RRT

Mechanical ventilation for the treatment of acute respiratory failure is intended to support respiration until an individual is able to completely assume the work of breathing. For the treatment of chronic respiratory insufficiency, the goals of this support change to that of relief of dyspnea and the reversal of alveolar hypoventilation and cor pulmonale. These latter circumstances, which lead to continuation of mechanical ventilation in the home, can be discussed from four viewpoints, as shown in Table 1.

GOALS OF HOME CARE

The success of home care can only be determined if the preestablished goals of care are met during the actual process of the delivery of care. To illustrate this point, we might examine a brief case report of a patient with motor neuron disease. At the age of 56, he retired early because of fatigue. A year later, he developed respiratory failure from diaphragmatic weakness due to motor neuron disease. The institution of mechanical ventilation at night permitted him to be rehabilitated to the point of being ambulatory during daytime hours for about 15 months. However, soon thereafter he became totally ventilatory-dependent and quadriplegic. The initial goals of rehabilitation changed when he required dependent care delivered by skilled nurses in the home. In analyzing our preparation of patients and families for home care, it is apparent that a patient's diagnosis alone cannot define the goals of care. Thus, we classify all patients as requiring either rehabilitative care or custodial (dependent) care. In doing so, we find that physiologic defects follow the classification and that ultimately the resources required to deliver the care can be predicted. This experience is summarized in Table 2. By the same token, however, it is important to keep in mind that the classification of a patient may change from one category to another.

At the same time that one considers home care for the ventilatory-dependent patient, contraindications to home care should be considered. These are listed in Table 3. We strongly recommend against

hospital caregivers' pursuing home care out of sole concern for the hospital administration's running out of the financial resources required for continued care. By the same token, home care should not be considered an ideal alternative to hospital or institutional care because "there's no place better than home." Further emotional recommendations, such as a person's right to die at home should be avoided. Home care providers and vendors should not be forced to take on the care of patients for the aforementioned reasons. Most important is the need for patients and primary caregivers to arrive freely at a decision to continue ventilator care in the home. Home care should not be considered an option for patient management of the terminally ill patient who has been placed inappropriately on mechanical ventilation. Finally, the hospital support team, the home care vendor, and home care service agencies assume a responsibility only to facilitate home care and not to assume primary responsibility for the care of the patient.

RESOURCES REQUIRED FOR HOME CARE

Successful home care requires proper equipment and adequate support personnel to achieve the goals outlined in Table 2. Equipment for home care with positive pressure ventilation and other such devices is reviewed elsewhere. Support personnel range from the equipment vendor to hospital social worker and primary home caregiver, as listed in Table 4.

As expected, patients who use mechanical ventilation to facilitate the rehabilitation process require fewer resources than the patient receiving custodial (dependent) care. Of major importance is that those patients in the latter category can be expected to require some type of skilled nursing care during the course of ventilatory dependency. This is particularly true when the primary caregivers require rest or approach the so-called "burn-out" phase. These events should be anticipated and handled appropriately by the prescribing physician, who should proactively recommend periods of relief for the primary caregiver. Prescription of skilled nursing care in the home or admission to a respite care center would be in order.

Equipment vendors should ensure that patients have adequate disposable supplies in the home, but not an expensive inventory. We recommend a 2- to 4-week supply of disposables. If a patient is totally ventilator-dependent, a second reserve ventilator should be kept in the home. One novel approach used by some vendors is to place a ventilator from their inventory in the home and not charge the patient unless

**TABLE 1   Principal Areas for Consideration for Successful
Home Care Ventilation**

The goals of care (Table 2).
Technical and human resources required for delivery of care (Table 4).
Technical interface between patient and equipment.
Physiologic and psychological follow-up of patient and primary caregivers
   (Table 5).

TABLE 2   Goals of Care

Rehabilitative Care	Custodial Care
Participation in his or her own care	Patient comfort in the ICU. ICU discharge
Extended periods of spontaneous ventilation	Continued comfort outside of the ICU (hospital or home)
Ventilator free for the entire day	Family and patient acceptance of permanent debilitation
Patient's mobility outside the home	Adequate home care to guarantee maximum physical comfort
Return to previous routines and employment	Stabilization of the domestic situation for patient and primary caregivers

Diseases Corresponding to Care Categories	
Kyphoscoliosis	Amyotrophic lateral sclerosis
Alveolar hypoventilation	Muscular dystrophy (Duschenne)
Diaphragmatic paralysis	Quadriplegia due to traumatic injury
Post heart surgery	
Acid maltase deficiency	
Old thoracoplasty	Chronic obstructive lung disease (emphysema)

TABLE 3   Contraindications to Home Care

Altered mental status (dementia, cerebral vascular accident, anoxic
   encephalopathy)
End-stage pulmonary fibrosis
End-stage liver, kidney, or cardiac disease
Underlying malignancy or hematological malignancy
Unwilling or inappropriate primary caregivers

TABLE 4   Responsibilities of the Home Care Team

Physician—Coordinates entire home care team. Prescribes services and
   equipment.
Home care respiratory therapist—Assesses patient and equipment in the
   home (employment by hospital and/or equipment vendor)
Nurse—Evaluates and directs patient care in the home (employment by
   hospital, home care agency, or visiting agency)
Social worker—Evaluates patient and family adjustment to home care. Assists
   with the processing of ever-present claim forms and assessments
Psychiatrist—Evaluates family adjustment to home care setting. Identifies
   family-patient conflicts
Home health aide—Assists primary caregiver in the delivery of care

it is placed into use. The ventilator should be located close to the bedside with proper settings "dialed-in" and ready for use. The caregivers should only be required to turn on the machine and connect the circuit and appropriate oxygen bleed-in. The same vendors should also ensure that all equipment is checked monthly and that preventive maintenance schedules are instituted.

Beyond equipment resources, human resources must also be available. We recommend that patients be no further than 35 miles or 45 minutes from technical support, provided either by a home care agency or by a durable medical equipment supplier. This distance or time is recommended to ensure proper technical interface between patient and ventilator. A list of priority telephone numbers, including ambulance service, hospital emergency room, electric company, equipment vendor, home care nurses, respiratory therapists, and physician should be kept by all telephones.

TECHNICAL INTERFACE BETWEEN VENTILATOR AND PATIENT

A positive pressure device, often with supplemental oxygen, delivers ventilation via a tracheostomy tube. Thus, the technical interface between patient and ventilator can be analyzed by discussion about ventilators and tracheostomy.

The tracheostomy itself should be performed well in advance of anticipation of home discharge. Because of the long-term requirements, recommendations should be made to the consulting surgeon that the tracheostomy stoma be of the permanent type. This is done usually by "tucking" the skin flaps down near the anterior surface of the trachea and pulling a ring of anterior tracheal tissue upward to create a cutaneotracheal fistula. It is easy to have this foresight when seeing rehabilitative care patients. On the other hand, with the more debilitated custodial care patients, stoma revision may be required if a permanent tracheostomy is not done. In the event that none of these procedures is followed, the caregivers should anticipate problems with stomal infection, bleeding, fibrosis, granulation tissue, and difficulty with tracheostomy tube changes. Care can be taken to minimize such problems by meticulous stoma care, (i.e., frequent dressing changes to keep the stoma site dry). We also recommend a light coating of zinc oxide ointment for chronically irritated skin around the stoma site. Additionally, we recommend that the tracheostomy tube be changed every 2 to 3 weeks. More frequent changes guarantee easier changes in the future. Should a stomal infection occur, it is usually manifested by thick secretions coming from around the stoma site, and irritation of the adjacent skin. We recommend treatment with a broad spectrum antibiotic and have found that cultures of the secretions contribute little to the outcome of the treatment. If tracheostomy tube changes become too difficult, we recommend surgical revision of the stoma site.

Some consideration should be given to the type of tracheostomy tube to be used. For the patient in the rehabilitative category, one possibility is the fenestrated type of tube that can be plugged to facilitate speech. Another possibility is the use of an oversized cuffless tube with fenestration. Speech may be possible by plugging the tube.

Ventilation with minimal air leak with this type of tube is accomplished by learning glottic relaxation and closure during sleep. This can be accomplished by training patients to allow the posterior pharynx and tongue voluntarily to relax to the point of upper airway obstruction. We have found that this voluntary maneuver, with practice, can take place involuntarily during sleep. A third possibility is using either type of these tubes to accomplish ventilation at night and substituting a plug or button in the stoma during the day. This latter technique has proven superior because it reduces resistance to airflow in the upper airway. Exercise tolerance, speech, and self-image are improved. Patients are taught to change the tubes themselves. Our experience is that such individuals become as competent as the most experienced practitioners of tracheostomy tube changes.

On the other hand, the patient in the custodial care category will be more debilitated and more susceptible to aspiration of oral secretions even if the cuff of the tube remains inflated. Thus, any patients with problems of excess secretions or with incompetent glottic function (as in neuromuscular disease) should use a foam-cuffed tube (Kamen-Wilkenson tracheostomy tube). We have found that this type of cuff is longer and better conforms to the shape of the trachea. This markedly reduces the incidence of excess oral secretions being aspirated. It should be pointed out, however, that for those patients without this problem, using the cuffless tube with glottic closure should be attempted.

With this technique, when speech is desired, the tidal volume on the ventilator can be increased to permit a controlled air leak, which will facilitate speech. We also recommend that the family members, primary caregivers, or appropriate nurses or therapists learn the technique of tracheostomy change in the home. We prefer to teach the primary caregivers; those who have learned proper technique have not encountered problems with tube change, bleeding, or infection.

The ventilator interface should be designed to facilitate achieving the goals of care. The basic premise employed is that the patient uses the ventilator to completely take over the function of the respiratory muscles. We usually recommend a tidal volume of 12 to 15 cc per kilogram and a rate slower than 12 per minute, as this tends to satisfy the patient's desire for air. Although the open intermittent mandatory ventilation (IMV) system mode is usually selected, we select mechanical rates so the patient receives full support of ventilation when on the ventilator, but is capable of spontaneous ventilation if the ventilatory drive increases.

Many patients (especially those requiring ventilation for neuromuscular or chest wall disease rather than lung disease) oxygenate adequately on room air and so do not require supplemental lung oxygen. One principal exception is the patient with chronic obstructive lung disease. Under these circumstances, supplemental oxygen is added to guarantee a P_{O_2} of

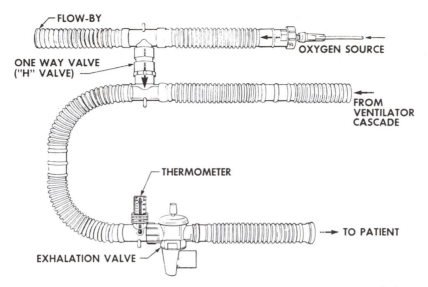

Figure 1 Ventilation is directed from the cascade. The "flow-by" may be used as a reservoir for spontaneous breathing by leaving it open to air. Otherwise, it may be directed to the piston intake port of the ventilator to maintain consistent inspired oxygen concentration.

70. This number is desired, as it most likely guarantees that the goals of relieving symptoms can be met. One pitfall to avoid with the open IMV system is neglecting to provide supplemental oxygen for spontaneously generated breathing. We have seen patients become agitated and breathe rapidly through the open system and miss the benefit of the supplemental oxygen delivered through the ventilator. This problem can be overcome by using an oxygen source connected into the ventilator piston air intake and an open IMV assembly. (This set-up may also be referred to as an "H" assembly, as shown in Fig. 1). Support of oxygenation with end-expiratory pressure is seldom required, and if so, one should seriously question the patient's stability and the appropriateness of home care.

We have found that only patients in the rehabilitative category are suitable candidates for weaning in the home. Such patients are those with diaphragmatic paralysis following heart surgery who require night-time ventilation to prevent recurrent respiratory failure and to guarantee proper rest at night to facilitate the rehabilitation process. When symptoms of orthopnea have disappeared and patients recover more than 50 percent of their vital capacity, we recommend that they merely begin sleeping off the ventilator, and if within a month there are no signs of cor pulmonale or symptoms of alveolar hypoventilation, the trachea is decannulated. We have found no other circumstances under which home weaning is appropriate. It should be emphasized that the decision to discontinue mechanical ventilation should be prescribed by the physician. The patient should be ambulatory and at a level of activity equivalent to the pre-ventilator state.

Close monitoring, although usually not necessary, should be decided on an individual basis.

PHYSIOLOGIC AND PSYCHOLOGICAL EVALUATION OF PATIENT AND OF PRIMARY CAREGIVERS

Rehabilitative Care

Once again we can return to the theme of the types of care delivered. For the patient in the rehabilitative category, we recommend a follow-up physician visit 1, 3, and 6 months after discharge, and yearly thereafter (Table 5). This is usually done in the outpatient department, with careful attention to the patient's activity history to determine if self-care and daily living activity levels have been reached. We find that patients in this category achieve this level within the first 6 months after discharge. Finally, we recommend that patients return to work if employment possibilities exist.

We measure spirometry and negative inspiratory forces at each visit to monitor stability of respiratory muscles. The stability of arterial blood gases should be established before hospital discharge. In addition, patients with diaphragmatic paralysis have vital capacity measured in the sitting and supine positions.

We further recommend that the home care supplier visit the patient in the home monthly for the first 3 months and every 3 months thereafter. The ventilator should be checked for parameters and alarm settings, and the patient should be questioned about adherence to maintenance of the machine and proper cleaning of the circuits. It is also recommended that the vendor maintain proper preventive maintenance schedules for the patient's equipment.

For the most part, we have not found it necessary to culture tracheal secretions or circuits on a routine basis. In addition, there is little place for oximetry or capnography measurements if the patient maintains a physiologic level of function equivalent to the events of daily living. Home care vendors should become experienced in observing the home environment for cleanliness; the general mood of the patient and family members; the signs of cor pulmonale and symptoms of alveolar hypoventilation; and adherence to prescribed respiratory therapy routines.

In this category, the most common problems include stomal infection, difficult tracheostomy tube change, and return of pre-ventilator symptoms. Stomal infections are usually due to poor tracheostomy hygiene and are easily rectified, as described above; if recurrent, ventilator circuits or the valve on manual resuscitator bags should be inspected to be sure that they have been properly cleaned. Tracheostomy tube change can be difficult if the stoma is fibrosed, which requires stomal revision every 2 to 3 years unless the cutaneotracheal fistula type of stoma is created. The return of pre-ventilator symptoms is usually due to ventilator circuit leak or patient attempts to wean completely off mechanical ventilation. We have found that patients in this category frequently recover to the point that they assume that mechanical ventilation at night is no longer necessary. Such attempts result in return of pre-ventilator signs and symptoms within 1 month.

Some other practical points include recommending influenza vaccination yearly, though we do not routinely recommend the pneumococcal vaccine (Pneumovax). If a patient develops an upper respiratory tract infection with thickening or discoloration of sputum, a course of an oral broad-spectrum antibiotic is in order.

Custodial Care

Patients in the custodial category may require a feeding gastrostomy or jejunostomy for nutritional support. Generally, the tubes used disintegrate over time, especially those with balloons on the distal end. In order to avoid disruption of the balloon and the tube falling out of the stoma, we recommend that the tube be changed once a month. We have also found that jejunostomy tube location is associated with fewer problems of nausea, vomiting, and aspiration of feedings. The same type of care given to the tracheostomy stoma should be given to the feeding tube stoma.

Maintenance of nutritional status is also important to guard against the development of bedsores. We do not routinely monitor the adequacy of visceral protein stores, but one may want to monitor nutritional intake, particularly for patients who are receiving feedings by gastrostomy or jejunostomy tubes.

TABLE 5 Assessments According to Types of Care

Rehabilitative Care	Custodial Care
1st month	1st month
a) Documentation of the level of physiological and psychological function	a) Tracheostomy change every 3 weeks
b) Examination of tracheostomy stoma Auscultation of the lungs and heart Examination of the lower extremities for edema	b) Gastrostomy or jejunostomy tube change monthly
c) Vital capacity. Negative inspiratory force (stability of arterial blood gases should be established before discharge)	c) Examination of tracheostomy stoma Vital signs. Physical examination of chest, abdomen, and skin
d) Ventilator circuit check. Review of patient's use and maintenance of equipment	d) Ventilator circuit check. Equipment use and maintenance by primary caregiver
	e) Observe patient and family members for signs of anger, fear depression, anxiety, or resentment
	f) Oximetry
2nd month	2nd month
a–d above	a–f above
3rd month	3rd month
a–d above	a–f above
6th month	6th month
a–d above	a–f above
12th month	12th month
a & b above	a–f above. Complete history and physical examination by physician
Thereafter	Thereafter
Influenza vaccine may be given each year as appropriate. Items a–d every 6 months for a year and then yearly	Assessments a–f above every 3 months and yearly examinations

With proper nutritional support and careful attention to frequent position change in bed, bedsores are seldom a problem. We have noted several situations in which persistent bedsores, recurrent carbuncle development, or *Candida* infection in skin folds should lead one to test further for evidence of diabetes mellitus.

At the present time, there are few facilities in the country where respite care is possible. If possible, patients and family members may get some relief from the constant daily stress of chronic care in the home. It is our impression that if the discipline of patient care in the home is to grow, some type of respite care will be required. For the future, we must also be mindful that ventilator-dependent patients have the potential to outlive their primary caregivers. Thus, a long-term care facility must also be available for contingencies.

We would be remiss if no mention were made about the burdens on patient care teams. Although these individuals leave their jobs behind at the end of a work day, patients and families depend upon them 24 hours a day. All must make efforts to guard against fatigue, emotional indifference, and anger. Patients and family members in the home care setting should be encouraged to become as independent as possible from the hospital discharge team. If this is not possible, then perhaps home care is not appropriate. The home care team may feel frustrated or helpless if the rigid discharge protocols are not followed. The rule of thumb to follow is that if patients are content and not in life-threatening situations, then the care is probably satisfactory. The principal psychological burden of the team is getting patients and families to accept the finality of the debilitation causing ventilator dependency.

Custodial care patients usually require more medications than rehabilitative care patients. The categories usually include sedation, analgesia, stool softeners, and bronchodilator therapy. The only patients who require bronchodilator therapy are those with chronic obstructive lung disease. We have found few exceptions to this rule. Sedation of these patients may be required to facilitate ventilator interface. We have also added hydrocodone therapy to relieve the sensation of dyspnea, which also smooths out interaction with the ventilator. In patients with severe lung hyperinflation, we have also seen anasarca develop and require rehospitalization and vigorous diuretic therapy. A weight gain in excess of five pounds per week usually heralds such a problem. At this point, daily doses of diuretic therapy are required. Under these circumstances, we do recommend monthly measurements of oxygen saturation by pulse oximetry to ensure that oxygenation is adequate.

Patients receiving custodial care are usually ventilator-dependent for more than 20 hours per day. Most deteriorate to levels of minimal activity and require the presence of a primary caregiver almost constantly. We recommend monthly ventilator checks for parameter and alarm settings. Patient assessment should be similar to that of the rehabilitative patient (see Table 5). The signs or symptoms of tachypnea, dyspnea, or cor pulmonale suggest some alteration in patient-ventilator interface. Problems with the tracheostomy tube, ventilator circuit, or ventilator should be actively monitored. Unlike for rehabilitative care patients, pulse oximetry readings are suggested for custodial care patients every 3 months, or when a patient is complaining of dyspnea over and above his baseline condition. In addition to the monthly visits by equipment suppliers, frequent visits by home care nursing agencies are also recommended to assess the quality of patient care delivered by primary caregivers. It should be emphasized that these caregivers assume a 24-hour a day task and should be observed for signs of anger, fatigue, or emotional indifference. Our experience is that the primary caregiver who displays no signs of such emotional strain is a rare exception. Almost invariably we recommend the support of hired attendants, be they skilled nurses or appropriately trained individuals, to lessen the family burden. Furthermore, we have found that most caregivers welcome relief by alternative caregivers. This ultimate requirement for outside hired help may frequently make the cost of home care for the custodial care patient more expensive than for long-term institutional care.

We especially emphasize that all members of the patient care team should learn about family conflicts and problems. Frequently, complaints about ventilator interface or vague symptoms about altered physiologic condition may be related to emotional strife rather than to a change in the physiologic condition. In these situations, the prehospital-discharge psychiatric evaluation of the patient and family will prove to be invaluable. We recommend that social services maintain open files on patients and encourage family members to voice problems to them. Many times patients or family members are more likely to express concerns to a social worker than to a physician. Physician visits are recommended every 3 months for the first year and every 6 months to a year thereafter. Although this frequency is minimal, more frequent contact, at least by telephone, is psychologically beneficial to patients and caregivers.

Finally, one is likely to encounter custodial care patients who will die at home on the ventilator. Our own experience has been that patients appear to develop fever and thick secretions and become withdrawn. In the final days, hallucinations are common, and caregivers are mistaken for relatives who have died. Although this is anecdotal experience, such observations should give rise to discussions with family members about keeping the patient comfortable at home. If necessary, hospice services in the home should be recommended. In the end, we have found that the physician is expected to pronounce the patient dead and discontinue mechanical ventilation when appropriate.

The concept of ventilator management in the home is not new. The signs and symptoms of alveolar hypoventilation remain the same, but the diseases have changed. By the same token, our society has changed. These changes emphasize that the medical community can no longer assume total responsibility for the care of the long-term ventilator patient. We must teach appropriate patients and families to become independent caregivers. The medical community itself, and society in general, are responsible for the facilitation of this quest for independence. We must be additionally responsible to the point of not forcing home care on patients and families who do not want it or cannot assume it.

Suggested Reading

Fisher DA, Prentice WS. Feasibility of home care for certain respiratory-dependent restrictive or obstructive lung disease patients. Chest 1982; 82:739–743.

Garay SM, Turino GM, Goldring RM. Sustained reversal of chronic hypercapnia in patients with alveolar hypoventilation syndromes. Long-term maintenance with noninvasive nocturnal mechanical ventilation. Am J Med 1981; 70:269–274.

Hoeppner VH, Cockcroft DW, Dosman JA, Cotton DJ. Nighttime ventilation improves respiratory failure in secondary kyphoscoliosis. Am Rev Respir Dis 1984; 129:240–243.

Make B, Gilmartin M, Brody JS, Snider GL. Rehabilitation of ventilator-dependent subjects with lung diseases. The concept and initial experience. Chest 1984; 86(3):358–365.

Sivak ED, Streib EW. Management of hypoventilation in motor neuron disease presenting with respiratory insufficiency. Ann Neurol 1980; 7:188–191.

Sivak ED, Gipson WT, Hanson MR. Long-term management of respiratory failure in amyotrophic lateral sclerosis. Ann Neurol 1982; 12:18–23.

Sivak ED, Cordasco EM, Gipson WT. Pulmonary mechanical ventilation at home: a reasonable and less expensive alternative. Respir Care 1983; 28(1):42–49.

Sivak ED, Cordasco EM, Gipson WT, Stelmach K. Clinical considerations in the implementation of home care ventilation: observations in 24 patients. Cleve Clin Q 1983; 50:219–225.

Sivak ED, Razavi M, Groves LK, Loop FD. Long-term management of diaphragmatic paralysis complicating prosthetic valve replacement. Crit Care Med 1983; 11(6):438–440.

Sivak ED. Long-term management of the ventilator-dependent patient: preparation for home care. Cleve Clin Q 1985; 52:307–311.

Sivak ED, Cordasco EM, Gipson WT, Mehta A. Home care ventilation: the Cleveland Clinic experience from 1977 to 1985. Respir Care 1986; 31(4):294–302.

Spaingard ML, Frates RC, Harrison GM, Carter RE, Jefferson LS. Home positive-pressure ventilation. Twenty years' experience. Chest 1983; 84:376–382.

White KD, Perez PA. Your ventilator patient can go home again. Nursing 1986; 16(12):54–56.

PATIENT MANAGEMENT APPROACHES

STABLE CHRONIC BRONCHITIS AND EMPHYSEMA (COPD)

THOMAS L. PETTY, M.D.

The management of stable chronic bronchitis and emphysema, together called chronic obstructive pulmonary disease (COPD), is a challenge for the primary care physician, the respiratory therapist, the nurse, and the physical therapist, all of whom may be involved in the care of growing numbers of patients who suffer chronic cough and unrelenting dyspnea. Data from the National Health Survey estimate that nearly 20 million Americans have various degrees of COPD, and the numbers seem to be increasing. Now that all underlying causes of death are listed in most states, the true statistics of emphysema mortality are becoming known. In 1984 there were at least 70,000 deaths from COPD in the United States.

COPD is a family clustering disease that is related to smoking and that worsens with age. The fact of airflow obstruction as measured by simple spirometry and the rate of decline of ventilatory function are potent prognostic indicators in this disease spectrum. An improvement in airflow in response to the use of bronchoactive drugs also predicts better survival than if reversibility cannot be achieved by any of the pharmacologic agents described in this chapter. I will briefly present a systematic approach to the assessment and the management of patients with various degrees of chronic stable COPD. I offer to the practitioner a pragmatic approach that should be useful in most patients.

ASSESSMENT

The development of chronic airflow obstruction in chronic bronchitis and emphysema is now clearly a problem that clusters in families. Thus, the family history of chronic airflow obstruction is an important indicator of the likelihood of airflow obstruction in any patient. Airflow obstruction is also related more closely to smoking than to any other factor. Therefore, recording the age of onset of smoking, the number of years of smoking, and the amount consumed daily is important. Ventilatory function in children who smoke is now known to be lower than in nonsmoking children of the same age. This suggests an adverse effect of tobacco smoke on lung growth. An assessment of ventilatory function as an indicator of the degree of severity of airflow obstruction is of paramount importance in judging the prognosis of all patients with chronic cough and expectoration. The availability of simple, accurate, dry, direct recording office spirometers makes simple measurements of forced vital capacity (FVC) and forced expiratory volume in one second (FEV_1) practical and highly useful. These measurements are the key indicators of volume and of flow, respectively, and are the only tests that are needed to estimate prognosis and to evaluate the response to therapy.

MANAGEMENT

Smoking Cessation

Smoking cessation is by far the most important intervention that can alter the course of COPD. Thus, an effort toward behavioral modification leading to smoking cessation should be made. The newly available nicotine-containing gum (Nicorette) may help to counteract the addictive features of nicotine as part of an overall smoking cessation program. The value of smoking cessation on the course and the prognosis of disease has been well-established. Susceptible smokers demonstrating premature loss of ventilatory function who stopped smoking before the age of 50 and who had relatively good remaining ventilatory function showed a rate of loss of ventilatory function equivalent to the age-related rate after they stopped, compared to the continued accelerated loss of ventilatory function in those who continued to smoke. Even patients who stopped smoking at age 65 with severe ventilatory function impairment and who averaged only 30 percent of the predicted FEV_1 for age 25 had a better survival than those who continued to smoke. Thus, there can be no doubt that discontinuance of smoking is the fundamental therapy for chronic bronchitis and/or emphysema.

Vaccines

The use of influenza virus vaccine is recommended by the Center for Disease Control; this vaccine is believed to provide a substantial degree of protection against common strains of influenza that can cause devastating illness in patients with COPD. When there is insufficient time to offer vaccine during epidemics, the use of oral amantadine or rimantadine offers substantial protection. These drugs are also likely to shorten the course of an exacerbation of chronic bronchitis caused by influenza if given when symptoms first appear. Whether or not pneumococcal vaccine offers significant benefit to patients with COPD is debatable. Newer vaccine preparations have introduced an increased number of antigenetic strains (from 14 to 23). It is my belief that both influenza virus vaccine and pneumococcal vaccine are valuable in the treatment of COPD, and they can be given simultaneously. Influenza virus vaccine should be given each fall if epidemics are predicted, and because of the antigenic shift of the organism, repeated yearly vaccination is recommended. According to current opinion, polyvalent pneumococcal vaccine should be given only once in a lifetime.

Bronchodilators

Bronchodilators are widely used in patients who demonstrate at least a small degree of reversibility of airflow obstruction as judged by simple office spirometry. At least a 15 percent improvement over baseline FEV_1 probably should be considered significant improvement. The systematic treatment of the nonspecific bronchial hyperreactivity that may accompany COPD could possibly prevent accelerated losses in lung function over time. The first step in bronchodilator management is the use of an inhaled beta-adrenergic agonist aerosol delivered by a metered-dose device (MDI). Increasing numbers of more selective, longer-acting preparations are now available. These preparations are listed in Table 1, along with older agents.

The proper use of a metered-dose aerosol is probably as effective as any method of bronchodilator administration. Nonetheless, some physicians still prefer to use beta-adrenergic agonist aerosols via pump-driven nebulizers. Table 2 lists selected solutions for use in powered nebulizers.

Proper Use of MDI Bronchodilators

Unfortunately, few patients, and even few physicians, know and apply the most advantageous method of using a MDI. Having the mouth open and providing a space between the mouthpiece of the device and the patient allows for the evaporation of the surrounding propellant, at least to a degree. Aerosol particles reach the conducting airways and are deposited by basically two processes. These processes include impaction in the larger airways and gravitational sedimentation of the smaller airways. Both of these steps require time. Larger particles impact more readily than small particles. According to all available data, the process of gravitational sedimentation, if successful, requires slow inhalation, a pause at the end of inspiration, and slow exhalation against pursed lips for best results. Probably 10 seconds should be allowed for the full process of inhalation. Two, three, or more inhalations should be continued until relief is achieved. Under-dosing is likely the reason for poor degrees of bronchodilatation in some patients.

Anticholinergics are also time tested drugs that provide potent bronchodilitation by the inhaled route. Atropine has been used as a medicine for over 100 years, and ipratropium has recently been released. Additional atropine derivatives are being studied, such as atropine methylnitrate and glycopyrrolate, both of which are fairly widely used in Europe. Anticholinergics work mostly in large airways in contradistinction to beta agonists, which exert their effect throughout the tracheal bronchial tree. In addition, the time of onset to bronchodilatation from anticholinergics is 30 to 60 minutes as opposed to only a few minutes with the inhaled beta agonists. In fact, both inhaled beta agonists and anticholinergics are quite compatible and complement the action of each other. In Europe and elsewhere, beta agonists and anticholinergics are commonly used in the same metered-dose inhaler.

Theophyllines are widely used for bronchodilatation (Table 3). Theophyllines are also known to improve respiratory muscle function and to prevent or reduce respiratory muscle fatigue in states of severe chronic airflow obstruction. Both beta-adrenergic agonists and theophyllines can improve mucociliary

---

TABLE 1   Selected Bronchodilator Aerosols (Metered-Dose Device)

Beta Agonists
 Nonprescription
  epinephrine (Bronkaid, Primatene)
 Prescription
  albuterol (Proventil, Ventolin)
  bitolterol (Tornalate)
  isoetharine (Bronkometer)
  isoproterenol (Isuprel)
  metaproterenol (Alupent, Metaprel)
  terbutaline (Brethaire)
Anticholinergics

TABLE 2   Selected Solutions for Nebulizers

Albuterol (Proventil or Ventolin)
Isoetharine (Bronkosol or generic)
Isoproterenol (Isuprel or generic)
Metaproperenol (Alupent, Metaprel, or generic)
Metaproterenol (Alupent)

TABLE 3   Common Oral Products That are Time Release Theophylline

Short Acting Products* (usually taken three or four times a day)
 Aminophylline (generic)
 Choledyl
 Theophylline USP
Long Acting Products (usually taken twice a day)
 Choledyl SA
 Constant T
 Respbid
 Slo-bid
 Theo-Dur
 Theovent
Ultra Long Acting Products (usually taken once a day)
 Theo-24
 Uniphyl

*Among others

clearance, but the clinical significance of this fact is not known. The availability of ultra long lasting theophyllines, which can be given once a day to persons with normal clearance rates, adds a new dimension in patient compliance.

Corticosteroids

Corticosteroids are well-known to be useful in the treatment of exacerbations of chronic bronchitis that result in acute respiratory failure. One controlled clinical trial has demonstrated objective improvement in airflow from corticosteroids as compared to placebo. Even patients considered to have irreversible airflow obstruction may respond to oral corticosteroids. Thus, most physicians, including myself, believe that a short-term trial of corticosteroids should be offered to nearly every patient with chronic airflow obstruction on a trial basis for approximately 2 weeks. A single morning dose of 40 mg of prednisone, guided by symptoms and spirometric measurements, identifies those patients with significant degrees of reversible airflow obstruction. Inhaled corticosteroids are not usually as effective as oral drugs in steroid-responsive patients. When there is no objective improvement, steroids can simply be stopped after a 2-week therapeutic trial. Tapering is not necessary in these patients. For those patients with chronically significant improvement, strategies are required to capitalize on benefits and also to minimize long-term side effects, such as osteopenia and eye complications, i.e., the acceleration of cataract formation in some patients and the aggravation of glaucoma.

Once complete control is achieved, some steroid responsive patients only require short bursts for exacerbations because the healing of the inflamed mucosa may return an important barrier against provocation from certain agents, such as inhaled cold air, dust, and irritants. When corticosteroids are given only in short courses of 5 to 7 days, longterm steroid side effects can usually be minimized. If chronic long-term steroids are required for both objective and subjective benefit, I try to use either a small morning dose of prednisone in the range of 5 to 15 mg or an alternate daily dose of 10 to 20 mg of prednisone. I prefer prednisone to the longer acting preparations to allow for some degree of responsiveness of the pituitary adrenal axis, even if these doses are used on a daily basis. When inhaled corticosteroids are sufficient for control, their use is preferable. Much smaller doses are deposited in the lung and very little is absorbed. An increased number of inhaled steroid preparations is available as summarized in Table 4.

Antibiotics

Antibiotics are probably the most widely used pharmacologic agents in the treatment of exacerbations of chronic bronchitis. Whereas the initial insult resulting in increased cough and expectoration is likely to be viral, the fact of later bacterial invasion in many patients is also well established. However, a bacterial pathogen is not found in many patients. *Streptococcus pneumoniae* and *Haemophilus influenzae* species are the most commonly cultured organisms. In addition, *Mycoplasma* is occasionally present, and the possibility of anaerobes must be considered. The culture of expectorated sputum is not necessary in most cases because purulent sputum may not accurately reveal the infecting pathogen. In some cases, this pathogen is a virus and rarely a mycoplasma. Oral antimicro-

TABLE 4   Inhaled Corticosteroid Preparations Currently Available

Pharmaceutical Name	Trade Name
Beclomethasone	Becotide, Vanceril
Flunisolide	AeroBid
Triamcinolone	Azmacort

bials can be selected on epidemiologic grounds, based on a knowledge of the organisms that are usually present. Table 5 lists the antibiotics in roughly their order of usage. These antimicrobials are empirically effective in reducing the symptom complex of chronic bronchitis exacerbations.

Special mention of chloramphenicol is in order because of the fears of devastating hematologic complications (i.e., aplastic anemia). In fact, these complications are exceedingly rare, occurring in roughly one in 10,000 to 40,000 prescriptions. Since chloramphenicol remains the drug of choice for *Haemophilus* species and since chloramphenicol is often effective against pneumococcus and highly effective against anaerobes, its use, when other antimicrobials are ineffective, is entirely appropriate. Chloramphenicol has been found to be superior to ampicillin in patients with severe exacerbations of chronic bronchitis. Trimethoprim with sulfamethoxazole (Bactrim or Septra) is also effective in the treatment and the prevention of purulent exacerbations of chronic bronchitis and is generally my first choice in antimicrobial management. The effectiveness of tetracycline in acute exacerbations of bronchitis in hospitalized patients with chronic bronchitis has been seriously questioned in a recent double-blind controlled clinical trial.

Controversy still surrounds the role of bacterial infection in the pathogenesis of chronic obstructive pulmonary disease (COPD). Seemingly, repeated viral and bacterial invasion with infection of the conducting airways could participate in chronic airway narrowing and perhaps could also do damage to the surrounding alveolar walls via release of proteases and/or free radicles from polymorphonuclear leukocytes that respond to the invading organisms.

A growing body of evidence relates childhood respiratory infections to the later development of chronic bronchitis with airflow obstruction. Repeated childhood infections could be a marker of the patient with inadequate natural antimicrobial defense mechanisms. An alternate hypothesis is that early and subtle injury of the lungs makes later infection more likely. Bronchial reactivity may follow viral illnesses in children. This bronchial hyperreactivity may persist into adult life and perhaps could become a factor in progressive airflow obstruction.

The impact of repeated infections on the course and the prognosis of adults with COPD is not certain. Some patients suffer step losses in ventilatory function following bronchopulmonary infections, thus suggesting major damage to the airways, but this pattern of disease progress is not common. The use of antimicrobials can shorten the symptomatic period of exacerbations of chronic bronchitis. Some evidence exists that the prophylactic use of antimicrobials reduces the frequency of winter exacerbations in patients who often suffer from acute attacks of purulent bronchitis. However, no controlled clinical trial has shown a favorable influence in the long-term course and the prognosis by the use of antimicrobials. Nonetheless, the weight of clinical experience and the high likelihood of improving the symptom complex in acute attacks have helped to establish the widespread use of antimicrobial agents for episodes of acute purulent bronchitis. It is my practice to institute a 7 to 10 day course of antimicrobials for each episode on empiric grounds. Sputum culture and sensitivity tests are not found useful in this context.

A SYSTEMATIC APPROACH TO THERAPY

No chapter can define all of the strategies of therapy that apply to every patient. A combination of smoking cessation, influenza virus, and pneumococcal vaccines is the most effective preventive approach available. The systematic use of inhaled and oral bronchodilators, and corticosteroids when indicated, and of antimicrobials constitutes effective therapy for most patients.

Today I begin almost all patients on an inhaled beta agonist taken three or four times a day, and more often if symptomatic relief requires. The use of inhaled beta agonists frequently throughout the day is perfectly reasonable in view of the almost miniscule amount that is actually deposited in a lung, i.e., only about 10 percent of each actuation. This dose would be 20 μg from a metered dose of 200 μg. It seems incredible that we are so parsimonious about our use

TABLE 5 **Common Antimicrobial (Antibiotic) Drugs Used for Exacerbations of Chronic Bronchitis**

Name	Usual Dose	Side Effects
Ampicillin	250 or 500 mg four times a day	rash, diarrhea
Trimethoprim-sulfa (Bactrim and Septra)	1 capsule twice a day 80 mg trimethoprim; 400 mg sulfamethoxazole	rare gastrointestinal upset 160 mg trimethoprim; 800 mg sulfamethoxazole
Tetracycline	250 mg four times a day—some other preparations once a day	stomach upset, diarrhea, vaginal yeast infections
Erythromycin	250 or 500 mg four times a day	stomach upset
Chloramphenicol	250 to 500 mg four times a day	rare GI upset, mild anemia (common), aplastic anemia (rare)

of inhaled beta agonists, while, at the same time, many physicians freely prescribe the same oral product, i.e., 4,000 to 5,000 µg, three or four times a day! Thus, it stands to reason that, from the tiny amount delivered and deposited in a lung from each actuation, even if a metered dose inhaler were used 20 times per day, the dose delivered would be no more than that in a single tablet, which is completely absorbed and delivered throughout the body!

At the same time I generally employ a once-a-day theophylline at bedtime. Patients can frequently remember to take their medications just before retiring. I most commonly use Uniphyl or Theo-24 for the advantage of increased compliance compared to the shorter acting preparations, which require more frequent dosing. In fact, in my own controlled clinical trials of Uniphyl, I found slightly better pulmonary function and blood levels with once-a-day Uniphyl compared to a previously used twice daily product, Theo-Dur. The strategy of the regular use of a metered dose inhaler throughout the day and the limitation of theophylline to evening dosing provides an extremely practical regime. If other therapies are required, I use prednisone, as stated previously, usually in the morning. This strategy separates the use of prednisone, which has a different purpose, from the evening bronchodilating Uniphyl (or an alternative theophylline). If multiple inhaled agents are used, these are given morning, noon, and night, which is sufficient for anticholinergics (if required) and corticosteroids. Inhaled, corticosteroids are nicely employed on a twice daily basis. Thus, the only agent the patient must carry for use throughout the day is the beta agonist inhaler for immediate bronchodilatation and symptomatic relief.

OTHER THERAPIES

Pulmonary rehabilitation techniques are useful in patients with severe airflow obstruction. Breathing retraining, physical reconditioning, and oxygen all play their roles. That oxygen can alter and improve survival and quality of life is no longer in doubt, based on two multicenter trials in both the United Kingdom and North America.

FUTURE TRENDS

More needs to be learned about the role of childhood chest infections and of exposure to tobacco, both actively and passively, as a prelude to the development of chronic bronchitis with airflow obstruction.

The early identification of patients with airflow abnormalities also predicts those who will become the respiratory cripples of the future. Although no controlled trials have proved this, it is likely that the early identification and the management of patients via smoking cessation and the use of bronchodilating aerosol to combat nonspecific bronchial hyperreactivity, known to be present probably in 15 to 20 percent of patients with early stages of disease, might well forestall or curtail the premature loss of ventilatory function that results in premature morbidity and mortality. At this writing, controlled clinical trials to test this hypothesis are underway, sponsored by the National Heart, Lung, and Blood Institute. In any case, I believe that, on a regular basis as maintenance management for patients with all stages of COPD, it is appropriate to offer, not only symptomatic management, but specific pharmacologically oriented therapy that is designed to improve airflow and to deal with bacterial invasion.

Suggested Reading

Albert RK, Martin TR, Lewis SW. Controlled trial of methylprednisolone in patients with chronic bronchitis and acute respiratory insufficiency. Ann Intern Med 1980; 92:753–758.

Anthonisen NR, Manfreda J, Warren CPW, et al. Antibiotic therapy in exacerbations of chronic obstructive pulmonary disease. Ann Intern Med 1987; 106:196–204.

Aubier M, DeTroyer A, Sampson M, et al. Aminophylline improves diaphragmatic contractility. N Engl J Med 1981; 305:249–252.

CDC Report: Update: Pneumococcal polysaccharide vaccine usage—United States. JAMA 1984; 251:3071–3075.

Mendella LA, Manfreda J, Warren CPW, et al. Steroid response in stable chronic obstructive pulmonary disease. Ann Intern Med 1982; 96:17–21.

Newhouse MT, Dolovich MB. Control of asthma by aerosols. N Engl J Med 1986; 315:870–874.

Peto R, Speizer FE, Cochrane AL, et al. The relevance in adults of airflow obstruction, but not of mucus hypersecretion, to mortality from chronic lung disease: results from 20 years of prospective observation. Am Rev Respir Dis 1983; 128:491–500.

Petty TL, Nett LM. The history of long-term oxygen therapy. Respir Care 1983; 28:859–865.

Ramsdell JW, Nachtwe FJ, Moser KM. Bronchial hyperreactivity in chronic obstructive bronchitis. Am Rev Respir Dis 1982; 126:829–852.

Report of the Surgeon General. Chronic obstructive lung disease. Public Health Service 1984; 84-50205:501–534.

Report of the Surgeon General. The health consequences of smoking. Public Health Service 1984; 84-50205:187–218.

Riddiough MA, Sisk JE, Bell JC. Influenza vaccination (cost effectiveness and public policy). JAMA 1983; 249:3189–3195.

Tager FB, Munez A, Rosner B, et al. Longitudinal analysis of the effects of cigarette smoking in children. Chest 1984; 85:8S.

Tager FB, Speizer FE. Role of infection in chronic bronchitis. N Engl J Med 1975; 292:563–571.

EXACERBATIONS OF CHRONIC OBSTRUCTIVE PULMONARY DISEASE: PHARMACOLOGIC MANAGEMENT

GEORGE G. BURTON, M.D.

Care of the patient with persistent or recurrent limitation of pulmonary airflow occupies a large portion of the respiratory clinician's workday. Exacerbations of chronic obstructive pulmonary disease (COPD) are heralded by worsening cough, change in sputum production or character, and dyspnea, alone or in combination, and may range in severity from a mild nuisance to life-threatening acute-on-chronic respiratory failure.

Exacerbations of the constellation of diseases known as COPD reflect the fact that some aspects of its pathophysiology are reversible: bronchospasm, inflammation, frank infection of airways and lung parenchyma, and mucous obstruction. Some COPD patients (perhaps 70 percent) do have some reversible elements to their airflow obstruction. Although this may be called the "asthmatic component" of COPD, the usual biologic markers of immunologically mediated hypersensitivity may not be present, and not all such patients may demonstrate improvement with bronchodilator therapy in the pulmonary function laboratory. An intelligent approach to therapy of exacerbations of COPD capitalizes on the presumed reversibility of a perhaps small, but clinically important, portion of airflow obstruction in such patients. Not reversible are the effects brought about by loss of pulmonary elastic recoil and alveolar capillary membrane surface area (in emphysema) and fibrotic distortion of airways (in chronic bronchitis).

When queried as to his or her condition, the patient suffering from exacerbation of COPD often responds with a terse "worse!" This may indicate that the cough and dyspnea are more severe, and "attacks" may last longer or be more frequent. Because repeated performance of even simple pulmonary function testing is not usually practical, it becomes important to ascertain precisely what the patient means by "worse" or "better" if the effects of therapy are to be correctly evaluated.

A useful strategy for treatment of exacerbations of COPD must include not only the many *types* of respiratory care modalities and medications, but the *timing* of their implementation as well. In addition, appropriate decisions as to the appropriate physical *site* of the interventions must be made: home, physician's office, emergency room, or hospital.

CONDITIONS THAT EXACERBATE THE SYMPTOMS OF COPD

Physicians tend to favor etiologic (and diagnostic) hypotheses that explain all of the patient's symptoms under one umbrella. Indeed, stable COPD alone can explain cough, breathlessness, fatigue, depression, weakness, lack of appetite, and even chest pain. However, given the age, family history, smoking and industrial exposure history, and medication use (and abuse) of patients with COPD, other legitimate comorbidities—a term born in the age of the diagnosis-related groups (DRGs)—must be considered (Table 1). The presence of infection (acute bronchitis or pneumonia) is perhaps the most common exacerbating factor of COPD, but it is by no means the only one.

PATIENT ASSESSMENT

Clinical assessment of the patient whose COPD is in exacerbation includes that of the possible comorbidities and is beyond the scope of this chapter (see Suggested Reading). Correct assessment of the severity of the patient's condition is as critical as is precision in the diagnosis of the exacerbating condition.

I tell my previously stable COPD patients *to call my office* for new instructions or medications (1) with any fever over 100° F (37.8° C) or any fever with chills, (2) after 2 days of temperature elevation greater than 1° F above their normal baseline, (3) with any nausea, vomiting, or diarrhea, and (4) with worsening dyspnea of more than 3 days' duration, refractory to the Backup Home Program described later in this chapter.

I ask my patients to *come to the office or emergency room* for evaluation if there is no improvement after therapy is added (e.g., antibiotics, steroids, or diuretics) or if there is any unrelieved dyspnea, hemoptysis, chest pain, change in mentation (especially agitation or confusion), or syncope. A thorough physical examination is then performed. In the office, evaluation of such patients usually includes an arterial blood gas analysis, a serum theophylline level (if the patient is on a theophylline-containing oral broncho-

TABLE 1 Comorbid Conditions that Present as Exacerbations of COPD

Condition	Common Clinical Symptoms	Diagnostic Laboratory Tests	Treatment
Acute bronchitis	Productive cough, increased dyspnea, substernal discomfort, purulent sputum	Leukocytosis, sputum, Wright's, and Gram's stain	Antibiotics, systemic and airway hydration (see text)
Pneumonia	Fever, productive cough, pleuritic chest pain	As above, plus chest radiograph and blood cultures	As above. If toxic or in impending respiratory failure, hospitalize
Asthmatic bronchoconstriction	Increased cough, dyspnea, wheeze	Increased blood and sputum eosinophil count, elevated IgE in bronchial asthma	Corticosteroids (see text), avoidance of causative agent if possible, desensitization when indicated, sodium cromolyn
Medication errors and noncompliance, tobacco smoke exposure; industrial smoke and fume exposure; failure to comply with exercise conditioning regime	Progressive dyspnea, "worsening" (see text)	Persistent eosinophilia, nontherapeutic serum theophylline levels, presence of CoHb, work history	Patient and family education, use of intelligent caregivers, job modification, closer work with pulmonary rehabilitation team
Malnutrition or weight gain	Weakness, weight loss or gain	Weight, characteristic blood chemistry and hematologic abnormalities	Nutrition counseling, dietary supplementation as indicated
Pneumothorax	Acute dyspnea, chest pain, syncope	Chest radiograph	Hospitalization, thoracotomy tube to suction
Acute myocardial infarction and/or congestive heart failure (CHF)	Increasing dyspnea, may not have typical anginal chest	ECG, chest radiograph (may not be typical; see text), cardiac enzymes	Hospitalization for cardiovascular monitoring
Pulmonary embolism and infarction	Acute dyspnea, hemoptysis (in infarction)	Chest radiograph, ventilation-perfusion lung scan (may be difficult to interpret), pulmonary angiogram	Anticoagulation or thrombolysis
Bronchogenic carcinoma	Weight loss, recurrent pneumonia, hemoptysis, chest pain	Chest radiograph, computed tomography (CT) scan, sputum cytology, bronchoscopy	Thoractomy and resection (if possible), radiation, chemotherapy

dilator medication), a circulating (absolute) eosinophil count, and, if indicated, a chest radiograph. Simple office spirometry may be done as well to determine deviation from prior baseline measurements. A sputum Gram's stain and culture may also be performed.

On the basis of these determinations, a decision is made regarding *hospitalization*. I generally decide to hospitalize patients who are dehydrated or who will need intravenous medications, patients with acute respiratory failure (respiratory acidosis and oxygen-refractory hypoxemia), those who are aged or senile, those who demonstrate radiographic infiltrates, and a few in whom medication errors have occurred. I also frequently hospitalize acutely ill patients who need new respiratory care devices at this point in their illness, such as medication nebulizers, chest percussors, apnea alarms, nasal continuous positive airway pressure (CPAP) devices, and cuirass-type shell ventilators. Rarely, patients who lack adequate personnel support services at home may need to be hospitalized as well, although not for that reason alone.

I rely heavily on our pulmonary rehabilitation team for both inpatient and outpatient teaching, and all the "touch-up" teaching is performed by them. My patients have come to rely on this group of health professionals as much as on our office nursing staff for assistance.

BACKUP HOME PROGRAM

Much has been written about the elements of good comprehensive respiratory care programs for COPD patients. Until relatively recently, it has seemed to me that "more was better," and the most complicated programs were touted as superior. I am happy to see that a plea for simplicity is now being heard. Most initial regimens now consist of an inhaled beta-agonist bronchodilator and a once- or twice-a-day ultra-long-acting theophylline-containing bronchodilator. In most patients with an asthmatic component, and as a last-ditch therapeutic trial in others, corticosteroids (inhaled or oral) are used.

I have found it helpful to have my patients share in their own prescription dosing by allowing them to increase the intensity of their bronchial hygiene program during times of symptom worsening (Table 2). I have yet to regret a decision to allow a reliable, intelligent patient to modify his therapeutic regimen in such a fashion. Indeed, it is generally the patient who rigidly holds to a regimen that was prescribed for stable COPD in the face of clinical deterioration that we see the next morning in the emergency room or the ICU.

INITIAL IN-HOSPITAL THERAPY OF THE ACUTELY ILL COPD PATIENT

The data base on which therapy is initiated will probably have been obtained in the office or emergency room, as discussed above. If not, it will need to be quickly assessed on admission to the hospital. The COPD patient with acute-on-chronic respiratory failure represents a medical emergency in which much must be accomplished simultaneously and quickly. In such circumstances, errors of omission occur more frequently than do errors of commission. We have found that the use of physician "standing orders" has been helpful in this connection. The physician initiating care of the patient may delete or insert additional orders as clinically indicated.

Oxygen therapy and ventilator support of gas exchange are discussed elsewhere in this volume. Pharmacologic management of acutely ill COPD patients involves the use of antibiotics, bronchodilators, mucolytics, corticosteroids, antiarrhythmic agents, and diuretics.

Antibiotic Therapy

Infectious exacerbations of COPD are commonly heralded by worsening cough, dyspnea, and an increase in sputum viscosity and purulence. Fever, leukocytosis, bandemia, and radiographic abnormalities may or may not be present, particularly early in the course of the exacerbation. The Health Care Financing Administration (HCFA) has appropriately assigned roughly equivalent DRG weights to pneumonia and acute bronchitis, suggesting that the morbidity of the two conditions is similar. With the possible exception of lobe- or segment-targeted chest physical therapy in the resolution phase of pneumonia, the treatment of the two conditions is also similar, if not identical.

The effectiveness of antibiotic therapy in exacerbations of COPD is difficult to evaluate, but a recent study has shown an advantage of antibiotic therapy over placebo in patients who presented with the symptoms listed above. The incidence of side effects was low in both treated and placebo groups, and the cost of antibiotic (a 10-day course of either trimethoprim–sulfamethoxazole, amoxicillin, or doxycycline) was not excessive. The benefits (i.e., shorter exacerbations and lower rates of deterioration) are complemented by low cost to make the use of antibiotics in infectious exacerbations of COPD attractive to most practitioners, no matter how empiric the data may be. As of now, there seems to be no clear antibiotic of choice for bronchitic exacerbations of COPD.

If pneumonia is present, initial antibiotic selection is based on the presumed exposure site: was the infection community- or hospital-acquired? In order of frequency, *Streptococcus pneumoniae* and *Legionella* species, followed by staphylococci, *Haemophilus influenzae*, and *Klebsiella* are the most common community-acquired pathogens. *Chlamydia* and *Mycoplasma* infections must also be considered. Because it is often impossible to determine the exact etiologic agent with certainty an initial management strategy based on the law of averages is necessary, pending the results of sputum microbiologic studies, blood cultures and, when indicated, serologic studies.

TABLE 2 Patient-Initiated Backup Program for Exacerbations of COPD

Bronchodilator therapy
  May increase use of MDI to q1–2h if observed by educated caregiver
  May use one aminophylline suppository (250–500 mg) or 15 ml (80 mg) of aminophylline elixir q4h × 2 days
Systemic hydration
  Force fluids of choice until urine is colorless
Corticosteroids
  May double maintenance dosage (up to 50 mg/qd of prednisone) for 2 days. If not improved, call office
Oxygen
  May use continuously; may turn up by 1.0 L/min (to maximum of 2 L/min) when up and about
Exercise conditioning
  May discontinue conditioning program for several days if too weak or dyspneic
Diuretics
  May increase daily dose by 50% for 7 days, as needed for peripheral edema

Pneumococcal pneumonia in COPD patients occurs more frequently in winter and in older patients and often begins by "crisis" with acute onset of fever, chills, and cough productive of rusty-brown and yellow sputum. There may have been an antecedent upper respiratory infection as well. The radiologic infiltrate of pneumococcal pneumonia in COPD is nonspecific, i.e., the "classic" lobar infiltrate rate seen in patients without COPD may not be present. If pneumococcal pneumonia is suggested, penicillin is the drug of choice, with erythromycin as an alternative in patients with penicillin allergy.

In patients with nonpneumococcal pneumonia, a distinction must be made between the remaining bacterial (*Haemophilus,* staphylococcal, and enteric bacillary) pneumonias and the nonbacterial types. Nonbacterial pneumonias are more indolent, with gradual onset of flulike symptoms: headache, low grade fever (to 38.5° C), chills, muscle aches, anorexia, nausea, and nonproductive irritating cough. The physical findings are diffuse, as are the pneumonic infiltrates.

Risk factors for *Legionella pneumonia* include male gender, age over 50 years, and immunosuppressive therapy; thus our COPD patients are readily included. With a virus-like prodrome, diarrhea, confusion, abnormal liver function tests, hypophosphatemia, and lymphocytosis, appropriate workup for *Legionella* should be pursued. Erythromycin is the drug of choice. Erythromycin is the drug of choice in mycoplasmal pneumonia as well, and I use this agent whenever I suspect either *Mycoplasma* or *Legionella* infection.

Aspiration pneumonia is not uncommon in patients with COPD, who are frequently afflicted with peptic ulcer disease and hiatal hernia as well. The presence of putrid-smelling sputum and the formation of abscesses or empyema should alert the clinician to this possibility. Aminoglycoside therapy, combined with anaerobic coverage (e.g., penicillin or clindamycin) may be indicated.

Bronchodilator Therapy

Patients ill enough to be hospitalized with exacerbations of COPD normally receive parenteral (intravenous or subcutaneous) bronchodilator therapy. Unless the patient gives evidence of theophylline toxicity, aminophylline may be started with a "maintenance dose" at a rate of 0.5 to 0.6 mg per kilogram per hour IV. A loading dose of 5 to 6 mg per kilogram of aminophylline will need to be given if the patient has not previously been receiving theophylline-containing bronchodilator medication. I have recently been impressed with the prompt bronchodilator effects of subcutaneous terbutaline, 0.25 mg subcutaneously, as well. This dose may be repeated in 15 to 20 minutes if improvement does not occur.

A theophylline level should be obtained in the emergency room or upon admission. Many patients prove to have inadequate serum theophylline levels and thus less than optimal effect from the basic pharmacologic agent. Adequate bronchodilation is achieved at serum levels of 10 to 20 μg per milliliter, though some workers report the optimal therapeutic range to be between 5 to 15 μg per milliliter.

Inhaled aerosolized bronchodilators should be used as well, either from a metered dose inhaler (MDI) or from an air-powered medication nebulizer. The in-hospital utility of patient-administered MDI therapy has recently been demonstrated. I use an every-2-hour × 4 dosing schedule for the first 8 hours, tapering back to an every-6- to 8-hour schedule as clinical improvement occurs.

Mucolytic Therapy

Systemic hydration represents the most efficacious form of mucolysis. Bland aerosol therapy and pharmacologic mucolysis (iodides, acetylcysteine) are discussed in other chapters, and are not reviewed here. My approach consists of intravenous hydration at the rate of 100 to 120 ml per hour × 8 hours, if no evidence of left-sided congestive heart failure (CHF) is present. The presence of right-sided heart failure (cor pulmonale) is not a contraindication to parenteral hydration.

The effects of bland aerosol therapy are difficult to evaluate. The results from systemic hydration and pharmacologic mucolysis, on the other hand, are more predictable, especially when combined with vigorous chest physical therapy, cough training, and if indicated, airway suctioning.

Corticosteroid Therapy

As stated earlier, some patients with COPD have a steroid-sensitive, asthmatic component to their condition. In such individuals, use of intravenous corticosteroids may be helpful during severe exacerbations. Although there are little data to support specific effective dosing regimens, there appears to be consensus that 75 to 125 mg of methylprednisone every 6 hours should be given in the first 24 hours, tapering back to a maintenance dose 9 to 12 days thereafter. In my opinion, aerosolized corticosteroids have little place in the pharmacologic management of hospitalized COPD patients in exacerbation.

Diuretic Therapy

It is beyond the scope of this chapter to discuss diuretic therapy in detail. However, most pulmonary physicians have seen patients who demonstrate both left-sided CHF and COPD, and appropriate treatment of one condition often improves the other. The usual chest radiographic signs of CHF are obscure in patients with COPD, and the diagnosis must often be made on other grounds. Review of serial films is helpful. In seriously ill patients, measurement of the pulmonary capillary wedge pressure may be required.

To protect against fluid overload, daily patient weights and intake and output records should be kept and reviewed. Patients with already high work of breathing produced by elevated airway resistance (COPD) certainly do not tolerate decreased pulmonary compliance (CHF) as well.

Suggested Reading

Anthonisen NR, Manfreda J, Warren CPW, et al. Antibiotic therapy in exacerbations of chronic obstructive pulmonary disease. Ann Intern Med 1987; 106:196–204.

Aubier M, Murciano D, Viires N, et al. Increased ventilation caused by improved diaphragmatic efficiency during aminophylline infusion. Am Rev Respir Dis 1983; 127:148–154.

Bryan C, Reynolds K. Bacteremic nosocomial pneumonia. Am Rev Respir Dis 1984; 129:668–671.

Donowitz GR, Mandell GL. Empiric therapy for pneumonia. Rev Infect Dis 1983; (Suppl 1):40–54.

Hill NS. Fluid and electrolyte considerations in diuretic therapy for hypertensive patients with chronic obstructive pulmonary disease. Arch Intern Med 1986; 146:129–133.

Hudson LD. Management of COPD–state of the art. Chest 1984; (Suppl 6):76–81.

Lode H. Initial therapy in pneumonia–clinical, radiographic, and laboratory data important for the choice. Am J Med 1986; 80:70–74.

Pines A. Successful treatment of respiratory tract infections in patients with chronic respiratory disease—how to make objective conclusions. J Antimicrob Chemother 1982; 9:165–168.

Theodore AC, Beer DJ. Pharmacotherapy of chronic obstructive pulmonary disease. Clin Chest Med 1986; 7:657–671.

Turino GM, Goldring RM, Heinemann HO. Water, electrolytes and acid-base relationships in chronic cor pulmonale. Prog Cardiovasc Dis 1970; 12:467–483.

EXACERBATION OF CHRONIC BRONCHITIS AND EMPHYSEMA: VENTILATORY MANAGEMENT

DAVID J. PIERSON, M.D.

Chronic obstructive pulmonary disease (COPD) is a clinical syndrome consisting of longstanding dyspnea and/or productive cough in combination with spirometrically demonstrated airflow obstruction, as seen predominantly in cigarette smokers in their 50s and beyond. This disorder can also be thought of pathophysiologically as a variable combination of emphysema, chronic bronchitis, and an element of "reversible airway obstruction"—asthma. The last of these, present to some extent in most patients with COPD, is the most directly treatable; however, because asthma is discussed in three other chapters in this book, I will not include it here.

Patients with COPD may require ventilatory support in a number of circumstances, notably, following cardiac or other surgical procedures. However, they generally do *not* require intubation and mechanical ventilation during acute exacerbations of their primary disease. With aggressive therapy using bronchodilators, corticosteroids, chest physiotherapy, and controlled oxygen administration, only one in ten to 20 such episodes should require these measures. This concept cannot be over-emphasized, because not only is mechanical ventilation largely unnecessary in COPD, it is also fraught with numerous, life-threatening hazards in this disorder.

GOALS OF MANAGEMENT

In light of the preceding, the first goal pertaining to ventilatory management in acute exacerbations of COPD is to avoid mechanical ventilation if at all possible. When this goal cannot be achieved, the clinician must concentrate on making the period of intubation and ventilation as short as possible. Patients with COPD are affected more adversely than other individuals by changes in acid-base, electrolyte, and nutritional status; thus, keeping these elements stable throughout the exacerbation constitutes another major goal.

The event, or process, precipitating the need for ventilatory support is an important determinant of how long this support will be necessary. Patients inadvertently over-sedated can usually be extubated in 4 to 6 hours or less, whereas recovery from an episode of gram-negative pneumonia may require many days of support.

The clinician should weigh the nature and the severity of the precipitating event when deciding whether or not to initiate mechanical ventilation. For example, ventilatory support may be appropriate in the setting of a spontaneous pneumothorax or an episode of acute bronchospasm not responding to initial therapy, but not when the patient is known to have been in inexorable decline for months, without a history of marked reversibility in previous acute episodes. Unfortunately, intubation and ventilation sometimes cannot be avoided for patients in the last category if they are previously unknown to the clinician who must make the decision in the heat of the moment, often in the setting of imminent respiratory arrest.

Although avoiding mechanical ventilation is an important goal, respiratory stimulant drugs, such as doxapram, should not be used for this purpose. These drugs increase the demands placed on the patient's ventilatory apparatus without augmenting the capacity to respond. Likewise, the notion that intubation can be forestalled by intermittent positive pressure breathing (IPPB) treatments has proven to be erroneous and to be fraught with unwarranted hazards for the patient.

INDICATIONS FOR ENDOTRACHEAL INTUBATION

Insertion of an endotracheal tube into the airway of a patient with COPD—even in the presence of a severe exacerbation—causes so much interference with cough, with mucociliary function, and with other airway functions, and so predisposes the patient to nosocomial infection, that intubation should be considered extremely carefully and should only be performed if unavoidable. If mechanical ventilation is indicated (see next section), then intubation must, of course, be done. Additional indications are essentially two: to protect the airway, as in acute epiglottitis or other threatened upper airway obstruction, and to clear airway secretions when other measures fail. This last indication rarely occurs in clinical practice.

Whether to intubate orally or nasally has long been controversial. Oral tubes are shorter, less sharply angled, and larger, so that suctioning is easier and airway resistance is lower; oral tubes are also harder to anchor at the mouth and are considerably more uncomfortable for an awake patient. Nasal tubes are better tolerated, but must be less than 8 mm in diameter, and, therefore, create greater airway resistance and more difficulty in suctioning; nasal tubes also may cause acute sinusitis and otitis media. I prefer nasotracheal intubation initially, unless insertion must be accomplished as an emergency procedure.

Is there a role for tracheostomy in the management of acute respiratory failure in severe COPD? Tracheostomy should only be necessary when truly prolonged (i.e., indefinite) mechanical ventilation is planned. Tracheostomy reduces anatomic deadspace, but robs the patient of speech. While the clinical importance of the former is unproven, the effect of the latter can be devastating.

INDICATIONS FOR MECHANICAL VENTILATION

Acute respiratory failure consists of impairment in tissue oxygenation and/or in CO_2 removal that occurs suddenly enough and is of sufficient severity to threaten the life of the individual. This physiologic state is usually accompanied by physical signs and symptoms—dyspnea, tachypnea, tachycardia, restlessness, confusion, and others—but all of these are nonspecific and are highly variable among individuals. Consequently, unless a patient is agonal or apneic, the presence and the severity of acute respiratory failure cannot be assessed accurately without arterial blood gas measurement, and sometimes hemodynamic data as well.

The need for intubation and ventilatory assistance in acute exacerbations of COPD requires the diagnosis of acute respiratory failure *plus* a pathophysiologic consideration of the possible reasons a patient might need these measures. This fact is crucial in view of the importance of avoiding mechanical ventilation in COPD.

Table 1 summarizes the six general categories of physiologic derangement that can require ventilatory assistance, along with the available means for assessing these categories. In most instances, two or more of the six conditions are present. If the patient's condition does not fit the conditions in Table 1, he or she should be observed without intubation and should be reassessed at frequent intervals.

It must be stressed that, in acute ventilatory failure (severe acute respiratory acidosis), the arterial pH, not the PCO_2, is important. Patients with arterial PCO_2 values of 50, 60, or even 80 mm Hg do not need to be ventilated if their pH values are above about 7.25 (because of compensatory metabolic alkalosis) and are not falling rapidly. Institution of mechanical ventilation, in such instances, frequently brings on acute alkalosis that increases, rather than diminishes, the threat to the patient's life.

The concept of "resting" a COPD patient in an acute exacerbation seems reasonable, but is extremely difficult to handle in practice. In addition, whether the respiratory muscles of these patients *should* be rested is far from clear. I rely heavily upon the assessments shown in Table 1, and hold off on intubation as long as these assessments permit, and as

TABLE 1   Indications for Mechanical Ventilation

Physiologic Mechanism	Best Indicators (Normal Values)	Values Indicating Need For Mechanical Ventilation
Inadequate alveolar ventilation	Arterial PCO_2 (36–44 mm Hg)	Acute increase from normal or from patient's baseline
	Arterial pH (7.36–7.44)	<7.25–7.30
Hypoxemia	Alveolar-to-arterial PO_2 gradient breathing 100% O_2 (25–65 mm Hg)	>350 mm Hg
	PaO_2/FiO_2 ratio (350–400 mm Hg)	<200 mm Hg
Inadequate lung expansion	Tidal volume (5–8 ml/kg)	<4–5 ml/kg
	Vital capacity (60–75 ml/kg)	<10 ml/kg
	Respiratory rate (12–20 breaths/min)	>35 breaths/min
Respiratory muscle weakness	Maximum inspiratory force (80–100 cm H_2O)	<25 cm H_2O
	Maximum voluntary ventilation (120–180 L/min)	<2 × resting ventilation requirement
	Vital capacity (60–75 ml/kg)	<10–15 ml/kg
Excessive work of breathing	Minute ventilation volume required to keep arterial PCO_2 normal (5–10 L/min)	>15–20 L/min
	Ratio of deadspace to tidal volume (25–40%)	>60%
	Respiratory rate (12–20 breaths/min)	>35 breaths/min
Unstable ventilatory drive	Breathing pattern; clinical setting	No readily available measurement

long as the patient can cooperate with bronchodilator administration and with other therapy.

Ventilator Settings

Diminution in expiratory airflow is the physiologic hallmark of COPD. In practical terms, air forced into the lungs under positive pressure returns more slowly than in individuals without airflow obstruction; if succeeding breaths are delivered before exhalation is complete, air is progressively trapped in the patient's lungs, where it can compromise cardiac function and can burst alveoli. To prevent these potentially fatal complications, several modifications must be made in the ventilator settings used for COPD patients as compared to the ventilator settings used for other clinical situations.

Tidal Volume

Spontaneously breathing individuals inhale 5 to 8 ml per kilogram with each quiet respiration. Tidal volumes of 12 to 15 ml per kilogram are commonly used during mechanical ventilation to prevent atelectasis and progressive hypoxemia. Alternatively, smaller, more "physiologic" breaths may be employed with occasional "sighs" of double or triple volume. Neither practice is safe in severe COPD, a condition in which atelectasis is of little concern in any event. Tidal volume should be about 10 ml per kilogram, and should be less in the presence of severe hyperinflation, and sighs should not be used because of the risk of alveolar rupture ("barotrauma").

Ventilator Mode

Whether patients with severe COPD should be ventilated with assist-control mechanical ventilation (AMV), with intermittent mandatory ventilation (IMV), or with one of their newer variations is a controversy the intensity of which sometimes approaches that of a holy war. Proponents of AMV and of other strategies to assume total ventilation of the patient's lungs feel that taking over the work of breathing while the patient is unable to meet all ventilatory needs is an important aspect of treatment, since respiratory muscle fatigue is assumed to be present in the face of greatly increased airway resistance. On the other hand, clinicians who advocate IMV believe that this mode, which obliges the patient to provide part of the required minute ventilation in order to avoid respiratory acidosis, prevents respiratory muscle atrophy and makes more sense teleologically.

I prefer to initiate mechanical ventilation by using AMV. If dyspnea and agitation result in rapid triggering of the ventilator and if the patient becomes alkalemic, I first assess and reassure the patient, making sure that there is no other cause for agitation (hypoxemia, pain, obstructed airway). Then I attempt to adjust inspiratory flow rate and other machine settings to better match the patient's desired pattern. If hyperventilation and agitation persist, I use sedation. These measures usually suffice, but if they do not, I try IMV; studies have shown, however, that using IMV routinely in preference to AMV does not decrease the frequency and the clinical severity of respiratory alkalosis.

Inspiratory Flow Rate

AMV does not abolish patient work during triggered breaths. Recent studies show that substantial effort may continue throughout each patient-initiated breath, but that this may be minimized by using rapid inspiratory flow rates (80 to 100 L per minute). Patients who are alert and dyspneic usually prefer such high inspiratory flows. In addition, maximizing the peak inspiratory flow provides more time for exhalation at any given respiratory rate and, thus, reduces the likelihood of air trapping and auto-PEEP (see following).

Respiratory Rate

The initial ventilator rate has to be empirical, with subsequent adjustment according to the results of arterial blood gas measurements. Ideally, arterial pH should be kept between 7.35 and 7.40, with hypercapnia essentially ignored for purposes of rate adjustment. The avoidance of hypocapnia and alkalemia should be a major goal.

Inspired Oxygen Concentration

Controlled oxygen therapy is of prime importance in the management of the spontaneously breathing COPD patient with a severe exacerbation. However, once the patient is intubated and placed on a ventilator, the clinician need not worry about suppressing hypoxic ventilatory drive. Hypoxemia in COPD is mainly attributable to ventilation:perfusion mismatching, which is readily corrected by supplemental oxygen, usually at inspired oxygen fractions (FiO_2s) well below 0.50. Oxygen toxicity is thus also not of clinical concern in these patients.

Preservation of hypoxic ventilatory drive, an important contributor to resting ventilation in some patients with severe COPD, becomes important again at the time of weaning. When the patient is asked to breathe spontaneously, PaO_2 should be kept between 55 and 65 mm Hg (saturation approximately 85 to 90 percent).

Although sedation may be required during the initial hours of ventilatory support, sedation should be reduced prior to weaning. I like to discontinue sedation, if possible, after 1 or 2 days, something much easier to do if patient comfort has been maximized using the ventilator adjustments and the other measures described previously.

Patients with COPD should be ventilated upright for as many hours in the day as possible. Lying flat is often distressing for such patients, and ventilatory mechanics are improved by moving from the supine to the fully seated position.

COMPLICATIONS OF MECHANICAL VENTILATION IN THE COPD PATIENT

While patients with COPD are subject to the same complications of intubation and mechanical ventilation as are other patients, these patients are particularly susceptible to some adverse effects. For example, because of their increased respiratory secretions, their ineffective cough, and their impaired mucociliary escalator, the further disruption of these functions by an endotracheal tube especially predisposes these patients to secretion retention and to bacterial infection. Intubation also interferes with eating, and this nutritional interruption can have severe consequences in these individuals.

"Auto-PEEP" is an important and an infrequently appreciated problem in the ventilatory management of patients with COPD. Auto-PEEP is the endogenous build-up of positive pressure at end-expiration that results from the incomplete emptying of the lungs prior to the next delivered positive pressure breath. Auto-PEEP's physiologic effects are the same as those of deliberately applied positive end-expiratory pressure (PEEP): increased intrathoracic pressure can reduce right ventricular filling and, thus, impair cardiac output, and air-trapping can overdistend and rupture alveoli, resulting in the rapid development of tension pneumothorax. Auto-PEEP is clinically inapparent and cannot be detected or quantitated unless specifically sought. However, auto-PEEP can be measured readily at the bedside by momentarily delaying delivery of the next breath, occluding the ventilator's expiratory line, and reading the pressure on the airway manometer at the moment at which the breath would have been delivered.

Auto-PEEP can be minimized in two ways. First, the inspiratory flow rate should be high (80 to 100 L per minute), thereby maximizing the expiratory time. Second, the inspiratory time can be further shortened and auto-PEEP correspondingly reduced if low-compressible-volume tubing is used. With conventional, high-volume circuits, a substantial amount of each delivered breath is compressed in the circuit, and in order to deliver the prescribed tidal volume to the patient, this delivered volume must be increased. As a result, inspiratory cycling time is increased and the time available for exhalation is reduced.

Another major hazard of mechanical ventilation in the patient with severe COPD is respiratory alkalosis from over-ventilation. Table 2 illustrates this complication, using typical values for pH, for PCO_2, and for serum bicarbonate (HCO_3). A patient with underlying chronic respiratory acidosis (chronic CO_2 retention) decompensates acutely and the arterial PCO_2 rises, producing acute acidemia and acute ventilatory failure. This patient's "normal" PCO_2 (as dictated by his ventilatory mechanics) is 55 mm Hg. When mechanical ventilation is initiated and a "normal" PCO_2 of 40 mm Hg is attained, the patient's established "compensatory" metabolic alkalosis is suddenly unopposed, and dangerous alkalemia results.

As Table 2 also shows, if the preceding situation is not promptly corrected, and if the same alveolar ventilation is allowed to continue for 2 or 3 days, the patient's kidneys "dump" the excessive bicarbonate, thus returning the arterial pH to normal in the face of a PCO_2 of 40 mm Hg. However, this now "fully normalized" situation, from the standpoint of arterial blood gas and serum bicarbonate values, is incompatible with the patient's underlying ventilatory mechanics. When asked to sustain the level of alveolar ventilation required to maintain a PCO_2 of 40 mm Hg during weaning, he again develops acute respiratory acidosis and "fails" weaning. This all-too-common sequence can be reversed only by allowing the PCO_2 to rise over several days, so that alveolar ventilation falls to a level that the patient can sustain indefinitely. Arterial pH is kept reasonably normal by reestablishment of the "compensatory" metabolic alkalosis.

WEANING FROM MECHANICAL VENTILATION

Discontinuation of ventilatory support may be approached in several ways, the two chief of which are a progressive diminution in the fraction of total

TABLE 2 Acute Respiratory Alkalosis* During Mechanical Ventilation

	Baseline Compensated State	Acute Respiratory Decompensation	Initial Values on Ventilator	Reestablished Compensated State After 2–3 Days
pH (units)	7.38	7.25	7.55	7.40
PCO_2 (mm Hg)	55	85	40	40
HCO_3 (mEq/L)	32	36	34	24

*A common adverse sequence during ventilator management of patients with acute ventilatory decompensation of severe COPD

minute ventilation provided by the ventilator (weaning with IMV), and an abrupt switch from total support to spontaneous breathing (traditional or "T-piece" weaning). I use the latter approach, guided by the principles summarized in Table 3.

Keeping in mind the first two goals of ventilatory management—to avoid mechanical ventilation, and if unavoidable, to keep the duration as brief as possible—the clinician should attempt to wean the patient as soon as the conditions in Table 3 are met. If, after several days of intensive management, the patient still fails to meet these conditions, a systematic examination of the physiologic mechanisms for this failure should be made.

By far the most common reasons for inability to meet weaning criteria are common, basic problems, not exotic disorders. Among the common problems are alkalosis (weaning is unlikely if the pH is above 7.50), excessive sedation, an excessively high ventilatory demand owing to high CO_2 production (from sepsis, agitation, or over-zealous hyperalimentation), and persistent severe airway obstruction (by bronchospasm, by secretions, or by a too-small endotracheal tube). Rare causes, such as hypophosphatemia, hypomagnesemia, myxedema, and primary disorders of muscles or of ventilatory drives, should be kept in mind, but should not be investigated until more common mechanisms have been excluded.

Failure of a patient to be "weanable" after several days of attempts should shift the focus of management to a more global, longer range plan. Failure to wean after prolonged mechanical ventilation is related less to the individual measurements listed in Table 3 than to the patient's over-all condition—the severity of the underlying disease, the number of organ systems affected, the intensity of support required (FiO_2, PEEP, minute ventilation), the nutritional state, and the mental status. Successful weaning requires careful attention to all these things, probably over several weeks, rather than simply repeating the weaning attempt every day.

Prolonged weaning is best accomplished by using brief periods of spontaneous breathing (on a separate, low-resistance T-piece circuit, rather than through the ventilator) interspersed with rest periods of complete ventilatory support. How long these respective intervals should be is entirely empirical, but patients should be permitted to rest for several hours between T-piece periods at first, and should be returned to the ventilator through the night. The periods of spontaneous ventilation are progressively lengthened, with reassurance, emotional support, and reliance on the patient's subjective response, rather than on repeated arterial blood gas samples. Weaning often occurs "by itself" if the patient's over-all condition can be improved, with a point reached at which it is obvious that the patient is able to wean successfully.

Recent years have seen much attention focused on the respiratory muscles during mechanical ventilation and weaning. Although less important, in my opinion, in patients who require only brief mechanical ventilation, respiratory muscle function is a main determinant of success or failure in long-term weaning. I consider the first task to be a reduction of the load on the ventilatory muscles (by improving respiratory mechanics). Pressure-support ventilation, which allows spontaneous initiation of breaths, but reduces the work required for a given tidal volume, may offer an advantage in this setting.

I strongly believe that whole-body exercise helps in weaning: patients who are able to get out of bed and to ambulate with assistance two or three times a day are more likely to wean than those who remain bed-ridden throughout their intensive care unit (ICU)

TABLE 3 Weaning from Mechanical Ventilation

Preset criteria satisfied, indicating readiness for weaning:
   Improvement in whatever precipitated acute exacerbation
   Acceptable supplemental oxygen requirement (50% or less)
   Minute ventilation required for normal or for baseline arterial P_{CO_2} not more than 10–12 L/min
   Adequate spontaneous ventilatory parameters:
      Spontaneous vital capacity at least 10 ml/kg
      Maximum inspiratory force at least 20–25 cm H_2O
      Maximum voluntary ventilation at least 2× resting ventilation requirement
Appropriate circumstances for weaning attempt present:
   Narcotics, tranquilizers, and sedatives eliminated or reduced
   Adequate personnel available for observation and for assistance
   Patient otherwise stable; no competing procedures or therapy
Airways clear of secretions
Patient sitting or in semi-upright position
Trial of spontaneous ventilation on T-piece* with inspired oxygen percentage the same as on ventilator
Continuous observation and reassurance of patient, with arterial blood gases checked after 20–30 minutes
T-piece trial continued as long as arterial P_{O_2} is at least 55 mm Hg (saturation 85%) and pH remains above 7.30
Extubation as soon as possible, assuming gas exchange is acceptable and patient is alert, can protect airway, and has no upper
   airway obstruction

*not through ventilator circuit, which increases work of breathing

stay. I personally have not been impressed with respiratory muscle exercises over and above sequential T-piece trials in the long-term weaning process.

Nutrition is another pertinent topic in ventilator management and, clearly, patients should not be allowed to starve under our care. Patients with severe COPD should also not be grossly overfed, especially with carbohydrate calories, since this overfeeding increases the demand placed on their ventilatory apparatus by boosting CO_2 production. A balanced mixture of protein, fat, and carbohydrate that provides around 2,500 calories per day to the average-sized patient would seem reasonable. I have not found that special "pulmonary" preparations offer a clinically evident advantage over other diets.

PROGNOSIS AND OUTCOME

Most patients (70 to 80 percent) survive an episode of acute respiratory failure complicating severe COPD, whether or not they are intubated and ventilated. However, the long-term outlook after such an episode is poor, with the intervals between successive exacerbations tending to shorten and the acute mortality tending to increase. Only about half the patients survive 2 years in most reported series.

For patients who ultimately stabilize in a ventilator-dependent state, long-term mechanical ventilation may be possible if the necessary family, social, and economic resources are available. However, only a small number of individuals with severe COPD can presently meet these criteria.

Suggested Reading

Hudson LD. Diagnosis and management of acute respiratory distress in patients on mechanical ventilators. In: Moser KM, Spragg RG, eds. Respiratory emergencies. 2nd ed. St. Louis: CV Mosby, 1982:201.

Luce JM, Tyler ML, Pierson DJ. Intensive respiratory care. Philadelphia: WB Saunders (Blue Books Series), 1984.

Marini JJ. Mechanical ventilation: taking the work out of breathing? Respir Care 1986; 31:695–702.

Petty TL. Critical care for chronic air-flow limitation: emphysema, chronic bronchitis, and cystic fibrosis. Semin Respir Med 1982; 3:263–274.

Pierson DJ. Indications for mechanical ventilation in acute respiratory failure. Respir Care 1983; 28:570–578.

Pierson DJ. Respiratory intensive care. Dallas: Daedalus Press (American Association for Respiratory Care), 1986.

Pierson DJ. Weaning from mechanical ventilation in acute respiratory failure: concepts, indications, and techniques. Respir Care 1983; 28:646–662.

Rosen RL. Acute respiratory failure and chronic obstructive lung disease. Med Clin North Am 1986; 70:895–907.

Scott LR, Benson MS, Pierson DJ. Effect of inspiratory flowrate and circuit compressible volume on auto-PEEP during mechanical ventilation. Respir Care 1986; 31:1075–1079.

Special issue. Continuing care of the ventilator-dependent patient. Respir Care 1986; 31:266–337.

STABLE ASTHMA

THEODORE W. MARCY, M.D.
RICHARD A. MATTHAY, M.D.

Asthma is a common disease that affects approximately 3 percent of the North American population. Despite its prevalence, there is no precise and universally accepted definition of asthma. Most physicians consider the diagnosis of asthma when patients have episodes of dyspnea, cough, or wheezing, and have evidence of reversible airway obstruction or of hyperreactivity of the airways to nonspecific stimuli. However, there is great heterogeneity in the clinical course and the severity of disease within this group of patients. While some individuals have infrequent symptoms that rarely require even over-the-counter medications, others have severe and unrelenting disease requiring large and often debilitating doses of corticosteroids. The onset of asthma can occur at any age and its cause is unpredictable, but older patients with new-onset asthma are often especially difficult to treat.

The pathogenesis of asthma is complex and is still not well-understood. Some patients have exacerbations of their asthma when exposed to specific antigens. That these patients often have a family or a personal history of allergic diseases suggests that immunologic mechanisms are primarily responsible for their asthma. Other patients have generalized airway hyperreactivity to nonspecific stimuli. These patients do not have a history of atopy, and their asthma does not appear to be attributable to immune mechanisms. Finally, many patients do not fit clearly into either one of these groups. Thus, asthma probably represents a clinical syndrome that is the final common outcome of several different pathogenic mechanisms. Despite the heterogeneity in asthma, all of these patients have the following common physiologic abnormalities that cause airway narrowing during an asthmatic exacerbation: (1) smooth muscle constriction, (2) mucus hypersecretion, (3) edema of bronchial epithelium, and (4) bronchial inflammation. Treatment strategies for asthma are aimed at preventing or decreasing the effect of these pathophysiologic components of airway narrowing.

THERAPEUTIC ARMAMENTARIUM (TABLE 1)

Beta Adrenergic Agonists

The binding of catecholamines to $beta_2$ receptors on the cell surface of bronchial smooth muscle causes muscle relaxation and bronchodilatation. In addition, catecholamines may increase ciliary clearance and reduce mediator release from mast cells and basophils. The different beta adrenergic agonist drugs that share structural similarity to catecholamines are the most important class of asthma medications and are the first line of medical therapy.

To avoid toxicity from the cardiovascular effects of catecholamine binding to the $beta_1$ receptors on the myocardium, the catecholamine structure is modified to provide drugs that are relatively $beta_2$ selective. Other modifications increase the duration of action. At present, there are several beta adrenergic medications available in the United States that share relative $beta_2$ selectivity and prolonged duration of action. Chronic administration of beta adrenergics does reduce the number of beta receptors, but the clinical effect of this is apparently small.

The newer $beta_2$ selective agents are relatively safe, and their limiting adverse effect is often accentuation of physiologic tremor, though other adverse effects (e.g., peripheral vasodilatation, decreased serum potassium, nausea, dizziness, and weakness, as well as $beta_1$ mediated tachycardia) can occur at higher doses. The toxicity of beta adrenergic agonists is less when they are inhaled than when they are orally or parenterally administered. Also, the onset of bronchodilatation occurs sooner (i.e., 3 to 6 minutes) after inhalation than after oral administration (30 minutes). For these reasons, inhaled beta adrenergics are preferred in stable asthma. However, orally administered beta adrenergics have the advantage of a longer duration of action, thus reducing the problems of compliance and inconvenience.

Methylxanthines

Theophylline and its salts, aminophylline and oxtriphylline, are used widely as orally administered bronchodilators. Originally, the mechanism by which theophylline caused bronchodilation was thought to be an inhibition of phosphodiesterase, which caused an accumulation of intracellular cyclic adenosine monophosphate (cAMP) with subsequent smooth muscle relaxation. However, several recent lines of evidence refute this concept. Some alternate theories

TABLE 1   Therapeutic Armamentarium for Stable Asthma

Drug (Trade Name)	Formulation	Dosage
Beta adrenergic agonist		
Metaproterenol (Alupent)	MDI* (650 µg/puff)	2 inhalations q4–6h
	Solution for nebulized (50 mg/ml)	0.2–0.3 ml in 3 ml saline q4–6h
	Syrup (10 mg/5 ml) or tablets (10, 20 mg)	10–20 mg p.o. t.i.d.–q.i.d.
Albuterol (Ventolin, Proventil)	MDI (90 µg/puff)	2 inhalations q4–6h
	Tablets (2 mg)	2–4 mg p.o. t.i.d.–q.i.d.
Terbutaline (Brethaire)	MDI (200 µg/puff)	2–3 inhalations q4–6h
	Tablets (2.5, 5 mg)	2.5–5 mg p.o. t.i.d.
Bitolterol Mesylate (Tornalate)	MDI (370 µg/puff)	2 inhalations q4–6h
Theophylline (Theo-Dur, Slow-Bid, etc.)	Sustained release tablets	Day 1–3: 100–200 mg b.i.d.
	Bead-filled capsules	Day 4–7: 200–300 mg b.i.d.
		Then adjust to maintain blood level of 10–20 µg/ml
	Once-a-day formulations	400–900 mg at 8:00 PM†
Cromolyn (Intal)	Spinhaler (20 mg capsules)	1 capsule inhaled q.i.d.
	MDI (1 mg/puff)	2 inhalations q.i.d.
	Solution for nebulizer (10 mg/ml)	2 ml with beta adrenergic q.i.d.
Corticosteroids		
Prednisone or equivalent	Tablets	15–40 mg every other day, or lowest daily dose possible
Beclomethasone (Vanceril)	MDI (50 µg/puff)	2–4 inhalations b.i.d.–q.i.d.
Flunisolide (AeroBid)	MDI (250 µg/puff)	2–4 inhalations b.i.d.
Triamcinolone (Azmacort)	MDI (100 µg/puff)	2–4 inhalations b.i.d.–q.i.d.

*Metered dose inhaler
†For use in selected patients with primarily early morning bronchospasm. Dosage should not be given within 1 hour of a meal.

are that (1) theophylline binds to adenosine receptors and blocks the bronchoconstrictive effects of adenosine, and (2) theophylline acts as an analogue of cAMP. However, the exact mechanism of bronchodilation remains unclear. In addition to bronchodilatation, theophylline also increases diaphragm strength, improves right and left heart function, and may increase mucociliary clearance.

Bronchodilatation appears to increase linearly to the logarithm of the theophylline blood level. This means that an increase in the blood level has diminishing therapeutic returns, but an increased likelihood of adverse effects, especially if the blood level rises over 20 µg per milliliter. In deciding on a theophylline dosage for an individual patient, one must account for individual differences in theophylline metabolism as well as for individual differences in bronchodilatory response to a given blood level. Interactions with other drugs must also be considered. Adverse effects include gastrointestinal symptoms, central nervous system irritability, diuresis, palpitations, and tachycardia. Fatal cardiac arrhythmias and seizures can occur at toxic levels above 40 µg per milliliter.

Cromolyn Sodium

Cromolyn (Intal) has no direct bronchodilator activity, but can prevent experimental allergen-induced asthma, presumably by stabilizing mast cells and preventing the release of the mediators of bronchocon-
striction. Cromolyn may also directly inhibit vagally-mediated reflex bronchospasm and may have indirect anti-inflammatory effects. These therapeutic benefits are achieved with almost no adverse effects. Cromolyn is a prophylactic drug that must be taken before exposure to bronchoconstrictive precipitants. The drug must be inhaled, either from a specially designed turbo inhaler (Spinhaler), from a recently released formulation in a metered dose inhaler (MDI), or from a compressed-air nebulizer.

Anticholinergics

Parasympathetic innervation of bronchial smooth muscle is probably responsible for resting bronchomotor tone and for reflex bronchoconstriction in response to nonspecific stimuli. Atropine competitively blocks acetylcholine at postganglionic receptors. When inhaled at a dose of 0.025 mg per kilogram in adults, atropine has a bronchodilatory effect in asthmatics that is about equivalent to that of beta adrenergic agonists. Unfortunately, atropine is easily absorbed across mucous membranes and has a number of adverse effects related to its antimuscarinic and anticholinergic properties, including tachycardia; inhibition of salivary, sweat, and nasal glands; urinary retention; and ileus. However, in contrast to previous concerns, anticholinergics do not appear to cause significant changes in mucus viscosity or mucociliary transport.

Ipratropium bromide (Atrovent), a quaternary ammonium derivative of atropine, has few of atropine's troublesome adverse effects, presumably because its more polar quaternary structure makes absorption insignificant. Ipratropium bromide in a metered dose inhaler has just been approved for use in the United States at a recommended dosage of 20 to 40 μg (one to two puffs) three times daily. In comparison to inhaled beta adrenergic agonists, ipratropium bromide has a later onset of maximal effect, a longer duration of action, and produces slightly less bronchodilation in asthmatic patients. The only adverse effect is its bitter taste. This drug may be especially helpful for patients who have cough as a primary symptom.

Corticosteroids

Corticosteroids have several actions that probably account for their therapeutic effect in asthma: potentiation of beta adrenergic responsiveness, inhibition of mucus production, and modulation of the inflammatory response. There is general agreement that corticosteroids are useful in acute exacerbations of asthma, but the role of steroids in chronic asthma is more controversial. Enthusiasm for chronic steroid use must be tempered by an appreciation of their long-term complications, which include serious adverse effects from hypercortisolism and from the inhibition of the hypothalamic-pituitary-adrenal axis.

Other Drugs

Current calcium-channel blockers (e.g., nifedipine [Procardia], diltiazem [Cardiazem], and verapamil [Calan]) have minimal bronchodilator activity, but may reduce airway hyperreactivity. Despite this, the clinical effect does not appear significant enough to warrant clinical use in asthma, though future calcium-channel blockers may play a role in asthma management.

Some centers advocate using the macrolide antibiotic troleandomycin (TAO) along with methylprednisolone in patients on high chronic steroid doses in order to reduce the required steroid dose. Adverse effects of TAO include hepatotoxicity and increased steroid side effects if the steroids are not tapered. Although the mechanism of action of TAO is not known, reduced hepatic metabolism of glucocorticoids is an attractive possibility. We are unimpressed that adding this drug to the antiasthma regimen leads to fewer adverse effects and await further clinical studies before using TAO in our patients.

Immunotherapy

Immunotherapy consists of administering small amounts of identified antigens regularly to patients who demonstrate allergic symptoms when exposed to these antigens. Proposed actions of immunotherapy in allergic disorders include (1) increasing serum and/or secretory immunoglobulin G and immunoglobulin A that block immunoglobulin E binding to mast cells, (2) decreasing immunoglobulin E, or (3) decreasing cell sensitivity.

Although immunotherapy is of proven effectiveness in allergic rhinitis, its role in asthma therapy is controversial. First, immunotherapy should only be effective in patients in whom asthma is caused by an allergic response to identifiable antigens. Most adult-onset asthmatics and patients with severe asthma lack evidence of an allergic etiology for their asthma. Second, the evidence that immunotherapy actually works in asthma is far from convincing, in part because of difficulties in selecting patients for these studies, in identifying the causative antigens, and in measuring the response to therapy. Finally, patients who have allergic asthma can be treated successfully by limiting their exposure to causative antigens or by using beta adrenergic agonists or cromolyn, often with less inconvenience than with immunotherapy. We use this latter approach. In patients with severe asthma, we believe that immunotherapy should only be done under a study protocol that permits further evaluation of immunotherapy's role in asthma therapy.

MANAGEMENT PRINCIPLES

Our general approach to the stable asthmatic is one of stepped care—increasing or decreasing the degree of therapeutic intervention according to the patient's condition at the time (Table 2). Our first step is to limit the patient's exposure to allergens or to nonspecific irritants. Specific recommendations are guided by a careful history that identifies when and where the patient experiences asthmatic exacerbations. If the asthma is of recent onset, we determine if there have been changes in ventilation or insulation at home, new pets or hobbies, or new medications, especially oral or ophthalmic beta blockers (e.g., Timoptic). In general, although patients should keep their homes free of smoke and dust, there is little added benefit from excessively compulsive house cleaning.

There is a group of asthmatics who have acute asthmatic responses to aspirin with or without associated rhinosinusitis, conjunctivitis, or urticaria. Some of these patients have the full-blown syndrome of aspirin sensitivity, asthma, and nasal polyps. Unfortunately, a clinical history of sensitivity is neither sensitive nor specific for this problem. Documentation of aspirin sensitivity requires detecting a fall in FEV_1 of greater than 25 percent in response to increments of oral aspirin. We perform this test in a laboratory with staff experienced with bronchoprovocation testing. These patients can also be sensitive to the structurally unrelated compounds of ibuprofen (e.g., Motrin), indomethacin (e.g., Indocin), and tartrazine yellow, a food dye. Avoidance of these compounds can be difficult. Desensitization can be safely achieved, but is temporary unless aspirin administration is continued indefinitely. In some patients, the degree of aspirin sensitivity correlates with the activity of the underlying asthma. Therefore, our approach in these patients is to treat their asthma optimally and to have the patient avoid aspirin and other nonsteroidal anti-inflammatory drugs. Cromolyn may also be useful in blunting the sensitivity to aspirin.

A few patients with chronic asthma have exacerbations of asthma when exposed to metabisulfites used as antioxidants by the food and beverage industries or by the pharmaceutical industry. Approximately 5 percent of patients with chronic asthma have been estimated to have this sensitivity. We consider this possibility in patients who have paradoxic bronchospasm in response to inhaled or parenteral medications or who have acute asthmatic exacerbations while eating.

Asthma can be caused by exposures to dusts, gases, fumes, or vapors in the workplace. We consider this possibility in patients who work with (1) textile dusts, (2) organophosphate insecticides, (3) noxious gases, such as chlorine, ammonia, or sulfur dioxide, (4) animal, plant, or bacterial proteins, (5) copolymerizing agents, such as the isocyanates, used in the plastics industry and in paints, or (6) wood dusts. If the patient's symptoms are temporally related to the work day or the work week and are absent during periods away from work, we try to document this relationship with peak flow rates or with spirometry before and after the work shift. The asthma may resolve if the patient wears a filtered mask, moves to a better ventilated area, or works at a different task. However, if the symptoms appear to result from occupational

exposure and do not respond to these maneuvers, we recommend alternative employment, since continued exposure can cause the asthma to become severe and unremitting.

If symptoms persist despite efforts to limit exposure to irritants or to allergens, we have the patient use an inhaled long-acting beta adrenergic agonist by a metered dose inhaler. Success with inhaled beta adrenergic agonists is highly dependent on an adequate technique of administration. For this reason, we recommend that a healthcare provider instruct the patient on proper MDI technique and observe the patient's technique. Despite proper instruction, some patients remain unable to use MDIs properly. We use one of the different types of spacer devices to improve drug delivery to the lower airway in such patients. Alternatively, although with far less convenience, we use compressed air-driven nebulizers, which eliminate the need to coordinate activation of the MDI with inhalation.

At first, we instruct the patient to use the beta adrenergic agonists as needed or before exposure to unavoidable irritants. In those patients with exercise-induced asthma, we try either a beta adrenergic agonist or cromolyn before exercise. Some patients benefit from regular administration of inhaled beta adrenergic agonists up to four times a day, although compliance to this schedule is difficult for even motivated patients. We reserve oral beta adrenergic agonists for patients who do not tolerate or cannot master inhalers.

When this regimen does not control symptoms adequately, our next step is to add theophylline in a sustained release formulation. We start with a low dose (200 to 400 mg a day in adults, or 12 to 16 mg per kilogram per day in patients under 25 kg) to minimize the risk of toxicity and to permit the development of

---

TABLE 2 Management of Stable Asthma

Step 1
  Avoidance of potential irritants/allergens
  Treat concurrent sinusitis or esophageal reflux
  Discontinue oral or ophthalmic beta blockers
  Consider occupational causes of asthma
  Consider aspirin or metabisulfite sensitivity
Step 2
  Inhaled beta adrenergic agonist
    (If not effective, try spacer device, then
      nebulized or oral beta adrenergic agonist)
Step 3
  Add oral theophylline
Step 4
  Trial of inhaled cromolyn
Step 5
  Add corticosteroids:
    Inhaled steroids begin when patient stable
    Taper oral steroids off, switch to alternate day therapy,
      or to lowest daily dose, as tolerated
As the patient improves, decrease therapy by a step.   •

tolerance to caffeine-like side effects. The patient is given instructions to increase the dose by 200 mg a day every 3 days to a dose of 800 mg a day in patients over 45 kg. Further alterations in dosage are made after measuring the serum concentration, doing spirometry, and inquiring about adverse effects.

The goal is to maintain an optimal blood level of 10 to 20 μg per milliliter without wide fluctuations in order to maximize benefit and minimize toxicity. Some patients do not tolerate a blood level in this range. In these patients, useful bronchodilatation can often be achieved at a better tolerated blood level of 5 to 10 μg per milliliter. The different formulations of theophylline vary in their method of slowing absorption. Despite advertising claims, there can be wide fluctuations in blood levels with slow-release products if taken at 12-hour intervals. In some patients, these medications must be given every 8 hours.

Recently, once-a-day formulations of theophylline (e.g., Theo-24 and Uniphyl) have become available. Their convenience improves patient compliance. Unfortunately, if taken within an hour of a meal, the theophylline in some of these formulations can be rapidly absorbed, thus leading to significant side effects. In addition, some of these once-a-day products do not maintain a sustained therapeutic blood level, especially in patients who are rapid metabolizers. Once-a-day formulations taken in the evening may be useful for patients who have bronchoconstriction in the morning. The peak blood level may then coincide with peak bronchoconstriction. However, we believe that there is not yet enough experience with these formulations to routinely recommend once daily dose forms for patients who require theophylline.

When patients continue to have exacerbations on optimal doses of theophylline and beta adrenergic agonists, we try cromolyn when the patient is stable. The aerosolized drug can act as an irritant and should not be given during an exacerbation. Our experience with the MDI formulation is limited at this time, so we still begin the patient on 20 mg of cromolyn administered four times a day by a Spinhaler. It is difficult to predict who will respond to the drug. Even with consistent administration four times a day, maximal effect may not be seen for 3 to 4 weeks. Also, cromolyn is expensive. For these reasons, cromolyn use has been limited, although given its high therapeutic ratio, the drug is probably underutilized in the United States. If there is a decrease in the frequency of exacerbations in the absence of other changes in medications, we continue cromolyn. Maintenance therapy on a twice daily schedule is sometimes sufficient.

Some patients still require short courses of oral corticosteroids for severe exacerbations of asthma. However, a few patients appear to be chronically "steroid dependent," since they have recurrences of severe symptoms as soon as they are tapered off corticosteroids. These are the patients at risk for adverse effects from hypercortisolism. The severity of these adverse effects can be reduced or eliminated by modifications in administration. Function of the hypothalamic-pituitary-adrenal axis is better preserved if a rapidly metabolized steroid, such as prednisone, prednisolone, or methylprednisolone, is used and if the steroid is administered once daily in the morning.

Alternate day therapy is associated with fewer adverse effects, although it is also less effective. We attempt to taper our patients to 40 mg of prednisone on alternate days—usually on the odd days of the month to make it easier for them to remember when to take the medication. The alternate day dose is then decreased gradually as tolerated.

Topically active corticosteroids like beclomethasone (Beclovent, Vanceril) and flunisolide (AeroBid) can be inhaled using an MDI. While inhaled corticosteroids are not effective for acute exacerbations of asthma, they may permit the tapering of oral steroids or the transition to alternate day administration in patients who are stable. Adverse effects of inhaled corticosteroids include oral candidiasis and dysphonia. These problems can be minimized if the patient gargles with water after each use. A spacer may improve delivery of the drug to the lower airway and may reduce deposition in the oral cavity. We recommend that the patient inhale two to three puffs of beclomethasone four times daily or up to four puffs of flunisolide twice daily, and that the inhaled steroid be used only after the beta adrenergic agonist inhaler. If the patient remains stable, the frequency of beclomethasone administration can be decreased to twice daily. High doses of an inhaled steroid—16 or more inhalations per day—can cause hypothalamic-pituitary-adrenal axis suppression. These patients may need stress doses of steroids (i.e., 150 to 300 mg of hydrocortisone, or equivalent) during acute illnesses.

Decisions on medication use are guided by the patient's symptoms, the physical examination, and the objective measures of airflow obstruction. We do spirometry on every office visit or emergency room visit. Some patients are sufficiently motivated to use a peak flow meter as an objective measure of air flow at home. This information can guide our decisions through telephone contacts with these patients and can help the patient know when an exacerbation is starting so that treatment for exacerbations can begin early.

SPECIAL PROBLEMS

Refractory Asthma

Some patients remain quite symptomatic despite optimal doses of bronchodilators and prolonged courses of oral corticosteroids. In these patients, we first consider whether the patients are compliant with the medications. Blood levels can document compliance with theophylline, but monitoring the use of other medications is harder. Family members are asked to assist the patient in remembering to take the medications.

We also reconsider whether asthma is the correct diagnosis. For example, upper airway obstruction from a variety of causes can present with similar symptoms, but often has a characteristic pattern on a flow-volume loop. Drugs such as nitrofurantoin and the sulfonamides can cause pulmonary eosinophilia with dyspnea and wheezing. The complete differential diagnosis of wheezing conditions is beyond the scope of this chapter, but we favor considering these other diagnostic possibilities in patients with refractory asthma.

Patients with asthma can be difficult to treat if they have chronic or acute sinus problems. Patients with symptoms of sinusitis and asthma should be treated with decongestants and antibiotics. If necessary, they should be referred to an otorhinolaryngologist. Asthma may be exacerbated by gastroesophageal reflex, perhaps from actual aspiration of stomach contents or from vagal reflexes stimulated by afferent nerves in the esophagus. In refractory patients, a trial of antireflux maneuvers and antacids is worthwhile, even if there are no clear symptoms of reflux.

Asthma in Pregnancy

Asthma occurs in approximately 1 percent of pregnant women. Severe uncontrolled asthma can be a considerable risk to the mother and the fetus, thereby causing increased perinatal morbidity and mortality and, occasionally, maternal death. However, asthma management during pregnancy must balance the risks of uncontrolled asthma to the mother and the fetus against the potential teratogenic risk of asthma medications. Unfortunately, data on the teratogenic effects of asthma drugs are often anecdotal, limited to animal studies, or lacking entirely.

Our approach to the pregnant asthmatic is similar to that in other asthma patients. In addition to the usual measures of allergen and irritant avoidance, we use antireflux maneuvers and sometimes antacids to limit the esophageal reflux that can occur with increased frequency during pregnancy. Specific drugs that we avoid because of possible or known fetal risk include tetracyclines, sulfonamides, iodides (included in cough preparations), phenylpropanolamine, phenylephrine, brompheniramine, and dextromethorphan.

In mild or intermittent asthma with pregnancy, we use inhaled beta adrenergic agonists as needed. We do not use cromolyn because 8 percent of the drug is absorbed into the systemic circulation and experience with it during pregnancy is limited. The use of beta adrenergic agonists during pregnancy appears to be safe, but these drugs should be avoided (if possible) at term because they inhibit uterine contractions. If asthma symptoms continue, theophylline is added in low doses and then increased as necessary. When optimal doses of theophylline and beta adrenergic agonists are insufficient, we first try inhaled beclomethasone (up to 16 inhalations a day). Oral corticosteroids can sometimes be avoided with this approach. However, if the asthma is severe we use oral prednisone—the preferred corticosteroid because of its high maternal-to-fetal ratio of serum concentration. The duration and dosage is kept as low as possible, but not at the expense of control of symptoms. If steroids are used during pregnancy, stress doses of hydrocortisone should be given on the day of delivery and until there is no evidence of puerperal complications.

We do not discourage our patients from breastfeeding, since most asthma drugs do not reach significant levels in breast milk. However, erythromycin and tetracycline should not be prescribed to lactating mothers.

Suggested Reading

Anonymous. Drugs for asthma. In: Abramowicz M, ed. Med Lett 1987; 29:11–16.

Baily WC, ed. Symposium on asthma. Clin Chest Med 1984; 5(4):555–713.

Brooks SM. Occupational asthma. In: Weiss EB, Segal MS, Stein M, eds. Bronchial asthma: mechanisms and therapeutics. Boston: Little, Brown, 1985:461.

Lichtenstein LM. An evaluation of the role of immunotherapy in asthma. Am Rev Respir Dis 1978; 117:191–197.

Pleskow WW, Stevenson DD, Mathison DA, Simon RA, Schatz M, Zeiger RS. Aspirin-sensitive rhinosinusitis/asthma: spectrum of adverse reactions to aspirin. J Allergy Clin Immunol 1983; 71:574–579.

Spector SL. Advantages and disadvantages of 24-hour theophylline. J Allergy Clin Immunol 1985; 76:302–311.

Stablein JJ, Lockey RF. Managing asthma during pregnancy. Compr Ther 1984; 10:45–52.

Ziment I, Popa V, eds. Symposium on respiratory pharmacology. Clin Chest Med 1986; 7(3):311–518.

ACUTE EXACERBATIONS OF ASTHMA AND STATUS ASTHMATICUS: PHARMACOLOGIC MANAGEMENT

CHRISTOPHER H. FANTA, M.D.

Most adults with asthma experience their illness as a chronic disease punctuated by acute flares. For some, the chronic phase of asthma is asymptomatic, and their acute exacerbations may be transient wheezing and chest tightness following, for example, strenuous exertion. For others, the disease manifests as frequent, perhaps daily, symptoms, and acute exacerbations may be life-threatening events of asphyxiation with hypercapnic respiratory failure. Even the patient with no or with minimal symptoms on a daily basis may, on occasion, suffer severe acute attacks of asthma that necessitate emergency care. These acute attacks are a major cause of the morbidity of asthma—they disrupt the orderly fabric of patients' lives, are often terrifying, and require noxious treatments—and they constitute the substrate of asthma deaths. Approximately 3,000 deaths attributable to asthma occur each year in the United States, and the rate appears to be increasing.

The general truism that the best therapeutic approach to disease is prevention certainly pertains to asthma. Although acute exacerbations of asthma are unavoidable in many, perhaps most, cases, many attacks that progress to life-threatening severity could be prevented if treated early and aggressively enough. Inadequate treatment is thought to be the cause of most asthma deaths. Causes of delayed or of insufficient treatment for exacerbations of asthma include (1) failure of the patient to recognize the severity of his or her attacks, (2) failure to seek prompt medical attention for a severe attack, either because of excessive reliance on self-treatment at home or because of inaccessible health care services, and (3) failure of the treating physician to recognize the seriousness of the patient's acute attack and to respond appropriately. If prescribed soon enough, an intensification of the patient's bronchodilator regimen or a short course of corticosteroids can often abort an increase in asthmatic symptoms and preclude the need for emergency care.

PATIENT ASSESSMENT

For the most part, a patient's respiratory distress (that is, rapid breathing, anxiety, and sense of not "getting enough air") suffices to indicate a severe attack of asthma. However, there is variability in the response to acute airflow obstruction, and it is not always possible to judge accurately the severity of an asthmatic exacerbation simply on the basis of a patient's apparent distress. Clinical clues that have, if present, been useful in alerting the physician to the presence of severe disease include use of the accessory muscles of inspiration (e.g., the sternocleidomastoid muscles), an accentuated fall in systolic blood pressure on inspiration (pulsus paradoxus), refusal to recline on the examining table or stretcher because of worsening dyspnea if not seated upright, and paradoxical inward movement of the lower anterior chest wall during inspiration (Table 1). In general, the presence of these physical findings predicts severe airflow obstruction (forced expiratory volume [FEV_1] less than 1.0 to 1.25 L or less than 25 to 30 percent of normal value).

A more direct approach to assessing the severity of an exacerbation of asthma is to measure lung function by spirometry or peak expiratory flow determination. The degree of the airflow obstruction as given by the FEV_1 or peak expiratory flow rate (PEFR) is the best determinant of the severity of an attack. In general, a patient with an acute flare of asthma will require hospitalization if, despite intensive treatment, the FEV_1 remains less than 35 to 40 percent of the predicted value. With an FEV_1 less that 25 percent of the predicted value, the patient is at risk for respiratory failure. Measurement of spirometry or peak flow will identify this patient at high risk, whereas accessory muscle use and pulsus paradoxus may be absent, and significant hypoxemia and hypercapnia may likewise not be present. Measurement of lung function can be made quickly and without undue stress in all but the most critically ill patients by using modern portable electronic spirometers or simple peak flow meters. A particularly useful time to make these measurements is after the first hour of intensive bronchodilator therapy, since the initial response helps to predict the likelihood of continued improvement over the next several hours of treatment.

DIFFERENTIAL DIAGNOSIS

Although the differential diagnosis of wheezing and shortness of breath is relatively broad, the acute

TABLE 1   Assessment of Acute Asthma

Clinical clues to severe obstruction
  Use of accessory respiratory muscles
  Paradoxical pulse
  Inability to lie supine owing to breathlessness
  Paradoxical inward movement of the lower
    portion of anterior chest wall during inspiration
Objective measures of disease severity
  Peak flow determination (PEFR)
  Spirometry (FEV_1)
  Arterial blood gases
    (If hypoxemia is suspected or
    if the FEV_1 or PEFR is $\leq 25\%$ of predicted)
Differential diagnosis
  Acute exacerbation of COPD
  Upper airway obstruction
  Congestive heart failure
  Pulmonary embolism

asthmatic attack rarely poses a diagnostic dilemma (see Table 1). Especially in the younger age group (e.g., less than 40 years old) where the prevalence of cardiac disease, of chronic obstructive pulmonary disease, and of pulmonary embolism is low, the diagnosis of asthma is usually straightforward and is often offered by the patient at presentation. Rarely, a focal upper airway obstruction may mimic asthma, and the stridor of acute epiglottitis may occasionally be mistaken for asthmatic wheezing. However, one can usually distinguish wheezing caused by upper airway obstruction by its monophonic quality, its fixed position in the respiratory cycle, and its site of maximal intensity in the tracheal area. In this circumstance, if the diagnosis of upper airway obstruction were overlooked, initial treatment for asthma would probably not cause any serious adverse outcomes. Although congestive heart failure may manifest with wheezing, giving rise to the misnomer "cardiac asthma," there

are usually adequate clues both by history (e.g., orthopnea, chest pain, prior history of cardiac disease) and physical examination (e.g., jugular venous distention, cardiac enlargement, third heart sound, inspiratory rales on chest exam) to indicate the correct diagnosis. Diffuse wheezing mimicking asthma has also been reported in acute pulmonary embolism, but this presentation is sufficiently rare so as not to cause diagnostic concern.

INITIAL TREATMENT

The major goal of the pharmacologic management of acute asthma (Table 2) is the prompt relief of airflow obstruction. The causes of the airflow obstruction in asthma are multiple, including tracheobronchial smooth muscle constriction, airway wall edema and inflammation, and intraluminal secretions and inflammatory "debris." Of these components, the one most susceptible to rapid reversal is the airway smooth muscle constriction, and this of course is the primary target of bronchodilator therapy.

Choice of Bronchodilators

The most potent bronchodilators in the setting of acute exacerbations of asthma are the sympathomimetic drugs. Available for use in the emergency care of asthma are epinephrine and terbutaline by the subcutaneous route and isoproterenol (e.g., Isuprel), isoetharine (e.g., Bronkosol), and metaproterenol (e.g., Alupent) by inhalation. Aerosolized albuterol (e.g., Ventolin, Proventil) has recently joined this list of inhaled agents. Both isoproterenol and terbutaline have also been administered intravenously, but concern over potential cardiac injury, especially with intravenous

TABLE 2   Treatment Guidelines in Acute Asthma

Initial bronchodilator treatment
  Inhaled beta-adrenergic agonists every 20–30 min for three or four doses
                           or
  Subcutaneous epinephrine every 20–30 min for three or four doses
Treatment for persistent airflow obstruction ("status asthmaticus")
  Inhaled beta-adrenergic agonists every 1–2 hours
  Intravenous aminophylline
  Intravenous corticosteroids
  Subcutaneous beta-adrenergic agonists, in some patients
Ancillary measures
  Antibiotics for fever and sputum purulence
  Supplemental oxygen for:
    Documented hypoxemia
    FEV_1 or PEFR $\leq 50\%$ of predicted value in patients >45 years old
Measures of uncertain benefit
  Hydration
  Inhaled saline mists
  Chest physiotherapy
  Expectorants
  Mucolytics

isoproterenol, has precluded this route of administration in routine care.

Epinephrine

There is widespread experience with the use of subcutaneous epinephrine for acute asthma. The bronchodilator response (and also the incidence of side effects) is dose-dependent. A standard dose is 0.3 mg, and some physicians have advocated an increase in dose to as much as 0.5 mg in persons weighing more than 75 kg. The onset of action of subcutaneous epinephrine is rapid (within a few minutes). Repetitive injections spaced every 20 to 30 minutes produce additional bronchodilation with each dose up to at least three doses. Thus, a reasonable protocol for the acute management of severe asthma might utilize subcutaneous epinephrine 0.3 mg every 20 minutes for three doses. When given in this manner, epinephrine induces 3 to 4 times the bronchodilation achieved with intravenous aminophylline given as a bolus followed by continuous infusion. Although side effects such as heart pounding, tremor, and a nervous sensation are common, repetitive doses of epinephrine are well tolerated hemodynamically: on average, blood pressure falls slightly and heart rate remains unchanged. Large increases in heart rate that lead to significant tachycardia occur, but are uncommon. The safety of this regimen has been repeatedly demonstrated in young persons with asthma; it has not been shown to be safe, however, in persons over 45 years of age or in persons with known heart disease.

Inhaled Sympathomimetics

For many years there has been a widely-held belief that inhaled sympathomimetics would not be effective in the most severely obstructed patients with asthma, because of the presumption that deposition of the drug would be limited to the upper airways. This notion has not been borne out in clinical trials. In fact, inhaled sympathomimetics given in repeated doses offer an attractive alternative to parenteral epinephrine: the inhalational route produces comparable bronchodilation, is equally potent even in the most severely obstructed patients, and requires no painful injections. A simple hand-held nebulizer device can be used to produce a wet aerosol. We routinely use isoetharine (1 percent) 0.5 cc or isoproterenol (0.5 percent) 0.5 cc in 2.0 cc of normal saline every 20 to 30 minutes for three doses. Others have preferred metaproterenol (5 percent) 0.3 cc. As with epinephrine, most patients experience unpleasant side effects as a result of systemic adrenergic stimulation, but, on average, blood pressure and heart rate do not increase significantly.

Many asthmatic patients take inhaled and/or oral sympathomimetics on a regular basis and may have suffered an acute exacerbation of their disease despite frequent use of their isoproterenol, isoetharine, or metaproterenol metered-dose inhalers. Have these patients developed sympathomimetic tolerance, such that they now might be expected to be resistant to sympathomimetic use in an emergency room setting? The answer appears to be no. In a study by Rossing and colleagues of 96 patients treated in an emergency room for acute flares of their asthma, the response to treatment with inhaled isoproterenol or subcutaneous epinephrine was the same among those patients who had been using inhaled and/or oral sympathomimetics prior to presentation as it was among those who had not taken any sympathomimetics. It is likely that any tolerance to beta-adrenergic stimulation that may develop can be overcome by the large doses of medication that are delivered in the acute treatment.

Aminophylline

For many years, intravenous aminophylline has been a popular treatment for acute asthmatic attacks. Recently, however, the bronchodilator potency of aminophylline in acute airflow obstruction has come under close scrutiny. As noted above, even when given in full loading doses so as to achieve therapeutic blood levels, aminophylline effects only modest bronchodilation, considerably less than can be achieved with repetitive doses of a sympathomimetic. In addition, many patients who present for emergency treatment are already taking a theophylline preparation. In these patients, in order to avoid toxic blood levels, the loading dose of aminophylline must be reduced, further limiting the utility of methylxanthines in the initial phase of therapy.

A number of investigators have examined the role of intravenous aminophylline in combination with sympathomimetics in the emergency room treatment of acute asthmatic attacks. Based on in vitro data and studies in stable asthma with mild to moderate airflow obstruction, an additive or perhaps synergistic effect of the two types of drugs might have been anticipated. However, the empiric observation has been repeatedly made that in the initial 1 to 2 hours of emergency treatment aminophylline adds little, if any, bronchodilation to sympathomimetics given in large, repetitive doses, as described above. One study found that only the adverse side effects were additive. Thus, contrary to widespread practice patterns, the insertion of an intravenous catheter for the purpose of delivering an intravenous bolus of aminophylline is not an important part of the initial care of the acutely ill asthmatic patient.

Anticholinergic Drugs

Recently, there has been a resurgence of interest in atropine and its congeners in the treatment of asthma. One of the quaternary ammonium congeners of atropine, ipratroprium bromide (Atrovent), has recently become available in this country for use by metered-dose inhaler. Another, atropine methonitrate, will soon be available in this dose form. Both will probably also become available for delivery by wet aerosol. These synthetic derivatives of atropine have the advantages over atropine sulfate of poor systemic absorption across the respiratory tract mucosa and no evident impairment of mucociliary clearance. Their potential role in the acute relief of airflow obstruction remains to be fully elucidated. Studies with aerosolized atropine sulfate, however, have been disappointing. In patients presenting to an emergency room for treatment of their acute exacerbation of asthma, atropine sulfate in large doses (6.4 mg total) was found to be a weak bronchodilator over the initial 80 minutes of treatment and added no further bronchodilation to inhaled metaproterenol when given sequentially.

Corticosteroids

Finally, corticosteroids have little or no intrinsic bronchodilator (i.e., airway smooth muscle relaxant) activity. They have been used in combination with bronchodilators to speed the rate of resolution of acute airflow obstruction. Although there has been some recent debate on this matter, it appears that corticosteroids, even when given intravenously in doses as large as 1 gram of hydrocortisone, do not cause a more rapid improvement in lung function beyond that achieved with hourly doses of inhaled sympathomimetics alone over the first 6 hours of treatment. Although steroids play a crucial role in the treatment of severe attacks of asthma, as will be discussed, their benefit cannot be anticipated in the initial phase of treatment in the emergency room.

STATUS ASTHMATICUS

After the first 60 to 90 minutes of treatment during which three doses of sympathomimetics have been administered, many patients will be ready for discharge home. Others will have some residual wheezing but will have improved sufficiently that subsequent discharge home can be anticipated after a period of additional bronchodilator therapy in the emergency room. Still others will remain severely obstructed despite the initial aggressive treatment; they will have persistent symptoms and possibly still be acutely distressed. It would seem appropriate to refer to this last group of patients as having "status asthmaticus." In our experience very few patients among this last group will show clinically significant improvement over the next several hours despite continued intensive bronchodilator therapy. That is, there is a subpopulation of patients with acute asthma who will have only lim-

ited improvement after initial therapy aimed at airway smooth muscle relaxation and, in these patients with "status asthmaticus," continued intensive bronchodilator therapy generally achieves little further relief of airflow obstruction over the ensuing 4 to 6 hours.

In the patient with persistent wheezing after the initial 60- to 90-minute treatment period, the severity of the airflow obstruction may be difficult to assess on clinical grounds alone. For this reason, measurement of lung function by spirometry or peak expiratory flow measurement becomes particularly important at this juncture. An FEV_1 or PEFR determination of less than 40 percent of the predicted value after repeated administration of a sympathomimetic according to the schedule described above indicates a patient in "status." It is likely (though unproven) that airway inflammation and mucus plugging are major contributors to the continued airflow obstruction in this patient, and therapy directed primarily at airway smooth muscle relaxation may not correct these abnormalities. It can be anticipated that this patient will probably require a prolonged course of treatment and quite possibly hospital admission. Furthermore, it is to this patient that corticosteroids should be given, because of their anticipated beneficial effect approximately 6 to 12 hours following administration. Finally, pulmonary function measurement after the initial treatment period will help to identify those asthmatic patients at risk for respiratory failure. If the FEV_1 or PEFR is less than 25 percent of the predicted value, arterial blood gases should be drawn. In the absence of sedatives or respiratory depressants, only patients with expiratory flow limitation of this severity will manifest hypercapnia.

MANAGEMENT BEYOND THE INITIAL PHASE OF TREATMENT

The optimal bronchodilator regimen and schedule for patients who require additional treatment beyond the initial 60 to 90 minutes has not been completely determined. We feel that hourly inhaled sympathomimetics should be the mainstay of any regimen; when the patient is no longer in acute distress the frequency of administration of the inhaled beta-adrenergic agonists can be reduced. Most patients hospitalized with asthma also receive an intravenous infusion of aminophylline. The bronchodilator effect of the methylxanthines probably comes into play when the frequency of sympathomimetic dosing is reduced—for instance, if the patient is able to sleep uninterrupted for several hours. Whether oral theophyllines might be manipulated in such a way as to provide comparable theophylline levels throughout the day as are achieved with continuous intravenous infusions of aminophylline is yet to be determined. In the patient failing to respond to methylxanthines and inhaled beta-agonists, subcutaneous sympathomimetics are often added: for example, terbutaline 0.25 mg every 4 to 6 hours. It is worth reemphasizing that this aggressive bronchodilator regimen has been found to be safe only in asthmatic patients 45 years old or younger who have no concomitant cardiovascular disease.

In the absence of a specific contraindication, all patients with asthma admitted to the hospital because of refractory airway obstruction should receive corticosteroids. Patients treated with steroids in addition to bronchodilators on average improve more rapidly than those treated with bronchodilators alone. In one study, five of nine hospitalized patients treated with bronchodilators alone had no improvement or actually worsened despite 24 hours of therapy, whereas all of the 11 steroid-treated patients improved. The optimal dose of steroids is unknown. Two popular regimens are methylprednisolone (e.g., Solumedrol) 125 mg by intravenous bolus every 6 hours, and hydrocortisone (e.g., Solucortef) 2 mg per kilogram intravenous bolus followed by 0.5 mg per kilogram per hour by continuous infusion. A recent provocative study indicated that oral prednisolone given in divided doses to a total of 75 mg over 24 hours was equally as effective as larger intravenous doses.

Corticosteroids also play an important role in patients who are discharged home from the emergency room. A short course (1 to 3 weeks) of steroids has been shown to decrease the rate of subsequent relapses to the emergency room with recurrent asthmatic symptoms. In general, it is a good practice to intensify the out-patient regimen of the asthmatic patient at the time of discharge home. After all, the bronchodilator medications administered in the emergency room have durations of action of only a few hours. If the patient returns to the same environment on the same medications as at the time of the acute attack, recurrent airway obstruction would not be surprising. If the acute attack developed despite use of a reasonable bronchodilator regimen of theophylline and sympathomimetics, then addition of a short course of prednisone or prednisolone is warranted. Other subgroups that might particularly benefit from steroids at discharge from the emergency room include patients already taking low doses of oral steroids at presentation and patients sent home with borderline lung function, that is, an FEV_1 or PEFR less than 60 percent of normal value (assuming a normal value for FEV_1 or PEFR when well).

ANCILLARY TREATMENT MEASURES

A variety of ancillary measures are often used to treat the acutely ill asthmatic patient, many aimed at alleviating the mucous plugging that contributes so importantly to the pathophysiology of airflow obstruction. One need only watch a patient cough again and again, struggling to expectorate seemingly endless amounts of thick, viscid mucus, to appreciate that the goal of these therapies is worthwhile. However, none has sound scientific footing upon which to justify its routine practice. Thus, hydration with large volumes of fluids, inhaled mists of water or saline, chest percussion or vibration, expectorants (such as potassium iodide solutions), and mucolytics (such as acetylcysteine, or Mucomyst) have never been convincingly documented to hasten clearance of airway secretions in acute attacks of asthma. Nor are they totally innocuous forms of therapy, since at least some may have an irritant effect and trigger bronchospasm. The routine use of antibiotics is also of questionable value, since even among those attacks of asthma precipitated by respiratory tract infection the majority are thought to be viral in etiology. We have generally reserved antibiotics for the febrile patient with sputum purulence, recognizing that even then we are probably overtreating many patients who do not have bacterial or mycoplasmal infections.

Supplemental Oxygen

It is surprisingly difficult to provide guidelines for the use of supplemental oxygen in the acutely ill asthmatic patient. Although it is easy to suggest that any patient with an arterial oxygen tension (PaO_2) of less than 60 to 65 mm Hg be given humidified low-flow oxygen by nasal cannulae, it is probably not necessary for every patient to have arterial blood gases drawn, and the PaO_2 correlates poorly with measures of airflow obstruction, such as FEV_1. This would be an inconsequential matter were it not that, for many persons with asthma, an arterial puncture is the most traumatic aspect of their care and one that sometimes makes them delay seeking needed medical attention. Furthermore, because a patient's status tends to fluctuate over time, multiple blood gas determinations would be necessary. Oximetry offers a painless alternative for identifying patients who would benefit from supplemental oxygen, but these devices may not be widely available. A reasonable compromise might be the following: patients under age 45 years without cardiovascular disease require supplemental oxygen only for documented hypoxemia (arterial blood gases drawn if the FEV_1 or PEFR is less than or equal to 25 percent of the predicted value, because of the risk of hypercapnia at this level of obstruction); patients over age 45 years, because of their higher risk of occult cardiovascular disease, should receive supplemental oxygen until the FEV_1 exceeds 50 to 60 percent of the predicted value, unless adequate oxygenation breathing room air has been demonstrated.

Suggested Reading

Feil SB, Swartz MA, Glanz K, Francis ME. Efficacy of short-term corticosteroid therapy in outpatient treatment of acute bronchial asthma. Am J Med 1983; 75:259–262.

Harrison BDW, Stokes TC, Hart GJ, Vaughan DA, Ali NJ, Robinson AA. Need for intravenous hydrocortisone in addition to oral prednisolone in patients admitted to hospital with severe asthma without ventilatory failure. Lancet 1986; 1:181–184.

Karpel JP, Appel D, Breidbart D, Fusco MJ. A comparison of atropine sulfate and metaproterenol sulfate in the emergency treatment of asthma. Am Rev Respir Dis 1986; 133:727–729.

Fanta CH, Rossing TH, McFadden ER Jr. Glucocorticoids in acute asthma: a critical controlled trial. Am J Med 1983; 74:845–851.

Rossing TH, Fanta CH, Goldstein DH, Snapper JR, McFadden ER Jr. Emergency therapy of asthma: comparison of the acute effects of parenteral and inhaled sympathomimetics and infused aminophylline. Am Rev Respir Dis 1980; 122:365–371.

Rossing TH, Fanta CH, McFadden ER Jr. Effect of outpatient treatment of asthma with beta agonists on the response to sympathomimetics in an emergency room. Am J Med 1983; 75:781–783.

Siegel D, Sheppard D, Gelb A, Weinberg PF. Aminophylline increases the toxicity but not the efficacy of an inhaled beta-adrenergic agonist in the treatment of acute exacerbations of asthma. Am Rev Respir Dis 1985; 132:283–286.

STATUS ASTHMATICUS: VENTILATORY MANAGEMENT

STEVEN R. DUNCAN, M.D.
THOMAS A. RAFFIN, M.D.

Mechanical ventilation can be life saving for those patients with status asthmaticus who are moribund at presentation, progressively deteriorate despite vigorous therapy, or suffer from therapeutic misadventures of omission (undertreatment) or commission (administration of sedatives). Assisted ventilation improves the pulmonary gas exchange of asthmatics in respiratory failure. More importantly, patient work of breathing is relieved, and fatigued muscles of respiration are allowed to rest and recover. Mechanical ventilation is supportive, in effect buying time until pharmacologic therapy controls and reverses the airflow obstruction. Ventilator management of the patient with status asthmaticus is often exceedingly complex and fraught with potential complications. Moreover, there are few systematic, controlled trials to guide therapy rationally; the literature abounds with anecdotal and often contradictory reports.

This chapter presents an approach to ventilator management in status asthmaticus based on clinical experience, critical review of the literature, and theoretic considerations. General guidelines and potential pitfalls that should facilitate practical clinical treatment are outlined.

INTUBATION

Indications for Intubation

In status asthmaticus, criteria that mandate emergent intubation and initiation of assisted ventilation under virtually all circumstances are obtundation, cardiorespiratory arrest, or life-threatening arrhythmia. In less extreme cases, the indications for intubation are neither absolute nor universally agreed upon. Initial arterial blood gas measurements and various clinical parameters observed prior to instituting bronchodilator therapy are generally weak predictors of subsequent response. Decisions should be guided by trends in the patient's course while undergoing therapy rather than reliance on predetermined criteria. Pharmacologic treatment should be maximal dur-

ing this early phase in order to avoid intubation if possible.

Nonetheless, if intubation is seemingly inevitable despite maximal therapy, it is clearly a mistake to delay until the patient is moribund. In most cases, the criteria listed in Table 1, tempered by clinical judgment, are indications for intubation.

Preintubation Maneuvers

If circumstances permit, a few simple maneuvers prior to intubation of the asthmatic patient may decrease complications. Careful explanation and reassurance too often are neglected but can assuage the tremendous anxiety seen in these patients and enlist their cooperation as much as possible. Repletion of an intravascular volume deficit may lessen the hypotension often seen with the initiation of mechanical ventilation. If possible, previous evacuation of stomach contents by nasogastric tube can reduce the risk of aspiration during intubation. Parasympathetic irritant receptors in the glottis and trachea that provoke bronchoconstriction are often stimulated during intubation. This reflex can be attenuated by premedication with atropine, given as a nebulized solution in saline (1 to 2 mg) or parenterally (0.5 mg). Preoxygenation with 100 percent oxygen by face mask decreases the incidence of hypoxemia during intubation. Suppression of hypoxemic respiratory drive is not a significant concern in status asthmaticus unless severe chronic obstructive lung disease is also present.

Intubation Technique

Awake nasotracheal intubation is the preferred technique in asthmatic patients. This procedure is almost always tolerated using 4 percent cocaine topical anesthesia and requires minimal or no sedation. Spontaneous breathing is maintained, and aspiration of gastric contents is less likely than during oral intubation. Nasotracheal tubes are more readily tolerated by patients and are more easily secured than oral tubes. Their disadvantages, when compared with oral endotracheal tubes, are their greater propensity to obstruct by bending, their generally smaller diameter, and their tendency to cause purulent sinusitis. The nasotracheal route is obviously contraindicated in the presence of nasal polyps, thrombocytopenia, or coagulation abnormalities. This method of intubation cannot be safely and reliably performed in the absence of spontaneous ventilation.

Oral intubation is the method of choice when rapid

**TABLE 1   Intubation Criteria for Patients
with Status Asthmaticus**

Mandatory criteria
    Mental status deterioration
    Life-threatening arrhythmia
    Cardiac or respiratory arrest
Elective criteria (to be applied during the course of therapy)
    Progressive acidosis (pH < 7.20–7.25)
    Increasing Pco_2 (> 60–65 mm Hg)
    Refractory hypoxemia (Po_2 < 55 with maximal supplemental FiO_2)
    Decreasing breath sounds (especially with absent wheezing)
    Worsening fatigue
    Increasing agitation or anxiety

airway control is urgently needed or when the nasotracheal route is contraindicated. Ideally, oral intubation should be performed using only lidocaine topical anesthesia and light sedation. Spontaneous ventilation diminishes or ceases with heavy sedation and paralysis. Asthmatics are often difficult or impossible to ventilate adequately using a bag-mask system because of their inordinate airway resistance. A failed or prolonged intubation can result in respiratory arrest. In reality, however, many asthmatic patients are too tachypneic, agitated, and confused to tolerate oral intubation without profound sedation and paralysis. Forced intubation under inadequate anesthesia can seriously exacerbate bronchospasm by stimulation of upper airway irritant receptors.

Regardless of the route of intubation, an endotracheal tube with an internal diameter of 8 mm is the desired minimal size. Smaller tubes disproportionately increase airway resistance, hinder suctioning and secretion clearance, and preclude bronchoscopy (although this procedure is seldom indicated in acute asthmatics). The endotracheal tube should have a soft, low-pressure, high-volume cuff. A chest film after intubation is mandatory to confirm correct tube placement.

Sedation

Sedation can be safely achieved and titrated to effect by the use of small incremental doses of midazolam (Versed), a short-acting benzodiazepine. A prudent dose is 1 to 2 mg given intravenously repeated at 3 to 4 minute intervals until the desired effect is achieved. Sedation can be subsequently maintained at an appropriate level by titration of a continuous infusion of midazolam at 1 to 5 mg per hour. Compared with diazepam (Valium), midazolam offers more rapid onset, less phlebitis, better amnesia, and, most importantly, a much shorter elimination half-life. Drug accumulation and untoward prolonged sedation are thereby minimized. Alternatively, the synthetic narcotic fentanyl (Sublimaze), in increments of 50 μg

IV, can be used during intubation or to provide continuous sedation by infusion (at 2 to 5 μg per kilogram per hour). Fentanyl, like midazolam, has rapid onset, is short-acting, and is associated with minimal cardiovascular effects. A specific although fortunately rare side effect is sudden onset of chest wall rigidity. In this instance ventilation is virtually impossible unless neuromuscular blockers or naloxone is administered.

Common sedative-hypnotic drugs to avoid using in asthmatics include thiopental and morphine. Thiopental lowers the threshold for laryngospasm and bronchospasm. Morphine is a strong histamine releaser that can theoretically exacerbate bronchospasm. More important, morphine may precipitate exaggerated hypotension, especially in the presence of intravascular volume depletion.

Asthmatics are particularly susceptible to depression of respiratory drive by even low doses of sedatives. It should be emphasized that sedatives are absolutely contraindicated in these patients unless they are undergoing intubation or mechanical ventilation.

Paralyzing Agents

If neuromuscular paralysis is required, vecuronium (Norcuron) at 0.1 mg per kilogram IV is a reasonable choice because it has remarkably few side effects. This drug has a relatively prolonged duration of action of approximately 30 to 45 minutes, which markedly increases the risk of respiratory arrest with a failed intubation. Facility with endotracheal intubation is a prerequisite to the use of neuromuscular blockers. Succinylcholine has the definite advantage of being much shorter-acting (about 5 minutes), but it can worsen bronchospasm by histamine release and cholinergic receptor agonism. Pancuronium has seen wide clinical use in status asthmaticus but can aggravate the often already marked tachycardia of these patients. Tubocurarine, metocurine, and atracurium are histamine releasers and should not be used in asthmatics.

VENTILATOR MANAGEMENT

Therapy must be individualized in order to provide adequate alveolar ventilation without producing deleterious intrathoracic pressures. Manipulation of ventilator parameters may minimize creation of high pressures and their adverse sequelae. However, complex mechanisms are involved in asthmatics, and minor changes of ventilator settings can result in unforeseen effects. For example, decreasing the inspiratory flow rate will have the desired effect of lowering peak airway pressure, but expiratory time is then shortened, and air trapping may thereby increase, resulting in increased mean airway and pleural pressures. Fundamental understanding of the interplay between mechanical ventilation and generation of intrathoracic pressures is essential for rational ventilator management.

Airway Pressure

Airway pressure in ventilated asthmatics is most readily and commonly assessed in terms of peak inflation pressure (PIP), also referred to as peak inspiratory pressure, or peak airway pressure (PAP). PIP is a product of the total airflow resistance of ventilator tubing, endotracheal tube, and conducting airways as well as a reflection of compliance characteristics of the lungs and chest wall. In the presence of constant airway resistance and chest compliance, PIP is a function of inspiratory flow rate and minute ventilation. PIP is directly correlated with delivered tidal volume size and indirectly correlated with rate (via the mechanism of air trapping).

Ventilation of asthmatics often requires tremendous PIP to overcome the increased forces of resistance (airflow obstruction) and elastance (poor pulmonary compliance because of hyperinflation). PIP greater than 50 to 60 cm H_2O in nonasthmatic patients has been shown to be associated with an inordinate incidence of barotrauma (pneumothorax, pneumomediastinum, subcutaneous emphysema, and pneumoperitoneum). In several series up to 20 percent of ventilated asthmatics developed pulmonary barotrauma, which can rapidly evolve into tension pneumothorax. Although it is still controversial, many authorities advise manipulation of ventilator parameters (inspiratory flow rate or minute ventilation or both) in the treatment of status asthmaticus to maintain PIP at less than 50 cm H_2O.

Air Trapping

Air trapping in asthmatics is the result of severe obstruction to expiratory airflow. Because expiration is markedly prolonged, alveoli have insufficient time to empty completely during exhalation prior to the next spontaneous inspiration or machine-delivered breath. As with PIP, air trapping is also directly related to increases of minute ventilation. A larger tidal volume may increase airway caliber, which reduces airflow obstruction but generates a greater volume of gas to expire. An increase of the respiratory rate allows less time between breaths for expiration. Air trapping produces deleterious consequences by increasing both lung volume (hyperinflation) and alveolar pressure ("autoPEEP" or "intrinsic" PEEP).

Hyperinflation in ventilated asthmatics is usually obvious. The thorax appears hyperexpanded, and the diaphragms are flattened (and shortened) on chest films. Shortened diaphragms are at a considerable mechanical disadvantage. Energy expenditure of breathing is increased, resulting in respiratory muscle fatigue or failure. Air trapping overdistends alveoli, which increases dead space and minute ventilation requirements. Lung compliance is worsened, which further raises PIP. The increased pulmonary artery resistance and right ventricular afterload associated with hyperinflation may result in a deleterious compromise of cardiac output. Air trapping can be quantitated by measurement of expired volumes or by serial chest circumference determinations.

Alveolar pressure cannot decrease to atmospheric pressure before the next machine-delivered breath if expiratory time is inadequate. This occult pressure (autoPEEP) is functionally identical to installation of a PEEP valve on the expiratory circuit of the ventilator; alveolar pressure remains positive throughout the respiratory cycle with transmission of pressure to the pleural and intravascular spaces. AutoPEEP exacerbates the hemodynamic consequences and barotrauma of high PIP. The propensity to autoPEEP is a direct function of the degree of airway obstruction and the amount of minute ventilation. AutoPEEP is a common but infrequently appreciated phenomenon. Neither the presence nor the magnitude of autoPEEP is apparent during usual ventilator monitoring. AutoPEEP can be demonstrated and quantitated on the ventilator manometer by briefly occluding the expiratory circuit at end-exhalation immediately prior to inspiration.

Pleural Pressure

Pleural pressure is increased in ventilated asthmatics because of the cumulative transmission of airway pressure and autoPEEP. Cardiac output may fall in the presence of increased pleural pressure, primarily as a result of impediment to venous return. In extreme cases, the reduction of cardiac output may result in profound hypotension and shock. This hemodynamic collapse is most frequently seen in asthmatics shortly after initiation of mechanical ventilation. Pleural pressure can be reduced and hemodynamic sequelae minimized by measures that reduce airway pressures and autoPEEP.

VENTILATOR SETTINGS

Type

Volume or time-cycled ventilators are best able to meet the demands of asthmatic patients. Pressure-cycled ventilators should not be used in adults because delivered tidal volume will fluctuate with changes in chest compliance and airway obstruction. High frequency jet ventilators are seemingly unable to deliver adequate tidal volume in the presence of severe airway obstruction.

Mode

With the initiation of mechanical ventilation, patients should be heavily sedated and, if necessary, paralyzed until spontaneous ventilation ceases. There are several reasons to do so during this critical period: (1) patient-ventilator dyssynchrony is avoided and chest wall compliance is improved, thereby minimizing peak airway and intrathoracic pressure, (2) CO_2 production is lessened, which decreases minute ventilation requirement, and (3) fatigued muscles of respiration are allowed to rest. Both assist-control (AMV) or intermittent mechanical (IMV) modes, with appropriately set rates, function as controlled ventilation (CMV) in patients not making spontaneous breathing efforts. There is never an indication for actually setting the machine mode on CMV; if patient anesthesia lightens and spontaneous ventilation is attempted, the discomfort and resulting agitation can be extreme. In later stages, as asthma remits, sedation is decreased and patients are allowed to spontaneously ventilate or initiate breaths. There are no clinical data that clearly document superiority of either the IMV or the AMV mode. Hence, the most appropriate mode is that with which the intensive care unit team has the greatest familiarity.

Fractional Inspired Oxygen Concentration (FiO₂)

An initial FiO_2 of 0.90 is recommended. Only rare asthmatic patients cannot be adequately oxygenated with moderately increased FiO_2; thus, there is little to be gained by initially using 100 percent as opposed to 90 percent oxygen. The additional FiO_2 increment does little to increase the arterial O_2 content but promotes absorption atelectasis. Subsequent decrements of FiO_2 are titrated to maintain arterial Po_2 in the range of 70 to 80 mm Hg. Continuous oximetric monitoring with finger or ear lobe probes may provide an additional margin of safety and decrease the frequency of blood gas measurements.

Minute Ventilation (V̇E): Tidal Volume (VT) and Rate (R)

Ventilation of asthmatics is initiated with a rate of 10 and a tidal volume of 10 ml per kilogram body weight. Minute ventilation (V̇E) is purposely somewhat less than that used in patients with other causes of respiratory failure. The reduction of V̇E may minimize early adverse effects of high intrathoracic pressures. Subsequent adjustment is determined on the basis of pH and Pco_2 of arterial blood gases, PIP, and air trapping (Fig. 1). When minute ventilation needs augmentation, initial preference should be given to increases of rate rather than tidal volume. This approach helps to control PIP at a reasonable level, although air trapping may result as expiratory time is shortened.

In ideal circumstances the Pco_2 should be slowly reduced by about 10 mm per hour while maintaining peak airway pressure at less than 50 to 60 cm H_2O. An overzealous, too rapid change of pH needlessly exposes patients to possible electrolyte shifts, arrhythmias, and seizures. In practice even a slow reduction of Pco_2 is usually initially impossible to achieve without producing extraordinarily high PIPs. If PIPs are greater than 50 cm H_2O or in the presence of autoPEEP with hemodynamic compromise, controlled hypoventilation should be tolerated during the first few hours of ventilation. By purposely allowing the Pco_2 to remain elevated, the V̇E requirement is thereby reduced. This reduction of V̇E results in favorable decreases of PIP, mean airway pressure, hyperinflation, and autoPEEP. Hypercarbia is generally not harmful as long as the pH is maintained in the range of 7.22 to 7.25 or greater. However, a more acidotic pH is associated with unacceptable risks of arrhythmias, depression of myocardial function, and vasomotor derangement. Likewise, beta-agonist bronchodilators may lose therapeutic efficacy in a severely acidotic environment. Of secondary concern is the cerebral vasodilating effect of hypercarbia. The increased cerebral blood flow could deleteriously raise intracranial pressure. This effect may be marked in the presence of impeded cerebral venous flow due to high intrathoracic pressures. The Pco_2 should be maintained at less than 70 mm Hg if otherwise feasible, although some groups will tolerate prolonged hypercarbia of up to 90 mm Hg. Later, as airflow obstruction remits with therapy, the V̇E can be increased and Pco_2 normalized without generation of extraordinary airway pressures.

In difficult situations in which pH and Pco_2 cannot be protected at adequate levels without generation of high inflation pressures, the real risks of acidosis

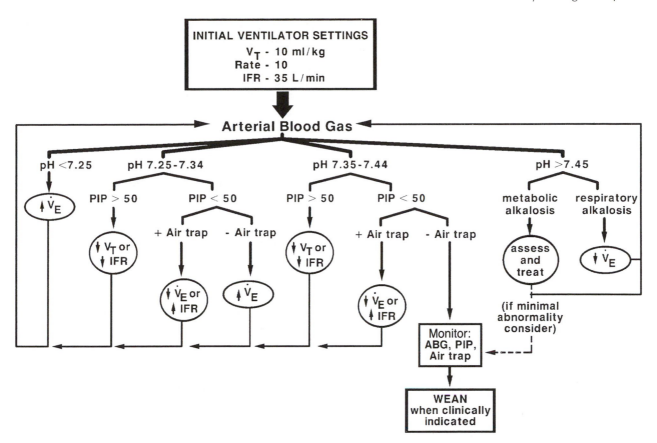

Figure 1 Algorithm for adjustment of ventilation in status asthmaticus. This protocal is intended as a guide to therapy until arterial blood gases and clinical findings normalize. Conservative values are given and should be considered approximate. However, no predetermined plan is a substitute for clinical judgment and individualized therapy. Key: V_T = tidal volume; IFR = inspiratory flow rate; V_E = minute ventilation; PIP = peak inflation pressure (cm H_2O); air trap = auto-PEEP (greater than 15 cm H_2O, especially when associated with refractory hemodynamic compromise).

The logic of this algorithm is based on the following three postulates. First, assuming arterial Po_2 is adequate (see text for further details), the overwhelmingly highest priority of assisted ventilation is maintainence of the pH in a safe range (approximately 7.25 to 7.49). The second priority is avoidance of barotrauma and hemodynamic compromise by keeping PIP at safe levels (less than 50 to 60 cm H_2O). Third, after ventilator adjustment for pH and PIP, attention should be directed to reduction of hyperinflation (air trap) as determined by quantitation of auto-PEEP.

For example; the initial arterial blood gas reading, after initiation of ventilation at the prescribed settings, showed that the pH was 7.31 and the Pco_2 46; but the PIP was 65. Although the pH was adequate under the circumstances, a reduction of V_T to lower PIP was indicated. Subsequent arterial blood gas measurement showed pH 7.28, Pco_2 53, the PIP was 48, auto-PEEP was 10, and clinical indices of cardiac output were adequate. No further ventilator adjustment was therefore necessary. After several hours of continued bronchodilator and sedative therapy, the PIP decreased, which allowed an increase of V_E by both V_T and rate. Arterial blood gases now showed a pH of 7.36, Pco_2 of 45, and the PIP was 46. However, the arterial blood pressure became marginally low, the urine output decreased, and these changes were resistant to intravascular volume expansion. The presence of significant auto-PEEP (23 cm) was confirmed. Sequential increases in inspiratory flow rate and reduction of V_E resulted in hemodynamic improvement, a pH of 7.30, and an unchanged PIP. The next day the patient's bronchospasm improved, permitting stepwise increments of V_E and IFR without producing inordinately high PIP or auto-PEEP. A trial of spontaneous T-piece breathing was clinically uneventful. During the T-piece trial with FIO_2 0.30, there was minimal residual wheezing and arterial blood gas readings revealed pH 7.42, Pco_2 38, and Po_2 83. The patient was extubated shortly thereafter.

outweigh potential problems of barotrauma, and the minute ventilation must be increased. An exception would possibly be the case of simultaneous worsening of acidosis, high airway pressures, and profound refractory hypotension (presumably due to the increased intrathoracic pressure). In this situation, low doses of sodium bicarbonate may maintain blood pH without the need for increasing minute ventilation, but there are potential serious side effects of this therapy (see below).

Inspiratory Flow Rate

Ventilator parameters should optimize expiratory time with low inspiratory-to-expiratory ratios (1:2 to 1:4) to lessen air trapping. Besides adjustment of minute ventilation, the primary determinant of expiratory time that can be manipulated on most ventilators is the inspiratory flow rate. Inspiratory time decreases as inspiratory flow rate increases. The greater proportion of respiratory cycle time allotted for expiration results in more complete alveolar emptying.

Other theoretic considerations warrant the use of high inspiratory flow rates. Increased inspiratory flow rate in the presence of airflow obstruction has been demonstrated to benefit pulmonary gas exchange and compliance. The work of breathing is inversely correlated with inspiratory flow rate in patients who are spontaneously breathing (IMV) or initiating ventilator breaths (AMV).

However, practical considerations of the higher PIP generated as flow increases temper use of maximal inspiratory flow rates. In practice, the inspiratory flow rate should initially be set at about 35 to 40 L per minute. After stabilization of the patient with an appropriate minute ventilation, the inspiratory flow rate is titrated upwards while monitoring airway pressures.

Positive End-Expiratory Pressure (PEEP)

According to conventional wisdom, asthmatic patients should be ventilated with no added PEEP. PEEP could augment already excessively large functional residual capacity, further increase intrathoracic pressure, and may worsen the risks of pulmonary barotrauma. Almost all ventilated asthmatics can be adequately oxygenated using only modest increments of FIO_2 without PEEP. However, there are preliminary reports that suggest PEEP may be beneficial in refractory status asthmaticus (see below).

MANAGEMENT OF REFRACTORY PATIENTS

Additional maneuvers or therapies may be tried when ventilated asthmatics progressively deteriorate despite treatment, or ventilation with even high inflation pressures is difficult. Data to support these modalities are primarily anecdotal, and in most cases these therapies have additional associated risks. As such, their use should probably be limited to extreme situations.

Isoproterenol

This nonselective beta-agonist given as a continuous infusion has been reported to be beneficial in treatment of severe bronchospasm. Most clinical experience is with asthmatic children. Few recent reports advocate the use of this agent in adults. Potentially deleterious severe chronotropic effects (in patients often already tachycardic), ventricular arrhythmogenicity, and hypotension resulting from vasodilatation should preclude its use except in situations in which patients are moribund.

Anesthetic Agents

Several inhalational agents have bronchodilating properties and have been widely, if sporadically, used in treatment of severe status asthmaticus. Ether and halothane have documented efficacy. Unfortunately, the former is quite explosive, and the latter is liable to cause arrhythmias, especially with concomitant use of beta-agonists and methylxanthines. Halothane does appear to be an effective bronchodilator in the presence of severe acidosis, which may be a useful property in dire situations. Enflurane, and more recently isoflurane, have been used with some success. Isoflurane, in particular, has several potential advantages and may ultimately be shown to be the anesthetic agent of choice for refractory bronchospasm. All anesthetic gases can depress myocardial function, and most additionally lower blood pressure by vasodilation. Parenteral ketamine has been advocated for use in asthmatics because of its desirable anesthetic and bronchodilating properties. The latter effect may be due to release of endogenous catecholamines. Clinical experience is limited largely because of concerns of profound dysphoria, and there are reports that the drug may release histamine in some patients.

Sodium Bicarbonate

The use of bicarbonate as an acid buffer in status asthmaticus has been advocated in small uncontrolled series. Bicarbonate can support the pH in acceptable ranges while permitting a reduction of $\dot{V}E$. However, this therapy has potentially severe adverse effects. CO_2 is generated by bicarbonate administration ($HCO_3 + H^+ \rightarrow CO_2 + H_2O$). Cell membranes and the blood-brain barrier do not impede diffusion of CO_2 but are relatively impermeable to bicarbonate ion. Although the blood pH may be corrected, the intracellular and cerebrospinal fluid PCO_2 is increased, and the pH in these compartments is paradoxically made more acidic. The myocardium and brain are particularly sensitive to intracellular acidosis. Additionally, the large amount of sodium administered could result in volume overload or hyperosmotic states. Bicarbonate administration can also dangerously exacerbate preexisting hypokalemia.

Respiratory acidosis should be corrected by increasing ventilation. In those rare situations in which the pH is falling uncorrectably, judicious bicarbonate therapy may be justified. Similarly, an argument could be made supporting the use of bicarbonate in the presence of lactic (metabolic) acidosis. However, it may be more prudent to minimize lactate production by augmenting oxygen delivery (cardiac output × arterial O_2 content) or lessening oxygen consumption or both.

Lowering CO_2 Production ($\dot{V}CO_2$)

Measures to lower CO_2 prediction are in general quite safe, but unfortunately therapeutic gains are often minimal. Fever, if present, should be treated with acetaminophen or cooling blankets. Shivering, which markedly increases $\dot{V}CO_2$, must be vigorously treated and may require muscle paralysis. Heavy sedation and paralysis decrease O_2 consumption and CO_2 production and should be used liberally during initial ventilator management. Reduction of caloric intake, especially carbohydrates, may appreciably lower $\dot{V}CO_2$.

PEEP

The traditional dogma that use of PEEP is unwarranted in status asthmaticus has been outlined. However, recent anecdotal reports and preliminary investigations suggest PEEP may decrease airway pressure and improve pulmonary mechanics during ventilation of patients with airflow obstruction (including asthma). The putative mechanism may be a lung volume-related increase in airway caliber resulting in reduction of airway resistance. Alveolar emptying is facilitated, thereby decreasing the air trapping and auto-PEEP. Although we cannot unequivocally recommend the use of PEEP in status asthmaticus, it would not seem entirely unreasonable to attempt judicious trials in severe refractory cases. PEEP could be applied in increments of 2.5 to 5.0 cm H_2O while carefully monitoring hemodynamics, PIP, arterial blood gases, and end-exhalation occlusion pressures (auto-PEEP). The optimal applied PEEP must be individualized but may be approximately 50 percent of the amount of autoPEEP initially present.

Bronchoscopic Lavage

There are no controlled trials that support the use of bronchoscopic lavage in acute asthma. There are several potential complications: severe bronchospasm may be precipitated; hypoxemia and hypercarbia are usually worsened; marked expiratory obstruction distal to the instrument creates high local PEEP that may promote lung disruption; and risk of pulmonary infection is increased. We consider the procedure contraindicated in these patients in the absence of very specific indications, e.g., lobar atelectasis refractory to chest physiotherapy or suspected foreign body aspiration.

Extracorporeal Membrane Oxygenation (ECMO)

ECMO has been reported as life saving in an otherwise moribund asthmatic patient. ECMO has not been shown to alter outcome of adult respiratory distress syndrome (ARDS), but the situation in status asthmaticus may be considerably different. Compared with patients with ARDS, asthmatics requiring mechanical ventilation do not often have multisystem failure, and their disease is amenable to specific therapy within a few days. ECMO is not devoid of potential problems, notably, complications related to vascular access, anticoagulation, trauma to circulating blood cells and platelets, and equipment malfunction. However, in those institutions with ECMO capability and expertise, its use in status asthmaticus should be considered in extraordinary circumstances.

ANCILLARY THERAPY

Chest Physiotherapy

Chest percussion can exacerbate bronchospasm in acute asthma. Consequently, it should not be routinely employed in the absence of lobar or segmental atelectasis or unless excessive secretions cannot otherwise be cleared. Postural drainage to promote secretion clearance can worsen hypoxemia, but this problem is not likely to be of clinical significance with supplemental FIO_2 in ventilated asthmatics. This otherwise benign maneuver may be of some benefit by promoting drainage of secretions into the central airways, where they can be suctioned or expectorated. Gentle suctioning should be performed as necessary to remove often copious secretions. Prior lavage with 10 ml of isotonic saline down the endotracheal tube may aid removal of viscous secretions and mucus plugs. Pretreatment with 5 to 10 ml of 1 percent lidocaine, also administered via endotracheal tube, may minimize reflex bronchospasm and cough.

Humidification of inspired gas by mist may assist expulsion of mucus plugs and clearance of secretions. Ultrasonic nebulizers have reportedly exacerbated bronchospasm and should probably be avoided during the initial therapy of asthma. However, some anecdotal experience suggests a possible benefit of ultrasonic nebulizers after several days of optimal therapy. Although mucolytic agents have some proponents, they have not been shown to be beneficial in controlled trials, and they conceivably may worsen bronchospasm.

Volume Repletion

As previously mentioned, at presentation asthmatics are often intravascularly volume-depleted. Correction of volume deficit may ameliorate hemodynamic sequelae of mechanical ventilation and is probably in aid to pulmonary secretion liquefaction. However, caution should be exercised to avoid overly vigorous repletion. Lung water is often significantly increased in asthmatics due to tremendous pressure gradients across the pulmonary interstitium. Frank volume overload will result in further increases in lung H_2O and cause impairment of gas exchange and worsening compliance. Pulmonary artery catheterization may rarely be required in complicated cases. Central venous pressure monitoring is often misleading because of complex hemodynamics whereby right-sided heart pressures poorly reflect the situation in the left ventricle.

Electrolytes

Hypokalemia is often associated with severe asthma and is probably caused by the effects of stress on renal tubular function and the mineralocorticoid action of steroid therapy. Hyponatremia is frequently present and is attributed to inappropriate secretion of antidiuretic hormone. Obviously, electrolyte abnormalities should be corrected, with the arrhythmogenicity of hypokalemia being a particular concern.

Infection Control

Preexisting pulmonary bacterial infection should obviously be assessed by clinical and radiologic features, and if present, the etiologic agent should be appropriately identified and treated. There is no justification for prophylactic administration of antibiotics. Routine sputum cultures in intubated patients in the absence of a specific indication of infection are most likely to yield misleading information.

Nosocomial pneumonia develops in a significant number of intubated asthmatics and is associated with markedly increased mortality. Aseptic airway care is of paramount importance for prevention.

Daily chest films should be obtained to assess endotracheal tube position, to exclude pneumothorax, and to facilitate early identification of pulmonary parenchymal infiltrates.

Gastrointestinal Hemorrhage Prophylaxis

Stress gastritis appears to be frequent in mechanically ventilated asthmatics. The etiology is probably multifactoral: decreased arterial perfusion of gastric mucosa, increased venous congestion, and ulcerogenic effects of high-dose steroids. Gastric bleeding can largely be prevented by the frequent administration via nasogastric tube of antacids titrated to raise gastric pH to higher than 3.5.

Pulmonary Embolus Prevention

Acutely ill, immobile, ventilated asthmatics with central venous congestion may be at greatly increased risk for the development of deep vein thrombosis and consequent pulmonary emboli. We advocate the use of "minidose" heparin (5,000 U subcutaneously every 12 hours) in ventilated asthmatics, although there are no directly applicable supporting data. Contraindications include active gastrointestinal bleeding or acute cerebrovascular accidents.

COMPLICATIONS

Complications related to or resulting from mechanical ventilation are frequent in status asthmaticus. Overall mortality from several noncomparable series ranges from 0 to 38 percent, the average is approximately 10 percent. Hypoxic brain injury appears responsible for about 30 percent of deaths; presumably most hypoxemic episodes occurred prior to initiation of ventilation. Ventilator failure, including inadvertent extubation, accounts for many preventable deaths.

Unique complications may result from the high intrathoracic pressures generated by mechanical ventilation of asthmatics. Pneumothorax is a feared complication, although the frequency with which barotrauma contributes directly to patient demise has not been clearly defined. Clinicians should be alert for sudden hemodynamic or respiratory deterioration, especially when accompanied by worsening PIP. Other possible etiologies in this situation are exacerbation of bronchospasm, pulmonary edema, ventilator tubing or endotracheal tube problems, including acute obstruction with secretions or mucus plugs, and less likely, pulmonary embolus. Cardiocirculatory collapse is frequent, and like pulmonary barotrauma, may often be preventable by zealous attention to and manipulation of ventilator parameters that minimize intrathoracic pressures.

Other causes of morbidity, notably nosocomial infection and endotracheal tube trauma, are common to all mechanically ventilated patients. Their discussion is beyond the scope of this article.

WEANING

Weaning patients with asthma from mechanical ventilation is as much an art as a science. The primary determinant of weaning success is reversal of the underlying airflow obstruction. Serious weaning attempts should not be undertaken until bronchospasm

TABLE 2   Guidelines for Weaning

Weaning criteria
    Overall clinical status improving
    Hemodynamically stable
    Clear or improving chest x-ray findings
    Afebrile
    P_{O_2} greater than 60 mm Hg with F_{IO_2} less than 0.50
    pH and P_{CO_2} normal
    Spontaneous vital capacity greater than 10 ml/kg
    Negative inspiratory pressure lower than -20 cm H_2O
    Spontaneous tidal volume greater than 5 ml/kg
Extubation criteria
    Includes the criteria listed above and the following:
        Trial of spontaneous ventilation with maintenance of blood gases and
        stable respiratory rate, blood pressure, and pulse
    Patient is sufficiently alert to protect airway and clear secretions

is well under control as attested to by minimal wheezing and good spontaneous air movement. These patients usually can be weaned without difficulty if the asthma is adequately controlled; in comparison to patients with most other causes of acute respiratory failure, asthmatic patients are generally younger and stronger and often have been ventilated for shorter periods (3 to 5 day average). It is often difficult to determine if residual bronchospasm is due to airway irritation from the endotracheal tube. A good response to gentle sedation or lidocaine via endotracheal tube suggests that bronchospasm may be lessened by extubation, but these maneuvers are no substitute for astute assessment. Occasionally patients with bronchospasm that has been exacerbated by endotracheal tube irritation or severe anxiety or both are most readily weaned and extubated after very light sedation. Low-dose continuous IV infusion of midazolam is particularly suitable. Sedation can be gently titrated, effects wear off rapidly after discontinuation of the drug, and respiratory drive suppression is minimal when midazolam is administered as a continuous infusion.

Attention to general details of patient care will facilitate weaning success. Weaning and extubation should be performed early in the day when more personnel are available for monitoring and emergent intervention. Prior to weaning attempts, patients should be well rested and as free as possible from the effects of sedatives. They should be euvolemic with electrolytes in normal ranges, especially those minerals that have a direct effect on muscle function (potassium, magnesium, calcium, and phosphate). Patients should have reasonably good nutritional status prior to weaning. Enteral or parenteral nutrition therapy should be provided if ventilation is prolonged for more than a few days or catabolic stresses (infection, sepsis) are present.

Knowing when to wean patients from mechanical ventilation requires clinical judgment and experience. The criteria listed in Table 2 are guidelines for weaning and subsequent extubation.

Suggested Reading

Dales RE, Mont PW. Use of mechanical ventilation in adults with severe asthma. Can Med Assoc J 1984; 130:391–395.

Darioli R, Perret C. Mechanical controlled hypoventilation in status asthmaticus. Am Rev Respir Dis 1984; 129:385–387.

Don H. Management of status asthmaticus in adults. In: Gershwin ME, ed. Bronchial asthma. 2nd ed. Orlando: Grune & Stratton, 1986:469.

Luksza AR, Smith P. Coakley J, et al. Acute severe asthma treated by mechanical ventilation: 10 years' experience from a district general hospital. Thorax 1986; 41:459–463.

Pepe DE, Marini JJ. Occult positive end-expiratory pressure in mechanically ventilated patients with airflow obstruction. Am Rev Respir Dis 1982; 126:166–170.

Raffin TA, Roberts P. The prevention and treatment of status asthmaticus. Hosp Prac 1982; 17:80N–80Z.

Scoggin CH, Sahn SA, Petty TL. Status asthmaticus. A nine-year experience. JAMA 1977; 238:1158–1162.

Webb AK, Bilton AH, Hanson GC. Severe bronchial asthma requiring ventilation. A review of 20 cases and advice on management. Postgrad Med J 1979; 55:161–170.

PNEUMONIA

MICHAEL S. NIEDERMAN, M.D.

Despite the recent emergence of new antibiotics, sophisticated diagnostic methods, and sleuth-like epidemiologists, pneumonia remains a common, confusing, and unconquered medical malady. In recent years we have seen the appearance of "new" pathogens for pneumonia (e.g., *Legionella, Chlamydia*), so that all pneumonias are no longer pneumococcal. With increasing exposure to antibiotics, microorganisms have become resistant to certain therapeutic agents, and an appropriate choice of antibiotics is not always simple. Although serologic, immunologic, and new bacteriologic techniques are available to study specimens collected both invasively and noninvasively, it is frequently difficult to establish a precise etiologic diagnosis of pneumonia. Finally, as medical care has advanced, patients are living longer, and with more complicated illnesses and host impairments, causing the incidence of lung infection to rise sharply in certain patient groups.

Not all individuals share the same risk of developing lower respiratory tract infection. The nature of an individual's general health, as reflected by the place of residence (home, hospital, or institution) and any known chronic illness, is a particularly important determinant of his or her likelihood of becoming ill with pneumonia. Two particularly high-risk groups are the elderly and those in the hospital. Whereas less than 1 percent of otherwise normal, healthy individuals develop pneumonia yearly, the noninstitutionalized elderly have an annual pneumonia incidence of between 2.5 and 4.4 percent. The incidence is even higher when an elderly individual is ill enough to require a chronic care facility or hospital. Yearly, 6.8 to 11.4 percent of all nursing home residents develop pneumonia, and at any one time 2.1 percent of all such individuals harbor pneumonia. In the hospital, the elderly have a threefold greater incidence of nosocomial pneumonia than younger patients, and overall, as many as 1.6 percent of all hospital admissions in this population are complicated by lower respiratory tract infection.

When pneumonia develops in a hospitalized patient, it should be viewed as an opportunistic occurrence that appears in those individuals who have the most serious underlying medical conditions. Although nosocomial infection may be seen in only 2 percent of hospitalized patients without an underlying fatal illness, it complicates the hospital course of nearly one-quarter of individuals with a known fatal illness. Among patients in an intensive care unit, the incidence of hospital-acquired pneumonia varies from 10 to 70 percent, depending on the population studied. One group at particularly high risk is patients with the adult respiratory distress syndrome (ARDS); as many as 70 percent of affected individuals develop pneumonia. Like the incidence data, the mortality implications of pneumonia vary according to the general health of the affected person. In the general population, pneumonia from all causes has about a 10 to 15 percent mortality rate. In contrast, the elderly have a 20 percent mortality rate from pneumonia, whereas those with ARDS and pneumonia have up to a 70 percent mortality.

APPROACH TO THE THERAPY OF PNEUMONIA

In approaching the treatment of pneumonia, two basic questions must first be answered: (1) does the patient *have* a lower respiratory tract infection? If so, (2) what is the most likely etiologic agent? Once it is established that the patient has pneumonia and not bronchitis, airway colonization, or some other parenchymal lung process, a decision to treat can be made. And once this decision is reached, an idea about etiology will allow for the most specific therapy available.

In the otherwise healthy patient with community-acquired pneumonia, the disease is typically heralded by the presence of chills, pleuritic chest pain, purulent cough, sputum, and tachypnea. Although viral and atypical pneumonias may manifest with a prodromal illness and dry cough in contrast to the more classic features of bacterial pneumonia, both types of infection appear as distinct clinical events. This pattern of illness often leads to evaluation by chest radiology, which then confirms the presence of a parenchymal lung infection. Recognition of the presence of pneumonia is often far more difficult in the elderly and in those with preexisting parenchymal lung disease.

The presence of coexisting disease states and medications and the altered physiology of aging and acute illness make the recognition of pneumonia a difficult task in some patients. For example, when the elderly patient develops pneumonia, classic signs and symptoms may be replaced by lethargy, confusion, or exacerbation or a preexisting condition. More than 10 percent of bacteremic elderly patients may not have fever, so that this cardinal sign of infection is not always reliable. Compared with younger patients, those over age 65 have rigors and pleuritic chest pain less frequently and are more often confused when they develop pneumococcal pneumonia.

In critically ill patients with ARDS, recognition that nosocomial pneumonia has developed is similarly difficult. Traditional clues to the presence of pneumonia, such as fever, purulent sputum, leukocytosis, new infiltrate on chest roentgenogram, and the clinical response to antibiotic therapy may not be of help in the patient with ARDS. Independent of the presence of pneumonia, patients with ARDS can have fever, leukocytosis, lung infiltrates, and gram-negative bacteria in the sputum. In one large series of patients with ARDS, one-third of all pneumonia patients were not treated because they were not thought to be infected, whereas one-fifth of uninfected patients were incorrectly treated for pneumonia. With these data in mind, it is clear that pneumonia will be recognized only with a high index of suspicion (but occasionally overdiagnosed) in high-risk patients with coexisting illnesses.

Once it is established that a patient has pneumonia, specific antibiotic therapy can be instituted and is directed at the most likely etiologic agents. The spectrum of possible causes varies according to the state of a patient's general health and the respiratory tract host defenses. In certain specific hosts, characteristic organisms are found and should be suspected to be the cause of pneumonia and treated. For example, alcoholics frequently have *Klebsiella* infections; those with chronic bronchitis may be infected with *Haemophilus influenzae;* patients with cystic fibrosis often harbor *Pseudomonas aeruginosa* or *Staphylococcus aureus;* patients with secondary post-influenza pneumonia are infected by *Staphylococcus aureus, Streptococcus pneumoniae,* or *Haemophilus influenzae;* and patients with known aspiration can develop cavitary pneumonias with anaerobic organisms.

In Table 1, the bacterial organisms causing pneumonia are listed in decreasing order of frequency based on place of residence. From this list, it is clear that community-acquired infection is most common with pneumococcus, *Mycoplasma pneumoniae,* or *Legionella pneumophila,* whereas hospital-acquired infection is most common with enteric gram-negative bacteria. One group that does not always follow this scheme is the elderly, in whom enteric gram-negative organisms can cause 20 to 40 percent of all community-acquired pneumonias. Although the true incidence of viral pneumonia in the community is unknown and not included in the table, it has been estimated that one-quarter to one-third of all pneumonias are of this type.

Frequently it is necessary to treat pneumonia according to an epidemiologic approach, choosing an antibiotic regimen that treats all likely pathogens for a given patient in a given situation. In this instance, the data in Table 1 will be useful. However, an attempt at collecting respiratory tract secretions and establishing a specific etiologic diagnosis is preferred. Although it is beyond the scope of this chapter to discuss an approach to diagnostic methods for pneumonia, respiratory secretions may be sampled by collecting expectorated sputum, suctioned sputum, induced sputum, bronchoscopic lung washings, bronchial secretions with a bronchoscopic-protected catheter brush, bronchial secretions with a transthoracic needle, or lung tissue with a bronchoscopic or surgical lung biopsy. The availability of serologic methods allows for the sampling of serum to establish a cause for lung infection, but these methods are often slow in providing an answer.

For most patients, the collection of sputum is the primary diagnostic test applied to find the cause of the pneumonia. Only in certain selected instances, when sputum is unavailable and empiric therapy is more risky than invasive procedures is bronchoscopy, lung aspiration, or lung biopsy employed. The use of sputum

TABLE 1 Bacterial Pathogens Causing Pneumonia in Descending Order of Frequency

Community-Acquired	*Hospital-Acquired*
Streptococcus pneumoniae	Enteric gram-negative bacilli,
*Mycoplasma pneumoniae**	including *Klebsiella pneumoniae,*
Legionella pneumophila	*Escherichia coli, Pseudomonas*
Haemophilus influenzae	*aeruginosa*
Enteric gram-negative bacilli,	
including *Klebsiella pneumoniae*	
Chlamydia trachomatis (TWAR)*	*Staphylococcus aureus*
Aspiration (including anaerobes)	*Haemophilus influenzae*
Staphylococcus aureus	*Streptococcus pneumoniae*
	Aspiration, including anaerobes
	Legionella pneumophila

*Although these organisms are not strictly bacteria, they are amenable to antibiotic therapy and thus included in this list.

in the diagnosis of pneumonia has several problems. Some patients are so weak or dehydrated that they cannot expectorate sputum, as is frequently the case with the elderly. Even when sputum is available, its analysis may lead to an incorrect approach. In one study of elderly patients with pneumonia, only one-quarter of sputum cultures led to a correct etiologic diagnosis. Similarly, when Gram's stains were analyzed in patients known to have pneumococcal pneumonia, only one-half of the samples had characteristic lancet-shaped diplococci. In the elderly and in hospitalized patients, the analysis of sputum cultures is complicated by the frequent presence of gram-negative bacillary colonization of both the oropharynx and the tracheobronchial tree. Colonization, or the presence of bacteria without invasive infection, can be seen in the oropharynx of elderly and hospitalized patients in direct relation to their underlying degree of illness. For example, up to 37 percent of the institutionalized elderly and 73 percent of moribund hospitalized patients harbor gram-negative bacilli in their oropharynx. When sputum is collected by expectoration through such a colonized oropharynx, interpretation of the culture result may be misleading. In mechanically ventilated patients, up to 75 percent have gram-negative organisms colonizing their tracheobronchial trees, and thus the finding of such bacteria in a tracheal aspirate is of unknown significance.

Considering the pitfalls in establishing a specific etiologic diagnosis of pneumonia, it appears that a judicious combination of epidemiologic analysis with a critical review of sputum culture results, when available, will lead to the most effective antimicrobial approach. In the future, more liberal use of bronchoscopy with a protected specimen brush, may be used in mechanically ventilated patients suspected of having pneumonia. In some preliminary studies, the use of this technique, along with quantitative culture methods, has been able to distinguish infection from colonization in patients with an endotracheal tube in place.

THERAPEUTIC MEASURES

The mainstay of therapy for pneumonia is the use of antibiotics directed at the probable responsible pathogens. Depending on the severity of illness, such drugs can be given orally or intravenously, in or out of the hospital. This therapy can be viewed as specific, in contrast to other nonspecific adjunctive measures. These nonorganism-directed, supportive therapies for pneumonia include supplemental oxygen, intraveous hydration, mechanical ventilation, chest physical therapy, mucolytic and mucokinetic agents, bronchodilators, and bronchoscopy. Some of these supportive measures are of unproven value, and the

decision about their use must be individualized to specific patient needs.

Need For Hospitalization

Patients with pneumonia should be hospitalized if they require supplemental oxygen (arterial oxygen tension less than 60 mm Hg on room air), intravenous hydration, or have extensive infiltration on their chest x-ray film (multilobe involvement or lobar consolidation). Patients with serious coexisting illness, such as congestive heart failure, diabetes, neuromuscular disease, chronic lung disease, or renal failure, should be considered for hospital admission even in the absence of obviously serious infection. In such individuals, their underlying conditions can further decompensate with infection, or the pneumonia itself may appear less severe than it actually is and may rapidly progress from mild to severe. In the presence of severe and extensive infection, antibiotics are best given intravenously, and this requires hospitalization. In addition, certain specific organisms, such as *Pseudomonas aeruginosa,* can be effectively treated with antibiotics that can only be given parenterally. Other indications for hospitalization include impending hypercarbic respiratory failure, need for assistance in expectorating large volumes of sputum, lobar atelectasis, and signs of metastatic spread of infection (e.g., empyema, meningitis, endocarditis).

Antibiotic Therapy

If the collection of respiratory secretions leads to a precise etiologic diagnosis, or if other cultures (blood, pleural fluid) yield a particular organism, then therapy can be quite narrow and specific. When such material is not available, epidemiologic clues can be used and are often quite accurate in narrowing down the possible etiologic agents. For example, when a young patient without any known medical problems develops an acute lobar pneumonia in the community, pneumococcus, *Mycoplasma pneumoniae,* and *Legionella pneumophila* are the most likely etiologic agents, and therapy with erythromycin (Erythrocin) would be appropriate. If a sputum Gram's stain from the same patient showed lancet-shaped diplococci suggesting pneumococcal infection, therapy could be further narrowed to the use of penicillin.

When an exact bacterial etiology is established or highly suspect in a patient with pneumonia, an organism-directed approach to antibiotic therapy is applied. *Streptococcus pneumoniae* infection is best treated with penicillin G, but erythromycin can be substituted in the penicillin-allergic patient. *Legionella pneumophila* is treated with erythromycin (Erythrocin) in doses of 2 to 4 g per day orally or intravenously. Seriously ill patients with this type of infection should receive the higher dosage intravenously. *Haemophilus influenzae* is usually sensitive to ampicillin, but certain communities have encountered resistant organisms. Other active agents against this organism include second- and third-generation cephalosporins, chloramphenicol (Chloromycetin), tetracycline (Achromycin), and trimethoprim-sulfamethoxazole (Bactrim, Septra). *Staphylococcus aureus* is usually treated with a penicillinase-resistant penicillin such as nafcillin (Nafcil, Unipen) or oxacillin (Prostaphlin), but first-generation cephalosporins and vancomycin (Vancocin) may also be used. Anaerobic aspiration pneumonias or lung abscesses are effectively eradicated with penicillin in most cases, but clindamycin (Cleocin) may be required when *Bacteroides fragilis* is present. Some of the newer cephalosporins have also been designed to be effective against anaerobes.

The therapy of enteric gram-negative bacilli varies depending on the actual organism being treated. The most common pathogens in this group are *Klebsiella pneumoniae, Escherichia coli,* and *Pseudomonas aeruginosa.* Generally an aminoglycoside, a third-generation cephalosporin, or a semisynthetic penicillin is indicated to treat gram-negative infection. When *Pseudomonas aeruginosa* is being treated, a second agent should be added to achieve synergism and to assure the best bacteriologic outcome. Serious infection with *Klebsiella pneumoniae* may also be more effectively treated with such a synergistic combination. In these circumstances, the primary antibiotic is usually an aminoglycoside, whereas the second agent can be a broad-spectrum penicillin such as ticarcillan (Ticar) piperacillin (Pipracil), or azlocillin (Azlin); a third-generation cephalosporin such as cefoperazone (Cefobid), ceftazidime (Fortaz), or ceftizoxime (Cefizox); or, in the patient who is allergic to penicillins and cephalosporins, trimethoprim-sulfamethoxazole.

When an exact etiologic diagnosis cannot be established, therapy must be selected on the basis of epidemiologic and clinical parameters. Since the place of residence of a patient and the presence of any coexisting illness will influence the type of pathogen present, empiric therapy is based on this type of information. The use of empiric therapy is based on the assumption that no diagnostic culture material is available. This approach is fraught with the problems of using multiple antibiotics, the omission of some likely pathogens, and the use of potentially nephrotoxic combinations. A suggested scheme for the empiric therapy of pneumonia is outlined in Table 2. Therapy for community-acquired pneumonia in individuals without host defense impairment is directed against *Streptococcus pneumoniae* and *Legionella pneumophila.* When host impairments are present, such

TABLE 2   Empiric Antibiotic Therapy of Pneumonia

	Putative Pathogens Treated
Community acquired	
No Host Impairment	
Erythromycin, 1 g IV every 6 hours or doxycycline, 100 mg IV every 12 hours	*Streptococcus pneumoniae, Legionella pneumophila, Mycoplasma pneumoniae*
Host Impairment	
Erythromycin, as above	*Streptococcus pneumoniae, Legionella pneumophila,* enteric gram-negative bacilli (except some *Pseudomonas* species), *Haemophilus influenzae,* most *Staphylococcus aureus*
Plus	
Cefoperazone,* 2 g IV every 12 hours, or trimethoprim-sulfamethoxazole,† 2 vials IV every 6 hours	
Institution or hospital acquired	
Aminoglycoside,† gentamicin, 1.75 mg/kg IV, loading dose, followed by 1.5 mg/kg every 8 hours; or amikacin 7.5 mg/kg every 12 hours	Enteric gram-negative bacilli (including *Pseudomonas aeruginosa*)
Plus cefoperazone* or trimethoprim-sulfamethoxazole†	*Haemophilus influenzae, Streptococcus pneumoniae,* gram-negative synergism
Plus erythromycin‡	*Legionella pneumophila*
Postinfluenza	
Cefotaxime*† 2 g every 8 hours	*Haemophilus influenzae, Staphylococcus aureus, Streptococcus pneumoniae,* enteric gram-negative bacilli

*Other third-generation cephalosporins can be used.
†Reduce dosage in renal insufficiency.
‡If *Legionella pneumophila* is highly suspect.

as advanced age or immunosuppressive therapy, coverage for enteric gram-negative bacilli is added. Patients receiving chemotherapy who have neutropenia must have adequate anti-*Pseudomonas* coverage. When pneumonia develops in an individual who is hospitalized or confined to a nursing-home, therapy is geared toward enteric gram-negative bacteria (including *Pseudomonas aeruginosa*), *Haemophilus influenzae,* pneumococcus, and *Legionella.* The patient who develops pneumonia after influenza may be treated with a third-generation cephalosporin that has activity against *Haemophilus influenzae, Staphylococcus aureus,* and pneumococcus.

Certain precautions should be employed when using antibiotics for lung infection. In patients who have a reduction in body water and lean body mass along with an increase in body fat, such as the elderly, there may be a relative rise in blood and tissue levels of drugs administered on a dose per body weight basis. When serum albumin is reduced, more drug can diffuse into tissues, especially if the drug is ordinarily protein-bound. Such an effect would be seen with the cephalosporins, oxacillin, and many penicillins, whereas aminoglycosides have little binding to albumin and their levels are not greatly affected by changes in serum albumin. Drug dosages must be adjusted in the presence of liver or renal dysfunction when excretion occurs by these routes. Drugs excreted by the liver include nafcillin, ampicillin (Omnipen), erythromycin, and chloramphenicol. Renally cleared drugs include penicillins, aminoglycosides, and some cephalosporins. To ensure the best patient outcome with the minimum toxicity, aminoglycoside therapy should be accompanied by monitoring of serum levels. In one study, a reduced survival with gram-negative pneumonia was seen in patients who had low peak serum aminoglycoside concentrations. On the other hand, nephrotoxicity can occur if the dose is too high.

The penetration of antibiotics into sputum is highly variable, and often sputum antibiotic levels are lower than serum levels. For example, ampicillin achieves 3 percent of serum levels in bronchial secretions, some cephalosporins reach 25 percent of serum levels, erythromycin reaches 40 percent of serum levels, and the aminoglycosides reach anywhere from 27 to 65 percent of serum levels. In the presence of lung inflammation, bronchial concentrations of antibiotics may reach higher levels. Although the clinical relevance of bronchial penetration of antibiotics is not fully known, it is possible that higher local levels of antibiotic than can be achieved with intravenous therapy are required to achieve a good therapeutic outcome. If this is the case, then there may be a rationale for using topical antibiotics to treat pneumonia.

Local application of antibiotics can be achieved by aerosolization or direct intratracheal injection. Both routes give adequate bronchial levels of drug and good distribution. Direct injection can only be used in the presence of an endotracheal tube or tracheostomy but may be able to achieve higher concentrations than aerosol therapy in infected areas. A patient who receives a direct tracheal injection of antibiotic is placed in the lateral decubitus position with the infected lung down, and the drug is generally distributed to only the infected lung, whereas aerosol therapy reaches both the healthy and the infected lung. Endobronchial antibiotics may induce bronchospasm, but they are not absorbed systemically to a large extent and thus concomitant intravenous therapy does not need to be modified. Less systemic absorption of aminoglycosides occurs after aerosol therapy than after direct inoculation. Although clinical studies documenting the efficacy of endotracheal antibiotics for established infection are limited, they may be helpful to patients with cystic fibrosis and those with severe gram-negative pneumonias, including those caused by *Pseudomonas aeruginosa.* Currently, this mode of therapy is probably best reserved as a supplemental approach to be used only in patients with severe gram-negative pneumonia that has not responded to conventional therapy. The use of endotracheal antibiotics to prevent pneumonia may also have some merit.

If the decision is made to use antibiotics via the endobronchial route, all patients should be pretreated with an inhaled bronchodilator, and the medication should be given in intervals of every 4 to 8 hours. In any therapy session, the total dose should be contained in a 2- to 10-ml volume. The most commonly nebulized drugs are polymyxin and the aminoglycosides; penicillins are rarely used for fear that they might induce hypersensitivity. Gentamicin (Garamycin) is given in doses of 5 to 120 mg per treatment and polymyxin is given in doses of 5 to 50 mg. When therapy is initiated, a therapist should monitor the patient closely for bronchospasm, using a small test dose and then advancing to a full dose if there is no patient intolerance. Particular caution, especially with the polymyxins, should be exercised when an asthmatic patient is treated.

Oxygen Therapy and Mechanical Ventilation

When pneumonia is complicated by arterial hypoxemia, supplemental oxygen is required. Temporary improvements in oxygenation can be achieved in patients with unilateral infection if the unaffected lung is positioned in a gravity-dependent position. This maneuver increases perfusion to the better ventilated lung and minimizes the shunt effect of the diseased lung. When hypoxemia is treated with supplemental oxygen, the goal should be to maintain an arterial oxygen tension of at least 60 mm Hg to ensure the hemoglobin is at least 90 percent saturated. If adequate oxygenation cannot be achieved without inducing respiratory acidosis, as can occur in some patients with chronic obstructive lung disease, then intubation and mechanical ventilation are required. If pneumonia is the precipitating cause of hypercarbic respiratory failure, intubation is indicated because reversal of the respiratory failure is likely once the pneumonia begins to clear. Other indications for mechanical ventilation in the patient with pneumonia are refractory hypoxemia (inability to maintain an arterial oxygen tension above 60 mm Hg with more than 50 percent supplemental oxygen) and inability to adequately clear the copious secretions associated with infection. In the latter instance, intubation provides access for deep tracheal suctioning and mechanical ventilation assures large tidal volumes, thus eliminating some areas of atelectasis.

When respiratory assistance devices are employed, specific measures must be taken to minimize the risk of their being contaminated and introducing secondary infection. This includes careful cleaning of equipment and the use of humidifying cascades that do not generate aerosols. In addition, personnel who handle these devices should wash their hands after every patient contact. The frequency with which respiratory tubing should be changed is not known precisely, but recent evidence suggests that changing every tubing 24 hours may not be superior to changing it every 48 hours. Tubing contamination poses its greatest risk if colonized water condensate is inadvertently washed back into the patient when the tubing is manipulated. Several studies have shown that patients can contaminate the tubing with their own endogenous colonizing flora and that these organisms can multiply to large numbers in the tubing condensate. If this condensate is washed into the patient as the tubing is moved about, a bolus intratracheal inoculation with bacteria can occur.

Chest Physiotherapy

Chest physiotherapy generally consists of a combination of several maneuvers aimed at promoting the clearance and expectoration of respiratory secretions. This "ketchup-bottle" approach to therapy can employ components of postural drainage, chest percussion, vibration, coughing, and the use of forced expiratory patterns.

Postural drainage is the use of various head-down positions to promote secretion drainage from dependent lung regions. This component of chest physiotherapy appears to be effective in increasing tracheobronchial mucociliary clearance, especially if more than a 15-degree head-down angle is used. Vigorous coughing is also effective in removing secretions, particularly those in the central airways. Data are conflicting as to whether percussion and vibration add

anything to the effect of coughing. Some evidence indicates that this therapy may supplement cough by acting primarily to move peripheral secretions into the central airways, where they can be expectorated. In patients with a depressed ability to cough, percussion and vibration may be particularly helpful. The use of one or two forced expirations from a normal or low lung volume, followed by a period of diaphragmatic breathing, may be another effective method to move secretions from peripheral lung regions to the central airways.

There are very few data that specifically evaluate the efficacy of chest physiotherapy for enhancing the resolution of pneumonia. One widely quoted study showed no efficacy for this modality in pneumonia patients, but the exclusion criteria of the study make the results difficult to apply to all patients. In that study, patients had scant respiratory secretions, and conditions associated with copious secretions (such as bronchiectasis, lung abscess, and cystic fibrosis) were not included. Furthermore, patients with depressed cough, such as those with recent stroke, were omitted, as were patients with hypercarbic respiratory failure. In other studies of patients with increased secretions, chest physiotherapy may have benefit for the pneumonia patient. The sum of all these data appears to be that pneumonia patients with copious secretions (more than 30 ml per day) or depressed cough ability should receive chest physiotherapy. This treatment should consist of postural drainage, forced expiration and cough, and when the latter is ineffective, percussion and vibration should be added.

Mucolytic and Mucokinetic Agents

Agents that affect the physical properties of mucus, reducing its viscosity and consistency, are defined as mucolytic. On the other hand, some therapies act to increase mucociliary clearance without altering the composition of the mucus, and these drugs can be viewed as mucokinetic. In reality, many drug therapies lead to both mucolytic and mucokinetic actions, so that there is considerable overlap between these two therapeutic modalities. In the treatment of pneumonia, no studies have shown an effective role for these agents. Nonetheless, their application would seem appropriate for the infected patient with thick, tenacious sputum that leads to retained secretions with or without atelectasis.

The most commonly employed mucolytic therapy is intravenous hydration. Patients with pneumonia may have increased respiratory water loss, which can be accentuated when fever is present. To preserve vital organ function and to liquefy secretions, vigorous systemic hydration is routinely employed. Respiratory tract hydration can also be achieved with bland aerosols of water and various concentrations of saline solution. When these therapies are given by means of a humidifier, little water actually reaches the lung, but with ultrasonic nebulizers, large amounts of liquid, enough to cause pulmonary edema, do reach the lower respiratory tract. Although the inhalation of pure water appears to have minimal effect on sputum viscosity, saline may lead to more marked alterations. Saline, particularly in hypertonic form, may liquefy secretions and stimulate a productive cough. At this time, there is no proven basis on which to recommend bland aerosol therapy for pneumonia, except that saline should probably be used as the routine diluent when other medications are nebulized into the bronchial tree.

Other available aerosolized mucolytics include N-acetylcysteine (Mucomyst), pancreatic dornase, trypsin, tyloxapol, and sodium bicarbonate. The most frequently used of these agents is probably N-acetylcysteine, which acts to disrupt disulfide bridges between mucoprotein strands. Although it can effectively reduce the viscosity of purulent sputum, it has no proven role in the treatment of lung infections and can induce bronchospasm and inhibit ciliary activity. At this time, its only use in the therapy of pneumonia would be for patients with known atelectasis due to retained secretions.

When N-acetylcysteine is given an inhaled bronchodilator should precede its administration. The drug is best administered by direct instillation of 1 to 2 ml of a 20 percent solution along with an equal volume of 2 to 5 percent sodium bicarbonate. Optimal activity occurs at alkaline pH, and little activity is preserved below a pH of 7.0. Contact with metals and rubber should be avoided, since these substances can lead to drug breakdown. If N-acetylcysteine is to be given via a nebulizer, again 2 ml, along with an equal volume of normal saline or sodium bicarbonate, is the recommended dose. Ultrasonic nebulization should not be used in the place of a routine nebulizer, as the mist may be too irritating.

A variety of pharmacologic agents can stimulate ciliary activity and serve as mucokinetics. Many of these agents are bronchodilators and should be used if pneumonia coexists with obstructive airway disease. When bronchodilators are used to relieve airway obstruction, secretions can be more effectively eliminated, and the mucokinetic action of these drugs will provide an additional theoretic benefit. However, in the absence of obstruction, these agents cannot be recommended for their mucokinetic effects alone, as there is no established role for their use in the therapy of lung infection. Bronchodilator drugs that enhance ciliary activity include beta agonists such as isoproterenol, terbutaline, and salbutamol; the theophyllines; and prednisolone. Other mucokinetics, include digitalis, potassium iodide, and acetylcholine.

Other Measures

When pneumonia is complicated by lobar atelectasis, especially in the absence of an air bronchogram, there may be central airway obstruction, and bronchoscopy may be indicated. If the central obstruction is the result of retained secretions, the bronchoscope can remove them, although chest physiotherapy may be just as effective. Bronchoscopy offers the advantage of rapid lung reexpansion in the physiologically compromised patient with atelectasis. In addition, when endobronchial obstruction appears on chest x-ray and the pneumonia is not resolving clinically, bronchoscopy is indicated to look for an aspirated foreign body or an obstructing endobronchial tumor. It must be recognized, however, that the radiologic resolution for pneumonia may be slow, especially in the immunocompromised patient, and bronchoscopy is only recommended if there is markedly delayed resolution (failure of the radiologic appearance to improve at all after 5 to 7 days) with signs of bronchial obstruction.

Other adjunctive measures that may speed the resolution of lung infection include the use of nutritional support and the elimination or dose reduction of immunosuppressive drugs (such as corticosteroids) when possible. Although hyperalimentation has not been investigated as a therapeutic modality for pneumonia, there are many studies showing impairment of pulmonary host defenses in the presence of malnutrition. In the future, we may find a benefit in using aggressive and early nutritional support of the patient with respiratory infection.

Suggested Reading

Graham WGB, Bradley DA. Efficacy of chest physiotherapy and intermittent positive-pressure breathing in the resolution of pneumonia. N Engl J Med 1978; 299:624–627.

Kiriloff LH, Owens GR, Rogers RM, Massocco MC. Does chest physical therapy work? Chest 1985; 88:436–444.

Niederman MS, Fein AM. The interaction of infection the adult respiratory distress syndrome. Crit Care Clin 1986; 2:471–495.

Verghese A, Berk SL. Bacterial pneumonia in the elderly. Medicine 1983; 62:271–285.

Wanner A, Rao A. Clinical indications for and effects of bland, mucolytic and antimicrobial aerosols. Am Rev Respir Dis 1980; 122:79–87.

MANAGEMENT OF ADULT RESPIRATORY DISTRESS SYNDROME (ARDS)

BARRY A. SHAPIRO, M.D.

Severe systemic insults commonly cause lung parenchymal dysfunction by means of multiple chemical mediators. Such parenchymal damage has been recently called acute lung injury (ALI), a spectrum that starts predominantly as endothelial cell malfunction that progresses to both epithelial and endothelial cell malfunction. Decreased compliance and hypoxemia are the two principal clinical concerns in ALI.

Altered endothelial cell permeability commonly is the first identifiable abnormality and results in an increased movement of water and colloid into the lung interstitium. This movement most commonly results in a noncardiogenic edema (NCE). The adult respiratory distress syndrome (ARDS) is morphologically described as diffuse cellular damage to both the endothelium and the epithelium.

Type 1 epithelial cells are relatively vulnerable to injury and have limited reparative capabilities. At least three sequelae of type 1 cell damage have been documented: (1) alveolar edema secondary to a breach in the normally water-tight alveolar epithelium, (2) atelectasis owing to impairment of the mechanisms normally assuring alveolar stability, and (3) decreased lung compliance owing to disruption of the surfactant layer, loss of normal "stretchability" of type 1 cells, and atelectasis.

Type 2 epithelial cells are the least susceptible to injury and have remarkable reparative capabilities. However, severe type 2 cell injury results in irreversible fibrosis of the gas exchange unit. Type 2 cells produce surfactant, and increased metabolic demands or direct insult to type 2 cells is believed to alter surfactant, thus resulting in severely decreased lung compliance and refractory hypoxemia.

CLINICAL DIAGNOSIS OF ALI

ALI refers to a clinical spectrum ranging from mild disease (pulmonary edema) to severe illness (ARDS). There appears to be general agreement that patients with multiple trauma, with sepsis, and with disseminated intravascular coagulopathy (DIC) are at high risk. Combinations of other physiologic insults (e.g., aspiration, drug injury, fat embolism, hypotension, interstitial pneumonia, multiple transfusions, operative procedures longer than 8 hours, and poor nutritional status) have been suggested as predisposing factors.

The more severe form of ALI—ARDS—is readily identified by the following: (1) a compatible clinical history and physical findings, (2) refractory hypoxemia (arterial Po_2 less than 60 mm Hg at an FiO_2 of 0.5 or higher), (3) a markedly diminished pulmonary compliance, and (4) a chest roentgenogram with diffuse bilateral parenchymal infiltrates. The less severe or earlier form of this pathology—noncardiogenic pulmonary edema—is more difficult to diagnose. The following features are reasonably reliable: (1) compatible clinical history, (2) FiO_2 of 0.35, or higher, required to maintain an arterial Po_2 greater than 60 mm Hg, (3) absence of chronic lung disease and cardiogenic edema, and (4) chest roentgenogram compatible with noncardiogenic edema and without pneumonic infiltrate or atelectasis.

TOXIC OXYGEN RADICALS AND ALI

Intracellular Biochemistry

Cellular metabolism involves the stepwise reduction of oxygen to water, with the addition of an electron at each step: step 1 produces a superoxide molecule (O_2^-); step 2 produces hydrogen peroxide (H_2O_2); step 3 produces an hydroxyl radical ($\cdot OH^-$); and step 4 produces water. The free radicals O_2^- and $\cdot OH^-$ are highly reactive molecules that tend to cause destructive and unregulated reactions of organic molecules. These free radicals are referred to as "toxic" oxygen radicals because they are capable of damaging cell membranes and mitochondria and of inactivating many cytoplasmic and nuclear enzymes. Mammalian cells contain enzyme systems that rapidly execute the stepwise reduction of oxygen, thereby preventing accumulation of toxic oxygen radicals. Intracellular hyperoxia is known to increase the rate of oxygen metabolism independently of energy demand.

ALVEOLAR HYPEROXIA AND ALI

Small mammals breathing 100 percent oxygen for even several days manifest ALI. These animals are known to rapidly deplete enzymes involved in oxygen reduction and, therefore to accumulate toxic oxygen radicals when hyperoxic. Lung endothelial cells are affected earlier and to a greater extent than epithelial cells.

Primates with normal lungs are known to have adequate enzyme reserves, which prevent accumulation of toxic oxygen radicals in hyperoxic conditions. In certain circumstances, preexistent cellular damage appears to diminish this reserve so that hyperoxic conditions may foster toxic oxygen radicals. The type 2 cell in primates is the most resistant to hyperoxia. As a result, human exposure to high inspired oxygen concentrations that do not damage type 2 cells may only cause noncardiogenic edema, whereas damage to type 2 cells may precipitate ARDS.

In persons with normal lungs, high alveolar oxygen tensions do not result in clinically significant abnormalities. However, previously damaged or stressed lung parenchyma may manifest significant abnormal function when confronted with alveolar oxygen tensions in excess of 250 Torr ($FiO_2 > 0.5$ ambient). There must be no doubt that inspired oxygen concentrations above 50 percent in critically ill patients are potentially damaging to the lung. The unanswered questions pertain to the extent and the relative importance of this damage when compared with other life-threatening processes affecting the patient and to whether FiO_2 below 0.5 may be damaging in some situations.

CHEMICALLY MEDIATED TOXIC OXYGEN RADICALS

Neutrophils, mononuclear cells, and macrophages are consistently found in the interstitium in ARDS. Polymorphonuclear leukocytes (PMNs) are closely associated with the inflammatory process, and their ability to adhere to endothelial cell membranes is believed important for migration from the vascular space. Platelet destruction results in fibrin thrombi (microembolization) that has been clearly documented in ARDS.

Activation of white blood cells (neutrophils, mononuclear cells, and macrophages) and fibrin thrombi is associated with the release of at least three groups of substances: (1) a platelet activating factor that promotes stasis of leukocytes and interstitial edema by activating blood complement factors, (2) leukotrienes (arachidonic acid metabolites) that increase adhesion to endothelial cells and increase vascular permeability, and (3) proteases that inactivate enzyme systems and produce toxic oxygen radicals.

PEEP THERAPY IN ALI

Specific therapy to prevent or to reverse the cellular damage of ALI is not yet available. Therefore, therapy must be aimed at treating the underlying pathology (sepsis, DIC, etc.) and maintaining oxygenation, while creating as beneficial a milieu as possible for lung repair. The best available evidence suggests that this milieu requires reexpansion of the lung and FiO_2 at or below 0.4. These goals are attainable through appropriate application of positive end-expiratory pressure (PEEP) therapy.

CLINICAL ENDPOINTS OF PEEP THERAPY

PEEP therapy is generally believed to benefit patients with acute lung injury because (1) arterial oxygenation is improved, (2) intrapulmonary physiologic shunting (QSP/QT) is reduced, (3) lung compliance (CL) is improved, and (4) inspired oxygen concentrations (FiO_2) can be reduced. However, the degree of PEEP therapy that provides the greatest benefit with the fewest nonbeneficial effects is difficult to define or to monitor clinically. To understand the various proposed "endpoints" for titrating PEEP therapy as they relate to ALI, it is necessary to review the seven factors most commonly studied:

1. Arterial oxygen tension (PaO_2). If we assume that hemoglobin content is constant, a low PaO_2 represents a significant deficiency in oxygen content (oxyhemoglobin plus dissolved oxygen). Improvement in PaO_2 up to 80 mm Hg reflects significant physiologic increases in oxygen content. A major goal of PEEP therapy is to improve arterial oxygen content.

2. Cardiac output (QT). This measurement requires a pulmonary artery catheter. In nonprimate models, the cardiac output is equal to or less than normal after injury, while in primates and in humans with ARDS the cardiac output is usually greater than normal. There is no clear explanation for this discrepancy.

3. Arterial-venous oxygen content difference ($C[a - v]O_2$). This calculation requires arterial and pulmonary arterial blood samples. It represents the volume of oxygen extracted from 100 ml of blood and is not necessarily reflective of total-body oxygen extraction per minute (VO_2). Acute stress has been demonstrated to cause cardiac output increases that outstrip increased oxygen demands, resulting in $C(a - v)O_2$ less than normal (3 to 4 volume percent). Untreated ARDS in humans usually produces $C(a - v)O_2$ less than 3.0 volume percent.

4. Oxygen delivery (O_2 DEL). This calculation is ten times the cardiac output multiplied by the arterial oxygen content. O_2 DEL is expressed as ml per minute and represents the total oxygen volume presented to the tissues per minute. O_2 DEL is decreased in ARDS.

5. Intrapulmonary physiologic shunting (QSP/QT).

This calculation requires the measurement of FiO_2 plus arterial and pulmonary artery blood samples. The physiologic shunt is dramatically increased in ARDS, usually greater than 30 percent.

6. Deadspace ventilation (*Vd*). Deadspace ventilation can be quantified by calculation of the deadspace to tidal volume ratio (*Vd/Vt*). This requires the collection of exhaled gases over a period of time and an arterial blood sample. Vd is increased in ARDS.

7. Lung compliance (CL). A reflection of total pulmonary compliance is available by calculating the effective static compliance (ESC). Lung compliance and ESC are severely diminished in patients with ARDS.

Extrapolation of available data in both animals and humans allows for these seven factors to be placed in the general schema depicted in Figure 1. The graphs represent preinjury levels, postinjury stabilized levels, and levels after incremental applications of PEEP therapy. It is assumed that the FiO_2 remains at 0.5, that the pH and Pco_2 remain acceptable, and that appropriate fluid therapy is administered. In our experience, in patients with ALI in whom intravascular volume and hemoglobin concentrations are appropriately maintained, the PEEP level at which a PaO_2 of 60 mm Hg is achieved with an FiO_2 of 0.4 or less corresponds to the classic PEEP endpoints of Optimal PEEP, Best PEEP, etc.

PRACTICAL APPROACH TO RESPIRATORY THERAPY IN ALI

The initiation of PEEP therapy should be seriously considered as soon as ALI is diagnosed. The primary goal of PEEP therapy in ALI is to accomplish adequate arterial oxygen content (with an adequate hemoglobin content this is achieved at arterial PO_2 greater than 60 mm Hg) at FiO_2 below 0.5 without significantly reducing cardiac output. This goal should provide adequate tissue oxygenation while avoiding potentially detrimental alveolar oxygen concentrations. I have found that an FiO_2 of 0.4 is an attainable and practical goal in most circumstances. Although PEEP is most consistently and reliably administered via endotracheal or tracheostomy tube, mask CPAP up to 15 cm H_2O PEEP is technically feasible and may prove beneficial in many patients who are not intubated. Patients with noncardiogenic edema usually show significant improvement in gas exchange with 5 to 15 cm H_2O PEEP, and most patients respond optimally with 10 cm H_2O PEEP. Others with ARDS are usually improved with 10 to 30 cm H_2O PEEP, and most of these patients manifest an optimal response between 10 and 20 cm H_2O PEEP. Positive

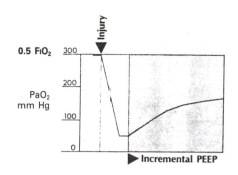

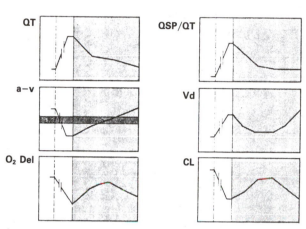

Figure 1 Graphic depiction of seven factors recommended for use as clinical monitors to determine the required level of PEEP therapy in humans with ARDS. Each graph represents the effects of increasing (left to right) PEEP level. QT = cardiac output. Unlike anesthetized animal models, which show a decreased cardiac output postinjury, humans respond to ARDS with a significantly increased cardiac output. $C(a − v)O_2$ = the arterial-mixed venous oxygen content difference. The horizontal gray band represents 3 to 4 volume percent. O_2 DEL = oxygen delivery expressed as ml per min (cardiac output × arterial oxygen context × 10). QSP/QT = physiologic intrapulmonary shunt; Vd = deadspace ventilation; CL = lung compliance.

end-expiratory pressure should be increased or decreased in increments of 3 to 5 cm H_2O, and the effects of these changes should be evaluated within 20 minutes. Positive pressure ventilation may be administered to normal lungs for prolonged periods without apparent lung damage; however, excessively high pressures can impair type 2 cell functions. When PEEP levels are not excessive, spontaneous ventilation results in better arterial oxygenation and less cardiovascular embarrassment. Most available data support the idea that spontaneous ventilation in conjunction with PEEP therapy enhances the pulmonary effects (increased transpulmonary pressures resulting in increased functional residual capacity [FRC]) while reducing detrimental effects on cardiac function (less rise in intrapleural pressures).

In my opinion, there are no absolute contraindications to the use of PEEP therapy in ALI. Data suggesting that clinically appropriate levels of PEEP can produce barotrauma are unconvincing. While patients requiring PEEP therapy for severe ALI (ARDS) have an increased incidence of barotrauma, this appears to be related to the severity of the parenchymal disease, rather than to the level of applied airway pressure therapy.

STEROID THERAPY FOR ALI

Steroids are known to decrease white blood cell adherence to endothelial cells and to stabilize cell wall membranes of type 2 cells when administered before the systemic insult. The role of steroids in the clinical management of ALI remains controversial. At best, steroid therapy appears to be helpful in preventing ALI after certain insults, such as fat embolization.

Fluid Therapy for ALI

One of the frustrations in treating NCE is the disappointing response to diuretics. In cardiogenic edema, diuresis provides reduction in microvascular pressures and thus decreases interstitial water. Diuresis does not decrease extravascular water (EVW) in NCE. Rather, vigorous diuresis may cause hypovolemia and thereby depress cardiac output.

The clinical problem of wet lung unresponsive to diuretic therapy is compounded by the need to maintain adequate vascular volume. Although relative hypervolemia should be avoided, it is not uncommon for ALI patients to require fluids to maintain euvolemia. The cardinal rule in managing ALI remains "adequate fluid administration with avoidance of vascular overload."

Positive end-expiratory pressure increases intrapleural pressure. This fact must be considered when interpreting central venous or pulmonary artery occlusion pressure (PAOP) measurements. The position of the catheter is important because it must lie in a constantly perfused area of lung to properly reflect pulmonary venous pressures. There is no advantage to removing the airway pressure before measuring pulmonary artery catheter pressures because this maneuver has been shown to give unreliable data. Measurements should always be made at end-exhalation. Variations in intrapleural pressure must be evaluated carefully and baselines established where appropriate. Remember that the trend reflected by these measurements is far more valuable than the absolute numbers. Common sense and sound clinical judgment must prevail.

The question of whether vascular volume should be maintained by colloid or by crystalloid infusion has attracted inordinate attention. Studies within the last 10 years have been equivocal and have led to the conclusion that, in most instances, there is little advantage to colloid therapy. Because ALI involves endothelial permeability abnormalities, colloids should not be expected to effectively remove water from the interstitium; in fact, colloids may worsen the edema. I believe that crystalloid solutions should be used to maintain vascular volume, unless a clear rationale for colloid therapy is present.

Suggested Reading

Fox RB, Hoidal JR, Brown DM, et al. Pulmonary inflammation due to oxygen toxicity: involvement of chemotactic factors and polymorphonuclear leukocytes. Am Rev Respir Dis 1981; 123:521–523.

Petty TL, Ashbaugh DG. The adult respiratory distress syndrome: clinical features, factors influencing prognosis and principles of management. Chest 1971; 60:233–239.

Shapiro BA, Cane RD. Fluid and electrolyte management in critical care. In: Askanazi J, Starker PM, Weissman C, eds. Pulmonary edema. Stoneham, MA: Butterworth Publishers, 1986:229.

Shapiro BA, Cane RD. Metabolic malfunction of the lung: non-cardiogenic edema and adult respiratory distress syndrome. Surg Annu 1981; 13:271–298.

Shapiro BA, Cane RD, Harrison RA. Positive end-expiratory pressure therapy in adults with special reference to acute lung injury: a review of the literature and suggested clinical correlations. Crit Care Med 1984; 12:127–141.

Shapiro BA, Harrison RA, Kacmarek RM, Cane RD. Clinical application of respiratory care. 3rd ed. Chicago: Year Book Medical Publishers, 1985.

SLEEP APNEA AND HYPOVENTILATION SYNDROMES

T. SCOTT JOHNSON, M.D.

This chapter will focus on the management of sleep apnea and of states of hypoventilation. These syndromes have in common a defective control of ventilation, either manifested during wakefulness by alveolar hypoventilation (elevated PCO_2) or during sleep by obstructive or central apneas. Specifically excluded from this discussion are patients with definable restrictive or obstructive lung diseases, such as chronic obstructive pulmonary disease (COPD), pulmonary fibrosis, or myasthenia gravis, which also may result in alveolar hypoventilation. Although many of the principles discussed will apply to these diseases, treatment directed towards the patient's major cause of lung dysfunction remains the first line approach to therapy in these conditions.

Considerable overlap exists between the clinical syndromes of hypoventilation and sleep apnea. For example, most patients who hypoventilate while awake exhibit disordered breathing during sleep. The converse is less frequent, however; only a rare patient with sleep apnea is found to exhibit daytime hypoventilation. Some predisposing conditions, such as hypothyroidism, can lead to hypoventilation, to sleep apnea, or to both. Finally, many of the therapeutic options can be applied to either condition.

DIAGNOSIS

A diagnosis of hypoventilation syndrome is made when an arterial blood gas sample that is drawn when the patient is awake demonstrates an elevated PCO_2, and when there is no intrinsic pulmonary disease, neuromuscular weakness, or chest wall deformity to account for the hypercapnia. Mild diaphragmatic weakness from neuromuscular disease may be extremely occult and therefore difficult to distinguish from idiopathic hypoventilation. Other treatable primary causes should be sought and excluded as well, such as metabolic alkalosis, hypothyroidism, or overuse of sedatives or narcotics. Many of the patients are morbidly obese (obesity-hypoventilation syndrome). The disturbance in ventilatory control can be established in the pulmonary function laboratory by demonstrating an abnormally low ventilatory response to hypoxia or to hypercapnia. A less rigorous, but easily performed bedside test involves having the patient voluntarily hyperventilate and then measuring pre- and post-hyperventilation blood gases. The ability to reduce the PCO_2 by at least 10 torr strongly suggests that a defect in central ventilatory control exists.

Patients are usually suspected of having sleep apnea on the basis of excessive daytime sleepiness or of nocturnal sleep disturbance. Observations by a bed partner of restless sleep, loud snoring, or pauses in breathing lend strong support to the clinical diagnosis. A nocturnal polysomnogram should then be performed, both to establish the diagnosis and its severity and to make the crucial distinction between central and obstructive forms of sleep apnea. Further testing may be necessary to determine if any underlying endocrine, neurologic, or upper airway obstructive disease is present (Table 1). Cephalometric roentgenograms and an ear, nose and throat (ENT) examination are usually required. The majority of patients are found, after such evaluations, to be middle-aged men with "idiopathic" obstructive sleep apnea. Approximately 50 percent of them are obese, and many exhibit anatomic narrowing of the upper airway.

TREATMENT

Based on the preceding considerations, therapy must first be directed towards any treatable underlying condition. However, only a minority of patients are found to have a treatable underlying cause. The remaining approaches are based on the presumed pathogenesis of a decreased central drive (as with central sleep apnea or with hypoventilation syndromes) and/or a structural or a functional obstruction of the upper airway (obstructive sleep apnea). The following therapies are not mutually exclusive and, in fact, are frequently used in some combination.

Weight Loss

Weight loss is associated with an amelioration of symptoms for the obese-hypoventilating patient and for the patient with obstructive sleep apnea. Exact mechanisms are unclear. Loss of fat from around the neck and from within the pharyngeal structures may improve upper airway patency. Reduction of abdominal and chest wall mass may improve respiratory mechanics. Ventilatory drive may increase following weight loss. Often, only modest weight reduction is

305

sufficient to achieve the desired effect. The obvious problem with weight reduction is that only a small percentage of patients can comply. Another problem is that weight reduction cannot provide immediate results for the symptomatic patient. Despite these drawbacks, weight loss should be recommended as part of a comprehensive treatment program for all obese patients and even for nonobese patients with obstructive sleep apnea.

Medications

Acetazolamide

Acetazolamide (Diamox) is a carbonic anhydrase inhibitor that leads to a nonanion gap metabolic acidosis through the loss of sodium, potassium, and bicarbonate in the urine. Respiratory stimulation ensues, owing to the acid pH bathing the central medullary chemoreceptors. The actual ventilatory response in any individual patient is difficult to predict. Some patients exhibit marked decrease from their baseline PCO_2 and others register little change. Consequently, obtaining arterial blood gas levels is imperative, both before treatment and after a few days of treatment with this agent. Acetazolamide should be used cautiously in patients who have respiratory acidosis before treatment to be sure they do not become dangerously acidemic. This agent has been most successful in managing central sleep apnea. Occasionally, there is a benefit to patients with idiopathic hypoventilation. Acetazolamide has no role in the treatment of obstructive sleep apnea. This drug is safe and relatively inexpensive (approximately $10 per month). Absorption is rapid from the gastrointestinal tract and excretion is by the kidney. The usual dose is 250 mg four times a day. From 1 to 2 weeks is required before the maximal effect is seen. The main side effects are paresthesias and occasional drowsiness, and these effects tend to wane as drug use continues.

Medroxyprogesterone Acetate

Medroxyprogesterone acetate (Provera) has been used successfully in hypoventilation syndromes (especially with obesity) and in both central and obstructive sleep apnea. Effect is achieved through action on central chemoreceptors and it heightens both hypercapnic and hypoxic respiratory drives. Patients with obesity-hypoventilation and those patients with sleep apnea who exhibit the full-blown pickwickian syndrome (obesity, excessive sleepiness, hypercapnia, and cor pulmonale) seem to have the best response to this drug. Patients with snoring and with mild to moderate obstructive sleep apnea do not respond favorably to this drug and may, in fact, experience more severe upper airway obstruction owing to the increased negative force of inspiration. The standard dose of medroxyprogesterone acetate is 20 mg three times per day. This dose can be increased to 40 mg three times a day, although this is rarely necessary. An effect is manifested within 4 to 7 days; usually the PCO_2 falls by 5 to 10 torr. In those patients who respond, central and/or obstructive apneas decrease. Excessive daytime somnolence and cor pulmonale improve. This drug has been used sublingually, but is absorbed through the gut. Provera is rapidly metabolized by the liver and excreted by both the liver and the kidney. There are few side effects, but some patients do complain of impotence. The main drawback to use is the expense. The average cost for a one-month course of treatment is over $75. Other measures, such as weight loss or nasal continuous positive airway pressure (CPAP), are commonly used in conjunction with Provera.

Protriptyline

Protriptyline (Vivactil) is the only drug for sleep apnea that has been subjected to a controlled, double-blind trial. Total apnea time for obstructive sleep apnea was reduced primarily by the curtailment of the quantity of rapid eye movement (REM) sleep. Since apneas are more frequent and of longer duration dur-

TABLE 1   Conditions Associated With Sleep Apnea

Central	Obstructive
Arnold-Chiari malformation	Hypothyroidism
Cardiac failure	Acromegaly
Poliomyelitis	Testosterone administration
Encephalitis	Micrognathia/retrognathia
Brain stem tumor	Pierre Robin syndrome
Brain stem infarction	Posterior fossa disease
Cervical cordotomy	Adenotonsillar hypertrophy
Idiopathic	Shy-Drager syndrome
Aging (?)	Myotonic dystrophy
	Nasal obstruction
	Parkinson's disease (?)
	Aging (?)

ing REM sleep, the reduction of REM improves breathing during sleep. The drug may also increase upper airway patency by augmenting the tone of upper airway muscles. This agent is a tricyclic antidepressant and shares the properties common to this class of medications. Protriptyline is one of the least sedating of these agents, and in fact, most patients feel more alert during the daytime while taking it. Bed partners often report that the patient is snoring less. Unfortunately, this drug causes frequent side effects, especially among middle-aged men in whom sleep apnea most commonly presents. Particularly bothersome are the anticholinergic side effects, such as constipation and urinary retention. Impotence has been reported. These problems, as well as alternative treatments for obstructive sleep apnea, have limited the use of this agent to a small number of patients. This drug deserves consideration in the unusual patient with both narcolepsy and sleep apnea because it is especially effective in narcolepsy. Also, protriptyline is worth trying in the patient with mild to moderate obstructive sleep apnea who does not desire surgery, is not overweight, and does not want to utilize nasal CPAP.

Oxygen Therapy

Oxygen therapy is a two-edged sword in the management of hypoventilation and of sleep apnea. While treating the hypoxemia, oxygen carries the potential of diminishing an already attenuated respiratory drive in the patient with hypoventilation and therefore can lead to further CO_2 retention and narcosis. In the patient with sleep apnea, oxygen tends to increase the mean oxygen saturation, but usually prolongs the apneas as well. In a small number of patients (who cannot be identified beforehand by available clinical criteria), oxygen may actually decrease the frequency of apneas, but this needs to be verified in the controlled setting of the sleep laboratory prior to institution in the home. Generally, oxygen has been administered during sleep via nasal prongs at a rate of between 2 and 4 L per minute. There are no known sequelae of oxygen used in this fashion.

Surgery

A variety of surgical approaches have been utilized in the management of hypoventilation and of sleep apnea. One approach to be mentioned simply in passing is surgery to treat obesity for the morbidly obese patient. In recent years, this surgery has been largely confined to gastric stapling or plication. A high rate of complications is common to all types of surgery in these patients. Those complications related to specific procedures will be mentioned later, but in general,

these patients tolerate surgery poorly because of respiratory problems, such as difficult intubation, ventilatory depression attributable to sedatives, postoperative pneumonia, pulmonary embolism, and respiratory failure. Consequently, all surgical procedures should be undertaken extremely cautiously in these precarious patients.

Tracheostomy to treat obstructive sleep apnea has lost favor in recent years. However, this procedure still remains the most definitive treatment for this condition and results in nearly 100 percent success in restoring normal breathing and sleep within a matter of days after the operation. Because of its success, tracheostomy must be considered the gold standard treatment for obstructive sleep apnea. Unfortunately, there are far too many complications for widespread use. These complications include a high frequency of stomal infections, stomal hemorrhage, and tracheal stenosis. Furthermore, patients object to the stigmata of a chronic tracheostomy. If tracheostomy is deemed necessary, an uncuffed, fenestrated tube with an inner diameter of 5 to 7 mm is most appropriate. Alternatives to the standard tracheostomy tube include various buttons or Silastic cannulae that protrude minimally into the trachea and that are flush with the skin (e.g., Olympus tracheostomy button). Both types of appliance are closed during the daytime to allow normal speech and breathing and are opened at night to bypass the upper airway obstruction. The advent of other measures, particularly nasal CPAP, has diminished the role of tracheostomy in managing patients with severe obstructive sleep apnea complicated by life-threatening heart failure, malignancy arrhythmias, or dangerous and disabling daytime somnolence.

Surgical revision of the upper airway continues to evolve and shows promise for the management of obstructive sleep apnea. For the past 5 years, uvulopalatopharyngoplasty (or a variant thereof) has been the most widely performed operation for the surgical treatment of obstructive sleep apnea. This procedure involves the removal of the uvula and a portion of the soft palate. The tonsils are removed and redundant mucosa is trimmed from the lateral and posterior walls of the pharynx. Often this procedure is combined with a nasal septoplasty. As many as 80 percent of patients undergoing this procedure experience an improvement in symptoms. Snoring is often completely alleviated. However, fewer than 50 percent are improved as judged by objective polysomnographic criteria. Complications are infrequent and include nasopharyngeal stenosis, nasal regurgitation of fluids, and throat discomfort. At this point, better selection criteria and perhaps some refinement in this operation are apparently still needed.

A minority of patients can be successfully treated with a less extensive procedure on the upper airway, such as nasal septoplasty or tonsillectomy-adenoidectomy alone. Likewise, more complex procedures, such as mandibular advancement or mandibulo-maxillary reconstruction, have successfully eliminated sleep apnea in selected patients, especially those with definable jaw abnormalities. Recent studies suggest that these latter approaches may be more widely applied in the future.

Mechanical Devices

Over 200 patents have been granted by the United States Patent Office for antisnoring devices. Attempts also have been made to control sleep apnea using mechanical devices.

The most successful approach to date has been the application of nasal continuous positive airway pressure (CPAP) (see the chapter on *Mask and Nasal Continuous Positive Airway Pressure*). With this device, a high-flow blower motor delivers room air through a hose to a soft plastic mask that fits tightly around the nose. A positive end-expiratory pressure (PEEP) valve is used to establish a positive pressure in the system of from 5 to 15 cm H_2O. A positive pressure is thus created in the pharynx that offsets the negative pressure of inspiration and, in the simplest fashion, provides a pneumatic splint to maintain the patency of the otherwise obstructing upper airway. This device is commercially available and has FDA approval for treating sleep apnea. The patient must be studied in a sleep laboratory in order to establish the effectiveness and to determine the pressure necessary to maintain upper airway patency. Only rarely is nasal CPAP unsuccessful in eliminating obstructive sleep apnea. Anecdotally, nasal CPAP also may be effective in some cases of central sleep apnea, though reasons for its effectiveness are unclear. Some theoretical complications, such as hypotension and barotrauma, have not been observed in clinical practice. Perhaps the biggest problem is simply maintaining patient compliance. A diligent and responsive home care company that spends the initial time educating the patient can be extremely helpful in achieving a high rate of compliance. Also, patients who have successfully employed nasal CPAP often volunteer to provide support to the novice user. Other minor complications include nasal drying and irritation, annoyance from the noise level of the blower, and sleep fragmentation. Pressure on the upper teeth may change the patient's bite. Despite these problems, an acceptance rate of 75 to 80 percent can be expected. Long-term studies have indicated that the motivated patient can wear this device indefinitely with excellent results. Nasal CPAP can also provide support for a period of time while other therapeutic modalities, such as weight loss, are being undertaken.

Sleeping position can greatly influence the severity of obstructive sleep apnea in some patients. Lying on the side or in a semirecumbent position may reduce the snoring and apneic events. Sleeping in a reclining chair can reduce mild sleep apnea. Devices to keep patients from lying on their back (which is usually the worst position for obstruction) have included tennis or squash balls sewn into the backs of pajama shirts or electronic sensors that ring a bell when the supine position is assumed. Although based on a sound principle and quite simple, these devices generally have had limited success, but may be worth trying in individuals.

The overwhelming majority of patients with obstructive apnea breathe quite effectively during sleep if the obstruction is alleviated with CPAP, with upper airway surgery, or with tracheostomy. For the rare patient who exhibits severe central sleep apnea after correction of the upper airway, or for patients with primary central sleep apnea or with hypoventilation syndrome who do not respond to respiratory stimulants, a diaphragmatic pacer can be used. The pacing unit is a radio frequency (RF) receiver that is implanted subcutaneously and attached to an electrode that stimulates the ipsilateral phrenic nerve. The energy for pacing is obtained from an external RF transmitter that is placed over the skin where the receiving unit lies. The patient usually must have a permanent tracheostomy. When the patient goes to sleep, the external RF transmitter is turned on and the tracheostomy opened. In most cases, pacing of one hemidiaphragm is sufficient to provide adequate alveolar ventilation during sleep.

THERAPEUTIC STRATEGIES

Given that no controlled or comparative trials are available to guide the clinician in applying the preceding therapeutic alternatives, one must exercise judgment and must undertake empiric trials in each patient. An approach can be formulated based on the available literature and on personal experience. In the following discussion, assume that any primary underlying disease has been excluded or treated (see Table 1).

First, consider obstructive sleep apnea syndrome, since it is the most common of these diseases. Mild cases (up to 100 apneas per 8 hours of sleep) can be treated with weight loss. Revision of the upper airway can be considered, especially if loud snoring that disrupts the spouse is the major complaint. If excessive daytime somnolence is paramount, a trial of protriptyline is warranted. Nasal CPAP can be tried, but is less likely to be of benefit in the mildly affected patient since this procedure is intrinsically disrupting to sleep. Finally, institution of treatment is not imperative but the disease likely will progress with time.

Moderate obstructive sleep apnea (100 to 250 apneas per night) demands more aggressive management, particularly if complications such as hypertension are present. Again, weight loss is urged, but is often insufficient by itself. Nasal CPAP or upper airway revision are the most useful therapies in this situation. I tend to institute nasal CPAP and to simultaneously refer the patient to a skilled surgeon interested in this problem. While the patient is adjusting to CPAP and determining if this therapy is going to be beneficial, he or she can consult with the surgeon. Then the three of us can review the options and decide whether to pursue surgery, to continue CPAP, or both. Needless to say, the patient's wishes figure prominently in this process, since there are no data to strongly favor one approach over another. Severe obstructive sleep apnea (over 250 apneas per night) should be managed similarly, but with consideration of tracheostomy in the rare patient with refractory heart failure, with malignant arrhythmias, or with disabling excessive daytime somnolence that has not responded to more conservative measures. Upright or lateral posture during sleep can be tried in any of the preceding situations, but is less likely to be tolerated by the mildly affected patient and is often insufficient for the severely affected patient.

The obesity-hypoventilation syndrome is usually associated with obstructive sleep apnea and should be treated like severe sleep apnea, except that weight loss is especially emphasized. Also, these patients benefit from Provera and from upright posture during sleep. Except for tracheostomy for the most direly ill, surgery is best postponed because of the excessive risk that these patients present. If obstructive apneas are absent, then a program of weight loss, Provera, and low flow nocturnal oxygen is indicated.

Acetazolamide is the drug of choice for the patient with predominantly central sleep apnea. There may be a role for nasal CPAP in these patients, but this is still being assessed. For the extreme case, consideration must be given to nocturnal support, either with a diaphragmatic pacer or with any of the other negative or positive pressure ventilation devices available.

Suggested Reading

Brownell LG, West P, Sweatman P, Acres JC, Kryger M. Protriptyline in obstructive sleep apnea. N Engl J Med 1982; 307:1037–1042.

Fujita S, Conway W, Zorich F, Roth T. Surgical correction of anatomic abnormalities in obstructive sleep apnea: uvulopalatopharyngoplasty. Otolaryngol Head Neck Surg 1981; 89:923–934.

Gastaut H, Tassinari CA, Duron B. Polygraphic study of the episodic diurnal and nocturnal (hypnic and respiratory) manifestations of the pickwick syndrome. Brain Res 1966; 2:167–186.

Guilleminault C, Tilkian A, Dement WC. The sleep apnea syndromes. Annu Rev Med 1976; 27:465–484.

Remmers JE, deGroot WJ, Sauerland EK, et al. Pathogenesis of airway occlusion during sleep. J Appl Physiol 1978; 44:931–938.

Smith PL, Avram RG, Meyers DA, Haponik EF, Bleecker ER. Weight loss in mildly to moderately obese patients with obstructive sleep apnea. Ann Intern Med 1985; 103:850–855.

Strohl KP, Cherniack NS, Gothe B. Physiologic basis of therapy for sleep apnea. Am Rev Respir Dis 1986; 134:791–802.

Sullivan CE, Berthon-Jones M, Issa FG, Eves L. Reversal of obstructive sleep apnea by continuous positive airway pressure applied through the nares. Lancet 1981; 1:862–865.

Sutton FD, Zwillich CW, Creager CE, et al. Progesterone for outpatient treatment of pickwickian syndrome. Ann Intern Med 1975; 83:476–479.

CHEST TRAUMA

RONALD A. HARRISON, M.D.

Evaluating and treating the chest trauma patient require early attention to the basic principles of resuscitation—airway, breathing, and cardiovascular function—for successful patient outcome. It has been estimated that approximately 25 percent of deaths associated with motor vehicle accidents are secondary to severe chest trauma, many primarily related to inadequate airway, ventilatory, and/or circulatory function. This discussion concentrates on the more commonly encountered injuries and on basic principles that have proven to be extremely beneficial in caring for these patients.

AIRWAY FUNCTION

The patient with an inadequate airway is a common problem that requires immediate attention. Treatment is more complex when the patient also has major facial injuries, because edema and bloody secretions in the oropharynx and nasopharynx increase the difficulty of establishing an endotracheal airway. Also, if the patient has a cervical spinal cord injury, the limited ability to manipulate the head and neck adds to the problem of airway access. Therefore, when a compromised airway is suspected, it is wise to intervene early and establish an artificial airway before significant cardiopulmonary decompensation. The choice of type of airway—whether oral or nasal endotracheal tube versus cricothyroidotomy or tracheostomy tube—depends on the patient's extent of injuries, clinical status, and the individual clinician's expertise. Under most circumstances, my first choice would be to place an oral endotracheal tube under direct vision. In this setting, the ability to skillfully use a fiberoptic laryngoscope is indispensable.

VENTILATORY AND RESPIRATORY FUNCTION

Evaluating breathing capability requires assessing both mechanical and alveolar ventilation and oxygenation status. Simple spirometric measurements of the patient's ventilatory pattern (the product of respiratory frequency and average tidal volume) provide the clinician with a quantitative assessment of the energy expenditure related to the mechanical work of breathing. If the patient is cooperative and can perform a forced vital capacity maneuver, this will give some measure of his or her mechanical ventilatory reserve. It is extremely important to correlate the quantitative mechanical measurements with the patient's type of breathing pattern. In other words, the presence of a diaphragmatic breathing pattern, use of accessory muscles of respiration, forced exhalation, a discoordinate breathing pattern, or paradoxical chest wall movements need to be documented and correlated with the patient's other injuries. The significance of these findings often becomes more obvious in conjunction with other clinical findings. Assessing the adequacy of alveolar (effective) ventilation requires a PCO_2 value obtained from arterial blood gas analysis. The status of alveolar ventilation is even more important in patients with head injuries, because hypercapnia increases cerebral blood flow with a resultant rise in intracranial pressure.

An absolute minimum evaluation of the patient's oxygenation status requires an assessment of arterial PO_2 and oxygen content, which are primarily a reflection of hemoglobin content, and FIO_2. Therefore, it is essential to use oxygen administration systems that provide a consistent FIO_2, i.e., a high flow oxygen delivery system. Only then is it possible for the clinician to reliably correlate changes in arterial oxygen tensions with the patient's clinical state.

CARDIOVASCULAR FUNCTION

Finally, circulatory function is most frequently compromised because of an absolute hypovolemia due to acute blood loss. Besides major blood loss associated with chest injuries, other anatomic areas associated with significant blood loss include vascular injuries in the abdominal cavity and those associated with fractures of the pelvis and femora. The magnitude of external cutaneous blood loss, especially that related to head and neck injuries, is frequently difficult to determine. It is important to remember that previously healthy individuals can acutely lose up to 20 percent of their blood volume with minimal changes in resting baseline cardiovascular parameters. However, if such patients are given narcotics for pain relief, an anesthetic, or even positioned semiupright without adequate volume replacement, the result can be a precipitous deterioration in cardiovascular function. Unless it is contraindicated, the patient can temporarily be placed in a modified reverse Trendelenburg's position. The presence or absence of orthostatic hypotension is a valid assessment of the blood vascular volume to vascular space relationship. The placement of at least two large-bore (preferably no. 14 gauge) intravenous catheters as peripheral and central venous lines is an extremely important early step in treating the chest trauma patient with suspected major blood loss.

CHEST TRAUMA ASSOCIATED WITH MAJOR BLOOD LOSS

Several vascular injuries in the chest will result in significant blood loss and death if unrecognized or improperly treated. Major blood loss associated with a closed hemothorax results in compromise of both cardiovascular and ventilatory function. Standard treatment consists of placement of an anterior chest tube in the midclavicular line at the second rib interspace to remove air, and a posterior chest tube in the midaxillary line at the seventh or eighth rib interspace to remove fluid. If profuse bleeding continues following drainage and reexpansion of the lung, one should suspect a bleeding diathesis most often secondary to decreased platelets, or laceration of a major pulmonary or systemic artery requiring an emergency thoracotomy and definitive surgery. For example, a rupture of the thoracic aorta, or one of its major branches, is a common injury associated with major blood loss in chest trauma. In the majority of cases, this entity is associated with a relatively increased arterial blood pressure in the upper extremities and a widening of the superior mediastinum on chest films. Confirmation of the diagnosis, including localization of the injury, is readily accomplished with aortography.

Before definitive surgical treatment, many chest trauma patients require extensive radiologic evaluation, including computerized tomographic scanning and angiographic studies. Invariably, this necessitates transfer of the patient to areas less than ideal for continued resuscitation and cardiopulmonary monitoring. It is, therefore, imperative to ensure that an adequate airway is present, ventilation or ventilatory support is appropriate, and adequate intravenous access and invasive monitoring lines and equipment are properly functioning before sending the patient for these diagnostic procedures. It is also important that personnel adequately trained in cardiopulmonary physiology and monitoring accompany the patient throughout the procedures.

CHEST TRAUMA CAUSING INADEQUATE MYOCARDIAL PUMP FUNCTION

Nonpenetrating blunt trauma can produce major injuries to cardiovascular structures, along with lung tissue damage. The responsible physical forces include compression-decompression phenomena, sudden acceleration-deceleration actions, and blast or concussive forces. The most frequent cause of nonpenetrating blunt trauma is a motor vehicle accident. Some injuries, such as cardiac rupture or laceration, carry a higher incidence of mortality even with recognition and immediate treatment.

Two common blunt trauma injuries involving the heart and pericardial sac—myocardial contusion and acute cardiac tamponade—merit additional discussion.

Myocardial Contusion

Confirming a diagnosis of myocardial contusion is frequently difficult, since most of the findings and diagnostic tests are not specific to this entity. When sternal fractures or contusions overlying the sternum or precordium are present, the clinician's index of suspicion should be increased. Electrocardiographic changes are highly variable and include nonspecific S-T segment and T-wave changes and the presence of atrial and ventricular ectopic activity. In rare cases, myocardial contusion has been associated with ventricular fibrillation or asystole. Hemodynamic evaluation in patients with myocardial contusion has documented a transient decrease in left ventricular function. Laboratory studies are not always definitive but support the diagnosis when there are significant increases in the myocardial component of serum creatine phosphokinase values. Echocardiography and other diagnostic procedures, such as radionuclide imaging, are often used to help arrive at the diagnosis. Fortunately, myocardial contusion is not usually life-threatening, and its physiologic effects are generally self-limited. Initially, however, careful monitoring of cardiac function is required to treat the aforementioned complications if they arise.

Cardiac Tamponade

Cardiac tamponade is potentially a more serious life-threatening problem than myocardial contusion. It is obviously not the amount of blood loss per se that results in cardiovascular compromise, but the blood loss in a confined space—the pericardial sac. The diagnostic hallmarks include increased venous pressure, decreased arterial pressure, quiet heart tones on auscultation, tachycardia, and pulsus paradoxus. The most readily recognizable sign of cardiac tamponade in the trauma patient is distended neck veins. With catheterization of the heart, the diagnosis is confirmed by the observation that all diastolic pressures within various heart chambers approach the same value. Contrary to traditional thinking, an increase in pulsus paradoxus—an accentuation of that normally observed with respiration—is not a reliable diagnostic sign. Unfortunately, chest film findings of a symmetrically enlarged heart or "water-bottle" silhouette are not always present in the patient with pericardial effusion and tamponade. The preferred short-term treatment in a life-threatening condition is a pericardial tap with removal of a small amount of blood, which can dramatically improve myocardial function. Other supportive techniques include using drugs that have positive inotropic and chronotropic effects on the heart. In addition, volume administration can be used to maximize preload or venous return to the heart. On the other hand, positive-pressure ventilation can have a marked deleterious effect, especially in the hypovolemic patient, because it is prone to decrease venous return to the right side of the heart.

CHEST TRAUMA AND LUNG PARENCHYMAL INJURY

The structural configuration of the pulmonary system makes it highly susceptible to injury both from wounds penetrating the chest wall and from blunt nonpenetrating trauma. In the former case, the degree of lung parenchymal injury tends to be more localized, but often pulmonary vascular injuries are more severe. On the other hand, in blunt trauma, the major insult is usually widespread damage to lung tissue with less tendency to major vascular injury and significant acute blood loss. The therapeutic implications of blunt trauma are that the more serious sequelae tend to be delayed in onset and require a prolonged recovery time. The classic example would be the fully developed acute lung injury (adult respiratory distress syndrome) due to pulmonary contusion. In the worst case, the patient presents with multiple penetrating wounds, major vascular damage, and extensive lung tissue injury from blunt trauma.

PULMONARY VEIN LACERATION

One of the major chest injuries produced by high velocity missiles or stab wounds is laceration of a pulmonary vessel. Laceration of a pulmonary vein, although not as serious as laceration of a pulmonary artery, is still associated with excessive hemoptysis. This can result in flooding of the airways with up to 300 to 400 ml of blood. If the patient has an intact coagulation system, the bleeding is usually self-limited. The immediate problem is to clear the obstructed airways and reestablish appropriate pulmonary gas exchange. Pulmonary vein laceration should not be confused with pulmonary lung contusion, in which the bronchial secretions are serosanguineous or appear as frothy blood-tinged sputum.

When there is major bleeding into the lower airways, it is essential to have a well-established airway to facilitate removal of the bloody secretions. It is just as important to actively support ventilation and use maximum concentrations of oxygen during this stabilization period. When the injury and bleeding are restricted to one side, it is helpful to use a double-lumen tube to separate the right and left lungs. This maneuver can significantly improve the overall ventilation and oxygenation status by maximizing gas transport in the unaffected lung. Unfortunately, this maneuver may not be easily accomplished in the chest trauma patient with concomitant upper airway injuries.

PNEUMOTHORAX AND TENSION PNEUMOTHORAX

Another serious complication of chest trauma is rupture of a branch of the tracheobronchial tree, resulting in a massive intrathoracic air leak. Here the ultimate concern is the development of a tension pneumothorax. A pneumothorax can be defined as an abnormal accumulation of air within a subcompartment in the thoracic cavity. This is usually the intrapleural space, mediastinum (pneumomediastinum), or, on occasion, the pericardial cavity (pneumopericardium). The progressive accumulation of air with increasing intrathoracic pressure adversely affects both pulmonary and myocardial functions. Eventually, this interferes with venous return through the great veins to the right side of the heart, which is the primary reason that tension pneumothorax is such an immediate life-threatening event. The one-way ball valve effect leading to progressive increase in intrathoracic pressure is greatly accelerated whenever positive-pressure ventilation is used. The classic signs of tension pneumothorax include decreased breath sounds and a hyper-resonant chest on percussion of the affected side, with mediastinal shift away from the affected side. Frequently, the cervical trachea is also displaced away from the affected side. Perhaps the most significant physical finding is the presence of subcutaneous emphysema. Radiologic findings of tension pneumothorax include increased space between the ribs, a depressed diaphragm on the affected side, and displacement of mediastinal structures to the unaffected side. Similarly, the presence of subcutaneous emphysema on chest film is compelling evidence for the diagnosis of tension pneumothorax. An important clinical dictum is that "when subcutaneous emphysema is present, as determined by either physical examination or chest x-ray film, it is imperative that the clinician rule out a tension pneumothorax." It is important to remember that tension pneumothorax is primarily life-threatening because of the precipitous cardiovascular collapse associated with compromised venous return. Thus, acute cardiovascular collapse, in combination with an inability to ventilate a patient who has a well-established airway, confirms the clinical diagnosis and demands immediate life-saving treatment.

Simply stated, the treatment is decompression of the intrathoracic cavity by opening the affected side of the chest to the atmosphere. The placement of a large-bore needle or catheter through a rib interspace may provide short-term relief until the chest can be adequately opened. The simplest technique to open the chest is to make a small midclavicular skin incision along the upper surface of the third rib, that is, the second rib interspace. This is immediately followed by inward forceful pressure with a blunt instrument until the chest cavity is penetrated. The placement of a chest tube is not the essential element in the immediate resuscitative treatment, and it can be placed along with a posterior chest tube under sterile conditions after the patient has been resuscitated.

If the patient again manifests cardiovascular instability shortly after these procedures and is difficult to ventilate, the possibility of bilateral tension pneumothorax must be considered. This condition obviously requires a mode of treatment similar to that just outlined. The placement of prophylactic chest tubes to prevent pneumothorax has not been shown to be beneficial to overall patient care and therefore is not routinely recommended. However, in the presence of subcutaneous emphysema on chest x-ray film in a patient who requires positive-pressure ventilation or positive end-expiratory pressure (PEEP) therapy, I believe it is prudent to have chest tubes electively placed, even without unequivocal demonstration of a pneumothorax on chest film.

RUPTURED ESOPHAGUS OR DIAPHRAGM

Some major chest trauma injuries do not usually cause an immediate life-threatening problem, except for unusual circumstances. For example, a ruptured esophagus is primarily associated with high long-term mortality if left surgically untreated because of the infectious complications of mediastinitis. A diagnosis of a ruptured diaphragm is easily determined when the visceral organs (gas bubbles) are present within the thoracic cavity on routine chest x-ray films. Radiologic diagnosis of ruptured diaphragm can be difficult, especially if it occurs on the right side. The presence of an abnormally high diaphragm, extraneous shadows, densities, and blurring of the dome of the diaphragm are characteristic findings. Although associated with some degree of respiratory distress and interference with gas exchange, a ruptured diaphragm does not usually cause immediate cardiopulmonary decompensation, unless there is massive herniation of intra-abdominal contents.

CRUSHED (FLAIL) CHEST INJURY

A common injury associated with blunt chest trauma is the crushed chest injury or flail chest syndrome. There are several different types of flail chest, based on the location of the fracture sites. They can be classified as an anterior or sternal flail chest, and a posterior and an anterolateral flail chest. The diagnosis of this injury is evident when "paradoxical chest wall movements" are observed. The inward movement of the free-floating chest wall segment during inspiration is accentuated by any factor, causing increased negative or subatmospheric intrapleural pressure. This is most commonly observed with increased patient ventilatory effort or any degree of airway obstruction. Correspondingly, the outward movement is exaggerated on forced exhalation. The anterior or sternal flail chest is most commonly encountered in hospitalized patients following chest massage during cardiac resuscitation. It is the result of either improperly applied or too vigorous compression over the anterior chest wall, causing bilateral disruption of several rib costochondral junctions. In many circumstances, this type of flail chest injury can be treated conservatively, requiring only analgesics for pain relief. Similarly, injuries causing a posterior flail chest wall generally require minimal treatment when the fracture sites are in close proximity to the vertebral bodies. The heavy paravertebral muscle layers overlying this section of the chest wall function to minimize paradoxical motion. The anterolateral flail chest is the most unstable and challenging chest wall injury to treat. In this situation, one fracture site occurs at the lateral acute angle of the ribs, since this portion of the rib is most vulnerable to excessive force. Most often, the second rib fracture site is either at the corresponding costochondral junction or at the anterior portion of the rib itself. This type of flail chest injury is generally more severe, since the magnitude of force applied to cause rib fractures also causes significantly greater injury to the underlying lung and vessels.

The immediate pathophysiologic effects of flail chest are related to increased work of breathing and ventilation-perfusion inequalities leading to interference with blood and tissue oxygenation. The patient is unable to effectively cough and deep breathe because of the unstable chest wall. This causes an accumulation of secretions and increased airway resistance, which accentuate the paradoxical chest wall movement. This eventually leads to collapse of alveoli, resulting in decreased lung compliance and ineffective gas exchange due to intrapulmonary shunting, invariably requiring increased ventilatory effort on the patient's part. Thus, a vicious positive feedback cycle is created in which the increased work of breathing eventually leads to acute ventilatory and respiratory failure. Even when the patient has adequate mechanical reserves to sustain ventilation during the acute phase, a common long-term complication of flail chest injuries is pneumonia. It is often not recognized until several days after the initial injury because of the recurrent problem of atelectasis.

Historically, several regimens have been successful in managing the patient with flail chest injuries. Initially, the most common approach involved external traction to the ribs in an attempt to stabilize the chest wall and prevent inward motion. For most patients this treatment modality was not very effective. However, successful treatment was greatly enhanced with either intubation or tracheostomy to establish a stable long-term airway and the use of positive-pressure ventilation. The use of mechanical ventilation with PEEP therapy has proved even more effective. The major benefits of this treatment regimen are adequate bronchial hygiene and the prevention of lung tissue collapse, thus avoiding atelectasis, associated hypoxemia, and pneumonia. Establishing a stable airway (whether by intubation or tracheostomy) is paramount to early effective support in those patients with extensive traumatic chest injuries. Control of pain is essential and has been best accomplished traditionally by using intermittent or continuous intravenous drip narcotic analgesics or intercostal blocks. Unfortunately, intercostal blocks require numerous injections along the multiple fractured sites and even with the use of long-acting local anesthetic agents (e.g., bupivacaine) need to be repeated every 10 to 12 hours. The thoracic epidural catheter is becoming more popular for long-term pain relief because it avoids the need for repeated injections into the fracture sites. This approach has proved effective with either long-acting local anesthetic agents or epidural narcotics. When this technique is used in conjunction with mask continuous positive airway pressure, it has obviated the need for ventilatory support, or even intubation or tracheostomy, in many less severe flail chest injury patients.

PULMONARY CONTUSION

Lung contusion is a major problem that is frequently associated with flail chest injury. Lung contusion is classically the result of blunt trauma, i.e., the compression-decompression injury, and it is a common injury in motor vehicle accidents, especially after the patient's chest strikes a rigid structure such as a steering wheel. It also occurs in blast injuries or blows to the chest after falls from various heights. It is important to realize that the lung parenchymal injury is often more severe when rib fractures are not present, since the applied force is primarily transmitted to the lung tissue. The pathophysiologic effects of lung contusion mimic those described for flail chest, although the onset of major physiologic abnormalities

is often delayed for up to 24 to 72 hours after the injury. There is a decrease in lung compliance and increase in work of breathing, both resulting in increased energy expenditures and oxygen consumption. Atelectasis is secondary to decreased surfactant, alveolar type II cell dysfunction, and increased pulmonary secretions that obstruct airways. The local tissue inflammatory response and disruption of pulmonary capillary membranes result in a noncardiogenic pulmonary edema. The result is a severe and refractory hypoxemia caused by a large physiologic shunt. When these patients have adequate mechanical reserves, hypercarbia and acute ventilatory failure are uncommon.

Combined Pulmonary Contusion and Crushed Chest Injury

The clinical management of lung contusion in combination with flail chest injury has traditionally included early intubation or tracheostomy, mechanical ventilation, and PEEP therapy. The relief of pain following adequate volume resuscitation is extremely important and can be achieved by using any of the techniques previously described. Maintaining excellent tracheobronchial hygiene is an essential element of care. Fiberoptic bronchoscopy has frequently been suggested as a way of effectively removing secretions. For the most part, it is no more effective than properly applied bronchial hygiene techniques, and its primary use remains for diagnostic purposes.

A controversy in the management of patients with pulmonary contusion concerns the amount and type of volume administration and manipulation of fluid balance. It is theoretically better to maintain the patient on a minimal volume intake and thus attempt to limit the extravasation of fluid into the impaired lung tissues. This technique is often quite successful in young patients with good myocardial function, but just as often it is ineffective in older patients with compromised myocardial reserves. This group of patients requires increased amounts of volume to maintain adequate preload and myocardial function during this period of stress. This inevitably results in some accumulation of excess fluid and colloid substances within the injured lung tissue. My particular preference concerning type of volume administered is to combine crystalloid fluids and whole blood or packed red cells as needed, while minimizing colloid solutions. The problem of lung water accumulation can be adequately managed with the judicious utilization of PEEP therapy or ventilatory support or both.

Respiratory Management of Pulmonary Contusion and Crushed Chest Injury

In general, the severity of injury can be used as a guide to determine the required respiratory support for patients with flail chest, lung contusion injuries, or both. The following general guidelines are helpful in deciding what support is appropriate. A tracheostomy can be avoided in those patients with good mechanical reserves who are likely to recover adequate gas exchange function over a period of 7 to 14 days. When a short-term artificial airway is required, a nasal or oral endotracheal tube is usually quite satisfactory. It is important to reemphasize that, in all traumatic chest injuries, it is essential to provide adequate pain relief to obtain the patient's cooperation. As epidural narcotic techniques become more familiar to clinicians, they are highly likely to become the preferred modality for analgesia. When a patient has only a mild to moderate flail chest segment, good mechanical reserves, and no significant lung contusion, an artificial airway is often not required to maintain adequate tracheal bronchial hygiene. Spontaneous ventilation in this patient group is the rule rather than the exception. As the chest trauma becomes more severe, such as that associated with significant lung contusion, more than three rib fractures, or an unstable anterolateral flail chest segment, the patient is at increased risk for serious complications. These patients are hypoxemic on room air or even low concentrations of administered oxygen and most often require oxygen concentrations greater than 50 percent. Although some patients in this group are still able to meet the increased energy demands associated with spontaneous ventilation, they all greatly benefit from early intubation,

partial ventilatory support, and appropriate application of PEEP therapy. In the most severe cases, when patients have extensive lung contusion and a severely unstable chest wall (exhibiting paradoxical respiratory motion with even minimal ventilatory efforts), total mechanical ventilatory support, PEEP therapy, and aggressive cardiopulmonary monitoring are the best treatment choices. Frequently, these are the patients who benefit from early tracheostomy, since their recovery time is predictably prolonged for more than 2 weeks. In my opinion, it is always best to err on the side of aggressive support, especially during the first 24 hours, if any uncertainty exists over the magnitude of the patient's injuries or any preexisting compromise of cardiopulmonary function.

Suggested Reading

Blaisdell FW, Trunkey DD, eds. Cervicothoracic trauma. New York: Thieme, 1986.

Daughtry DC, ed. Thoracic trauma. Boston: Little, Brown, 1980.

Gill W, Long WB. Shock trauma manual. Baltimore: Williams & Wilkins, 1979:52.

Kirsh MM, Sloan H. Blunt chest trauma: general principles of management. Boston: Little, Brown, 1977.

Lucas CE, Ledgerwood RM, Higgins RF, Weaver DW. Impaired pulmonary function after albumin resuscitation from shock. J Trauma 1980; 20:446–451.

Newman RJ, James IS. A prospective study of 413 consecutive car occupants with chest trauma. J Trauma 1984; 24:129–135.

Worthley LI. Thoracic epidural in the management of chest trauma. A study of 161 cases. Intensive Care Med 1985; 11:312–315.

SPINAL CORD INJURY

ROBERT BROWN, M.D., C.M.
STEVEN M. SCHARF, M.D. Ph.D.
STEPHEN C. MELIA, RRT

In spinal cord injury, dysfunction of the respiratory system is a major cause of morbidity and mortality. Age at injury, level of lesion, and extent of paralysis (complete or incomplete) are important determinants of survival, but none of these factors can be influenced therapeutically. Most of the respiratory complications of spinal cord injury can be attributed to respiratory muscle paralysis and retention of respiratory secretions, both of which are most severe in the acute phase of the injury and improve with time.

PATHOPHYSIOLOGY

Muscle Weakness

Crucial to a thorough understanding of current therapeutic methods and goals is an appreciation of the numerous effects of respiratory muscle paralysis (Table 1). With lesions above the phrenic motoneurons, i.e., above C3, all the primary ventilatory muscles are paralyzed and ventilation must be supported mechanically or by phrenic nerve pacing. Of the accessory muscles of inhalation, probably the sternocleidomastoid, scalenes, and hyoid are the most important. There are a few patients in whom the accessory muscles have been trained sufficiently to maintain ventilation for periods up to about 2 hours. If innervation of the diaphragm is spared, inhalation is limited owing to paralysis of the other major muscles of inhalation, classically considered to be the external intercostals. Recent evidence suggests that at low lung volumes the internal intercostals and parasternals may play a role in inhalation. Both tidal and forced exhalation are, essentially, passive in tetraplegia because the primary muscles of exhalation (internal intercostals and muscles of the abdominal wall) are paralyzed.

The paralysis of major muscles of inhalation results in a diminished total lung capacity. In chronic tetraplegics with functioning diaphragms this is, on the average, about 70 percent of predicted, depending, of course, on the level of the lesion. Paralysis of the major muscles of exhalation means that affected individuals cannot exhale substantially below functional residual capacity. The overall result is that these chronic tetraplegics have a vital capacity of roughly 50 percent of predicted, but the range is substantial and those with the higher levels tend to have the smaller vital capacities. Why do these muscle abnormalities and the associated limitations of inhalation and forced exhalation cause problems? From studies in dogs as well as in patients with polio and kyphoscoliosis, it is known that chronic low tidal volume breathing and failure to take deep breaths result in instability and ultimately collapse of peripheral airways of the lung. Normally, we avoid this by periodic sighs. Spinal cord–injured patients with a high level of injury may be so limited as to be unable to take breaths of normal size. In addition, many tetraplegics do not sigh, no matter what the level of their injury. Narrowed or collapsed peripheral airways cause increased airways resistance, atelectasis, increased work of breathing, and gas exchange problems, all of which must be the target of our therapeutic efforts. Also, paralysis of the rib cage muscles results in paradoxical inward motion of the upper rib cage during inhalation. The associated ventilation-perfusion mismatching adds to the gas exchange difficulties, in particular in the supine posture.

TABLE 1 Muscles of Respiration

	Muscles	Innervation	Principal Action
Primary	Diaphragm	C3–C5	Inspiratory
	External intercostals	T1–T12	Inspiratory
	Internal intercostals	T1–T12	Expiratory
	Oblique abdominal	T6–L1	Expiratory
Cervical accessory	Sternocleidomastoid	Brain stem, C1–C3	Inspiratory
	Infrahyoid	C1–C3	Inspiratory
	Trapezoid	C1–C4	Expiratory
	Scalenes	C4–C8	Expiratory
Other	Serratus anterior	C5–C7	Inspiratory
	Serratus posterior superior	T2–T5	Inspiratory
	Serratus posterior inferior	T9–T12	Expiratory
	Rectus abdominus	T6–T12	Expiratory

TABLE 2 **Acute or Early Phase Monitoring**

Function	Monitoring Frequency	Comments
Measure VC, MIP, VT, RR	On admission and q2h until stable, then q.d.	Monitor closely for deterioration of VC
ABG	On admission and p.r.n.	To assess need for supplementary O_2 and assisted ventilation
Auscultate chest	On admission and q4h	Note change
Assess need for assisted ventilation	On admission	Use ABG, VC, MIP, VT
Provide supplementary O_2	p.r.n.	Maintain adequate PO_2
Provide CPT with assisted cough	q4h and p.r.n.	Monitor sputum characteristics
Suction	p.r.n.	If unable to expectorate secretions
Provide nebulized bronchodilator	q4h	Treat bronchospasm and stimulate mucociliary clearance
Provide apnea monitor	On admission	Until stable
IPPB or incentive spirometry	q4h	Use mode that achieves greatest VT

Abbreviations: ABG, arterial blood gas; CPT, chest physiotherapy; MIP, maximal inspiratory pressure; IPPB, intermittent positive pressure breathing; RR, respiratory rate; VC, vital capacity; VT, tidal volume.

Retention of Secretions

We think that a very important factor in the genesis of respiratory failure in spinal cord injury is the paralysis of muscles of exhalation because this results in an ineffective cough and retention of even normally secreted respiratory mucus. The problem is considerably worse in the 10 to 15 percent of acute tetraplegics who have pulmonary secretions that are extraordinarily viscous and copious in amount. Retained secretions predispose patients to pneumonia, atelectasis, hypoxemia, and hypercarbia. Thus, removal of secretions is a major therapeutic goal.

ASSESSMENT OF DIAPHRAGMATIC FUNCTION

Physiological Parameters

The information provided above forms the substrate on which to base initial and follow-up assessment of the acute spinal cord-injured patient. In most ways, the preliminary assessment is similar to that of other patients who have or are at risk of developing respiratory failure. In this regard, history, physical examination, chest x-ray examination, and arterial blood gases are standard and important (Tables 2 and 3). Features worth stressing in the spinal cord injured are the following:

1. Assessment of diaphragm function
2. Measurement of respiratory muscle strength
3. Measurement of vital capacity

The higher and more complete the level, the worse the dysfunction of the respiratory muscles and the more likely the need for ventilatory assistance. This is particularly the case in the presence of diaphragmatic dysfunction (most such patients would not have survived without ventilatory assistance), which can be ascertained at the bedside by observations of motion

TABLE 3 **Patient Receiving Assisted Ventilation**

Function	Frequency	Comments
ABG	On admission and p.r.n.	Ensure proper ventilator settings
Check ventilator	q2h	Ensure operation, drain tubing
Measure VC, MIP, VT	On admission and q8h	Monitor for improvement or deterioration
Suction	q2h and p.r.n.	Monitor change in sputum characteristics
Provide tonsil tip suction	Continually	Hang near mouth for oral secretions
Provide nebulized bronchodilator	q4h and p.r.n.	Treat bronchospasm and stimulate mucociliary clearance
CPT with assisted cough	q4h	To aid in mobilization of secretions
Auscultate chest	q2h	Note changes
Assess ability to wean	q2h	Use ABG, VT, VC, MIP
Monitor etCO$_2$ during weaning	Continually	Use as an alarm for increase in PCO_2
Deflate cuff	When stable	To allow phonation
Arrange for portable ventilator	When stable	Psychological benefit of making patient mobile

Abbreviations: ABG, arterial blood gas; CPT, chest physiotherapy; etCO$_2$, end tidal carbon dioxide; MIP, maximal inspiratory pressure; VC, vital capacity; VT, tidal volume.

of different components of the respiratory system. During tidal inhalation, the rib cage and abdomen normally move outward, with descent of the diaphragm causing protrusion of the abdominal wall. In a tetraplegic with phrenic motoneurons spared, the abdomen moves outward and, owing to the absence of intercostals, the upper rib cage moves paradoxically inward during inhalation. Action in cervical accessory muscles of respiration can elevate the upper rib cage, but one should not expect to observe this during tidal breathing in an acutely injured patient. During inhalation, inward motion of the abdomen implies paralysis or fatigue of the diaphragm, cephalad motion of which is caused by the negative intrathoracic pressure generated by accessory muscles. Clinically, this diaphragm fatigue and inward abdominal motion is well known in nonparalyzed patients with severe airway obstruction or in association with problems related to weaning from assisted ventilation. We emphasize that the same physical signs are useful in paralyzed patients. In the acute tetraplegic, the accessory muscles should not be expected to generate sufficient pleural pressure to sustain ventilation, and so if ventilatory assistance is discontinued for assessment of diaphragmatic activity, the period should be brief.

Measurement of Respiratory Muscle Strength

Because from the respiratory function point of view we are dealing primarily with a disorder of the respiratory muscles, it is appropriate to regularly monitor respiratory muscle strength. At first, maximal inspiratory pressure (MIP) should be measured at functional residual capacity every 2 hours. Progressive diminution in MIP can occur rapidly over the first 12 to 24 hours and suggests that the spinal level of injury is rising, perhaps due to edema, hemorrhage, or instability of the vertebral fracture, and that ventilatory assistance may be needed. Once it is certain that the spinal level and MIP have stabilized, the measurement can be made daily and then weekly. The pressure recorded is effort dependent and thus maximal effort is required so that data can be compared properly. Also, the MIP is sensitive to body position, being greater in the supine posture in which functional residual capacity is reduced and the diaphragm lengthened, than it is in the upright posture in which the diaphragm is shorter. Maximal expiratory pressure (MEP) is also commonly monitored but is of lesser value, in particular in tetraplegics because paralysis of most of the muscles of exhalation makes exhalation almost passive.

Measurement of Vital Capacity

We think that the vital capacity is an excellent measurement to make in these patients. In that the vital capacity maneuver requires maximal use of muscles of inhalation and exhalation, it combines the features of both MIP and MEP. Reduction in vital capacity may not necessarily be due to alteration in respiratory muscle strength, however, and other causes such as atelectasis, pneumothorax, pleural effusion, and so on should be sought.

In the pathophysiology of respiratory dysfunction in spinal cord injury, we have emphasized the importance of diminished respiratory muscle strength. To improve respiratory muscle function, it would seem reasonable to attempt respiratory muscle training in these individuals. The topic of such training in different diseases is in various stages of evaluation at the present time. In chronic spinal cord-injured patients, we have demonstrated that training with a target (such as mean airway pressure) produces better results than does untargeted training, and we are currently assessing the effectiveness of respiratory muscle training in acute spinal cord injury.

Methods for Managing Bronchial Secretions and Atelectasis

Physical Therapy and Bronchoscopy

Experience with the spinal cord injured shows that assiduous monitoring for the problems related to mucus retention and chronic low tidal volume breathing and failure or inability to sigh (atelectasis, pneumonia, gas exchange abnormalities) is required in the management of these patients. This is easily accomplished in the usual manner with chest auscultation, oximetry, blood gas determination, and chest x-ray examination. Because effective cough is absent, keeping the airways as free from mucus as possible becomes the job of the therapist. Many patients require nasotracheal suctioning frequently, so it is absolutely essential to use nontraumatic techniques in order to prevent damage to vocal cords, trachea, carina, and main stem bronchi. Physical therapy methods are useful for clearing secretions in these patients. Chest clapping and postural drainage are standard, but assisted cough should also be performed and is perhaps of greatest value. The patients are asked to inhale maximally and hold their breath by relaxing against a closed glottis. Placing the hands on the abdomen just below the costal margins, the therapist then performs several vigorous thrusts to push the diaphragm cephalad and force gas out of the chest. The maneuver is coordinated with release of glottal closure by asking the patient to attempt to cough. A suction catheter should be available to remove material from the larynx and pharynx. Just how vigorous the thrusts should be is not known. Clearly, extra caution should be exercised in patients with recent abdominal trauma or surgery or with vascular prostheses. The importance of this is underscored by the recent report that this cough assist maneuver had caused disruption and migration of an inferior vena cava filter in one patient. Physical therapy may be so effective in relieving atelectasis that, if gas exchange is not an issue, we try it for 12 to 24 hours before bronchoscopic intervention. When necessary, the cough assist maneuver may be combined with fiberoptic bronchoscopy. During the maneuver, we have observed distal mucous plugs migrating mouthward (they can quickly be suctioned through the bronchoscope) and disappearing into distal airways again during the subsequent inhalation.

In patients receiving assisted ventilation, the cough assist maneuver can be initiated immediately following a deep ventilator-generated breath, perhaps to a pressure at the airway opening of about 35 cm H_2O. The presence of the endotracheal tube precludes glottal closure, and glottal closure is obviously not useful in the presence of a tracheostomy. Even so, the method is effective.

Drugs

Three classes of drugs are also used in the management of retained secretions. Aerosolized beta-agonist drugs are commonly administered to enhance mucociliary clearance, although the specific clinical benefit of this is not clear.

The use of mucolytic agents such as *N*-acetylcysteine is, at best, controversial and there is disagreement as to its effectiveness even among the authors of this chapter. Atropine, a parasympatholytic, is another agent about which there is controversy. It appears to be effective in reducing mucus secretion. However, its detractors argue that it "dries" the secretions and makes them more viscous. This claim has not been borne out by rheologic studies. To patients with mucus hypersecretion we commonly administer atropine by inhalation (0.8 mg atropine mixed with 1 ml sterile normal saline three to four times per day) and on occasion have noted an apparent salutary effect. We emphasize, however, that none of the drugs mentioned here, including atropine, has been subject to carefully controlled trials in spinal cord injury.

Assisted Deep Breaths and Other Mechanical Methods

In the patient not receiving assisted ventilation, the problem of chronic low tidal volume breathing is a difficult one, not only because breath size is limited owing to respiratory muscle impairment but also because, as noted above, many spinal cord-injured patients fail to sigh. Devices to encourage deep inhalation (e.g., incentive spirometer) may be effective but are needed most in those with a high spinal injury level, who, owing to immobilization and paralysis of upper limbs, are unable to use them unassisted. Such patients should be made aware of the need to inhale deeply 10 to 20 times per hour, a matter that should be emphasized and put into effect by nurses, physical therapists, and respiratory therapists on their frequent bedside visits. When vital capacity is less than about 25 percent of predicted, we recommend that patients regularly receive deep inhalations with an Ambu Bag connected to a mouthpiece or with an intermittent positive pressure breathing (IPPB) apparatus, even though its usefulness is questionable in other diseases such as chronic obstructive pulmonary disease.

Continuous positive airway pressure (CPAP) achieved with underwater seal or a valve may be used in nonintubated patients with recurrent atelectasis. Particular caution is required in patients with marked respiratory muscle weakness because positive pressure increases lung volume at end exhalation and thus shortens and further compromises the already weakened inspiratory muscles. As a result, inspiratory capacity and tidal volume may become dangerously small and thus we do not recommend use of CPAP in patients with severe reductions in vital capacity.

Assisted Ventilation

As in other diseases, indications for assisted ventilation in spinal cord injury are hypoxemia uncontrollable with oxygen administered by mask and unstable hypercarbia. Other chapters in the book deal with this level of intervention in the management of respiratory failure and include the use of diaphragm pacing in C1-C2 tetraplegics. Following, we stress several issues somewhat peculiar to patients with spinal cord injury, in particular at high levels.

We recommend that ventilator settings be chosen so that respiratory rate is slow (generally 6 to 10 breaths per minute) and tidal volume large (about 30 percent of predicted vital capacity or approximately 15 ml per kilogram ideal body weight) with regular sighs of about 500 ml greater than the tidal volume. The large volumes help avoid atelectasis and, in addition, satisfy these patients' commonly observed desire for large breaths. Why such patients feel uncomfortable with normal breath size is not clear but may be related to diminished sensory information about respiratory system volume because of paralysis of rib cage muscles. Be aware that carbon dioxide production is diminished in paralyzed individuals and thus the required alveolar ventilation may be less than ordinarily anticipated.

A further level of intervention to prevent recurrent atelectasis is the use of positive end-expiratory pressure (PEEP). High values of PEEP may cause decreased cardiac output and hypotension in any patient but this is a particularly thorny problem in tetraplegics in whom the normal sympathetic nervous system response to hypotension is absent. We have observed acute tetraplegics whose cardiac output was so strikingly diminished in response to PEEP that mixed venous oxygen tension fell to levels low enough to lead to systemic hypoxemia. Nasotracheal suctioning, endotracheal intubation, or even manipulation of balloon volume stimulates irritant receptors in the larynx and trachea and thereby elicits a vagal response producing bradycardia and hypotension. Again, the absence of a counteracting sympathetic response may allow the bradycardia and hypotension to be so severe as to cause syncope. Administration of atropine prior to manipulation of the airway may prevent the problem but, for patients requiring frequent suctioning, the total daily dose may be prohibitive and a temporary cardiac pacemaker may be necessary.

Last, once an acute spinal cord-injured patient requires assisted ventilation, it is common for the need to be prolonged and thus the risk for vocal cord and tracheal damage is great. Therefore, it is important to take extraordinary care at the time of intubation and to manage the tubing systems and balloon volumes appropriately. Movement of the tip of the endotracheal tube can be diminished by the use of the Morch swivel.

CHRONIC SPINAL CORD INJURY

In spinal cord injury a number of factors appear related to the transition from patients often difficult to manage and with a plethora of respiratory problems to patients whose major problems are no longer respiratory in nature. In addition to spinal damage there may have been other trauma that complicated respiratory function (head trauma, fractured ribs, etc.). Also, for unclear reasons, following the initial decrease, inspiratory muscle strength and vital capacity undergo progressive recovery and improvements of 50 percent over about 6 months may be expected. In addition, mucus hypersecretion usually stops within a few months. Those patients who have not needed or who have been successfully weaned from assisted ventilation usually need little in the way of respiratory therapy. Even patients who require chronic ventilator therapy are easier to manage because they are otherwise stable, often are young, and have normal lungs. The task of the respiratory therapist then becomes greatly simplified, consisting for the most part of ventilator checks and routine airway care unless intercurrent respiratory illness occurs.

Suggested Reading

Clough P, Lindenauer D, Hayes M, Zekany B. Guidelines for routine respiratory care of patients with spinal cord injury. Phys Ther 1986; 66:1395–1402.

DeTroyer A, Heilporn A. Respiratory mechanics in quadriplegia: the respiratory function of the intercostal muscles. Am Rev Respir Dis 1980; 122:591–600.

Fugl-Meyer AR. Effects of respiratory muscle paralysis in tetraplegic and paraplegic patients. Scand J Rehabil Med 1971; 3:141–150.

Haas A, Lowman EW, Bergofsky EH. Impairment of respiration after spinal cord injury. Arch Phys Med Rehabil 1965; 46:399–405.

McCool FD, Pichurko BM, Slutsky AS, et al. Changes in lung volume and rib cage configuration with abdominal binding in quadriplegia. J Appl Physiol 1986; 60:1198–1202.

McKinley AC, Auchinclosis JJ Jr, Gilbert R, Nicholas JJ. Pulmonary function, ventilatory control and respiratory complications in quadriplegia subjects. Am Rev Respir Dis 1969; 100:526–532.

McMichan JC, Luc M, Westbrook PR. Pulmonary dysfunction following traumatic quadriplegia: recognition, prevention and treatment. JAMA 1980; 242:528–531.

Pichurko B, McCool FD, Scanlon P, et al. Factors related to respiratory function recovery following acute quadriplegia. Am Rev Respir Dis 1985; 131(4):A337.

Stone DJ, Keltz H. The effect of respiratory muscle dysfunction on pulmonary function. Am Rev Respir Dis 1963; 88:621–629.

PREOPERATIVE PREPARATION OF THE PATIENT

JAMES K. STOLLER, M.D.

In evaluating the patient for upcoming surgery, several questions confront the respiratory care practitioner:

1. What are the anticipated respiratory effects of the upcoming surgery?
2. How likely are postoperative pulmonary complications to occur?
3. Will preoperative preparation or treatment lessen the risk of postoperative pulmonary complications?
4. If so, what type of perioperative respiratory care is recommended?

In addressing these questions, this chapter focuses on available strategies to lessen both the frequency and the severity of postoperative pulmonary complications, which include atelectasis, hypoxemia, and pneumonia.

POSTOPERATIVE PULMONARY FUNCTION CHANGES

Profound changes in pulmonary function commonly accompany abdominal and nonresectional thoracic surgical procedures. Features that determine the degree of postoperative pulmonary impairment include the type of incision (e.g., thoracic versus abdominal, upper abdominal versus lower abdominal) and its position (e.g., subcostal versus median upper abdominal). Both thoracic and upper abdominal incisions are associated with marked postoperative decreases in the compartments of lung volume, with changes most evident in the forced vital capacity (FVC) and functional residual capacity (FRC). As shown in Figure 1, after upper abdominal surgery the FVC may decline to 40 percent of its preoperative value on the day following surgery, with subsequent return to baseline over the course of the following 10 to 14 days. FRC may decline to 60 percent of its preoperative value, with gradual restoration to baseline by the seventh postoperative day. The decline in FRC is especially important, because the resulting atelectasis gives rise to physiologic shunt and associated declines in oxygenation. Arterial oxygen saturation, therefore,

also declines after upper abdominal surgery, and the changes generally parallel declines in FRC.

Pulmonary function changes after lower abdominal surgery are much less pronounced than after either upper abdominal or thoracic surgery, with milder decrements in the FVC (to approximately 60 percent of baseline) and little appreciable decline in FRC. Lung function changes after thoracic procedures resemble those following upper abdominal surgery and are similar after median sternotomy and thoracotomy, although median sternotomy is generally considered to be a less painful incision. Finally, in patients undergoing cholecystectomy, a subcostal incision is associated with smaller postoperative declines in FVC than is a midline incision, and postoperative pulmonary complications are less common following subcostal incisions.

Although some postoperative pulmonary impairment seems inevitable after thoracic and upper abdominal surgery (perhaps due to postoperative changes in diaphragm function and postanesthetic effects), postoperative impairment of pulmonary function can be minimized by careful attention to pain control. For example, intercostal nerve blocks with long-acting local anesthetics (e.g., 0.5 percent bupivacaine, with or without epinephrine) are associated with marked reduction in post-thoracotomy pain and with a smaller decline and more rapid recovery of postoperative pulmonary function. By the same token, epidural anesthetics have been helpful in managing patients with flail chest as well as those with a variety of thoracic and upper abdominal incisions. When possible, effective local anesthetic techniques are preferable to systemic narcotics, because hypoventilation can lead to atelectasis and resulting complications of hypoxemia and pulmonary infection.

RISK FACTORS FOR POSTOPERATIVE PULMONARY COMPLICATIONS

Decline in postoperative pulmonary function is only one of several risk factors for postoperative pulmonary complications like atelectasis, hypoxemia, and pulmonary infection. Other clinical features that increase the patient's risk include obesity, advanced age, type of anesthesia (general versus spinal), duration of surgery, baseline pulmonary dysfunction, and in high-risk patients, the absence of preoperative pulmonary treatment. In perhaps the most careful available assessment of preoperative predictors of postoperative pulmonary complications, Celli and co-workers have performed a discriminant function analysis of risk fac-

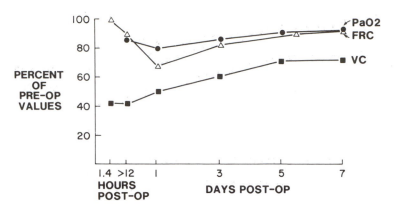

Figure 1 Changes in vital capacity, functional residual capacity, and arterial oxygen after upper abdominal surgery. (Reprinted with permission from the International Research Society. From Craig DB. Postoperative recovery of pulmonary function. Anesth Analg 1981; 60:46–52.)

tors and identified upper abdominal (versus other) surgery as the most potent risk, followed in descending order by the absence of perioperative respiratory therapy, increasing duration of surgery, increasing age, and obesity. The relative importance of baseline pulmonary dysfunction and of smoking status is probably underestimated in this series.

In assessing the patient preoperatively, the clinician appropriately focuses on remediable risk factors, which include active smoking, marked obesity, and pulmonary dysfunction. As mentioned, subcostal incisions are preferred when surgically possible, and in high-risk pulmonary patients, spinal anesthesia may be preferable to general anesthesia. For example, in evaluating the surgical outcome in 464 patients with moderate to severe chronic lung disease, Tarhan and colleagues reported that for comparable types of surgery, no patients receiving spinal or epidural anesthesia died from postoperative pulmonary complications, whereas the pulmonary mortality rate was 6.3 percent in patients receiving general anesthesia.

MANEUVERS TO PREVENT POSTOPERATIVE PULMONARY COMPLICATIONS

Other maneuvers to minimize postoperative complications include antibiotic and bronchodilator therapy, abstinence from smoking, and lung expansion with either chest physical therapy (e.g., deep breathing and coughing, postural drainage, percussion, vibration), or mechanical aids (i.e., incentive spirometry, intermittent positive pressure breathing [IPPB], or mask continuous positive airway pressure [CPAP]).

The incidence of postoperative pulmonary complications varies greatly among series (12 to 85.6 percent) because definitions of pulmonary complications

differ and because the compared patient groups, surgical management, and proficiency of the preventive maneuvers also differ. Although study conclusions vary too, the best-designed studies clearly demonstrate that perioperative preparation of high-risk patients (i.e., those with baseline pulmonary dysfunction and upper abdominal surgery) can help avert postoperative pulmonary complications. The evidence is less convincing that respiratory treatment benefits patients with good preoperative health undergoing nonemergent surgery, even for cholecystectomy.

Used alone or as part of an integrated program of respiratory care, chest physiotherapy can prevent postoperative pulmonary complications. The efficacy of chest physiotherapy as a stand-alone treatment was first demonstrated over 30 years ago when Thoren and colleagues observed fewer pulmonary complications in a treated group than in a comparable control group also undergoing cholecystectomy. The postoperative pulmonary complication rate was lowest (12 percent) when patients were given chest physiotherapy both pre- and postoperatively.

Although the efficacy of chest physiotherapy has been known for 3 decades, relatively little attention has been given to the contributions of individual components of a chest physiotherapy program, which include deep breathing and coughing, huffing, percussion, vibration, postural drainage, and early mobilization after surgery. Guidelines on the optimal frequency and duration of therapy are also unavailable, but several conclusions seem justified. First, chest physiotherapy is more effective when patients are supervised and actively encouraged than when they are simply reminded to breathe deeply and cough. As shown by Thoren, supervision should begin before surgery. Although the optimal intensity and duration of therapy have not been examined, it seems prudent to perform chest physiotherapy at least three times daily until the patient is mobile and able to reliably initiate deep breathing and coughing on his own.

Despite its demonstrated efficacy as a stand-alone modality, chest physiotherapy is incompletely effective in preventing postoperative pulmonary complications, which have been observed to occur in 12 to 71 percent of chest physiotherapy recipients. Over time, this observation has led many investigators to examine the role of various mechanical aids to lung expansion (e.g., incentive spirometry, IPPB, and mask CPAP), either alone or with chest physiotherapy, as means of further preventing pulmonary morbidity.

Blow bottles and IPPB enjoyed early enthusiasm in the 1960s and early 1970s but have since fallen into general disfavor. Blow bottles or variants (e.g., "blow gloves," in which the patient is encouraged to inflate a rubber glove by forcefully exhaling) appear to be physiologically misconceived, because atelectasis may be encouraged rather than prevented by an expiratory Valsalva maneuver. IPPB, although physiologically appealing as a way of promoting lung expansion, has generally proven disappointing in preventing postoperative pulmonary complications. However, having recognized prevailing opinions about these two therapies, it is noteworthy that carefully performed current studies do show that IPPB and blow bottles can be effective. Most notably, Celli and co-workers found both IPPB and blow gloves to be effective in preventing respiratory complications after cholecystectomy, and just as effective as more widely accepted maneuvers like enforced deep breathing plus coughing and incentive spirometry. These data and personal observations suggest that IPPB may still play a limited role in preventing or treating postoperative atelectasis. For example, thoracotomy patients who develop atelectasis after failure of preventive chest physiotherapy or incentive spirometry may benefit from either IPPB or mask CPAP. The added inconvenience, expense, and potential morbidity of mask CPAP (e.g., gastric distention or perforation, aspiration, and nasal necrosis) recommend IPPB as a first-line method. To assure maximal efficacy, the patient should be supervised by a respiratory care practitioner to assure delivery of acceptable volumes, ideally to total lung capacity.

Besides its role as a "salvage" procedure for patients who have failed chest physiotherapy or incentive spirometry, IPPB may also be a first-line preventive therapy for patients with either chest wall deformity (e.g., kyphoscoliosis) or weakness (e.g., neuromuscular disease) who are undergoing surgery. Mechanical difficulty may preclude spontaneous chest expansion in such patients, and IPPB (or mask CPAP) with attention to delivering adequate volumes seems justified.

The initial wave of enthusiasm for IPPB has been largely replaced by recent preferences for incentive spirometry, a technique in which the patient is encouraged to breathe deeply by observing a device (e.g., spirometer, a column with a floating ball, etc.) that displays and reinforces large inspiratory efforts (see chapter on *Incentive Spirometry*). Since its initial description by Bartlett in 1973, incentive spirometry has become the most widely used preventive technique in the United States, already surpassing the use of IPPB by 1976.

Although incentive spirometry may not be necessary in low-risk patients (e.g., patients assigned American Society of Anesthesiology classes 1 or 2), many studies have shown that incentive spirometry is an effective preventive maneuver for higher-risk patients undergoing chest or abdominal surgery. Besides being effective as a stand-alone method, incentive spirometry is suggested by some studies to be additively effective when used with chest physiotherapy. Dohi and Gold also observed that the combination of incentive spirometry and inhaled sympathomimetics was associated with fewer postoperative pulmonary complications than a regimen of IPPB and bronchodilators (29 percent vs. 57 percent). As with chest physiotherapy, however, maximum benefit from incentive spirometry is achieved when the patient is instructed preoperatively, is actively encouraged to participate, and is pain-free without oversedation.

As further discussed in the chapter *Mask and Nasal Continuous Positive Airway Pressure,* mask CPAP can effectively reverse postoperative atelectasis and hypoxemia and may avert intubation and mechanical ventilation in some rapidly reversible types of acute respiratory failure. Mask CPAP also appears to be an effective way of preventing postoperative pulmonary complications. Recent work has shown that mask CPAP (12 cm H_2O used for 3 hours a day over the first 5 postoperative days) more rapidly restores postoperative pulmonary dysfunction to baseline than does an enforced regimen of deep breathing and coughing given every 3 hours. Also, when compared with either encouraged deep breathing or with incentive spirometry, frequent mask CPAP therapy (7.5 to 15 cm H_2O given for up to 30 breaths hourly) more frequently restored the alveolar-arterial oxygen gradient and averted atelectasis. Although adverse effects of mask CPAP (e.g., gastric distension or rupture, nasal necrosis) are rare with intermittent use, they do occur, and in the absence of head-to-head comparisons of mask CPAP to IPPB for reversing atelectasis, a trial of IPPB may still be recommended first. The lower charges of IPPB therapy may further recommend this strategy, although a failure of IPPB should not interdict a mask CPAP trial.

In addition to these mechanical techniques for promoting lung expansion and clearance of secretions, several pharmacologic maneuvers have been examined, including perioperative antibiotics and bronchodilator therapy. Although antibiotics have been part of a multifaceted treatment program that successfully averts postoperative pulmonary complications, their distinctive contribution has been difficult to show. Except for one trial showing that perioperative treatment with a broad-spectrum antibiotic combination (penicillin and streptomycin) decreased postoperative pulmonary morbidity (Collins), studies of antibiotics have not shown decreased chest morbidity in treated patients. Regimens of ampicillin (500 mg IM 1 hour before surgery and every 8 hours thereafter for 5 days) and of penicillin (500,000 units every 6 hours for 1 day before and 5 days after surgery) have been ineffective, even in patients with baseline chronic bronchitis. Given this general lack of efficacy, the potential complications of antibiotics (i.e., selection of resistant strains, superinfection, and adverse drug reactions) weigh against their use as pulmonary prophylaxis. One possible exception is the patient with a preoperative flare-up of bronchiectasis, in whom aggressive chest physiotherapy, antibiotics, and inhaled bronchodilators does seem justified.

Although also part of successful overall perioperative treatment programs, bronchodilators too have been generally ineffective as stand-alone treatment to avert postoperative pulmonary complications. Most available studies have used inhaled sympathomimetic agents (e.g., isoproterenol), either alone or along with IPPB. Although little evidence supports using perioperative bronchodilators to prevent chest complications in patients with chronic airflow obstruction, special consideration should be given to asthmatics, in whom remaining preoperative airflow obstruction increases postoperative pulmonary risk. In such patients, aggressive preoperative bronchodilator therapy seems justified.

Because of potential toxic interactions with halothane (a preferred inhalational anesthetic for patients with bronchospasm), aminophylline is often avoided preoperatively in favor of short-term glucocorticoid infusions, which have been shown to accelerate restoration of FEV_1 in asthmatics. We favor an initial hydrocortisone (Solu-Cortef) infusion of 2 mg per kilogram, followed by a continuous delivery of 0.5 mg per kilogram per hour, the steroid regimen found effective in double-blind controlled trials of acute asthma treatment. Some evidence suggests that even larger steroid doses (e.g., methylprednisolone [Solu-Medrol] 125 mg every six hours) may be more effective.

ROLE OF SMOKING CESSATION PREOPERATIVELY

In the active smoker, stopping smoking before surgery has been shown to reduce the risk of postoperative pulmonary complications.

In addition to being implicated as a cause of lung cancer, cigarette smoking has other more acute cardiopulmonary effects that may increase surgical risk. These acute cardiovascular effects result from inhaling carbon monoxide and nicotine. Nicotine has chronotropic and pressor effects, and carbon monoxide compromises the oxygen carrying capacity of blood, the net effect of which is to lessen the patient's exercise capacity and response to cardiovascular stress. Although preoperative carboxyhemoglobin levels have not been found to predict pulmonary complications following surgery, it is clear that abstinence from smoking for even 12 hours can lower carboxyhemoglobin levels and enhance oxygen-carrying capacity. This observation itself would seem to justify at least short-term abstinence.

The adverse respiratory effects of smoking are equally profound. Smoking a single cigarette can cause acute increases in airway resistance, while habitual smoking commonly produces severe physiologic impairments including airflow obstruction, mucus hypersecretion, and impaired mucociliary clearance. That active smoking increases the risk of postoperative pulmonary complications was first shown by Morton in 1944; active smoking of at least 10 cigarettes per day was associated with a sixfold increase in postoperative bronchitis, atelectasis, or pneumonia as compared with a nonsmoking control group (58.3 percent versus 7.5 percent overall complication rate). Although estimates of the imposed risk have varied with differing study criteria in subsequent series, active smoking has proven a consistent risk factor for postoperative pulmonary morbidity.

Key questions about smoking in patients facing upcoming surgery include: (1) Is the pulmonary dysfunction reversible with abstinence? and, if so, (2) Over what time course is improvement expected, so that elective surgery can be scheduled to minimize smoking-associated risk?

Ample studies show that the adverse respiratory effects of smoking—symptoms of cough, breathlessness, spitting, and wheezing; airflow obstruction and impaired mucociliary clearance—are at least partially reversible with cessation of smoking, but current understanding of the time course of reversal remains incomplete. Perhaps the most rapid and profound improvement is noted in smoking-related symptoms. Within 1 month of stopping smoking, former smokers may experience marked improvement in cough and phlegm production. Alveolar macrophage adherence, which is also depressed in smokers, may also rapidly improve, reverting to normal by as soon as 1 week (and rarely longer than 1 month) after stopping. Alterations in circulating T cell populations (with an increased proportion of suppressor cells) occur in heavy smokers (greater than or equal to 50 pack-years) and may normalize with cessation, although normalization may not occur before 2 months of abstention.

Whether tracheobronchial clearance of secretions actually improves in former smokers remains controversial; any expected improvement will not be apparent after 1 week's abstinence and is only partially realized after 3 months.

Airflow obstruction is both more common and accelerated in active smokers than in patients who have never smoked or who have quit. Studies in smokers with sufficient airflow obstruction to compromise FEV_1 show that smoking cessation rarely improves FEV_1 but does slow its rate of decline compared to that of those who have never smoked. The one exception may be smokers who stop before age 35, in whom smoking cessation is associated with short-term increases of FEV_1 of approximately 25 ml per year. Despite the dim prospects that FEV_1 will improve with stopping smoking, quitting permits improvement in other parameters of airflow, particularly indicators of small airway obstruction. These include the ratios of closing volume to vital capacity (CV/VC), of closing capacity to total lung capacity (CC/TLC), the slope of the alveolar plateau of a nitrogen washout curve, and the volume of isoflow during helium-maximal expiratory flow maneuvers. These parameters are frequently abnormal in smokers at a time when FEV_1 is preserved, so it is not surprising that improvements in small airway function may be unaccompanied by improvements in FEV_1. Nevertheless, to the extent that they reflect impairment or unevenness of airflow in small airways, improvement in these parameters with smoking cessation does justify quitting before surgery.

The time course of pulmonary improvement after stopping smoking should determine the optimal period of abstention before elective surgery. Unfortunately, although data on the acute airflow effects of stopping smoking are sparse, most studies suggest that little change can be expected for at least several weeks after stopping. Although mild improvements in expiratory airflow at low lung volumes (e.g., FEF_{25}) may begin within a week of stopping smoking, most measures of small airway obstruction are barely changed before 1 month and may continue to show progressive improvement at 3 and 6 months after stopping smoking. Information on physiologic recovery after stopping smoking therefore suggests that patients should quit 1 to 2 months before elective surgery. A similar recommendation comes from a recent study of the impact of preoperative abstinence on the frequency of postoperative pulmonary complications. Among 456 patients undergoing coronary artery bypass graft surgery, Warner and colleagues found that the prevalence of postoperative pulmonary complications was the same among patients who never stopped smoking as among smokers who quit no sooner than 8 weeks preoperatively (45 to 62 percent), but declined substantially (to 15 to 20 percent) among patients who stopped smoking at least 8 weeks before surgery. Abstaining for more than 2 months (i.e., up to 1 year)

did not further reduce postoperative pulmonary risk.

Based on this information about physiologic recovery after smoking cessation and the effects of smoking cessation on postoperative morbidity, it seems reasonable to recommend 2 months of abstinence before elective surgery. Recognizing that this may often prove impossible or impractical, the promise of clearing nicotine and carboxyhemoglobin and the trend toward fewer complications with increasing duration of abstinence favor the longest possible (i.e., up to 2 months) smoking-free interval before surgery.

SUMMARY

Patients with clinical features associated with postoperative pulmonary complications (e.g., upper abdominal surgery, especially when accompanied by preoperative pulmonary dysfunction, active smoking, obesity, or advanced age) benefit from perioperative treatment to minimize this risk.

A variety of respiratory treatments have been proposed, and although none can completely avert postoperative pulmonary morbidity, most are effective. In addition to abstinence from smoking for 2 months before elective surgery, we recommend a regimen of chest physiotherapy (consisting of enforced deep breathing, coughing or huffing, and percussion and vibration) along with active use of an incentive spirometer. Instruction in using the incentive spirometer and in the chest physiotherapy regimen should begin before surgery, and these maneuvers should be administered by a respiratory care practitioner at least three times daily in the immediate postoperative period. Patients should be encouraged to use the incentive spirometer and to breathe deeply and cough as frequently as possible. Besides the enforced sessions, further casual reminders seem advisable. For patients whose compliance with this program is poor or who cannot breathe deeply (because of neuromuscular weakness or chest wall deformity), we favor addition of intermittent lung inflation, either by IPPB or by mask CPAP. In the absence of compelling data for the superiority of one technique over the other, the more modest expense and possibly lower morbidity of IPPB recommend it first.

Preoperative antibiotics have little role in minimizing pulmonary risk, with the possible exception of patients whose bronchiectasis has flared up. In such patients, aggressive chest physiotherapy (with emphasis on percussion, vibration, and postural drainage) should be administered along with antibiotics addressed at the likely airway flora (e.g., *Streptococcus pneumoniae* and *Haemophilus influenzae*, usually beta-lactamase negative).

Preoperative bronchodilator therapy can be reserved for patients suspected to have a reversible component of airflow obstruction, based either on spirometric evidence or on a clinical description of fluctuating airflow obstruction.

Suggested Reading

Celli BR, Rodriguez KS, Snider GL. A controlled trial of intermittent positive pressure breathing, incentive spirometry, and deep breathing exercises in preventing pulmonary complications after abdominal surgery. Am Rev Respir Dis 1984; 130:12–15.

Chodoff P, Margand PMS, Knowles CL. Short term abstinence from smoking: its place in preoperative preparation. Crit Care Med 1975; 3:131–133.

Collins CD, Darke CS, Knowelden J. Chest complications after upper abdominal surgery: their anticipation and prevention. Br Med J 1968; 1:401–406.

Craig DB. Postoperative recovery of pulmonary function. Anesth Analg 1981; 60:46–52.

Dohi S, Gold MI. Comparison of two methods of postoperative respiratory care. Chest 1978; 73:592–595.

Jones RM. Smoking before surgery: the case for stopping. Br Med J 1985; 290:1763–1764.

Kigin MS. Chest physical therapy for the postoperative or traumatic injury patient. Phys Ther 1981; 61:1724–1736.

Morton HJV, Camb DA. Tobacco smoking and pulmonary complications after operation. Lancet 1944; 1:368–370.

Tarhan S, Moffitt EA, Sessler AD, Douglas WW, Taylor WF. Risk of anesthesia and surgery in patients with chronic bronchitis and chronic obstructive pulmonary disease. Surgery 1973; 74:720–726.

Thoren L. Post-operative pulmonary complications. Observations on their prevention by means of physiotherapy. Acta Chir Scand 1964; 107:193–205.

Warner MA, Divertie MB, Tinker JH. Preoperative cessation of smoking and pulmonary complications in coronary artery bypass patients. Anesthesiology 1984; 60:380–383.

POSTOPERATIVE VENTILATORY MANAGEMENT

PHILIP G. BOYSEN, M.D.

There are two major reasons for which most patients require mechanical ventilation postoperatively. The majority of patients have normal underlying respiratory function but still require ventilatory support because of the effects of either the anesthetic technique or the surgery. Since the need for this respiratory support depends on the anesthetic technique, it is maintained until the effects of the agents used during anesthesia can either be metabolized or their effects reversed by specific antagonist agents. A smaller number of patients are ventilated because of compromised pulmonary or cardiovascular function. Those individuals with severe pulmonary dysfunction may actually require ventilation for 48 to 72 hours postoperatively to regain baseline function. Patients in this group include those individuals with chronic airway obstruction, patients with altered ventilatory drive or other neuromuscular abnormalities, and patients with upper airway obstruction. The most common of these situations are listed in Table 1.

The anesthetic agents most commonly involved in the alteration of postoperative pulmonary function are muscle relaxants, narcotics, and inhalational agents. For many types of surgery, including thoracic and abdominal surgery, adequate muscle relaxation necessitates the use of pharmacologic paralysis. Although a depolarizing agent such as succinylcholine is commonly used for anesthetic induction, during maintenance anesthesia agents such as pancuronium, vecuronium, and atracurium are more commonly used. At the termination of the surgical procedure and at the beginning of anesthetic emergence these agents are often reversed by receptor antagonists such as neostigmine or edrophonium (both in combination with atropine to block muscarinic effects). When reversal of a muscle relaxant is not feasible owing to the administration of high doses of these agents during surgery, the patient is mechanically ventilated until these agents are fully metabolized. Some patients may be transported to an intensive care unit without reversal of these agents because of some underlying contraindication. Whether the agents are allowed to metabolize or whether reversal agents are administered, residual paralysis is monitored by asking the patient to respond to commands (e.g., squeeze the cli-

nician's hand or maintain a headlift for 5 seconds). Objective physiological monitoring is provided by neuromuscular stimulation using a twitch monitor. Further analysis of respiratory function can be completed by instructing the patient to perform a vital capacity (VC) maneuver or by instructing the patient to perform an inspiration against an occluded airway or peak negative pressure (PNP). Finally, with reversal of muscle relaxants, patients should be able to maintain spontaneous breathing through the anesthetic circle with an adequate rate (6 to 9 per minute) and tidal volume (5 to 7 ml per kilogram).

When narcotics are administered either as a primary anesthetic technique in combination with nitrous oxide (N_2O) and oxygen or to augment anesthetic effect, these agents may additionally cause suppression of ventilation. Again, because of very high dosages used during anesthesia to maintain a stable hemodynamic state (such as in coronary artery bypass surgery), there is a prolonged effect that suppresses ventilatory drive. With smaller doses of narcotics a reversal can be accomplished using naloxone or a variety of other agents. During spontaneous breathing the patient is again monitored under direct observation while intubated, breathing through an anesthetic circle, and the respiratory rate and tidal volume are monitored. The narcotized patient typically breathes with a slow respiratory rate of approximately 6 to 9 breaths per minute and deep tidal volumes. In addition to clinical observation, many operating rooms now are equipped with either mass spectrophotometry or capnography such that the end-tidal carbon dioxide tension can be obtained from a sample of expired gas. Thus, the respiratory rate, tidal volume, and end-tidal CO_2 or the arterial carbon dioxide tension provide an assessment that would indicate whether the patient can maintain spontaneous ventilation.

Inhalational agents that are now commonly used uniformly suppress ventilatory drive. Even subanesthetic doses of these agents cause a significant shift of the carbon dioxide response curve, and this effect is compounded when narcotic agents have been used during the course of the anesthetic. In situations when mass spectrophotometry is available, the end-tidal concentration of anesthetic can be monitored in addition to the end-tidal carbon dioxide concentration. Most commonly, however, direct clinical information (with observation of an adequate spontaneous breathing rate and tidal volume) and response to stimulation indicate successful recovery from an anesthetic and provide information as to whether endotracheal extubation can be accomplished.

In patients in whom the thorax or the upper abdomen was the site of the surgical incision, there can be further difficulties with lung expansion in the early postoperative period. During emergence from anesthesia, particularly if pain is present, these patients breathe rapidly with very small tidal volumes. Deep inspiration can often be accomplished on examination, and the vital capacity is a direct index of the adequacy of lung expansion. When the patient fails to maintain adequate tidal volumes or fails to perform a deep inspiration periodically, there is a continued fall in the functional residual capacity (FRC) and a change in the lung-thorax compliance. In concert with these changes, there is subsequent hypoxemia because of the ventilation/perfusion abnormalities that result from the decrease in lung volume. Sustained maximal lung inflation becomes necessary to reverse these changes. A variety of techniques has been used to accomplish this during spontaneous breathing. In some patients, mechanical ventilation is necessary to provide lung expansion and to maintain a normal FRC and gas exchange during the early postoperative period.

The question of early versus late extubation following major surgical procedures has been studied. As concerns patients who have had major surgery for abdominal vascular reconstruction, there appears to be no major reason to provide routine mechanical ventilation in the postoperative state. If the patient is awake and responsive; if there are no residual effects of the muscle relaxants, narcotics, or inhalational anesthetics; and if the patient is hemodynamically stable and of near-normal body temperature, extubation can be accomplished without incident or further complications. The major reason to maintain ventilation in these patients again relates to the anesthetic technique employed and to the successful recovery from these agents. Additionally, hemodynamic stability is an important factor and is often the limiting factor that necessitates respiratory support. In those patients who are stable but ventilated "prophylactically" there is a tendency to use more sedatives and narcotics to maintain patient comfort during endotracheal intubation and mechanical ventilation, resulting in an increased incidence of complications due to these drugs and manipulation and instrumentation of the airway.

Similarly, the patient in whom coronary artery bypass surgery has been performed can usually be extubated once cardiovascular function is stabilized. High-dose narcotic techniques combined with muscle relaxants often necessitate continued mechanical ventilation for 12 to 15 hours postoperatively. If lower-dose narcotics have been combined with an inhalational agent, most of these patients can be extubated. In a prospective series of cardiac surgical procedures under inhalational anesthesia, 87 percent were extubated within 3 hours of the conclusion of the procedure, with a low incidence of reintubation. The 13 percent who required postoperative ventilation were characterized by an unstable hemodynamic status rather than respiratory dysfunction. Indices predicting the need for continued ventilation included a low mixed venous oxygen saturation or elevated left atrial pressure. Other authors have pointed out that evidence of dysfunction usually occurs during or after the operation and may not be predictable preoperatively. Another study randomized patients into an extubated group and a ventilated group once hemodynamic stability was achieved. Complications, cost, and sedative or narcotic dosing were higher in the ventilated group; intensive care unit (ICU) stay was the same. It thus appears that for the postoperative cardiac surgery patient who is hemodynamically stable, anesthetic technique determines the need for mechanical ventilation. If inhalational agents are used, extubation can be accomplished within hours.

TIDAL VOLUMES AND INTERMITTENT SIGHS

Early recommendations for ventilatory support were devised for neuromuscular respiratory failure during polio epidemics. These recommendations were based on observations made during spontaneous breathing and focused on CO_2 removal rather than oxygenation. The Radford nomogram suggested a tidal volume (V_T) of about 500 ml and rates of 12 to 15 per minute for adult males. Such a V_T is small by today's standards because of subsequent documentation of lower PaO_2 values than were found with delivery of large tidal breaths.

Since the above rates and volumes (4 to 8 ml per kilogram) were considered physiologic, and since during quiet breathing most people sigh between 6 and 10 times per hour, the same mechanism was suggested for positive pressure ventilation; i.e., intermittent use of a large breath, three times the average V_T. Since anesthetized patients did not sigh and a widened alveolar-to-arterial gradient and decreased lung compliance resulted, the intermittent artificial sigh seemed a reasonable way to reverse these abnormalities. This proved to be the case, and the mean PaO_2 rose by 150 mm Hg. Similar data were gathered in ICU patients.

Subsequent studies questioned the original comparison of spontaneous breathing versus breathing with positive pressure. It is now clear that hypoxemia and loss of compliance can be prevented without the use of the sigh mechanism if the V_T is 12 to 15 ml per kilogram. On the other hand, mechanical ventilation with V_T greater than 20 ml per kilogram has been associated with a high incidence of barotrauma, especially since positive end-expiratory pressure (PEEP) is often used in conjunction with mechanical ventilation. In practice, V_{TS} of 12 to 15 ml per kilogram have become standard in the management of both routine postoperative ventilation and acute respiratory failure. Smaller tidal volumes result in atelectasis and hypoxemia; larger volumes may cause barotrauma and cardiovascular compromise. Within such guidelines, there is no additional benefit from the addition of intermittent sighs. These devices are unnecessary and should be removed from anesthesia and postoperative ventilators.

INSPIRATORY FLOW PATTERN AND I:E RATIO

Because during quiet, spontaneous breathing normal individuals maintain a ratio of inspiration to expiration (I:E) of about 1:2, the same ratio was suggested during mechanical ventilation. The effects of prolonged inspiratory time on hemodynamic function further strengthened this recommendation. For many years it has been suggested that a prolonged inspiratory time, especially if followed by a pause at high lung volume, would result in improved distribution of ventilation and gas exchange. Modern ventilators, with microprocessor capabilities, allow manipulation of the I:E ratio, end-inspiratory pauses, and variation of the inspiratory flow wave.

Study of lung models would indicate that a slow inspiratory flow rate and end-inspiratory pause would improve distribution of inspired gas when there is variable resistance introduced into the system. With changes in compliance, there appears to be no advantage. These data have not been confirmed in humans with either normal lungs or acute respiratory dysfunction.

For the routine patient who is ventilated postoperatively these manipulations are superfluous. In addition, there may be adverse effects on gas exchange and hemodynamics. Prolongation of inspiratory time in the patient with chronic obstructive pulmonary disease (COPD) is limited because of encroachment on the expiratory time. Airflow obstruction during exhalation requires sufficient time to avoid gas trapping, hyperinflation, and increased deadspace ventilation. The result is a negative effect on gas exchange and the possibility of hemodynamic compromise. Thus, manipulation of inspiratory flow patterns is not of clinical importance in the patient with normal underlying lung function. During acute respiratory failure there may be some improvement in oxygenation and ventilation, but whether these modalities offer significant clinical benefit has yet to be determined, especially in view of potential adverse effects.

PaO_2/FiO_2

The target PaO_2 for the normal postoperative patient has not been established. In general, I recommend that the PaO_2 be maintained at 80 mm Hg or above, because at this level hemoglobin is adequately saturated. Conversely, however, in the patient with a pH of 7.40 and adequate hemoglobin, i.e., 15 g per deciliter, there is no obvious need to maintain the arterial oxygen tension over 100 mm Hg. In this situation, little is gained except an increase in dissolved oxygen, which is negligible in terms of overall gas exchange and oxygen delivery. Furthermore, if the patient is maintained at a higher FiO_2 there is the question of subsequent lung damage due to oxygen toxicity. We know that if the FiO_2 is maintained between 0.40 and 0.50 no serious side effects have been noted, even if these inspired oxygen concentrations are maintained over prolonged periods of time. At the other end of the spectrum, a very high FiO_2, especially an FiO_2 of 1.0, has been thought to result in absorption atelectasis and a marked decrease in lung volume over short periods of time such as 10 to 20 minutes. I feel that this problem is also negligible if the FiO_2 is maintained at 0.70 or below. I thus recommend beginning mechanical ventilation with an FiO_2 of 0.80 until cardiopulmonary stability has been established and then rapidly tapering this level based on arterial blood gas analysis.

Similarly, the consequences of transient hypoxemia are generally unknown. Arterial oxygen saturation (SaO_2) less than 80 percent is apparently of little consequence if the occurrence is transient and occasional. However, an SaO_2 less than 85 percent for 20 minutes has been shown to result in deficits in short-term memory. Little is known about hypoxemic episodes that are transient but repetitive. It is my opinion, however, that in the elderly patient or the patient with underlying ischemic heart disease, episodes that in other patients would be benign could result in severe consequences and may result in arrhythmias and sudden death. A noninvasive measurement of arterial oxygen saturation by oximetry may become even more important in the patient who undergoes early extubation and is breathing spontaneously. Clearly, during surgical anesthesia and in the early postoperative environment, oximetric technology has now become state of the art.

VENTILATOR MODE

Realizing that not every patient can be approached in the same manner, I nevertheless have formulated guidelines with which to initiate mechanical ventilation postoperatively. If we assume that we begin with a patient with normal lungs and that we are awaiting pharmacologic recovery from anesthetic agents and further assume that such a patient has no spontaneous respirations, we can begin as follows. First, I would administer a V_T of 12 to 15 ml per kilogram of body weight with a frequency of $7\frac{1}{2}$ to 8 breaths per minute. The I:E ratio from delivered ventilator breaths should be approximately 1:2. The FIO_2 would first be set at 0.80 and then lowered depending on assessment of oxygenation. CPAP would be maintained at 3 to 5 cm H_2O, which is the level designated as "physiologic PEEP" and should replace some of the distending pressure that has been lost following intubation of the airway. These values assume a V_D/V_T of approximately 0.50. Thus, with 8 L per minute total ventilation, one would provide 4 L per minute alveolar ventilation, a level that should be enough to maintain a normal adult male.

I typically use ventilators equipped to deliver intermittent mandatory ventilation (IMV). For early postoperative management this has been efficacious owing to its similarities to the anesthetic circle. The anesthetic circle allows spontaneous breathing with minimal inspiratory work through a system which provides at least 5 L of reservoir gas in an anesthesia bag. In addition to spontaneous breathing, a mechanical ventilator can deliver a positive pressure breath, or the anesthesiologist can pressurize the anesthesia bag by hand, similarly delivering a breath under positive pressure. Spontaneous breathing can be assessed by visual observation and palpation of the anesthesia reservoir bag during inhalation and by the assessment of measured V_T attained from the exhalation limb of the anesthetic circle. Thus, the conversion from mechanical ventilation to spontaneous breathing can be

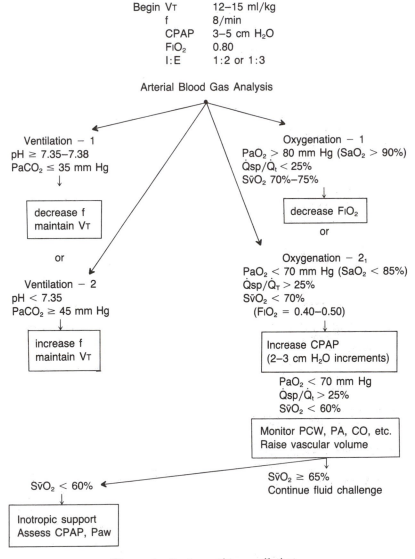

Begin V_T	12–15 ml/kg
f	8/min
CPAP	3–5 cm H_2O
FIO_2	0.80
I:E	1:2 or 1:3

Figure 1 Postoperative ventilation.

accomplished smoothly, and when spontaneous ventilation is initiated, one can assess the respiratory rate, tidal volume, and the breathing pattern. An IMV ventilator provides the same methods of assessment, and by clinical observation combined with objective data, the transition to spontaneous breathing should proceed smoothly and rapidly with eventual extubation of the patient's airway. In many recovery rooms, there is also instrumentation available to measure end-tidal carbon dioxide tension as this transition is accomplished. If clinically necessary, further information can be obtained by arterial blood analysis.

If we assume that there is underlying abnormal lung function, there are, in general, three choices of ventilator modes. These include IMV as mentioned above, controlled mechanical ventilation (CMV), and assisted mechanical ventilation (AMV). The need for controlled ventilation is assessed by the above outlined parameters. If IMV is chosen, it is important to choose a ventilator circuit that provides the possibility for unassisted breathing, but such spontaneous breathing should be unrestricted so that no flow-resistive work is performed during spontaneous inspiration. This implies a minimal fall in the airway pressure measured at the endotracheal tube during spontaneous breathing. If AMV is chosen, similar caution must be maintained. With this mode of ventilation, an inspiratory effort with a subsequent fall in airway pressure triggers the ventilator to deliver a positive pressure breath. Thus the sensitivity of the machine that initiates the positive pressure breath must be correctly adjusted to maintain early delivery of airflow and patient comfort. There must also be an adequate inspiratory flow rate that should exceed the patient's inspiratory flow rate once the mechanical breath is initiated. Although this provides greater patient comfort, it has now been well established that respiratory work is still performed while breathing through such systems and that this work is of a greater magnitude than previously

suspected. With AMV, an adequate tidal volume must be administered to achieve lung distention, whether the system is pressure or volume limited. Thus, if the machine delivers a volume-limited breath, pressure should be monitored, and if the machine is pressure limited, the exhaled volume must be monitored. For most postoperative patients, management can be achieved successfully with either ventilatory mode, depending on therapeutic objectives.

Monitoring during mechanical ventilation is similar to the monitoring techniques instituted in the operating room. These include the electrocardiogram for rhythm and rate, the arterial blood pressure either invasively or noninvasively, and body temperature. Visual assessment should be provided not only by physicians but, more importantly, by continuous observation by nursing and respiratory therapy personnel. Auscultation of the lungs is performed routinely in response to perceived alterations in clinical state. In many institutions, noninvasive techniques such as arterial oxygen saturation by oximetry and end-tidal carbon dioxide tensions are becoming widely available. These should provide an adequate assessment of both oxygenation and ventilation and are perceived as an extension of the clinical examination. A suggested outline for approaching postoperative mechanical ventilation is provided in Figure 1.

Suggested Readings

Culpepper J, Rinaldo J, Grenvik A, Rogers R. Effect of ventilator mode on tendency to respiratory alkalosis (abstract). Am Rev Respir Dis 1983; 127(4, part 2):104.

Hurlow RS, Hudson LD, Pierson DJ, Craig KC, Albert RK. Does IMV correct respiratory alkalosis in patients on AMV? (abstract). Chest 1982; 82:211.

Zwillich CW, Pierson DJ, Creagh CE, Sutton FD, Schatz E, Petty TL. Complications of assisted ventilation. A prospective study of 354 consecutive episodes. Am J Med 1974; 57:161–170.